Hair Cells: Regeneration, Repair and Death

Hair Cells: Regeneration, Repair and Death

Edited by Jacob Evans

STATES
ACADEMIC PRESS
www.statesacademicpress.com

States Academic Press,
109 South 5th Street,
Brooklyn, NY 11249, USA

Visit us on the World Wide Web at:
www.statesacademicpress.com

ISBN: 978-1-63989-249-5

Cataloging-in-Publication Data

Hair cells : regeneration, repair and death / edited by Jacob Evans.
p. cm.
Includes bibliographical references and index.
ISBN 978-1-63989-249-5
1. Hair cells. 2. Hair cells--Regeneration. 3. Cell death. I. Evans, Jacob.
RL91 .H35 2021
646.724--dc23

Table of Contents

Preface

The sensory receptors which belong to the vestibular and auditory systems of vertebrates are termed as hair cells. They are present within the ears. These cells are able to detect movement around them through mechanotransduction. In mammals, hair cells are located in the cochlea of the inner ear. These cells can be categorized into two types, the inner and outer hair cells. They are functionally and anatomically different from each other. The inner hair cells are responsible for converting the sound vibrations in the fluids of the cochlea into electrical signals which are then conveyed to the brain. They are unable to regenerate. Therefore, any injury or damage to them is permanent and can lead to a decrease in hearing sensitivity. This book covers in detail some existent theories and innovative concepts revolving around the regeneration, repair and death of hair cells. Its aim is to present researches that have transformed this discipline and aided its advancement. This book will help the readers in keeping pace with the rapid changes in this field.

The information contained in this book is the result of intensive hard work done by researchers in this field. All due efforts have been made to make this book serve as a complete guiding source for students and researchers. The topics in this book have been comprehensively explained to help readers understand the growing trends in the field.

I would like to thank the entire group of writers who made sincere efforts in this book and my family who supported me in my efforts of working on this book. I take this opportunity to thank all those who have been a guiding force throughout my life.

Editor

1

Early transcriptional response to aminoglycoside antibiotic suggests alternate pathways leading to apoptosis in sensory hair cells in the mouse inner ear

Litao Tao [1,2] *and Neil Segil* [1,2,3*]

[1] *Genetic, Molecular and Cellular Biology Program, University of Southern California, Los Angeles, CA, USA,* [2] *Department of Stem Cell Biology and Regenerative Medicine, University of Southern California, Los Angeles, CA, USA,* [3] *Department of Otolaryngology, University of Southern California, Los Angeles, CA, USA*

Edited by:
Andy Groves, Baylor College of Medicine, USA

Reviewed by:
Stefan Heller, Stanford University, USA
Mark E. Warchol, Washington University School of Medicine, USA
Lisa Cunningham, National Institutes of Health, USA

***Correspondence:**
Neil Segil, Department of Stem Cell Biology and Regenerative Medicine, University of Southern California, 1425 San Pablo Street, Los Angeles, CA 90033, USA
nsegil@med.usc.edu

Aminoglycoside antibiotics are "the drug of choice" for treating many bacterial infections, but their administration results in hearing loss in up to one fourth of the patients who receive them. Several biochemical pathways have been implicated in aminoglycoside antibiotic ototoxicity; however, little is known about how hair cells respond to aminoglycoside antibiotics at the transcriptome level. Here we have investigated the genome-wide response to the aminoglycoside antibiotic gentamicin. Using organotypic cultures of the perinatal organ of Corti, we performed RNA sequencing using cDNA libraries obtained from FACS-purified hair cells. Within 3 h of gentamicin treatment, the messenger RNA level of more than three thousand genes in hair cells changed significantly. Bioinformatic analysis of these changes highlighted several known signal transduction pathways, including the JNK pathway and the NF-κB pathway, in addition to genes involved in the stress response, apoptosis, cell cycle control, and DNA damage repair. In contrast, only 698 genes, mainly involved in cell cycle and metabolite biosynthetic processes, were significantly affected in the non-hair cell population. The gene expression profiles of hair cells in response to gentamicin share a considerable similarity with those previously observed in gentamicin-induced nephrotoxicity. Our findings suggest that previously observed early responses to gentamicin in hair cells in specific signaling pathways are reflected in changes in gene expression. Additionally, the observed changes in gene expression of cell cycle regulatory genes indicate a disruption of the postmitotic state, which may suggest an alternate pathway regulating gentamicin-induced apoptotic hair cell death. This work provides a more comprehensive view of aminoglycoside antibiotic ototoxicity, and thus contributes to identifying potential pathways or therapeutic targets to alleviate this important side effect of aminoglycoside antibiotics.

Keywords: sensory hair cells, aminoglycoside antibiotics, gentamicin, ototoxicity, RNA sequencing, differential gene expression

Introduction

Ototoxicity is a well-known side effect limiting the use of aminoglycoside antibiotics, with reported incidence of hearing loss between 2% and 25% of treated patients (Huth et al., 2011). Several biochemical mechanisms of aminoglycoside ototoxicity have been investigated, including production of reactive oxygen species (ROS) (Forge and Schacht, 2000), disruption of intracellular calcium storage (Matsui et al., 2004), and inhibition of cytoplasmic protein synthesis (Francis et al., 2013). Through biochemical assays, some pathways have also been identified as signaling pathways mediating aminoglycoside-induced hair cell death, such as the pro-apoptotic JNK pathway (Ylikoski et al., 2002) and the protective NF-κB pathway (Jiang et al., 2005). Based on observations made in organ cultures, a timeline of critical signaling events has been established. ROS production is induced shortly after aminoglycoside administration; the JNK pathway responds to drug treatment within 3 h; the intracellular calcium level is increased dramatically at around 4 h; cytochrome C is released into cytoplasm at around 12 h and apoptosis execution steps occur at around 18 h (Matsui et al., 2004).

The methods utilizing low-throughput biochemical assays have been instrumental in dissecting some of the sequelae of antibiotic treatment of hair cells. However, cells are complex systems that integrate input from multiple mechanisms and respond by adjusting multiple pathways simultaneously. High-throughput methods may help us gain a better understanding of the ototoxicity associated with aminoglycosides by providing a complex view of the response; among them, DNA microarray and antibody array experiments have been performed to profile the changes in the cochlea after ototoxic drug treatment at the transcriptional level and the protein level, respectively (Nagy et al., 2004; Jamesdaniel et al., 2008). However, whole cochlea samples were used in those studies, which consisted largely of many different non-hair cell populations in addition to hair cells, and the heterogeneity of the samples limited the interpretation of the results due to a low signal to noise ratio.

Here we have utilized RNA sequencing to investigate the early gene expression changes in hair cells induced by the aminoglycoside antibiotic gentamicin. Compared to microarray analysis, RNA sequencing is more accurate for analyzing expression levels, more informative for pathway analysis, and more powerful in exploiting unannotated genes (Wang et al., 2009). We made use of the Atoh1-GFP transgenic mice, whose fluorescent reporter under the control of the Atoh1 enhancer faithfully identifies hair cells (Lumpkin et al., 2003), to purify GFP+ hair cells by fluorescence-activated cell sorting (FACS) after a 3 h gentamicin treatment for a direct analysis of gene expression changes by RNA sequencing. We chose the 3 h time point because it was previously shown that signaling pathways have initiated a response to the drug, but the cell death process did not appear to be initiated (Matsui et al., 2004). We present analyses of the gene changes associated with several major pathways known to be dysregulated in response to aminoglycoside antibiotics.

Genome wide, 3709 genes, including those involved in a variety of pathways and cellular processes, were found to change significantly in hair cells after gentamicin treatment. Genes involved in the JNK pathway and the NF-κB pathway were differentially expressed in gentamicin-treated hair cells, which is consistent with previous findings that these pathways are important for aminoglycoside ototoxicity (Ylikoski et al., 2002; Jiang et al., 2005). Surprisingly, we did not observe a strong stress response at the transcriptional level at this early time point. Comparison of gentamicin-induced gene expression changes in hair cells and data from other cell lines and tissues, revealed a similarity between aminoglycoside-induced hair cell death and neuronal cell death, as well as a resemblance between aminoglycoside ototoxicity and nephrotoxicity. Additionally, genes involved in the cell cycle and DNA damage repair were also strongly affected by gentamicin at the transcriptional level, indicating a gentamicin-induced disruption of the postmitotic state, which may underlie an alternate pathway leading to hair cell death. In contrast, significantly fewer genes (698 genes) with altered expression after gentamicin treatment were present in the non-hair cell population at this time. Interestingly, expression of genes involved in cell cycle and metabolite biosynthesis pathways were significantly affected in this population. Analyses of our RNA sequencing data indicate that prior to severe oxidative stress, multiple events, including previously implicated activation of the JNK and the NF-κB pathways, and newly hypothesized disruption of the postmitotic state, occur in hair cells in response to aminoglycoside antibiotic treatment. Our work provides a comprehensive view of aminoglycoside ototoxicity, and our transcriptome data could be used to analyze other potential signaling pathways or biological processes mediating aminoglycoside-induced hair cell death which are not covered here.

Materials and Methods

Organotypic Culture, Drug Treatment, and FACS Sorting

Atoh1-GFP transgenic mice on CD-1 background (Lumpkin et al., 2003; available in the Jackson Laboratory but in different genomic background: B6.129S-Atoh1$^{tm4.1Hzo}$/J) were used for this study. All animal procedures and usage were approved by the IACUC committee in House Research Institute. Inner ears were collected from postnatal day 1 (P1) animals under sterile conditions and then transferred into ice cold Ca^{2+}- and Mg^{2+}-free PBS (Invitrogen), in which cochlea were further dissected under the microscope (Chen et al., 2002). The cochleae were mounted on polycarbonate membranes (13 mm diameter, 1.0 μm pore size, SPI supplies) floating on DMEM/F12 medium (Invitrogen) supplemented with 1% N2 (Gibco) and 100 U/ml penicillin (Sigma). Organ cultures were maintained under low oxygen conditions (37°C, 5% CO_2 and 5% O_2) overnight, and treated with gentamicin the next day.

To trace the accumulation of gentamicin in hair cells, Texas Red conjugated gentamicin (GTTR) was prepared as described in the literature (Steyger et al., 2003). 4.4 ml of gentamicin sulfate (Sigma; 50 mg/ml in K_2CO_3, pH 9) was mixed with 0.6 ml succinimidyl ester of Texas Red (Invitrogen; 2 mg/ml in dimethyl formamide), and then agitated overnight to produce a mixture of gentamicin and GTTR with an approximate 300:1 molar ratio. This GTTR mixture solution was diluted 1:100 with culture medium for treatment of organotypic cultures. After 30 min incubation, organs were fixed with 4% paraformaldehyde, cryosectioned and photographed by fluorescence microscopy.

To confirm the level of hair cell death induced by gentamicin, organ cultures were treated with 0.5 mM gentamicin for 3 h, and then gentamicin was washed out and replaced with fresh medium. GFP positive hair cells were photographed at 3 and 24 h timepoints (**Figure 1B**).

To purify hair cells for RNAseq, organs were digested with 0.05% Trypsin (Invitrogen) and 1 mg/ml Collagenase (Worthington) in PBS at 37°C for 8 min, then incubated with 10% FBS (Life Technologies) in PBS to stop enzymatic digestion. To make single cell suspensions, organs were triturated with a P200 pipette 300 times. The suspension was passed through a cell strainer (40 μm, BD Biosciences) before FACS purification. GFP-positive hair cells, as well as the GFP-negative non-hair cell population (non-hair cell cochlear epithelial cells included Deiters' cells, pillar cells, Hensen cells, cells in the GER, cells in the LER, and other cells constituting surrounding tissues) were purified on a BD FACS Aria II with a 100 μ nozzle. Cells with low-levels of GFP were excluded by stringent gating during FACS purification (**Figure 1C**). Quality control by FACS-resort, and by immunofluorescence for a hair cell marker (MyosinVI), indicated >95% purity. Sorted cells were collected directly into RNA lysis buffer (Zymo). At least 50,000 cells were collected for each sample, and three replicates were prepared for each condition.

RNA Sequencing, Reads Alignment, PCA and Differential Gene Expression

RNA was extracted from samples using the Zymo Quick-RNA Microprep kit, and then processed for library construction, using the Illumina True-Seq mRNA-seq kit. Six samples were barcoded, combined into one lane, and sequenced by Illumina Hi-Seq 2000 for single-end 50 cycles (50 bp reads). More than 30 million reads were obtained for each replicate. The reads were trimmed on both ends (quality score ≥25) and aligned against the mouse genome assembly mm10 using TopHat 2 in PartekFlow (Partek Inc.). Normalized read score for each gene was calculated considering total read numbers and gene length (reads per kilobase of transcript per million reads mapped, RPKM). Principal component analysis (PCA) was conducted in PartekFlow based on normalized read numbers for individual genes in each replicate. Differential gene expression was assessed by the embedded gene specific analysis (GSA) module in PartekFlow.

RNA sequence data was deposited into NCBI GEO database (GSE66775).

IPA Analysis

Differential gene expression datasets, including gene symbols, fold changes, p-values and total numbers of raw reads, were prepared for Ingenuity pathway analysis software (IPA, Version 21901358, Qiagen Inc.). The gene expression dataset from untreated and gentamicin-treated hair cells, and from untreated and treated non-hair cell samples, were analyzed by the IPA software. A filter of p-value less than 0.01, fold change greater than 1.2 (or less than −1.2), and total number of raw reads greater than 100 was applied, and core pathway analysis was conducted for each dataset. Canonical pathway analysis, diseases and function analysis, upstream regulator analysis, and network analysis were included in the core analysis with default settings.

Q-PCR Validation

The cDNA libraries for Q-PCR were made by qScript reverse transcriptase supermix (Quanta Biosciences) using RNA extracted from FACS purified cells as template. *Rpl19* was used as internal control for normalization. For validation purpose, four independent biological replicates were collected and analyzed by Q-PCR. Genes were chosen arbitrarily among the list of gentamicin-induced genes in hair cells. SYBR-Green (Applied Biosystems) was used to detect amplified double strand DNA on ViiA 7 machine (Applied Biosystems). Primer pairs used for Q-PCR were listed below. *Rpl19* forward 5′-GGTCTGGTTGGA TCCCAATG-3′, reverse 5′-CCCGGGAATGGACAGTCA-3′. *Atf2* forward 5′-CCGTTGCTATTCCTGCATCAA-3′, reverse 5′-TTGCTTCTGACTGGACTGGTT-3′. *Mapk8* forward 5′-AGC AGAAGCAAACGTGACAAC-3′, reverse 5′-GCTGCACACACT ATTCCTTGAG-3′. *Jun* forward 5′-CCTTCTACGACGATG CCCTC-3′, reverse 5′-GGTTCAAGGTCATGCTCTGTTT-3′. *Nfkb1* forward 5′-ATGGCAGACGATGATCCCTAC-3′, reverse 5′-TGTTGACAGTGGTATTTCTGGTG-3′. *Nfkbib* forward 5′-GCGGATGCCGATGAATGGT-3′, reverse 5′-TGACGTAGC CAAAGACTAAGGG-3′. *Chuk* forward 5′-GTCAGGACCGTG TTCTCAAGG-3′, reverse 5′-GCTTCTTTGATGTTACTGAGG GC-3′. *Gadd45g* forward 5′-GGGAAAGCACTGCACGAACT-3′, reverse 5′-AGCACGCAAAAGGTCACATTG-3′. *Klf11* forward 5′-CATGGACATTTGTGAGTCGATCC-3′, reverse 5′-CCTTTGGTAGATCAGGTGCAG-3′. *Ddit3* forward 5′-CTG GAAGCCTGGTATGAGGAT-3′, reverse 5′-CAGGGTCAAGAG TAGTGAAGGT-3′. *Bnip1* forward 5′-AGGCTATGCAGACT CTAGTCAG-3′, reverse 5′-CAGTTCTCGGCGGTTGTACT-3′. *Casp3* forward 5′-ATGGAGAACAACAAAACCTCAGT-3′, reverse 5′-TTGCTCCCATGTATGGTCTTTAC-3′. *Ccar1* forward 5′-AGATGAGTATGACCCAATGGAGG-3′, reverse 5′-CCTTGCAGTACCGGCTGAC-3′. *Ccnb2* forward 5′-GCC AAGAGCCATGTGACTATC-3′, reverse 5′-CAGAGCTGGTAC TTTGGTGTTC-3′. *Ccne2* forward 5′-ATGTCAAGACGCAGC CGTTTA-3′, reverse 5′-GCTGATTCCTCCAGACAGTACA-3′. *Ercc8* forward 5′-GAGGAAGATGAAGCTATGGAA-3′, reverse 5′-CTTCAGGGGTTTCTCTTTGTC-3′. *Rad52* forward 5′-CTT TGTTGGTGGGAAGTCTGT-3′, reverse 5′-CGGCTGCTAATG TACTCTGGAC-3′. *Apex2* forward 5′-GGATGGATGGCTTGC TCAGTA-3′, reverse 5′-ACTTCAGGGAGTAAGAAGGAGG-3′. *Alkbh3* forward 5′-GAGCCAGTCTGCTACTCAGC-3′, reverse 5′- AACACAAATTGTCGGTCACATTG-3′.

Results

Perinatal cochleae from Atoh1-GFP transgenic mice, cultured and treated with gentamicin, show that gentamicin accumulated

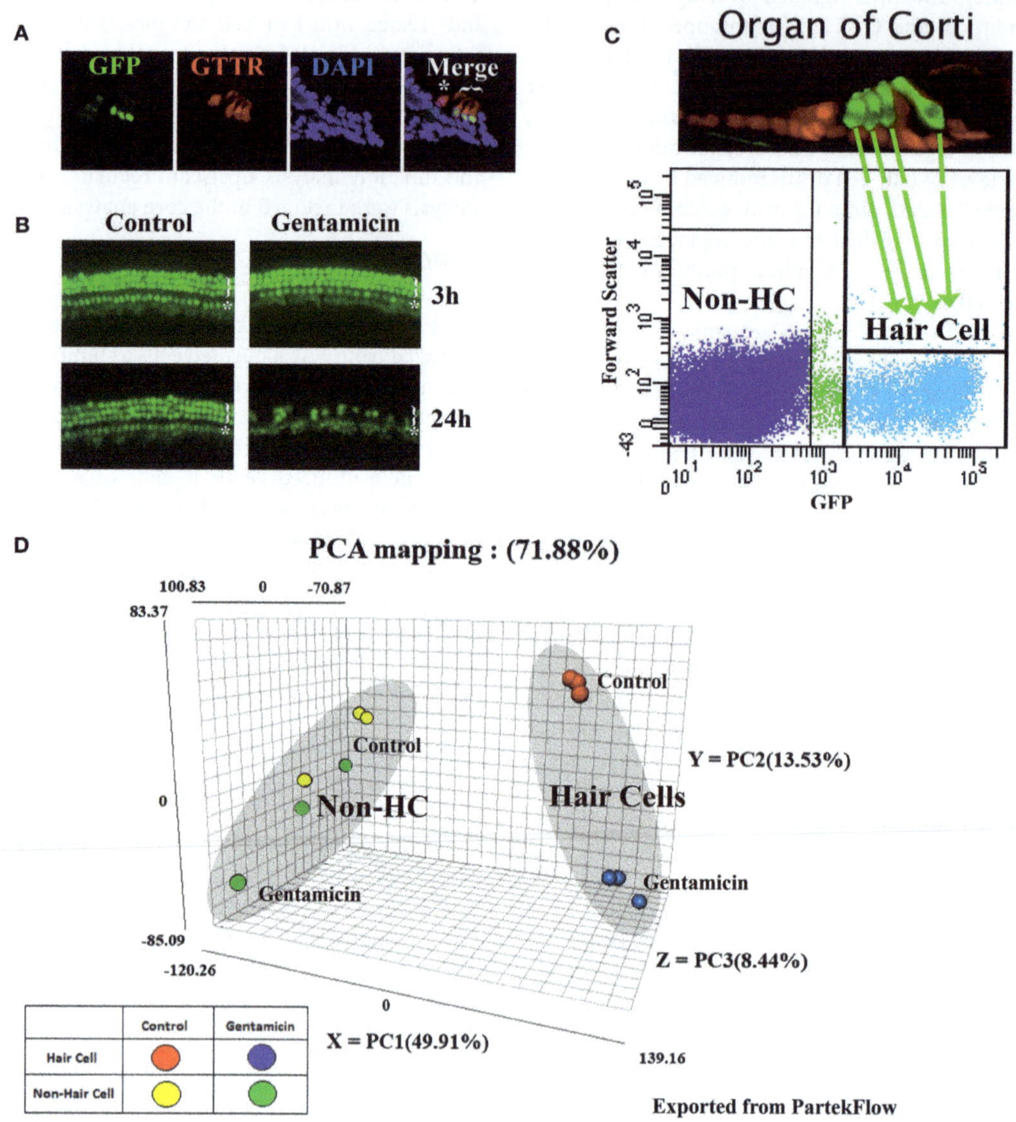

FIGURE 1 | Gentamicin-induced hair cell loss, and principal component analysis (PCA) of RNA sequencing datasets. (A) Gentamicin accumulates preferentially in hair cells in *in vitro* organ of Corti culture. Cross sections through cochlear explants from P1, Atoh1-GFP mice (Lumpkin et al., 2003), treated for 30 min with Texas Red conjugated gentamicin (GTTR). Star indicates the inner hair cell, and bracket indicates three outer hair cells. Cells with weak GFP under the inner hair cell are inner phalangeal cells. **(B)** Atoh1-GFP fluorescence in untreated and 0.5 mM gentamicin-treated organs at 3 and 24 h. There was no detectable hair cell loss at 3 h, but severe hair cell damage caused by gentamicin at 24 h. Star indicates a single row of inner hair cells and bracket indicates three partial rows of outer hair cells. **(C)** Scatter plot of Atoh1-GFP hair cell purification by FACS shows gate settings and diagram shows a P1 organ of Corti indicating hair cells (green) and supporting cells (red) (Chen and Segil, 1999). **(D)** PCA map showing the three most significant variances among samples. 78.88% of variance in the combined dataset is captured in the analysis; (49.91% in PC1-X axis, 13.53% in PC2-Y axis, and 8.44% on PC3-Z axis). Each dot represents one biological replicate.

specifically in hair cells, as indicated by the uptake of Texas-Red conjugated gentamicin (**Figure 1A**), and 91% (SD ± 7%; $n = 3$) of outer hair cells were killed by gentamicin at 24 h (**Figure 1B**). To investigate the early transcriptional response of hair cells to gentamicin, cultured cochleae were treated with gentamicin for 3 h, and immediately dissociated and FACS-sorted to obtain purified hair cell and non-hair cell samples (**Figure 1C**) for RNA sequencing. Since there is a low level of misexpression of GFP in inner phalangeal cells and probably in border cells, cells with low-level GFP expression were excluded by stringently gating GFP during FACS purification to minimize possible contamination. We validated the purity of the hair cell population by immunostaining, as more than 95% of purified GFP-positive cells stained positive for the hair cell marker MyoVI (data not shown). In addition, known hair cell specific genes, such as *Atoh1*, *Pou4f3*, *Myo6*, and *Myo7a*, have much greater normalized read numbers in hair cell samples than that in non-hair cell samples (**Table S1**), suggesting the high purity of our hair cell sample. The reliability of the RNA sequencing data was verified by Q-PCR analysis with primers specific for selected genes (**Figures 2A, 3A, 4A, 5A, 6A**).

Expression of 23420 genes was quantified and analyzed with the Negative Binomial, Poisson or Lognormal Linear distribution model (gene specific analysis algorithm provided by PartekFlow) (**Table S1**). After 3 h of gentamicin treatment, the mRNA level of 3709 genes in hair cells was significantly altered, with 1917 genes found to be up-regulated and 1792 genes down-regulated (p-value < 0.01, fold change > 1.2 or < -1.2, and raw reads ≥ 100). In contrast, significantly fewer genes (698) were found to be affected with the same criteria in the non-hair cell population, with 436 genes up-regulated and 262 genes down-regulated.

Principal Components Analysis

Principal components analysis (PCA) is a method for analyzing the variance in high dimensional datasets, and to present variance in a few dimensions for easier interpretation (Ringnér, 2008). The PCA analysis of our RNA sequencing data shows that 71.88% variance in the dataset was captured within the three most significant principal components (PCs): 49.91% in PC1 (X axis), 13.53% in PC2 (Y axis), and 8.44% in PC3 (Z axis) (**Figure 1D**). These PCs correspond to different cell types and different treatment conditions.

In the PCA map, each biological replicate of different experimental groups is represented by one dot (**Figure 1D**). PCA analysis indicates that the variance among the replicates of FACS-purified hair cells is low. Three untreated hair cell replicates cluster tightly in the PCA map (red dots), as do three gentamicin-treated hair cell replicates (blue dots) (**Figure 1D**). This tight clustering indicates low statistical variance between replicates, and likely stems from the low cellular heterogeneity among FACS-purified replicates. In contrast, both treated (green dots) and untreated (yellow dots) samples from the non-hair cell replicates, which include all other cells in our dissected epithelial preparations, are scattered in the PCA map (**Figure 1D**), indicating the higher statistical variance among replicates of the non-hair cell samples. Hair cell samples and the non-hair cell samples (**Figure 1D**, red vs. yellow) lie at the two ends of the most significant variance axis (PC1, X axis), suggesting that the hair cell gene expression profile is significantly different from the non-hair cell population. Along the second variance axis (PC2, Y axis), gentamicin-treated hair cell samples are separated from untreated hair cell samples (**Figure 1D**, blue vs. red), indicating the significant gene expression shift in hair cells caused by gentamicin treatment at the 3 h time point. In contrast, the non-hair cell samples are not separated by gentamicin treatment (**Figure 1D**, green vs. yellow), suggesting that the gentamicin-induced gene expression shift in the non-hair cell population was not as consistent as the one in hair cells. Together, the PCA results suggest that gentamicin treatment induced significant and consistent gene expression changes in hair cells.

Signaling Pathways and Biological Processes Affected by Gentamicin in Hair Cells

Gene expression in hair cells was affected significantly by gentamicin treatment at 3 h, as shown by the large number of deregulated genes and by the PCA results. To investigate the underlying biological pathways affected in hair cells upon gentamicin treatment, IPA software (Qiagen) was used to analyze affected signaling pathways after gentamicin treatment, and to compare our hair cell datasets with datasets derived from other cell lines and tissues. Pathways affected by gentamicin treatment at 3 h are listed in **Table S2**. Below we verify and discuss several of these pathways that have been reported to be important in aminoglycoside induced hair cell death, as well as proposing that elements of the cell cycle may provide an additional pathway, signaling apoptosis in hair cells.

Expression of JNK Pathway-Related Genes was Significantly Affected by Gentamicin

The JNK pathway has been strongly implicated in aminoglycoside-induced hair cell death. After aminoglycoside treatment, phosphorylation of JNK and c-Jun was observed in hair cells (Ylikoski et al., 2002), indicating activation of the JNK pathway. Furthermore, inhibition of the JNK pathway by pharmaceutical inhibitors has been shown to protect hair cells from aminoglycoside ototoxicity (Ylikoski et al., 2002), suggesting that JNK activation may be involved in mediating aminoglycoside-induced hair cell death.

Consistent with these findings, we observed changes in the expression of genes involved in JNK signaling pathways upon gentamicin treatment. We verified the expression changes of three genes in this pathway by Q-PCR, namely *Atf2*, *Mapk8* (*Jnk1*), and *Jun* (*c-Jun*) (**Figure 2A**). IPA pathway analysis revealed that the expression of JNK pathway-related genes was significantly affected in gentamicin-treated hair cells (p = 0.000001). As shown in **Figure 2B** (color coded, see legend), *Mapk8* (*Jnk1*) itself, in addition to several upstream and downstream factors including *Jun*, *Atf2*, *Nfatc1*, and *Elk1*, were changed at the transcriptional level in gentamicin-treated hair cells. Interestingly, the induction of *Jun* expression is regulated by phosphorylation of Jun itself, in an autoregulatory loop, by JNK (Angel et al., 1988); thus the increased mRNA expression of *Jun* indicates the likely activation of the JNK pathway. Transcriptional changes in other targets of Jun regulation are summarized in **Table S3**. The pattern of changed expression of JNK pathway-related genes is consistent with the timeline of critical signaling events for aminoglycoside-induced hair cell death, indicating that the JNK pathway is one of the early response pathways that are activated in hair cells after aminoglycoside treatment (Matsui et al., 2004).

Genes Involved in the NF-κB Pathway were Expressed Differentially after Gentamicin Treatment

Activation of the NF-κB pathway has been implicated as protective against aminoglycoside ototoxicity in several biochemical assays (Jiang et al., 2005). Aminoglycoside treatment has been shown to increase DNA binding activity of NF-κB, indicating activation of the NF-κB pathway by aminoglycoside antibiotics (Jiang et al., 2005). Additionally, reagents promoting NF-κB translocation into nuclei reportedly protect hair cells from aminoglycoside ototoxicity (Jiang et al., 2005).

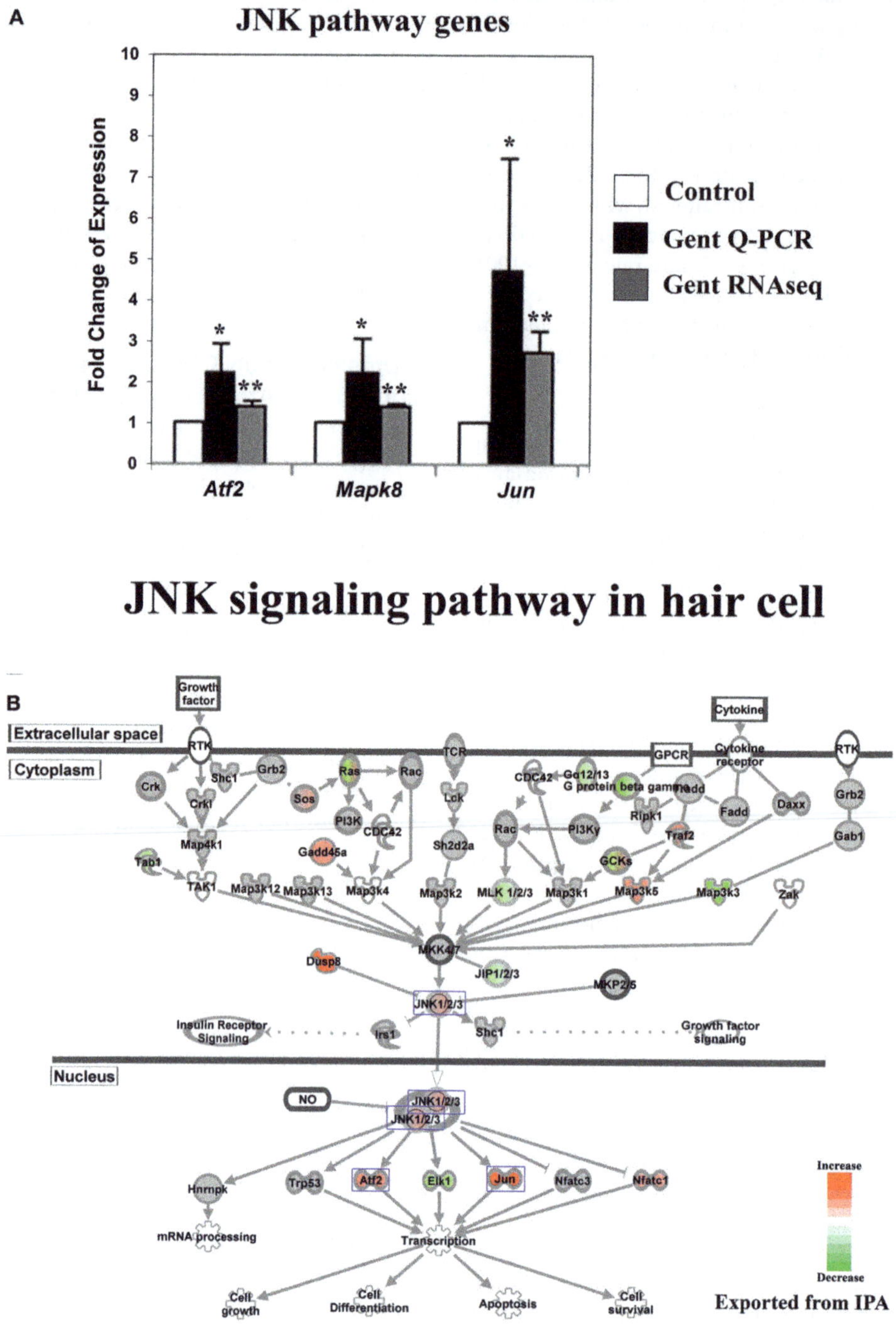

FIGURE 2 | Gentamicin-induced changes in expression of genes in the Jun-kinase (JNK) pathway. (A) Q-PCR results validating increased messenger RNA levels in hair cells after gentamicin treatment. Error bar, standard deviation: $^{*}p < 0.05$; $^{**}p < 0.01$. **(B)** The JNK signaling pathway with color-coded expression changes indicating significant transcriptional response to gentamicin. Only genes with significant expression changes are colored. Red, increased expression; green, decreased expression relative to control; half red-half green, indicates nodes with multiple genes with some genes upregulated and some genes downregulated. Genes validated and discussed in the text are boxed in the corresponding protein pathway diagrams.

Our RNA sequencing data show that the expression of genes involved in the NF-κB pathway was altered in hair cells after gentamicin treatment. Gentamicin-induced expression changes of *Nfkb1* (*p50*), *Nfkbib* (*Ikbb*), and *Chuk*(*Ikk1*) were verified by Q-PCR (**Figure 3A**). Fold changes based on RNA sequencing were smaller but remained highly significant ($p < 0.01$). In IPA pathway analysis, the NF-κB pathway was identified as a significantly affected pathway in gentamicin-treated hair cells ($p = 0.00004$). Expression changes of genes involved in the NF-κB pathway are shown in **Figure 3B**. Among these genes,

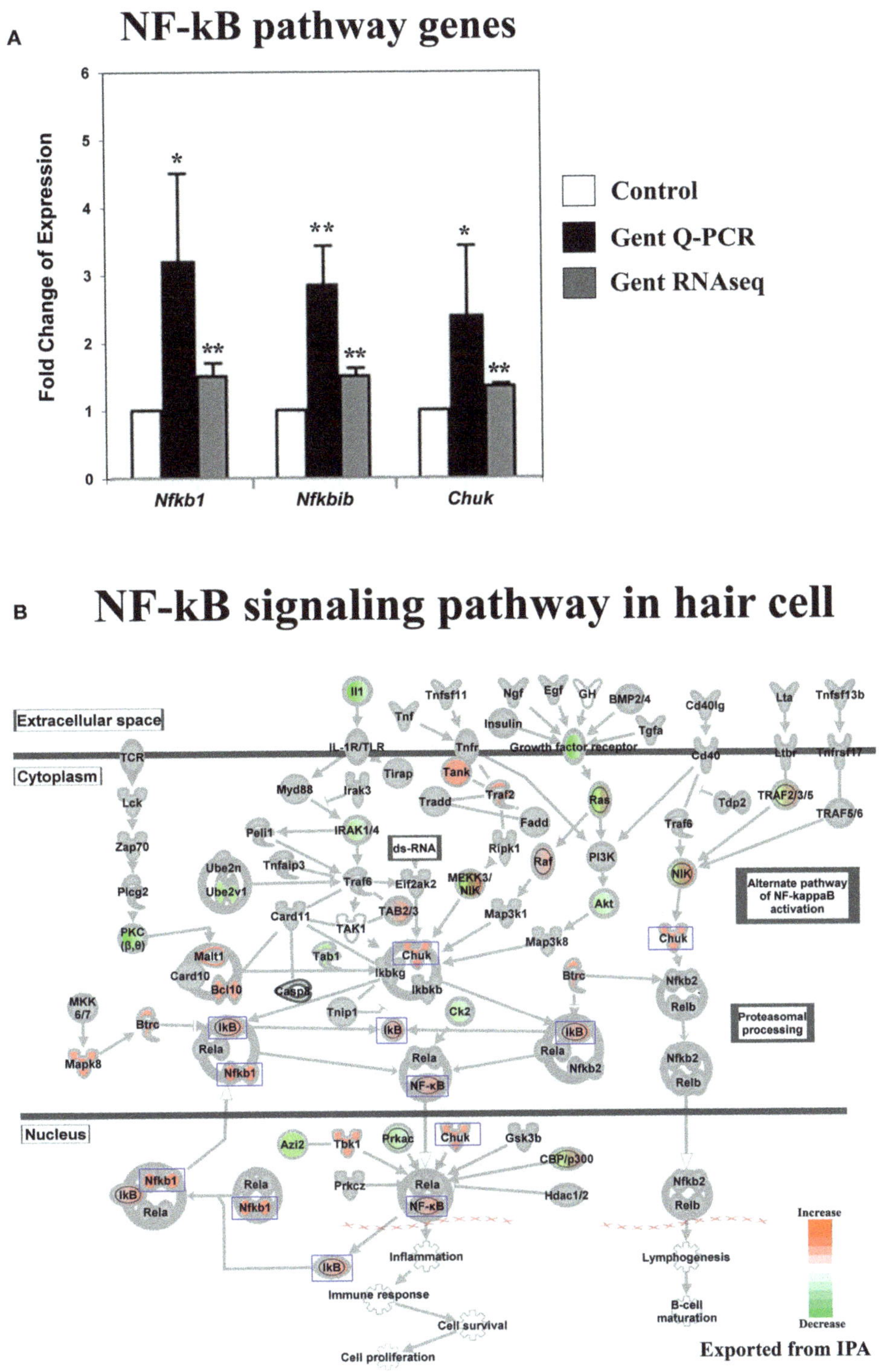

FIGURE 3 | Gentamicin-induced changes in expression of genes in the NF-κB pathway. (A) Q-PCR results validating increased messenger RNA levels in hair cells after gentamicin treatment. Error bar, standard deviation: $^*p < 0.05$; $^{**}p < 0.01$. **(B)** NF-κB pathway with color-coded expression changes suggesting early transcriptional response to gentamicin. Only genes with significant expression changes are colored. Red, increased expression; green, decreased expression relative to control; half red-half green, symbols for nodes consisting of multiple genes with some genes upregulated and some genes downregulated. Genes validated and discussed in the text are boxed in the corresponding protein pathway diagrams.

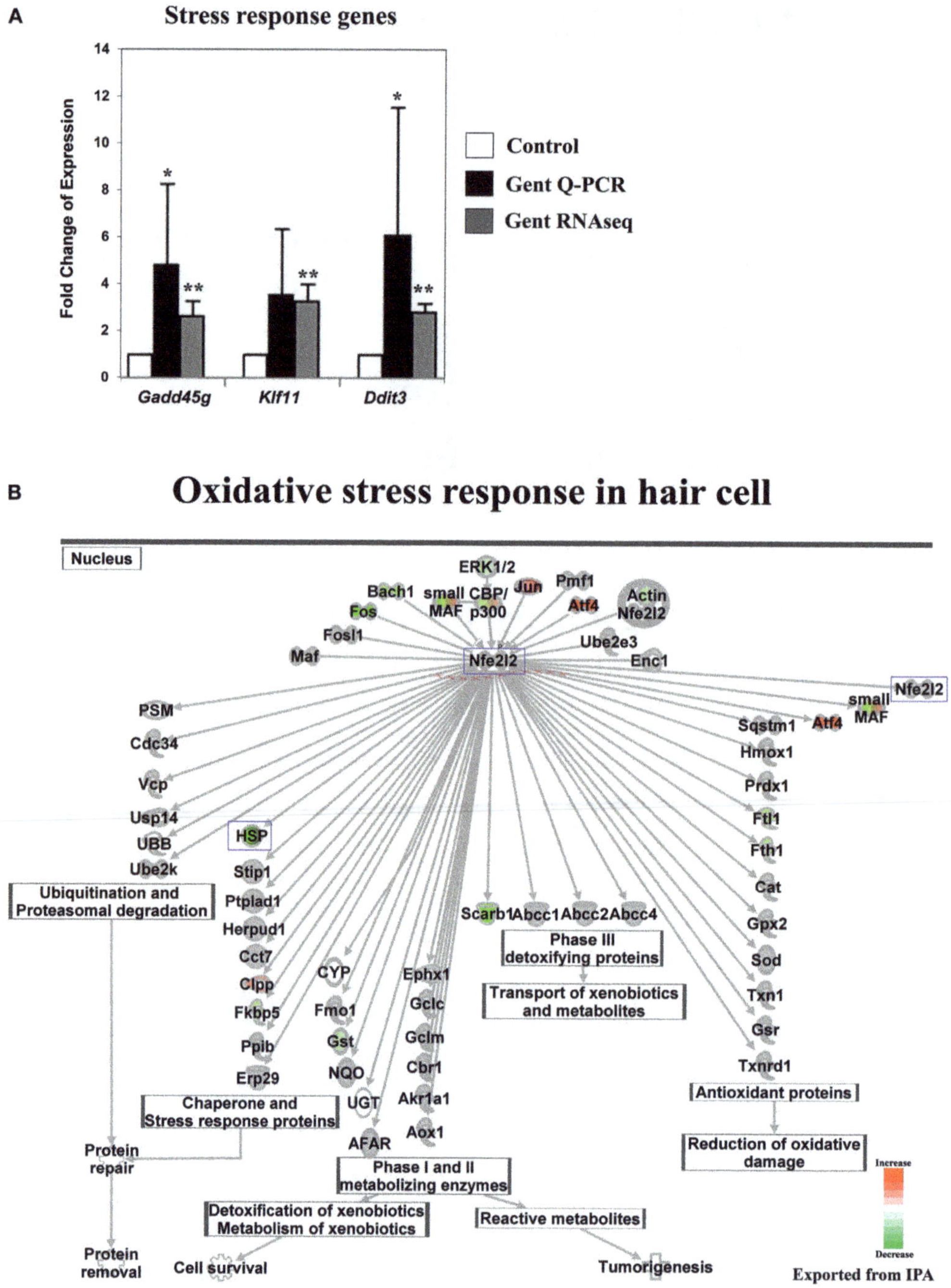

FIGURE 4 | Gentamicin-induced changes in expression of stress-response genes. (A) Q-PCR results validating increased messenger RNA levels in hair cells after gentamicin treatment. Error bar, standard deviation: $^{*}p < 0.1$; $^{**}p < 0.01$. **(B)** NRF2-mediated oxidative stress response network with color-coded expression shifts showing the absence of significant induction of oxidative stress response at the transcriptional level. Only genes with significant expression changes are color labeled. Red, increased expression; green, decreased expression relative to control; half red-half green, indicates nodes with multiple genes with some genes upregulated and some genes downregulated. Genes validated and discussed in the text are boxed in the corresponding protein pathway diagrams.

Nfkb1 and *Nfkbib* have been identified as target genes of NF-κB (Ten et al., 1992; Schreiber et al., 2006), and their increased expression strongly suggests the activation of the NF-κB pathway in gentamicin-treated hair cells. Transcriptional changes in other NF-κB targets are summarized in **Table S3**. Our expression data indicate that the NF-κB pathway, like the JNK pathway, is an early response pathway that is activated in hair cells by aminoglycosides.

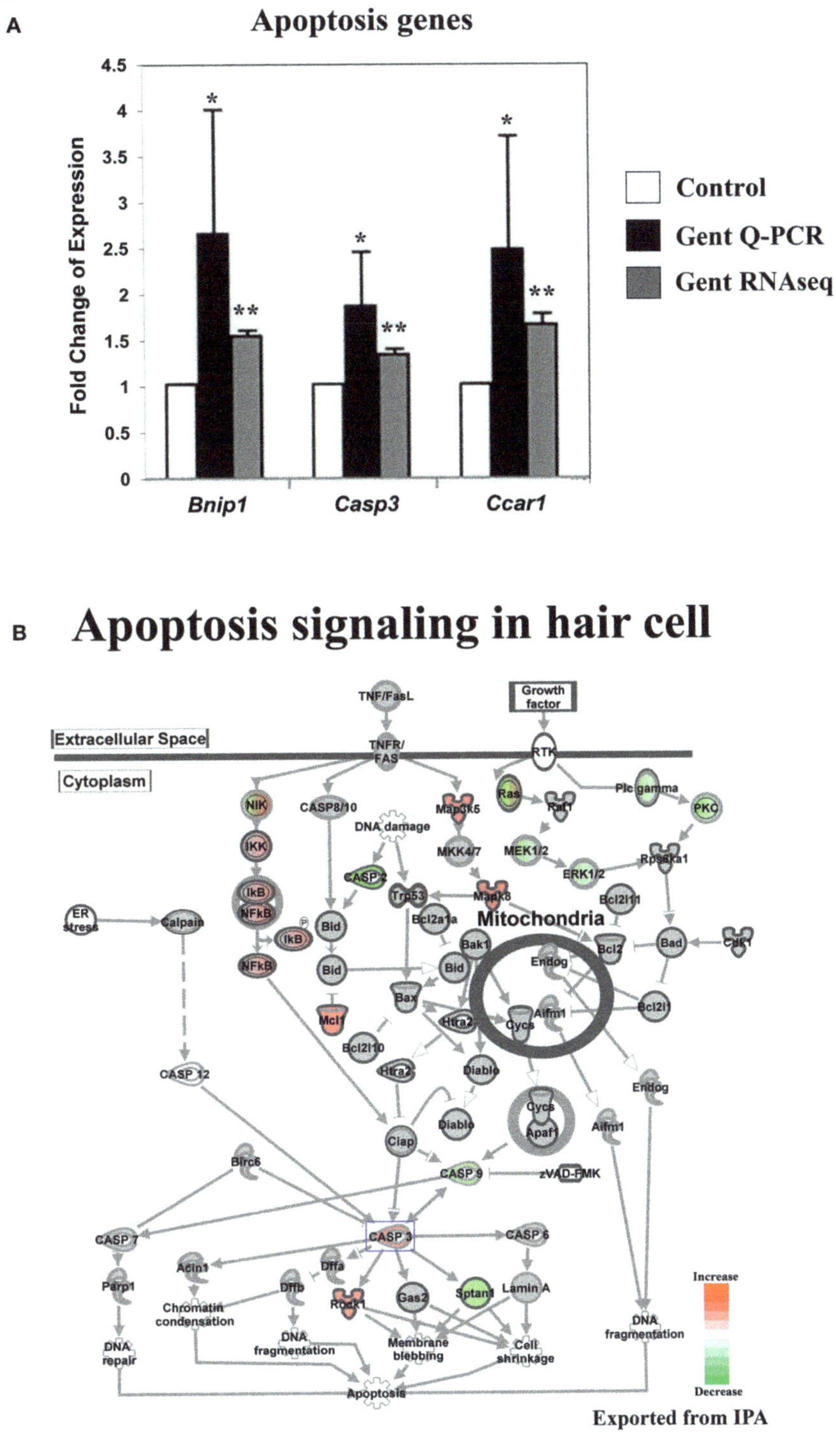

FIGURE 5 | Gentamicin-induced changes in expression of genes involved in apoptosis. (A) Q-PCR results validating increased messenger RNA levels in hair cells after gentamicin treatment. Error bar, standard deviation: $^{*}p < 0.05$; $^{**}p < 0.01$. **(B)** The apoptosis gene network with color-coded expression changes showing the absence of significant changes for apoptosis initiation and execution genes at transcriptional level. Only genes with significant expression changes are colored. Red, increased expression; green, decreased expression relative to control; half red-half green, indicates nodes with multiple genes with some genes upregulated and some genes downregulated. Genes validated and discussed in the text are boxed in the corresponding protein pathway diagrams.

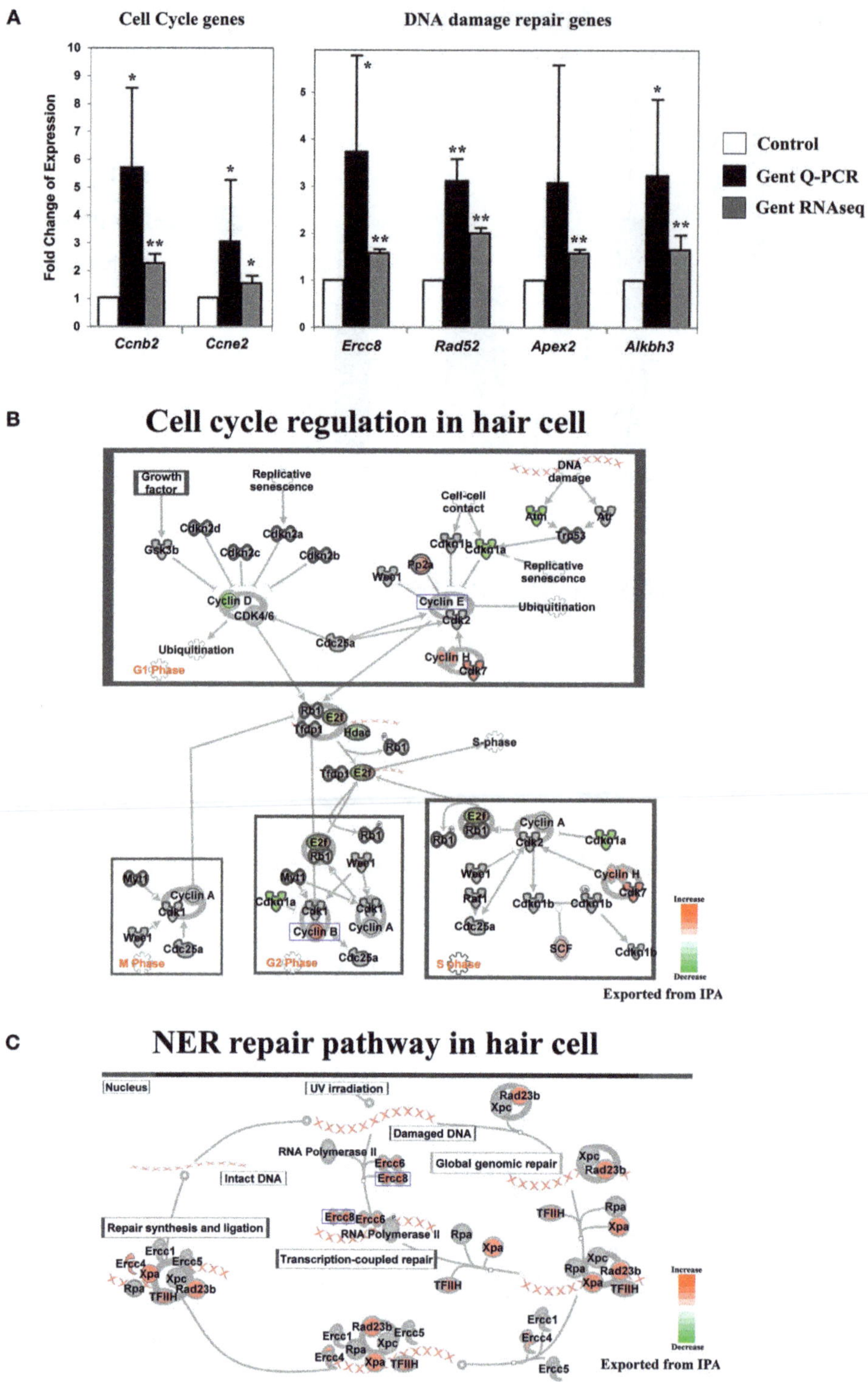

FIGURE 6 | Gentamicin-induced changes in expression of genes involved in cell cycle and DNA damage repair. (A) Q-PCR results validating increased messenger RNA levels of selected genes in hair cells after gentamicin treatment. These results confirm the up-regulation of cell cycle and DNA damage repair genes in gentamicin-treated hair cells. Error bar, standard deviation: $^*p < 0.05$; $^{**}p < 0.01$. **(B)** Cell cycle regulation network with color-coded expression changes suggesting affected cell cycle gene regulation by gentamicin. **(C)** Nucleotide excision repair (NER) network with color-coded expression changes showing significant induction of NER genes. Only genes with significant expression changes are colored. Red, increased expression; green, decreased expression relative to control; half red-half green, indicates nodes with multiple genes with some genes upregulated and some genes downregulated. Genes validated and discussed in the text are boxed in the corresponding protein pathway diagrams.

No Significant Stress Response was Observed at the Transcriptional Level for NRF2 Target Genes at the 3 h Time Point

The prevailing hypothesis of aminoglycoside ototoxicity holds that aminoglycoside-induced ROS production causes oxidative stress, which triggers apoptosis in hair cells. Cellular ROS levels are reported to increase within minutes of aminoglycoside administration *in vitro* (Hirose et al., 1997), and antioxidant reagents are shown to protect hair cells from aminoglyocside ototoxicity (Schacht, 1999). In addition, the oxidative stress response mediated by the transcription factor NRF2 (Nfe2l2) has been implicated in aminoglycoside ototoxicity (Hoshino et al., 2011). Therefore, a response to oxidative stress at the transcriptional level was expected. Surprisingly, although some genes upstream of the Nrf2-dependent oxidative stress pathway were upregulated in response to gentamicin at 3 h, the transcriptional key regulator Nrf2 (Nfe2l2), was not affected, nor were its well-studied transcriptional targets (Ma, 2013) (**Figure 4B** and **Table S3**). We interpret this to mean that at this early time point, the Nrf2 oxidative stress pathway has not been fully activated. One explanation for this might be that at the 3 h time point, aminoglycoside-induced ROS production had not increased to a level sufficient to overwhelm the highly-developed antioxidant system in hair cells, and this hypothesis is supported by the observation that after the initial disruption, a new balanced redox state indicated by stable NAD(P)H fluorescence is reached within 15 min post-gentamicin treatment (Schafer and Buettner, 2001; Tiede et al., 2009). Alternatively, the catastrophic oxidative stress may be caused by temporally downstream events such as mitochondrial dysfunction.

Another group of genes, which drew our attention because of a lack of early response, were those encoding heat shock proteins. Expression of these genes was not induced by gentamicin at 3 h, including the HspA group (*Hspa1a*, *Hspa1b*, *Hspa5,* and others), the HspB group (*Hspb1*, *Hspb2,* and others), the HspC group (*Hsp90aa1*, *Hsp90ab1,* and *Hsp90b1*), and other members in the HspD, HspE, and HspG groups (**Table S1**). Among Dnaj family members, which are involved in oxidative stress response, only *Dnaja2*, *Dnajb4*, and some *Dnajc* genes were expressed at slightly higher levels (**Table S1**). The absence of strong induction of heat shock protein genes suggests that hair cells had not launched a broad stress response at 3 h, and indicates that transcriptional changes in signaling pathways, such as the JNK and the NF-κB pathways, at this time point were not simply caused by dysregulation of general transcription under stress conditions.

Genes Involved in the Initiation and Execution of Apoptosis were not Significantly Affected at the Early Time Point

Aminoglycoside antibiotics are thought to induce hair cell death through an intrinsic mitochondrial apoptosis pathway (Forge and Li, 2000). Apoptosis is an active process that requires gene transcription and protein synthesis (Matsui et al., 2002). In contrast to genes involved in upstream pathways, such as the JNK and the NF-κB pathways, which regulate apoptosis and survival, genes involved in apoptosis initiation and execution were not significantly affected in gentamicin-treated hair cells at 3 h post treatment (**Figure 5B**). Although we observed up-regulation of *Casp3* expression and down-regulation of *Casp2* and *Casp9* expression, the majority of intrinsic mitochondrial apoptosis pathway-related genes remained unchanged, including pro- and anti-apoptosis Bcl2 family members (**Figure 5B**). The lack of significant induction of apoptosis factors at this relatively early time point is consistent with the critical events timeline of aminoglycoside-induced hair cell death (Matsui et al., 2004). We verified the expression changes of *Bnip1*, *Casp3* and *Ccar1* by Q-PCR (**Figure 5A**).

We analyzed the cell-type specific response by comparing gentamicin-induced expression changes in hair cells, with gene expression changes during cell death in fibroblasts, neurons, and kidneys (based on published literature as curated in the IPA data base). Like hair cells, neurons are terminally-differentiated, non-dividing cells, but pathways regulating neuronal cell apoptosis are well characterized. We also emphasized the kidney because nephrotoxicity is another well-known sequela to aminoglycoside antibiotics treatment. These comparisons in IPA revealed that gentamicin-induced gene expression changes in hair cells are significantly different from the dataset derived from fibroblasts ($p = 0.0000927$ and activation z-score -1.81) (activation z-score is a quantitative measure of how similar the hair cell dataset is to the "comparing dataset": larger positive number indicates there are more genes with expression changes in the same direction in both datasets, while larger negative number means there are more genes with changes in opposite direction between datasets; see **Table 1** caption), but similar to datasets of neuronal cell death ($p = 0.000280$ and activation z-score 0.312), and cell death of kidney cells ($p = 0.00576$ and activation z-score 0.664). The observed similarity between aminoglycoside-induced hair cell death and neuronal cell death is not surprising, as hair cells and neurons are related types of terminally differentiated, excitable cells. The similarity between hair cells and kidney cells in response to aminoglycoside-induced stress will be discussed in Section: "Similarity between aminoglycoside ototoxicity and nephrotoxicity" found below.

Gentamicin-Induced Changes in Cell Cycle and DNA Damage Repair Genes Indicate Disruption of the Postmitotic State

Another group of early response genes whose expression was significantly affected upon exposure to gentamicin includes those involved in cell cycle regulation and DNA damage repair. We verified several genes in this group, including *Ccnb2* (*Cyclin B2*), *Ccne2* (*Cyclin E2*), *Ercc8* (*Csa*), *Rad52*, *Apex2*, and *Alkbh3* (**Figure 6A**). Expression changes of genes involved in cell cycle regulation and nucleotide excision repair are shown in **Figures 6B,C**, respectively. Comparisons between gentamicin-induced gene expression changes and known transcription regulation of related genes during cell cycle or DNA damage repair are summarized in **Tables 2**, **3**, respectively. These data suggest that the postmitotic state of hair cells was disrupted following gentamicin treatment. Loss of control of the postmitotic state and re-entry into the cell cycle preceding neuronal cell apoptosis has been observed (Arendt, 2000), and inhibition of cell cycle re-entry by blocking CDK activity has

TABLE 1 | Comparison of the hair cell dataset with known expression changes during cell death in other tissues and cell types.

Comparing dataset	*p*-value	Activation z-score	# Genes
Cell death of kidney cells	5.76E-03	0.664	73
Cell death of kidney cell lines	1.09E-03	0.579	67
Neuronal cell death	2.80E-04	0.312	149
Cell death of brain cells	4.10E-04	0.024	63
Cell death of central nervous system cells	6.80E-04	0.015	66
Cell death of fibroblast cell lines	2.71E-04	−0.539	98
Cell death of cerebellar cortex cells	2.77E-05	−0.574	17
Cell death of tumor cell lines	4.70E-06	−0.656	331
Cell death of lymphoma cell lines	2.54E-03	−1.148	46
Cell death of fibroblasts	9.27E-05	−1.81	61

Selected entries are shown. The p-value, which is calculated using the right-tailed Fisher Exact Test by IPA, is a measure of the likelihood that the association between a set of focus genes in two datasets is due to random chance. Activation z-score is a quantitative measure of how similar the hair cell dataset is to the "comparing dataset": larger positive number indicates there are more genes with expression changes in the same direction in both datasets, while larger negative number means there are more genes with changes in opposite direction between datasets. # Genes indicates number of overlapping genes in the comparison.

TABLE 2 | Comparison of the hair cell dataset with known expression changes in datasets from different stages of cell cycle.

Comparing dataset	*p*-value	Activation z-score	# Genes
G2 phase	1.08E-06	0.964	69
G2/M phase	1.31E-03	0.507	46
Cell cycle progression	3.96E-07	0.199	237
Mitosis	2.51E-05	−0.075	112
G1 phase	6.42E-04	−0.401	86
G1/S phase transition	1.75E-03	−0.506	46
M phase	2.37E-04	−0.891	55
S phase	1.44E-04	−1.122	63
Interphase	9.91E-08	−1.334	160
Entry into interphase	4.35E-03	−1.523	35

Selected entries are shown.

been shown to protect neurons from apoptosis induced by certain drugs or stress (Kruman, 2004; Golsteyn, 2005). Consistent with these observations in neuronal cells, aberrant cell cycle re-entry, induced by knocking out *Cdkn1a (p21)* and *Cdkn2d (p19)*, leads to hair cell apoptosis (Laine et al., 2007). Inhibition of CDK2 activity also protects hair cells from gentamicin ototoxicity (Tao and Segil, unpublished data), suggesting that the cell cycle machinery plays a role in mediating hair cell death. Our RNA sequencing data showing transcriptional changes to cell cycle-related genes indicate a disruption of the postmitotic state, which supports the idea that loss of cell cycle control may underlie an additional pathway leading to hair cell death after gentamicin treatment.

Induction of DNA damage repair genes also supports the hypothesis that the postmitotic state is disrupted in hair cells after gentamicin treatment. It is plausible that the induction

TABLE 3 | Comparison of the hair cell dataset with known expression changes in genes associated with the DNA repair process.

Comparing dataset	*p*-value	Activation z-score	# Genes
Repair of DNA	7.05E-06	1.953	66
DNA damage response of cells	6.09E-05	0.343	43
DNA replication	7.48E-05	−0.523	61
Metabolism of DNA	6.37E-04	0.357	90
Excision repair	1.02E-03	2.756	20

of DNA repair genes by DNA damage is caused by elevated ROS levels after gentamicin treatment, but our experimental observations do not support this explanation. First, the absence of significant induction of oxidative stress response genes suggests that the ROS production had not reached a level sufficient to induce the change in known response genes. Second, we failed to detect DNA damage by immunostaining against phosphorylated Chk, or by comet assay (Tao and Segil, unpublished data). Third, we did not observe induction of DNA damage repair genes at the transcriptional level after treating the cochlea with the DNA-damaging agent cisplatin (Ng, Rainey and Segil, unpublished data). Based on these observations, we postulate that up-regulated expression of DNA damage repair genes is not triggered by gentamicin-induced DNA damage and ROS production, but rather is more likely to reflect a change in cell cycle status following gentamicin treatment.

Gene Expression Changes Induced by Gentamicin in the Non-Hair Cell Population

Hair cells are specifically marked by GFP in Atoh1-GFP transgenic mice (**Figure 1A**), thus the GFP negative population consists of supporting cells (Deiters' cells, pillar cells and Hensen cells), cells in the greater epithelial ridge, cells in the lesser epithelial ridge, and other cells constituting surrounding tissues (inner phalangeal cells were excluded by FACS, based on their low-level misexpression of GFP, **Figures 1A,C**). The number of genes whose expression was affected by gentamicin in non-hair cell samples is much smaller than that in hair cells. The PCA results (**Figure 1D**) also show that the non-hair cell population does not respond to gentamicin uniformly, probably as a result of high heterogeneity. Expression of genes involved in cholesterol synthesis, lipid synthesis, nucleotide metabolism, and other biosynthesis processes, was significantly induced after gentamicin treatment in this population (**Table 4**). In addition, expression of genes involved in DNA replication and cell cycle was significantly affected (**Table 4**). The gentamicin-induced gene expression pattern of the non-hair cell population suggests gentamicin-stimulated biosynthesis, and induced cell proliferation in this population.

In the presence of Texas-Red conjugated gentamicin (GTTR) in culture medium, hair cells had much higher GTTR fluorescence than other cell types (**Figure 1A**), suggesting that gentamicin preferentially accumulates in hair cells. However, hair cells and supporting cells form a mosaic linked by tight epithelial junctions and other cell-cell contacts (Gulley and Resse, 1976). Communication between hair cells and supporting cells

TABLE 4 | Comparison of non-hair cell dataset with known expression changes in biosynthesis and proliferation datasets.

Comparing dataset	*p*-value	Activation z-score	# Genes
Synthesis of sterol	4.76E-11	1.723	16
Synthesis of cholesterol	1.04E-10	1.937	14
Metabolism of cholesterol	3.01E-10	1.937	17
Steroid metabolism	1.38E-05	1.937	20
Steroidogenesis	2.79E-05	1.929	17
Synthesis of terpenoid	3.74E-05	2.075	20
Metabolism of terpenoid	5.42E-05	1.937	21
Metabolism of membrane lipid derivative	6.59E-05	1.66	25
Conversion of acyl-coenzyme A	9.34E-05	1.964	4
Proliferation of cells	3.80E-03	2.161	136

Selected entries are shown.

is continuous as a result of cell-cell contact, and changes in one cell type that result from the gentamicin treatment likely effect physiological change in the other. One such cell-cell signaling pathway significantly affected by gentamicin treatment in non-hair cells is the Notch signaling pathway. *Dll1* and *Jag2* are highly expressed as Notch ligands in hair cells, and *Hes1*, *Hes5*, *Hey1*, and *Hey2* are expressed in supporting cells as Notch target genes (Zine and de Ribaupierre, 2002; Doetzlhofer et al., 2009); after gentamicin treatment, expression of *Dll1* and *Jag2* were down-regulated in hair cells, and *Hes1*, *Hes5*, *Hey1*, and *Hey2* were also expressed at a lower level in the non-hair cell population (p = n.s. for *Hes* and *Hey* genes) (**Table S1**), indicating disrupted cell-cell signaling between hair cells and supporting cells. This observation supports the idea that the expression profile changes that we observe in the non-hair cell population may be brought about by changes in response to gentamicin in hair cells. However, we could not exclude the possibility that non-supporting cells in the GFP-negative population might be responding to gentamicin treatment directly at the transcriptional level.

Similarity between Aminoglycoside Ototoxicity and Nephrotoxicity

Nephrotoxicity is another side effect of aminoglycoside antibiotics, and several publications catalog the changes in response to aminoglycoside antibiotics (Oh et al., 2006; Ozaki et al., 2010). A statistical comparison of gentamicin-induced hair cell gene expression changes and transcriptional profiles after gentamicin treatment in kidney identified a significant overlap between gene expression changes in gentamicin-treated hair cells and kidneys (p = 8.02E-08). In the dataset obtained from kidney, 211 genes were identified by microarray that were significantly changed after gentamicin treatment (Ozaki et al., 2010), and there were 50 genes in our hair cell dataset that were changed in the same direction as they were in kidney (**Table 5**).

We further compared the underlying biological processes and pathways that were affected by gentamicin in kidney and in hair cells, based on the transcriptional changes. We observed similar changes in the expression of genes involved in ribosome biogenesis, RNA processing, and translation in gentamicin-treated kidney and hair cells (**Table 5**). In addition, up-regulation of expression at the *Jun* gene, and induction of DNA repair gene *Lig4* were observed in both hair cells and kidney. The similarity in transcriptional response to gentamicin between hair cells and kidney cells suggests that there may be some common mechanisms responsible for aminoglycoside ototoxicity and nephrotoxicity, such as translation inhibition.

Despite the aforementioned similarity, the expression of stress response genes differed greatly in gentamicin-treated kidney and hair cells. Expression of oxidative stress response genes and *Hsp* chaperone genes was collectively increased in gentamicin-treated kidney while expression of these genes was not induced in hair cells. The discrepancy might be based on the different time points of sample collection (3 h post-gentamicin treatment for hair cell sample vs. 7 days after treatment for kidney). It was difficult to directly compare the expression of proliferation genes in kidneys with that in hair cells, because the kidney is an organ consisting of heterogeneous cell populations, with both dividing cells and quiescent cells, whereas hair cells are postmitotic.

Discussion

The causes of hypersensitivity of hair cells to aminoglycoside antibiotics remain unclear, and the prevailing hypothesis of aminoglycoside ototoxicity holds that aminoglycosides induce high levels of ROS leading to apoptotic stimulation. Our purpose in this project was to characterize the hair cell response to aminoglycoside antibiotics at an early time following administration, before the changes associated with apoptosis were apparent. To this end, we analyzed the response of hair cells after 3 h of treatment with gentamicin. As indicated in **Figures 2**, **3**, the JNK pathway and the NF-κB pathway are early responders, with many active components of the pathways showing significant increases. In addition, early changes in cell cycle-related genes, and DNA damage repair genes, signaled the potential disruption of the postmitotic state. In contrast, genes of the apoptosis and stress response pathways remain relatively unchanged at this time point. The transcription profile of hair cells at the early time point suggests that prior to the detection of an ROS response at the transcriptional level, other changes occur that may lead to the stimulation of apoptotic pathways, such as the aforementioned JNK pathway, NF-κB pathway and postmitotic state disruption.

Aminoglycoside-induced ROS production (Hirose et al., 1997), the protective effect of antioxidants (Schacht, 1999), and the NRF2-mediated oxidative stress response (Hoshino et al., 2011), have all been implicated in aminoglycoside ototoxicity. However, we did not observe a significant induction of the transcriptional targets of NRF2 at 3 h in our *in vitro* system. In addition, expression of heat shock chaperons and other stress response genes were not significantly upregulated. These results suggest that, although ROS changes in hair cells are rapid, at 3 h after gentamicin treatment they have not reached a level sufficient to trigger a broad stress response at the transcriptional level. The catastrophic oxidative stress that triggers apoptosis might be caused by continuous ROS build up, or by subsequent events such as mitochondrial dysfunction.

TABLE 5 | Comparison of gentamicin-induced hair cell gene expression changes with gentamicin-induced expression changes in kidney.

Gene symbol	Function Annotation	*p*-value in HC dataset	Fold Change in HC dataset	Findings in nephrotoxicity	Consistent
Ppp1r10	Phosphatase	5.84E-06	4.524746	Upregulates	Yes
Ddit3	Transcription factor	2.62E-05	2.751878	Upregulates	Yes
Jun	Transcription factor	0.00245	2.732988	Upregulates	Yes
Ccnl1	RNA splicing	4.46E-06	2.482795	Upregulates	Yes
Gnl3	p53 pathway regulation	7E-06	2.127794	Upregulates	Yes
Chka	Phospholipid synthesis	6.28E-07	2.029311	Upregulates	Yes
Ddx39	RNA splicing	4.98E-06	1.991224	Upregulates	Yes
Nop58	Ribosome biogenesis	7.68E-08	1.941254	Upregulates	Yes
Ppp1r15a	Phosphatase	0.009454	1.739694	Upregulates	Yes
Kti12	Unkown	0.008232	1.649551	Upregulates	Yes
Ptbp1	RNA splicing	3.83E-05	1.636352	Upregulates	Yes
Eed	Transcription repressor	8.35E-06	1.601639	Upregulates	Yes
Eif2b2	Translation	3.21E-06	1.572336	Upregulates	Yes
Cul2	Ubiquitin ligase	7.77E-06	1.510931	Upregulates	Yes
Zfp622	Transcription regulator	4.77E-06	1.483148	Upregulates	Yes
Naa15	N-acetyltransferase	0.000102	1.461136	Upregulates	Yes
Smn1	RNA splicing	0.000161	1.45206	Upregulates	Yes
Phax	RNA export	0.006074	1.438425	Upregulates	Yes
Lig4	DNA repair	5.82E-05	1.41918	Upregulates	Yes
Azin1	Metabolism	0.001597	1.388636	Upregulates	Yes
Arf6	Ras superfamily	0.000976	1.388019	Upregulates	Yes
2310044G17Rik	Unkown	0.005972	1.37605	Upregulates	Yes
Eaf1	Transcription factor	0.000222	1.369313	Upregulates	Yes
Cdk13	Transcription elongation	0.000244	1.365288	Upregulates	Yes
Pafah1b1	Inactivates platelet-act. factor	0.000164	1.346669	Upregulates	Yes
Gfer	Growth factor	0.001933	1.324081	Upregulates	Yes
Pelo	Mitosis	0.000148	1.319478	Upregulates	Yes
Tsc22d1	Transcription regulator	0.000157	1.315102	Upregulates	Yes
Ddx50	RNA helicase	0.00147	1.313465	Upregulates	Yes
Gadd45a	MAPK pathway regulator	0.007003	1.30902	Upregulates	Yes
Tars	tRNA synthesis	0.001263	1.292011	Upregulates	Yes
Mdm2	p53 pathway regulation	0.005424	1.28435	Upregulates	Yes
Dnaja2	Chaperone	0.001429	1.282581	Upregulates	Yes
Eif2b4	Translation	0.001361	1.270756	Upregulates	Yes
Sfpq	RNA splicing	0.000749	1.252767	Upregulates	Yes
Cnksr3	Sodium transport	0.00051	1.240931	Upregulates	Yes
Cand1	Ubiquitin ligase	0.003349	1.215329	Upregulates	Yes
Mybbp1a	Transcription regulator	0.000956	1.214954	Upregulates	Yes
Ncl	Ribosome biogenesis	0.00327	1.206809	Upregulates	Yes
Decr2	Metabolism	0.003445	−1.21269	Downregulates	Yes
Asl	Urea cycle	0.000314	−1.27227	Downregulates	Yes
Acsl3	Metabolism	0.000638	−1.27564	Downregulates	Yes
Gstm1	Antioxidant	0.00249	−1.32453	Downregulates	Yes
S100a1	Calcium binding	0.006299	−1.37041	Downregulates	Yes
Abat	Metabolism	0.002967	−1.38497	Downregulates	Yes
Mrpl23	Mitochondrial ribosome	0.003565	−1.38508	Downregulates	Yes
Hacl1	Metabolism	0.002033	−1.43919	Downregulates	Yes
St6galnac3	Glycolipid synthesis	0.005244	−1.46649	Downregulates	Yes
Pcx	Metabolism	0.00279	−1.65712	Downregulates	Yes
Eef1a1	Translation	2.35E-05	−2.0177	Downregulates	Yes
Zfp354a	Unkown	0.001648	1.544937	Downregulates	No

(Continued)

TABLE 5 | Continued

Gene symbol	Function Annotation	*p*-value in HC dataset	Fold Change in HC dataset	Findings in nephrotoxicity	Consistent
Hyou1	Stress	0.002956	−1.22211	Upregulates	No
Nedd4	Ubiquitin ligase	2.45E-06	−1.27335	Upregulates	No
Ctsd	Protease	0.00174	−1.33383	Upregulates	No
Hspa5	Stress	0.004463	−1.3884	Upregulates	No
Calr	Calcium binding	0.000413	−1.4266	Upregulates	No
Hsp90b1	Chaperone	5.87E-05	−1.56328	Upregulates	No
Egr1	Transcription regulator	0.004467	−1.61013	Upregulates	No
Zfp36l1	Growth factor response	0.001571	−1.65211	Upregulates	No
Pdia4	Protein folding	0.002689	−1.72559	Upregulates	No
Tubb5	Cytoskeleton	0.001836	−2.0123	Upregulates	No
Spp1	Cell-matrix interaction	0.004118	−4.30391	Upregulates	No

Expression of genes involved in initiation and execution of apoptosis were not significantly induced at this early time point, which is consistent with the established timeline of hair cell apoptosis (Matsui et al., 2004), and in line with the absence of a strong stress response at the transcriptional level. Together, the data suggest that, at this relatively early time point, hair cells are not yet committed to apoptosis. However, we observed expression changes for genes in upstream signaling pathways regulating apoptosis and cell survival. Not surprisingly, comparison of the observed gentamicin-induced changes in hair cells, with those from cell death studies in other cell lines or tissues, revealed a significant similarity in response to stress.

The disruption of the postmitotic state of hair cells is indicated by expression changes of cell cycle-related genes, suggesting that postmitotic state disruption in dying hair cells is another potential mechanism regulating apoptosis in hair cells, similar to what has been reported in postmitiotic neurons. Cell cycle re-entry has been observed in neurons before neuronal cell death, especially in neurodegenerative diseases (Arendt, 2000). In the central nervous system, mature neurons with mutated genes involved in maintaining the postmitotic state (inactivation of $p19^{Ink4d}$ and $p27^{Kip1}$) lose control of the postmitotic state, re-enter the cell cycle, and eventually undergo apoptosis (Zindy et al., 1999). Activation of the cell cycle machinery is considered one of the mechanisms controlling programmed cell death in postmitotic neurons, either through direct regulation of apoptosis pathways, or through checkpoint activation (Kruman, 2004; Golsteyn, 2005). In the cochlea, aberrant cell cycle re-entry leads to hair cell apoptosis (Chen et al., 2003; Laine et al., 2007). Inhibition of CDK activity by pharmaceutical inhibitors or genetic mutations of CDK genes protect hair cells from aminoglycoside ototoxicity (Tao and Segil, unpublished data), suggesting that cell cycle machinery regulates hair cell death. This mechanism is also supported by our expression data. Genes involved in cell cycle progression, G2 phase, and G2/M were significantly affected at the transcriptional level (**Table 2**), indicating a disruption of the quiescent state of hair cells by gentamicin treatment.

Further evidence supporting the loss of cell cycle control mechanisms includes our observation that hair cells up-regulate the expression of DNA repair genes after gentamicin treatment. Although induction of DNA repair genes by gentamicin-induced DNA damage is a plausible explanation, the lack of strong oxidative stress response at the transcriptional level, failure of DNA damage detection in hair cells after gentamicin treatment (Tao and Segil, unpublished data), and unchanged DNA repair gene expression at the transcriptional level in hair cells after DNA damaging agent treatment (Ng, Rainey and Segil, unpublished data) together suggest that gentamicin-induced DNA repair gene expression is not responding to DNA damage, but may be responding to a form of "replicative stress" induced by the disruption of the postmitotic state, similar to that observed in neurons exiting the postmitotic state (Andrusiak et al., 2012). During final differentiation and withdrawal from cell cycle, many postmitotic cells, such as neurons, which need never replicate their genomes again and thus can resort to repairing only essential genes, down-regulate global genomic DNA repair and rely entirely on transcription-coupled repair to maintain actively transcribed genes (Nouspikel and Hanawalt, 2000). Based on the observation that hair cell homeostasis requires transcription-coupled repair for long-term survival (Nagtegaal et al., 2015), we postulate that DNA repair capacity is regulated during hair cell differentiation and cell cycle withdrawal. Thus, up-regulation of the expression of DNA repair genes may indicate disruption of the quiescent state and cell cycle control.

Taken together, our RNA sequencing data suggests that at 3 h, an early time point after gentamicin treatment, activation of the JNK and NF-κB signaling pathways and the disruption of the quiescent state, indicated by significant transcription changes, precede broad stress response and apoptosis initiation, and that these early responses may regulate aminoglycoside-induced hair cell death.

Acknowledgments

We would like to thank USC Epigenome Center for library construction and sequencing services, Jane Johnson for Atoh1-GFP transgenic mice, Yibu Chen and Meng Li in USC NML Bioinformatics Service Program for their help with PartekFlow and IPA applications, Juan F. Llamas and Welly Makmura for animal care, and Robert Rainey and Greta Segil for careful reading of the manuscript. This project was supported by funds from NIH Grant R01DC007173, the Sidgmore Family Foundation, and the Hearing Health Foundation.

Table S1 | Gentamicin-induced differential gene expression in hair cells and in the non-hair cell population.

Table S2 | IPA canonical pathways that were affected by gentamicin in hair cells (pathways discussed in text are highlighted in yellow).

Table S3 | Gentamicin-induced expression changes of transcriptional targets of Jun, Nfkb1 and NRF2 (Nfe2l2). Red, significantly upregulated target genes; green, significantly downregulated target genes.

References

Andrusiak, M. G., Vandenbosch, R., Park, D. S., and Slack, R. S. (2012). The retinoblastoma protein is essential for survival of postmitotic neurons. *J. Neurosci.* 32, 14809–14814. doi: 10.1523/JNEUROSCI.1912-12.2012

Angel, P., Hattori, K., Smeal, T., and Karin, M. (1988). The jun proto-oncogene is positively autoregulated by its product, Jun/AP-1. *Cell* 55, 875–885.

Arendt, T. (2000).Alzheimer's disease as a loss of differentiation control in a subset of neurons that retain immature features in the adult brain. *Neurobiol. Aging* 21, 783–796. doi: 10.1016/S0197-4580(00)00216-5

Chen, P., Johnson, J. E., Zoghbi, H. Y., and Segil, N. (2002). The role of Math1 in inner ear development: uncoupling the establishment of the sensory primordium from hair cell fate determination. *Development* 129, 2495–2505.

Chen, P., and Segil, N. (1999). p27(Kip1) links cell proliferation to morphogenesis in the developing organ of Corti. *Development* 126, 1581–1590.

Chen, P., Zindy, F., Abdala, C., Liu, F., Li, X., Roussel, M. F., et al. (2003). Progressive hearing loss in mice lacking the cyclin-dependent kinase inhibitor Ink4d. *Nat. Cell Biol.* 5, 422–426. doi: 10.1038/ncb976

Doetzlhofer, A., Basch, M. L., Ohyama, T., Gessler, M., Groves, A. K., Segil, N. et al. (2009). Hey2 regulation by FGF provides a Notch-independent mechanism for maintaining pillar cell fate in the organ of Corti. *Dev. Cell* 16, 58–69. doi: 10.1016/j.devcel.2008.11.008

Forge, A., and Li, L. (2000). Apoptotic death of hair cells in mammalian vestibular sensory epithelia. *Hear. Res.* 139, 97–115. doi: 10.1016/S0378-5955(99)00177-X

Forge, A., and Schacht, J. (2000). Aminoglycoside Antibiotics. *Audiol. Neurootol.* 5, 3–22. doi: 10.1159/000013861

Francis, S. P., Katz, J., Fanning, K. D., Harris, K. A., Nicholas, B. D., Lacy, M., et al. (2013). A novel role of cytosolic protein synthesis inhibition in aminoglycoside ototoxicity. *J. Neurosci.* 33, 3079–3093. doi: 10.1523/JNEUROSCI.3430-12.2013

Golsteyn, R. M. (2005). Cdk1 and Cdk2 complexes (cyclin dependent kinases) in apoptosis: a role beyond the cell cycle. *Cancer Lett.* 217, 129–138. doi: 10.1016/j.canlet.2004.08.005

Gulley, R. L., and Resse, T. S. (1976). Intercellular junctions in the reticular lamina of the organ of Corti. *J. Neurocytol.* 5, 479–507. doi: 10.1007/BF01181652

Hirose, K., Hockenbery, D. M., and Rubel, E. W. (1997). Reactive oxygen species in chick hair cells after gentamicin exposure *in vitro*. *Hear. Res.* 104, 1–14. doi: 10.1016/S0378-5955(96)00169-4

Hoshino, T., Tabuchi, K., Nishimura, B., Tanaka, S., Nakayama, M., Ishii, T., et al. (2011). Protective role of Nrf2 in age-related hearing loss and gentamicin ototoxicity. *Biochem. Biophys. Res. Commun.* 415, 94–98. doi: 10.1016/j.bbrc.2011.10.019

Huth, M. E., Ricci, A. J., and Cheng, A. G. (2011). Mechanisms of aminoglycoside ototoxicity and targets of hair cell protection. *Int. J. Otolaryngol.* 2011:937861. doi: 10.1155/2011/937861

Jamesdaniel, S., Ding, D., Kermany, M. H., Davidson, B. A., Knight, P. R. IIIrd., Salvi, R., et al. (2008). Proteomic analysis of the balance between survival and cell death responses in cisplatin-mediated ototoxicity. *J. Proteome Res.* 7, 3516–3524. doi: 10.1021/pr8002479

Jiang, H., Sha, S. H., and Schacht, J. (2005). NF-kappaB pathway protects cochlear hair cells from aminoglycoside-induced ototoxicity. *J. Neurosci. Res.* 79, 644–651. doi: 10.1002/jnr.20392

Kruman, I. I. (2004). Why do neurons enter the cell cycle? *Cell Cycle* 3, 769–773. doi: 10.4161/cc.3.6.901

Laine, H., Doetzlhofer, A., Mantela, J., Ylikoski, J., Laiho, M., Roussel, M. F., et al. (2007). p19(Ink4d) and p21(Cip1) collaborate to maintain the postmitotic state of auditory hair cells, their codeletion leading to DNA damage and p53-mediated apoptosis. *J. Neurosci.* 27, 1434–1444. doi: 10.1523/JNEUROSCI.4956-06.2007

Lumpkin, E. A., Collisson, T., Parab, P., Omer-Abdalla, A., Haeberle, H., Chen, P., et al. (2003). Math1-driven GFP expression in the developing nervous system of transgenic mice. *Gene Expr. Patterns* 3, 389–395. doi: 10.1016/S1567-133X(03)00089-9

Ma, Q. (2013). Role of Nrf2 in oxidative stress and toxicity. *Annu. Rev. Pharmacol. Toxicol.* 53, 401–426. doi: 10.1146/annurev-pharmtox-011112-140320

Matsui, J. I., Gale, J. E., and Warchol, M. E. (2004). Critical signaling events during the aminoglycoside-induced death of sensory hair cells *in vitro*. *J. Neurobiol.* 61, 250–266. doi: 10.1002/neu.20054

Matsui, J. I., Ogilvie, J. M., and Warchol, M. E. (2002). Inhibition of caspases prevents ototoxic and ongoing hair cell death. *J. Neurosci.* 22, 1218–1227.

Nagtegaal, A. P., Rainey, R. N., van der Pluijm, I., Brandt, R. M. C., van der Horst, G. T. J., Borst, J. G. G., et al. (2015). Cockayne syndrome group B (Csb) and group A (Csa) deficiencies predispose to hearing loss and cochlear hair cell degeneration in mice. *J. Neurosci.* 35, 4280–4286. doi: 10.1523/JNEUROSCI.5063-14.2015

Nagy, I., Bodmer, M., Brors, D., and Bodmer,.D. (2004). Early gene expression in the organ of Corti exposed to gentamicin. *Hear. Res.* 195, 1–8. doi: 10.1016/j.heares.2004.04.010

Nouspikel, T., and Hanawalt, P. C. (2000). Terminally differentiated human neurons repair transcribed genes but display attenuated global DNA repair and modulation of repair gene expression. *Mol. Cell Biol.* 20, 1562–1570. doi: 10.1128/MCB.20.5.1562-1570.2000

Oh, J. H., Park, H. J., Lim, J. S., Jeong, S. Y., Hwang, J. Y., Kim, Y. B., et al. (2006). Gene expression profiling of early renal toxicity induced by gentamicin in mice. *Mol. Cell Toxicol.* 2, 185–192. doi: 10.1002/jbt.20277

Ozaki, N., Matheis, K. A., Gamber, M., Feidl, T., Nolte, T., Kalkuhl, A., et al. (2010). Identification of genes involved in gentamicin-induced nephrotoxicity in rats – A toxicogenomic investigation. *Exp. Toxicol. Pathol.* 62, 555–566. doi: 10.1016/j.etp.2009.07.004

Ringnér, M. (2008). What is principal component analysis? *Nat. Biotechnol.* 26, 303–304. doi: 10.1038/nbt0308-303

Schacht, J. (1999). Antioxidant therapy attenuates aminoglycoside-induced hearing loss. *Ann. N. Y. Acad. Sci.* 884, 125–130.

Schafer, F. Q., and Buettner, G. R. (2001). Redox environment of the cell as viewed through the redox state of the glutathione disulfide/glutathione couple. *Free Radic. Biol. Med.* 30, 1191–1212. doi: 10.1016/S0891-5849(01)00480-4

Schreiber, J., Jenner, R. G., Murray, H. L., Gerber, G. K., Gifford, D. K., and Young, R. A. (2006). Coordinated binding of NF-kappaB family members in the response of human cells to lipopolysaccharide. *Proc. Natl. Acad. Sci. U.S.A.* 103, 5899–5904. doi: 10.1073/pnas.0510996103

Steyger, P. S., Peters, S. L., Rehling, J., Hordichok, A., and Dai, C. F. (2003). Uptake of gentamicin by bullfrog saccular hair cells *in vitro*. *J. Assoc. Res. Otolaryngol.* 4, 565–578. doi: 10.1007/s10162-003-4002-5

Ten, R. M., Paya, C. V., Israël, N., Le Bail, O., Mattei, M. G., Virelizier, J. L., et al. (1992). The characterization of the promoter of the gene encoding the p50 subunit of NF-kappa B indicates that it participates in its own regulation. *EMBO J.* 11, 195–203.

Tiede, L., Steyger, P. S., Nichols, M. G., and Hallworth, R. (2009). Metabolic imaging of the organ of corti–a window on cochlea bioenergetics. *Brain Res.* 1277, 37–41. doi: 10.1016/j.brainres.2009.02.052

Wang, Z., Gerstein, M., and Snyder, M. (2009). RNA-seq: a revolutionary tool for transcriptomics. *Nat. Rev. Genet.* 10, 57–63. doi: 10.1038/nrg2484

Ylikoski, J., Liang, X. Q., Virkkala, J., and Pirvola, U. (2002). Blockade of c-Jun N-terminal kinase pathway attenuates gentamicin-induced cochlear and vestibular hair cell death. *Hear. Res.* 166, 33–43. doi: 10.1016/S0378-5955(01)00388-4

Zindy, F., Cunningham, J. J., Sherr, C. J., Jogal, S., Smeyne, R. J., and Roussel, M. F. (1999). Postnatal neuronal proliferation in mice lacking Ink4d and Kip1 inhibitors of cyclin-dependent kinases. *Proc. Natl. Acad. Sci. U.S.A.* 96, 13462–13467.

Zine, A., and de Ribaupierre, F. (2002). Notch/Notch ligands and Math1 expression patterns in the organ of Corti of wild-type and Hes1 and Hes5 mutant mice. *Hear. Res.* 170, 22–31. doi: 10.1016/S0378-5955(02)00449-5

2

Local mechanisms for loud sound-enhanced aminoglycoside entry into outer hair cells

Hongzhe Li[1], Allan Kachelmeier[1], David N. Furness[2] and Peter S. Steyger[1]**

[1] Oregon Hearing Research Center, Oregon Health & Science University, Portland, OR, USA, [2] School of Life Sciences, Keele University, Staffordshire, UK

Edited by:
Andy Groves,
Baylor College of Medicine, USA

Reviewed by:
Hong-Bo Zhao,
University of Kentucky Medical Center, USA
Jenny Stone,
University of Washington, USA

***Correspondence:**
Hongzhe Li and Peter S. Steyger,
Oregon Hearing Research Center,
Oregon Health & Science University,
3181 SW Sam Jackson Park Road,
Portland, OR 97239, USA
Tel: (+1) 503-494-2935,
(+1) 503-494-1062,
Fax: (+1) 503-494-5656
liho@ohsu.edu;
steygerp@ohsu.edu

Loud sound exposure exacerbates aminoglycoside ototoxicity, increasing the risk of permanent hearing loss and degrading the quality of life in affected individuals. We previously reported that loud sound exposure induces temporary threshold shifts (TTS) and enhances uptake of aminoglycosides, like gentamicin, by cochlear outer hair cells (OHCs). Here, we explore mechanisms by which loud sound exposure and TTS could increase aminoglycoside uptake by OHCs that may underlie this form of ototoxic synergy. Mice were exposed to loud sound levels to induce TTS, and received fluorescently-tagged gentamicin (GTTR) for 30 min prior to fixation. The degree of TTS was assessed by comparing auditory brainstem responses (ABRs) before and after loud sound exposure. The number of tip links, which gate the GTTR-permeant mechanoelectrical transducer (MET) channels, was determined in OHC bundles, with or without exposure to loud sound, using scanning electron microscopy. We found wide-band noise (WBN) levels that induce TTS also enhance OHC uptake of GTTR compared to OHCs in control cochleae. In cochlear regions with TTS, the increase in OHC uptake of GTTR was significantly greater than in adjacent pillar cells. In control mice, we identified stereociliary tip links at ~50% of potential positions in OHC bundles. However, the number of OHC tip links was significantly reduced in mice that received WBN at levels capable of inducing TTS. These data suggest that GTTR uptake by OHCs during TTS occurs by increased permeation of surviving, mechanically-gated MET channels, and/or non-MET aminoglycoside-permeant channels activated following loud sound exposure. Loss of tip links would hyperpolarize hair cells and potentially increase drug uptake via aminoglycoside-permeant channels expressed by hair cells. The effect of TTS on aminoglycoside-permeant channel kinetics will shed new light on the mechanisms of loud sound-enhanced aminoglycoside uptake, and consequently on ototoxic synergy.

Keywords: aminoglycoside, GTTR, outer hair cells, ototoxicity, auditory function, cellular uptake

Introduction

Aminoglycoside antibiotics, like gentamicin and tobramycin, are clinically-essential antibiotics for treating life-threatening Gram-negative bacterial infections in premature babies or patients with cystic fibrosis, Gram-positive infections like tuberculosis, and protozoal infections (Durante-Mangoni et al., 2009; Zimmerman and Lahav, 2013). Despite their wide use, broad-spectrum bactericidal efficacy, and low cost, clinical dosing with aminoglycosides is limited by the risk of acute kidney damage and life-long hearing loss, with significant ramifications for quality of life (Forge and Schacht, 2000; Zimmerman and Lahav, 2013).

In the mammalian cochlea, auditory sensory cells, particularly outer hair cells (OHCs), are more susceptible to aminoglycoside-induced cytotoxicity than other cochlear cells, particularly at the base of the cochlea most sensitive to high frequency sound. Once these sensory cells are lost, they cannot be regenerated, leading to life-long hearing loss and deafness. Thus, extensive efforts are underway to ameliorate and prevent aminoglycoside-induced hair cell death.

Aminoglycosides can rapidly cross the blood-labyrinth barrier (BLB) into cochlear tissues and fluids (Tran Ba Huy et al., 1986; Li and Steyger, 2011), and enter hair cells through a number of routes. The best-characterized route is permeation through the mechanoelectrical transduction (MET) channel (Marcotti et al., 2005; Alharazneh et al., 2011). The MET channel is mechanically-gated by extracellular, heterodimeric tip links between adjacent stereocilia (Kazmierczak et al., 2007). Other mechanisms by which aminoglycosides can enter hair cells include endocytosis (Hashino and Shero, 1995), and permeation through other aminoglycoside-permeant cation channels expressed by hair cells, such as TRPV4 on apical membranes (Karasawa et al., 2008), or TRPA1 on basolateral membranes, of OHCs (Stepanyan et al., 2011).

In vitro studies show that when the MET channel is blocked, there is significantly reduced entry of aminoglycosides, or other organic cations such as FM1–43, into hair cells and reduced hair cell death (Gale et al., 2001; Marcotti et al., 2005; Wang and Steyger, 2009; Alharazneh et al., 2011), suggesting that the MET channel is a primary conduit for aminoglycoside entry into hair cells. Additionally, *in vitro* studies demonstrate that when tip links are broken or congenitally absent, hair cells show reduced uptake of aminoglycosides or FM1–43, and reduced drug-induced cytotoxicity (Seiler and Nicolson, 1999; Gale et al., 2001; Alharazneh et al., 2011; Vu et al., 2013). If extant tip links are broken, they can be regenerated within 24–48 h to restore MET function, and aminoglycoside uptake (Zhao et al., 1996; Vu et al., 2013). Tip link regeneration may represent one mechanism underlying temporary threshold shifts (TTS) in auditory perception (Zhao et al., 1996) following exposure to brief periods of intense sound such as explosions, gunfire, or loud music at rock concerts. The physiological effects of TTS also include transient reduction of endolymphatic potential (EP; Syka et al., 1981) and hair cell depolarization via purinergic receptors (Housley et al., 2013). Loud sound exposure has long been known to exacerbate aminoglycoside-induced ototoxicity in rodent studies (Brown et al., 1978; Gannon et al., 1979). We previously demonstrated that aminoglycoside exposure during moderate-to-intense sound exposure increases murine hair-cell uptake of fluorescently-tagged gentamicin (GTTR), elevating the risk of ototoxicity (Li et al., 2011). Experimentally, loud sound levels break tip links *in vivo* and close mechanically-gated MET channels (Husbands et al., 1999; Kurian et al., 2003; Sellick, 2007; Sellick et al., 2007) would be expected to reduce OHC uptake of aminoglycosides. This raises the question of how loud sound-enhanced GTTR uptake by OHCs occurs. To answer this question we conducted experiments to correlate the degree of tip link breakage in OHCs with uptake of GTTR. We found that loud sound-induced TTS was accompanied by a significantly decreased percentage of surviving OHC stereociliary tip links, while increasing OHC uptake of GTTR. This finding suggests that the tip link-gated MET channel is not the only conduit for GTTR entry into hair cells. We suggest several potential routes of entry for GTTR into hair cells in the presence of noise damage including changes in the MET channel following tip-link loss, endocytosis and basolateral channels, and further experimental hypotheses that if tested will shed new light on the mechanisms of loud sound-enhanced aminoglycoside uptake, and the ototoxic synergy between sound and aminoglycosides.

Material and Methods

Mice

To induce TTS, adult C57Bl/6 mice at 6–7 weeks of age with positive Preyer's reflex were exposed to wideband noise (WBN; 86, 91 or 96 dB SPL) for 6 h/day for 3 days (Li et al., 2011). Mice were then intra-peritoneally (*i.p.*) injected with fluorescently-conjugated gentamicin (GTTR, 2 mg/kg) dissolved in phosphate buffered saline (PBS, pH = 7.4) within 30 min of cessation of noise exposure on the 3rd day, to track gentamicin uptake as previously described (Li et al., 2011). Control animals without noise exposure also received GTTR. Thirty minutes after GTTR administration, all mice were deeply anesthetized, and cardiac-perfused with PBS, then 4% formaldehyde. Fixed cochlear tissues were excised and processed for confocal microscopy and fluorescence quantification (Wang and Steyger, 2009). The care and use of all animals reported in this study was approved by the Animal Care and Use Committee of Oregon Health and Science University (IACUC approval #IS00001801).

TTS Assessment

Mice were assessed by auditory brainstem response (ABR) measurements to determine the degree of TTS and time course of hearing recovery. Briefly, ABRs to 1 ms rise-time tone burst stimuli at 4, 8, 12, 16, 24 and 32 kHz, with 5 dB steps, were recorded and thresholds obtained for each ear, using an in-house system described previously (Mitchell et al., 1996). ABRs were obtained from both ears of each mouse the day before loud sound exposure (denoted as "pre" in **Figures 1A–C**), within 1 h ("day 0"), as well as one day ("day 1"), one week and two weeks after loud sound exposure was completed. Prior to ABR recording, mice were anesthetized *i.p.* with ketamine (65 mg/kg) and xylazine (13 mg/kg) and placed on a heating pad in a sound-proof, electrically isolated chamber. Needle electrodes were placed subcutaneously below the test ear, at the vertex, and with a ground on the claw. Each ear was

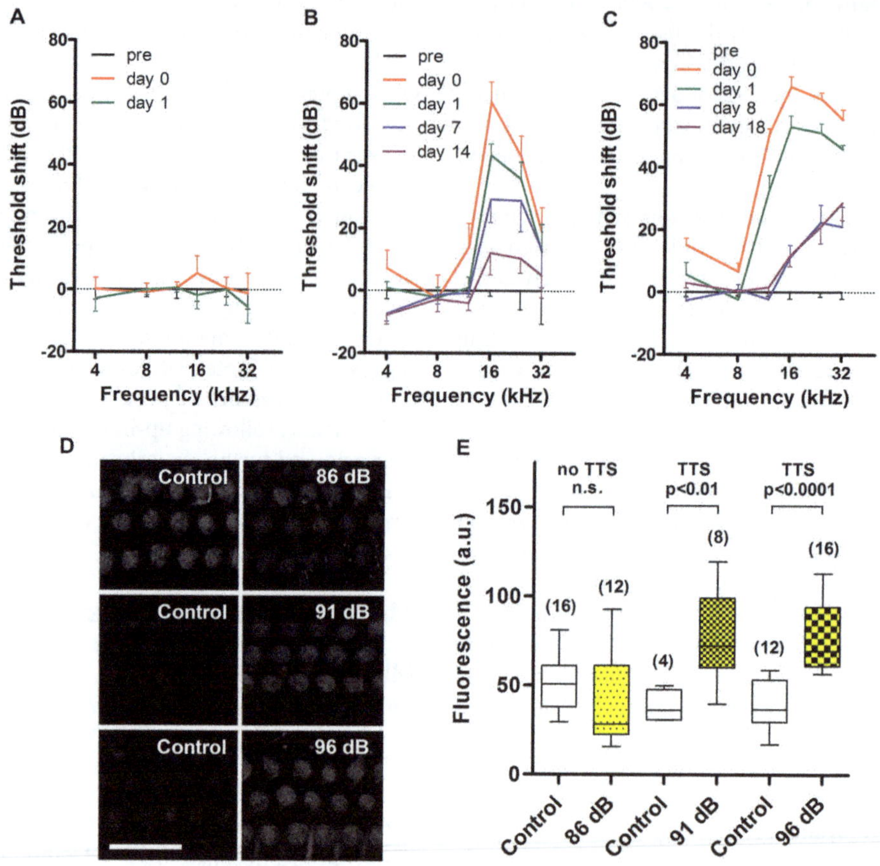

FIGURE 1 | Temporary threshold shifts (TTS) and sound-enhanced GTTR uptake by OHCs. (A) Prolonged wide-band noise (WBN) at 86 dB SPL for 18 h over 3 days did not induce TTS (n = 3 mice/6 ears tested), nor enhance GTTR uptake by OHCs from the mid-basal coil of the cochlea (**D**, top row). **(B, C)** Prolonged WBN at 91 and 96 dB SPL for 18 h over 3 days did induce TTS that was maximal immediately after sound exposure, and mostly recovered over the next two weeks. Note that some permanent threshold shifts were observed at 16, 24 and 32 kHz 2 weeks after exposure to 91 dB SPL (n = 3/6 ears), and were more protracted 18 days after 96 dB SPL (n = 4/8 ears). Sound-induced TTS was also manifested in a broader frequency range at 96 dB SPL (12–32 kHz in **C**) compared to 91 dB SPL (16–32 kHz in **B**). **(D)** TTS induced by 91 and 96 dB SPL WBN enhanced GTTR uptake by OHCs from the mid-basal coil of the cochlea (middle and bottom rows). Note that experiments at different levels of sound exposure were conducted independently of each other, thus GTTR uptake was only comparable within experiments, i.e., horizontally within rows in **(D)**. Scale bar = 25 μm. **(E)** Sound-enhanced uptake of GTTR was significantly elevated after exposure to 91 (n = 2 for control, 4 for sound exposure) and 96 dB SPL (n = 3 for control, 4 for sound exposure), using unpaired t test. GTTR uptake was not further elevated at 96 dB SPL in the mid-basal cochlear regions. For 86 dB SPL comparison, n = 2 for control, 4 for sound exposure. Box represents the 25 and 75 percentiles of each dataset, while whiskers represent the minimum and maximum of each dataset. Number with parenthesis above the whiskers is the number of images analyzed per experimental condition. n.s. = not significant.

stimulated separately with a closed tube sound delivery system sealed into the ear canal. ABR threshold was defined as the sound level at which the minimum identifiable ABR response occurred.

Imaging and Data Analysis

The intensity of GTTR fluorescence was measured in single plane images of OHCs and pillar cells obtained with confocal settings kept identical across experiments, and processed in Photoshop and FIJI (ImageJ) as described previously (Wang and Steyger, 2009). An additional cohort of mice, exposed to 91 dB SPL WBN, was cardiac-perfused with 2.5% glutaraldehyde in 0.1 M sodium cacodylate buffer, and cochlear tissues processed for field emission scanning electron microscopy (FESEM) using the osmium-thiocarbohydrazide impregnation method (Furness and Hackney, 1986). The number of stereociliary tips and visible tip links per hair bundle (10 bundles per OHC row) was counted at a mid-cochlear location corresponding to a frequency range of 12–16 kHz. Student's t-test and 1-way ANOVA with Tukey's *post hoc* comparisons test were used to determine any significant differences between treatment groups.

Results

Enhanced GTTR Uptake by OHCs in Cochlear Regions with TTS

We systematically measured the degree of TTS induced by 3 different sound levels and assessed ABR threshold at multiple time points after sound exposure. This allowed us to assess the degree of TTS and correlate the degree of TTS and GTTR uptake for each sound protocol. Since serial ABR measurements are required to determine the degree of TTS, an independent set of mice was examined to determine GTTR uptake for each sound protocol.

Prolonged wide-band noise (WBN) at 86 dB SPL for 18 h over 3 days did not induce TTS (**Figure 1A**). Prolonged WBN at 91 and 96 dB SPL did induce TTS (**Figures 1B,C**). Elevation in sound-induced TTS (>50 dB) was more prevalent over a broader frequency range after 96 dB SPL sound treatment (12–32 kHz, **Figure 1C**) than at 91 dB sound exposure (16–32 kHz, **Figure 1B**). Exposure to 96 dB SPL WBN also induced a smaller, yet significant, TTS (<20 dB) in the lower 4-kHz frequency region (**Figure 2B**) that was not evident after exposure at 91 dB SPL. This smaller TTS in the 4-kHz region after 96 dB SPL exposure (and also at the 12-kHz region after 91 dB SPL exposure) recovered quickly within 24 h. Recovery from major TTS, 12 kHz and above after 96 dB SPL exposure and 16 kHz and above after 91 dB SPL exposure, was longer, and recovery took up to 2 weeks, and some permanent threshold shifts were seen at 24 and 32 kHz after 96 dB SPL exposure.

Exposure to prolonged WBN at 86 dB SPL which did not induce TTS (**Figure 1A**) did not enhance GTTR uptake by OHCs in the mid-basal coil of the cochlea (**Figure 1D**). Prolonged exposure to WBN at 91 and 96 dB SPL that did induce TTS (**Figures 1B,C**) also enhanced GTTR uptake by OHCs in the mid-basal coil of the cochlea (**Figure 1D**). However, loud (91 dB SPL) sound-enhanced OHC uptake of GTTR in the mid-basal coil of the cochlea appeared not further increased after exposure to higher sound levels (96 dB SPL; **Figure 1E**).

Regions with Enhanced GTTR Uptake are Broader than Regions with Major Elevations in TTS

All OHCs in cochleae with 96 dB SPL-induced TTS exhibited greater GTTR fluorescence compared to OHCs from equivalent regions in control cochleae (**Figure 2A**). GTTR fluorescence intensity was assessed in OHCs from apical, middle, and basal coils, representing a frequency range of 4–6 kHz, 12–20 kHz, and 32–48 kHz respectively, as determined by a murine frequency-location map (Ou et al., 2000; Müller et al., 2005). This enabled comparison of the degree of enhanced GTTR uptake at various cochlear tonotopic locations. In apical, 4-kHz frequency cochlear regions, 96 dB SPL WBN induced a small TTS that was generally less than 20 dB (**Figure 2B**), but significantly enhanced OHC uptake of GTTR compared to OHCs from equivalent regions in control cochleae (**Figure 2C**). At basal, 12–32 kHz, cochlear regions, 96 dB SPL WBN induced threshold shifts up to 70 dB, and more statistically significant OHC uptake of GTTR than in OHCs from equivalent regions in control cochleae (**Figures 2B,C**).

Sound-Enhanced GTTR Uptake is More Robust in OHCs than in Pillar Cells

Previously we demonstrated that TTS increased cochlear uptake of GTTR, particularly in marginal cells adjacent to vasodilated

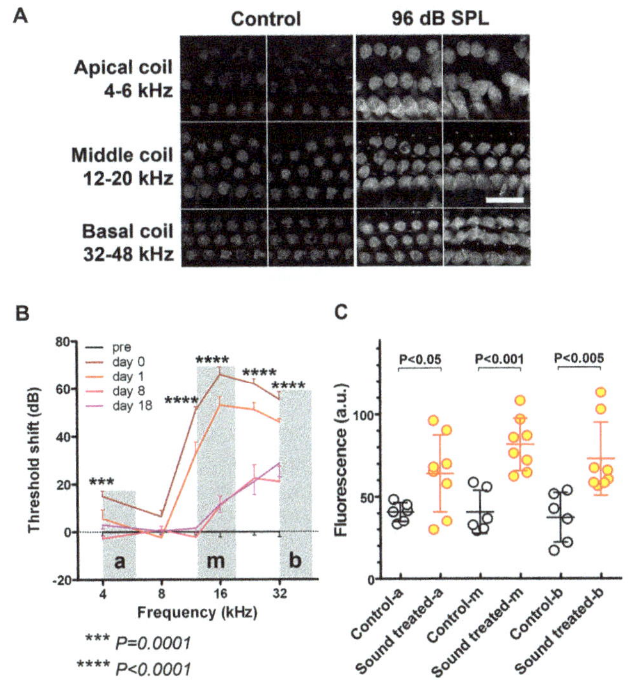

FIGURE 2 | Regions with sound-enhanced GTTR uptake correspond to regions with TTS. (A) GTTR fluorescence in OHCs from apical, middle, and basal coils, representing 4–6 kHz, 12–20 kHz, and 32–48 kHz respectively, determined by the murine frequency-place map ImageJ plug-in.[1] Scale bar = 25 μm. OHCs in loud sound-treated cochleae exhibited greater GTTR fluorescence compared to OHCs in all coils from control cochleae. **(B)** 96 dB SPL WBN resulted in a high-pass shaped TTS curve, minimal, yet significant, TTS at lower frequencies, i.e., 4–8 kHz, and TTS up to 70 dB at higher frequency regions, i.e., 12–32 kHz, using unpaired *t*-tests. "**a**", "**m**", and "**b**" depict apical, middle and basal cochlear regions respectively. Shaded areas depict cochlear regions where GTTR fluorescence was imaged and quantified. **(C)** WBN-induced sound-enhanced GTTR uptake is statistically significant at all examined frequency regions, using unpaired *t*-tests. Mean and s.d. are superimposed on each dataset.

capillaries in the *stria vascularis* (Li et al., 2011), which was also observed here (data not shown). In this experiment, we assessed whether major TTS is accompanied by enhanced uptake of GTTR in pillar cells (as a proxy for all supporting cells within the organ of Corti), or preferentially by OHCs, by comparing the relative increases in GTTR fluorescence after induction of TTS in OHCs and adjacent pillar cells. After exposure to prolonged WBN at 96 dB SPL, only a third of pillar cells displayed enhanced GTTR uptake, yet the majority of OHCs in the same region displayed enhanced GTTR uptake (**Figure 3A**; **Table 1**). A one-way ANOVA with *post hoc* Tukey's multiple comparison test revealed significant increases in GTTR fluorescence in OHCs, but not pillar cells, after loud sound exposure (**Table 1**). Data obtained from cochleae after prolonged sound exposure to 91 dB SPL presented a similar trend (**Figure 3B**; **Table 1**). This suggests

[1] http://www.masseyeandear.org/research/otolaryngology/investigators/laboratories/eaton-peabody-laboratories/epl-histology-resources/imagej-plugin-for-cochlear-frequency-mapping-in-whole-mounts/

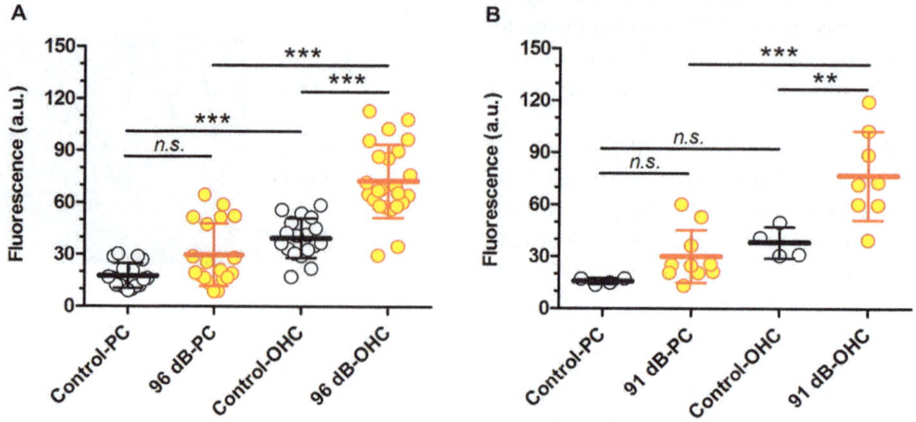

FIGURE 3 | Loud sound-enhanced GTTR uptake in two cell populations from the organ of Corti after 96 dB SPL (A) or 91 dB SPL (B) sound exposure. (A) Sound-enhanced GTTR fluorescence was observed in a fraction of pillar cells from the middle and basal cochlear regions of 2 out of 4 cochleae after exposure to WBN at 96 dB SPL for 18 h over 3 days. In contrast, enhanced GTTR fluorescence was observed in the majority of OHCs adjacent to pillar cells in the same regions. $n = 3$ for control cochleae, $n = 4$ for loud sound-treated cochleae; up to six sites were examined for each cochlea and averaged from at least 16 pillar cells or OHCs. **(B)** Sound-enhanced GTTR fluorescence was observed in a few pillar cells from the middle cochlear regions after exposure to WBN at 91 dB SPL for 18 h over 3 days. In contrast, enhanced GTTR fluorescence was observed in the majority of OHCs adjacent to pillar cells in the same regions. $n = 2$ for control cochleae, $n = 4$ for sound-treated cochleae; up to six sites examined for each cochlea and averaged from at least 9 pillar cells or OHCs. For both sound levels, sound-enhanced GTTR uptake is only statistically significant in OHC populations, using Tukey's multiple comparison test from one-way ANOVA. $^{***}p < 0.001$, $^{**}p < 0.01$, *n.s.* = not significant. Mean and s.d. are superimposed on each dataset.

TABLE 1 | Loud sound exposure induced greater GTTR uptake by OHCs compared to pillar cells.

		96 dB SPL			91 dB SPL*		
		N	Mean ± s.e.m.	Tukey's test[#]	*N*	Mean ± s.e.m.	Tukey's test[#]
OHCs	**Control**	18	39.49 ± 2.696	$p < 0.001$	4	38.13 ± 4.541	$p < 0.001$
	Sound-treated	24	72.70 ± 4.306		8	76.96 ± 9.068	
Pillar cells	**Control**	17	17.59 ± 1.740	$p > 0.05$ (n.s.)	4	15.70 ± 0.8995	$p > 0.05$ (n.s.)
	Sound-treated	19	29.87 ± 4.173		10	30.20 ± 4.803	

**Only cells from the middle coil of 91 dB SPL sound-exposed cochleae (and their respective controls) were imaged, while cells from apical, middle and basal cochlear regions of 96 dB SPL sound-exposed cochleae (and their respective controls) were imaged and GTTR fluorescence quantified (arbitrary unit). [#]Tukey's multiple comparison test from one-way ANOVA including all four conditions: Control-OHC, Sound-treated-OHC, Control-PC and Sound-treated-PC. $p < 0.05$ is significant. PC = Pillar cells. N = number of images, multiple cells per image were averaged.*

that OHCs appear to possess at least one mechanism that facilitates greater GTTR uptake compared to pillar cells.

Noise Exposure Reduces the Number of Tip Links

Scanning electron microscopy of OHCs with or without prolonged exposure to WBN at 91 dB SPL, revealed OHCs with a classic "V" or "W" stereociliary bundle (**Figures 4A,D**). In OHCs without exposure to WBN, tip-links between stereocilia of adjacent rows were clearly identifiable (**Figure 4B**). The percentage of tip links present in representative OHCs in the middle cochlear coil of control mice varied between OHC rows, ranging from 38% for the innermost row to 61% for the outermost row (**Figure 4C**; **Table 2**). Prolonged exposure to WBN at 91 dB SPL caused no obvious disarray of bundle morphology in OHCs from equivalent regions to those in control cochleae (**Figure 4D**). Nonetheless, substantially fewer tip links were observed in all three rows of OHCs in loud sound-exposed cochleae compared to OHCs from equivalent regions in control cochleae (**Figures 4E,F**; **Table 2**). This reduction in tip link survival was statistically significant for all three row-to-row comparisons using unpaired *t*-tests with Welch's correction ($p < 0.0001$).

Discussion

The present study has demonstrated that: (i) moderate-to-loud sound level exposures (91 and 96 dB WBN for 6 h per day over 3 consecutive days) that induce TTS also increase OHC uptake of ototoxic aminoglycosides (GTTR) *in vivo*; (ii) higher levels of sound exposure (96 dB SPL) increase the degree of TTS and widen the region of GTTR uptake; and (iii) tip link survival in the region of increased GTTR uptake is reduced significantly. In addition, pillar cell uptake of GTTR is not

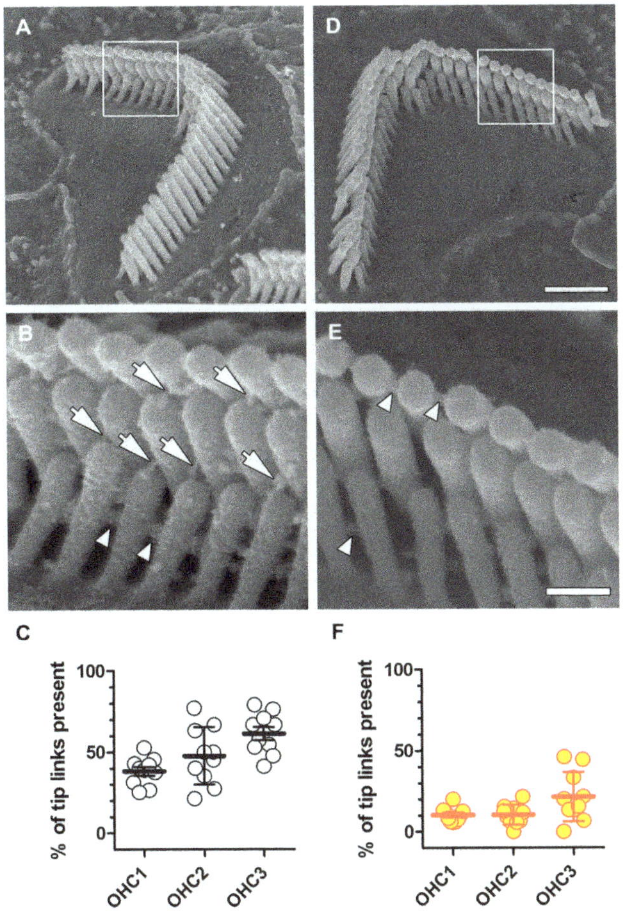

FIGURE 4 | Reduced tip-link survival after noise exposure. (A) A representative stereociliary bundle from the second OHC row in the middle coil of a control cochlea. Framed area is enlarged in **(B)**, arrows indicate identifiable tip links, and arrowheads point to identifiable side links. **(C)** The percentage of tip-links in OHC rows from the middle coil in a representative control mouse that survived processing for SEM is shown. Each symbol represents the percentage of tip-links observed in an individual OHC bundle (n = 10 per row), with mean and s.d. superimposed. **(D)** A representative stereociliary bundle from the third OHC row in the middle cochlear coil of a representative mouse exposed to WBN at 91 dB SPL for 18 h over 3 days displaying normal gross bundle morphology, but no visible tip links **(E)**, while lateral links between stereocilia of the same row are still present. **(F)** Following prolonged WBN at 91 dB SPL for 18 h, the percentage of tip-links surviving sound exposure and SEM processing are substantially reduced in all three OHC rows. Scale bar = 1.0 μm in **(D)** also applies to **(A)**. Scale bar = 250 nm in **(E)**, also applies to **(B)**.

significantly increased after loud sound exposure, suggesting that endolymph levels are statistically unchanged, and that increased OHC uptake of GTTR after loud sound exposure is hair cell-specific. These findings are clinically relevant as they provide additional evidence for a synergistic ototoxicity of loud sound exposure and aminoglycoside treatment (Gannon et al., 1979; Ryan and Bone, 1982). These findings also have implications for patients treated with aminoglycosides and (prior) exposure to high noise levels (Li and Steyger, 2009; Zimmerman and Lahav, 2013).

The findings have two additional implications. The first is that loss and regeneration of stereociliary tip links may explain loud sound-induced TTS. In organ of Corti explants, stereociliary tip links are regenerated 24–48 h after ablation, restoring functional kinetics and aminoglycoside permeability to MET channels (Indzhykulian et al., 2013; Vu et al., 2013). If this capability also exists *in vivo*, it may contribute to the recovery of auditory function from TTS in the 4 kHz region after 96 dB SPL WBN exposure. To test this hypothesis, it will be necessary to test whether the extent of tip-link loss and regeneration correlates with the degree of TTS and recovery observed in this region. Experiments to verify this are ongoing.

Other mechanisms besides loss of tip links could contribute to the TTS, including synaptic mechanisms (Chen et al., 2012; Liu et al., 2013), or a reduction (followed by recovery) in the EP (Syka et al., 1981; Ahmad et al., 2003). We used C57BL/6 mice that are resistant to changes in the EP after acoustic overstimulation (Ohlemiller and Gagnon, 2007), which reduced the contribution of EP loss allowing us to better evaluate the role of the organ of Corti in TTS.

The second major implication of these data is that GTTR uptake is enhanced in regions associated with TTS and significant loss of tip links. At first sight, this result is surprising as tip-link destruction would be predicted to *reduce* GTTR uptake. Tip links are required for gating the MET channels, and aminoglycosides enter hair cells through these channels when open. The critical evidence is that mutant hair cells lacking Pcdh15, one of the two main molecular components of the tip link, show substantially reduced tip-link numbers, and fail to load with aminoglycosides (Alagramam et al., 2011). Moreover, hair cells with double-homozygous mutations of the putative MET channel proteins TMC1 and TMC2, but with intact tip links, also fail to take up gentamicin (Kawashima et al., 2011; Pan et al., 2013). The calcium-binding site within the MET channel pore modulates MET channel conductance (Pan et al., 2012) and permeation by aminoglycosides. Increasing extracellular [Ca^{2+}] reduces aminoglycoside permeation of MET channels (Marcotti et al., 2005; Coffin et al., 2009; Wang and Steyger, 2009), and is manifested by greater hair cell survival (Coffin et al., 2009; Alharazneh et al., 2011). Conversely, lower [Ca^{2+}] increases MET channel conductance and aminoglycoside permeation, promoting hair cell death (Marcotti et al., 2005; Coffin et al., 2009; Alharazneh et al., 2011). With the loss of hair bundle tip-links gating the GTTR-permeant MET channels, we discuss below potential mechanisms that could facilitate this increased uptake of GTTR by OHCs after loud sound exposure.

Increased Driving Potential may Enhance GTTR Uptake through Fewer Active Channels

The loss of tip links will have complex physiological consequences on MET channel kinetics. The open probability of OHC MET channels is ~50% (Cody and Russell, 1987; Legan et al., 2005), any loss of tip links would reduce the gross standing current through the remaining tip link-gated MET channels, and increase the EP (Sellick et al., 2007). The effect would increase

TABLE 2 | Tip link numbers decreased in OHCs after 91 dB SPL sound exposure.

Control			91 dB SPL		
Animal ID	**Row**	**Mean % ± s.e.m.**	**Animal ID**	**Row**	**Mean % ± s.e.m.**
2	1	13.03 ± 3.541	5	1	3.061 ± 1.287
	2	42.04 ± 5.008		2	1.891 ± 0.9688
	3	44.97 ± 4.703		3	11.52 ± 1.673
	Overall	**33.35 ± 3.654**		Overall	**5.492 ± 1.092**
3	1	38.20 ± 2.720	6	1	10.25 ± 1.388
	2	47.51 ± 5.5		2	10.29 ± 1.921
	3	61.25 ± 3.947		3	21.41 ± 4.864
	Overall	**48.99 ± 2.951**		Overall	**13.98 ± 1.995**
4	1	38.46 ± 3.062	7	1	61.45 ± 6.571
	2	56.73 ± 3.150		2	47.88 ± 6.124
	3	68.12 ± 5.681		3	46.06 ± 6.046
	Overall	**54.44 ± 3.237**		Overall	**51.80 ± 3.709**

Ten hair bundles in each OHC row from the mid-cochlear region (12–16 kHz region) of each cochlea were examined (3 mice per group). The percentage of tip link survival was calculated as the number of visible tip links divided by identifiable stereociliary tips (bar the tallest row of stereocilia) × 100.

the driving force from endolymph into hair cells and increase the rate of GTTR entry into OHCs via aminoglycoside-permeant channels (Marcotti et al., 2005).

MET Channels may Still Permit Aminoglycoside Entry in the Absence of Tip Links

Although the identity of the MET channel remains uncertain, experimental evidence suggests that a mechanosensitive ion channel remains in hair cells lacking tip links through which aminoglycosides may still enter the cell. Meyer et al. (1998) recorded MET currents in isolated OHCs before and after tip link ablation using BAPTA and elastase. Since these currents were blocked by MET channel blockers including aminoglycosides, amiloride, and gadolinium, the loss of tip links could result in a tonically open channel.

In more recent studies of mice lacking tip link proteins, anomalous MET currents have been recorded in which the channels displayed reverse polarity, becoming open for hair bundle displacements in the normally negative direction (Alagramam et al., 2011). Similar results were obtained in TMC1/TMC2 double mutants, in normal mouse hair cells exposed to BAPTA and allowed to recover for several minutes (Kim et al., 2013), and in hair cells in which the bundle was severely mechanically damaged (Marcotti et al., 2014).

Two explanations have been posited to explain these data. The first is that a mechanically sensitive channel, for example a precursor of the MET channel itself, is unmasked in the hair-cell apex in these cases (Marcotti et al., 2014), or, alternatively, that the original MET channels are redistributed to a different part of the hair bundle where they still operate mechanically but in an abnormal, reversed fashion (Barr-Gillespie and Nicolson, 2013). One possible explanation, therefore, for the increased OHC uptake of GTTR despite reduced numbers of tip links is that some form of aminoglycoside-permeant MET channel or precursor allows aminoglycoside entry. However, this explanation is not consistent with the absence of aminoglycoside entry in TMC1/TMC2 double mutants or tip-link protein mutants, as noted earlier. The contribution of such unmasked or redistributed MET channels to GTTR uptake may not be substantial.

Other Routes of Aminoglycoside Entry

Basolateral Membrane Mechanisms

One candidate aminoglycoside-permeant cation channel residing in the basolateral membrane of OHCs is TRPA1 (Stepanyan et al., 2011). These channels are inflammatory, irritant, and oxidative stress sensors (Kwan et al., 2006) and, hence, could be activated following the stress of noise damage. TRPA1 channels have a pore diameter of 1.1 nm (Karashima et al., 2010), sufficient to allow permeation by aminoglycosides, and show agonist-induced dilation (to ~1.4 nm) and permeation by organic cations (Chen et al., 2009; Banke et al., 2010; Karashima et al., 2010). The TRPA1 agonist, 4-hydroxynonenal, is elevated after noise exposure and *in vitro* facilitates increased OHC uptake of GTTR (Yamashita et al., 2005; Stepanyan et al., 2011).

Another basolateral channel, the nicotinic acetylcholine receptor (nAChR), may provide another route for the sound-enhanced aminoglycoside uptake by OHCs (Luk et al., 2014). Efferent activation of nicotinic acetylcholine receptor (nAChR) channels induces a calcium influx that opens nearby Ca^{2+}-sensitive K^+ channels (Murthy et al., 2009; Lipovsek et al., 2012). Aminoglycosides block efferent activation of acetylcholine-induced Ca^{2+} and K^+ currents *in vitro* (Blanchet et al., 2000; Seluakumaran et al., 2008). There are 3 potential mechanisms by which activated nAChR channels may modulate OHC uptake of aminoglycosides: (1) through nAChR itself from perilymph; (2) through nearby Ca^{2+}-sensitive K^+ channels, such as SK2 (Murthy et al., 2009) and BK channels (Hafidi et al., 2005; Yu et al., 2014), although this would be against the efflux direction of the native cation (K^+) current; and (3) via hyperpolarization of OHCs by activating outward potassium current (Housley and Ashmore, 1991; Doi and Ohmori, 1993) that increases the driving force through apically-located aminoglycoside-permeant channels, including MET, as described above.

These mechanisms are dependent on aminoglycoside entry into the scala tympani, which has been demonstrated (Tran Ba Huy et al., 1986; Hirose et al., 2014). However, uptake of aminoglycosides by healthy, physiologically-functioning OHCs from the scala tympani is far slower than from systemically-delivered aminoglycosides via endolymph (Li and Steyger, 2011). Nonetheless, aminoglycoside uptake by OHCs from the perilymphatic scala tympani may represent a mechanism of synergistic ototoxicity by OHCs over longer time frames, or after damaging sound exposures (Stepanyan et al., 2011).

Endocytosis

Hair cells are also able to endocytose aminoglycosides into the apical cytoplasm (Hiel et al., 1993; Hashino et al., 1997; Alharazneh et al., 2011). However, concanavalin A or Dynosore, non-selective blockers of endocytosis, did not significantly alter the rate of GTTR uptake, nor protect hair cells against aminoglycoside cytotoxicity (Alharazneh et al., 2011). Although TTS could enhance endocytosis of aminoglycosides *in vivo* by hair cells, delipidation of cochlear tissues to unmask GTTR fluorescence will remove endosome-associated GTTR fluorescence, and alternative unmasking steps should be utilized to further test this hypothesis (Myrdal et al., 2005).

Summary

This study reveals one possible contributor to loud sound-induced TTS is the loss of tip links, for which tip link regeneration may underlie the functional recovery associated with TTS. Furthermore, this study shows increased OHC uptake of GTTR during TTS that may contribute to the synergistic ototoxicity of noise and aminoglycosides. Finally, the apparent discrepancy between tip link loss and enhanced GTTR uptake may be explained by the activation of one or more additional routes of aminoglycoside entry into hair cells during TTS.

Acknowledgments

Studies funded by NIH R03 DC011622 and W81XWH1410006 (HL), NIH R01 DC04555 (PSS) and P30 DC005983.

References

Ahmad, M., Bohne, B. A., and Harding, G. W. (2003). An *in vivo* tracer study of noise-induced damage to the reticular lamina. *Hear. Res.* 175, 82–100. doi: 10.1016/s0378-5955(02)00713-x

Alagramam, K. N., Goodyear, R. J., Geng, R., Furness, D. N., Van Aken, A. F., Marcotti, W., et al. (2011). Mutations in protocadherin 15 and cadherin 23 affect tip links and mechanotransduction in mammalian sensory hair cells. *PLoS One* 6:e19183. doi: 10.1371/journal.pone.0019183

Alharazneh, A., Luk, L., Huth, M., Monfared, A., Steyger, P. S., Cheng, A. G., et al. (2011). Functional hair cell mechanotransducer channels are required for aminoglycoside ototoxicity. *PLoS One* 6:e22347. doi: 10.1371/journal.pone.0022347

Banke, T. G., Chaplan, S. R., and Wickenden, A. D. (2010). Dynamic changes in the TRPA1 selectivity filter lead to progressive but reversible pore dilation. *Am. J. Physiol. Cell Physiol.* 298, C1457–C1468. doi: 10.1152/ajpcell.00489.2009

Barr-Gillespie, P. G., and Nicolson, T. (2013). Who needs tip links? Backwards transduction by hair cells. *J. Gen. Physiol.* 142, 481–486. doi: 10.1085/jgp.201311111

Blanchet, C., Erostegui, C., Sugasawa, M., and Dulon, D. (2000). Gentamicin blocks ACh-evoked K^+ current in guinea-pig outer hair cells by impairing Ca^{2+} entry at the cholinergic receptor. *J. Physiol.* 525(Pt. 3), 641–654. doi: 10.1111/j.1469-7793.2000.t01-1-00641.x

Brown, J. J., Brummett, R. E., Meikle, M. B., and Vernon, J. (1978). Combined effects of noise and neomycin. Cochlear changes in the guinea pig. *Acta Otolaryngol.* 86, 394–400. doi: 10.3109/00016487809107518

Chen, J., Kim, D., Bianchi, B. R., Cavanaugh, E. J., Faltynek, C. R., Kym, P. R., et al. (2009). Pore dilation occurs in TRPA1 but not in TRPM8 channels. *Mol. Pain* 5:3. doi: 10.1186/1744-8069-5-3

Chen, L., Xiong, S., Liu, Y., and Shang, X. (2012). Effect of different gentamicin dose on the plasticity of the ribbon synapses in cochlear inner hair cells of C57BL/6J mice. *Mol. Neurobiol.* 46, 487–494. doi: 10.1007/s12035-012-8312-7

Cody, A. R., and Russell, I. J. (1987). The response of hair cells in the basal turn of the guinea-pig cochlea to tones. *J. Physiol.* 383, 551–569.

Coffin, A. B., Reinhart, K. E., Owens, K. N., Raible, D. W., and Rubel, E. W. (2009). Extracellular divalent cations modulate aminoglycoside-induced hair cell death in the zebrafish lateral line. *Hear. Res.* 253, 42–51. doi: 10.1016/j.heares.2009.03.004

Doi, T., and Ohmori, H. (1993). Acetylcholine increases intracellular Ca^{2+} concentration and hyperpolarizes the guinea-pig outer hair cell. *Hear. Res.* 67, 179–188. doi: 10.1016/0378-5955(93)90245-v

Durante-Mangoni, E., Grammatikos, A., Utili, R., and Falagas, M. E. (2009). Do we still need the aminoglycosides? *Int. J. Antimicrob. Agents* 33, 201–205. doi: 10.1016/j.ijantimicag.2008.09.001

Forge, A., and Schacht, J. (2000). Aminoglycoside antibiotics. *Audiol. Neurootol.* 5, 3–22. doi: 10.1159/000013861

Gale, J. E., Marcotti, W., Kennedy, H. J., Kros, C. J., and Richardson, G. P. (2001). FM1-43 dye behaves as a permeant blocker of the hair-cell mechanotransducer channel. *J. Neurosci.* 21, 7013–7025.

Gannon, R. P., Tso, S. S., and Chung, D. Y. (1979). Interaction of kanamycin and noise exposure. *J. Laryngol. Otol.* 93, 341–347. doi: 10.1017/s0022215100087119

Hafidi, A., Beurg, M., and Dulon, D. (2005). Localization and developmental expression of BK channels in mammalian cochlear hair cells. *Neuroscience* 130, 475–484. doi: 10.1016/j.neuroscience.2004.09.038

Hashino, E., and Shero, M. (1995). Endocytosis of aminoglycoside antibiotics in sensory hair cells. *Brain Res.* 704, 135–140. doi: 10.1016/0006-8993(95)01198-6

Hashino, E., Shero, M., and Salvi, R. J. (1997). Lysosomal targeting and accumulation of aminoglycoside antibiotics in sensory hair cells. *Brain Res.* 777, 75–85. doi: 10.1016/s0006-8993(97)00977-3

Hiel, H., Erre, J. P., Aurousseau, C., Bouali, R., Dulon, D., and Aran, J. M. (1993). Gentamicin uptake by cochlear hair cells precedes hearing impairment during chronic treatment. *Audiology* 32, 78–87. doi: 10.3109/00206099309072930

Hirose, K., Hartsock, J. J., Johnson, S., Santi, P., and Salt, A. N. (2014). Systemic lipopolysaccharide compromises the blood-labyrinth barrier and increases entry of serum fluorescein into the perilymph. *J. Assoc. Res. Otolaryngol.* 15, 707–719. doi: 10.1007/s10162-014-0476-6

Housley, G. D., and Ashmore, J. F. (1991). Direct measurement of the action of acetylcholine on isolated outer hair cells of the guinea pig cochlea. *Proc. Biol. sci.* 244, 161–167. doi: 10.1098/rspb.1991.0065

Housley, G. D., Morton-Jones, R., Vlajkovic, S. M., Telang, R. S., Paramananthasivam, V., Tadros, S. F., et al. (2013). ATP-gated ion channels mediate adaptation to elevated sound levels. *Proc. Natl. Acad. Sci. U S A* 110, 7494–7499. doi: 10.1073/pnas.1222295110

Husbands, J. M., Steinberg, S. A., Kurian, R., and Saunders, J. C. (1999). Tip-link integrity on chick tall hair cell stereocilia following intense sound exposure. *Hear. Res.* 135, 135–145. doi: 10.1016/s0378-5955(99)00101-x

Indzhykulian, A. A., Stepanyan, R., Nelina, A., Spinelli, K. J., Ahmed, Z. M., Belyantseva, I. A., et al. (2013). Molecular remodeling of tip links underlies mechanosensory regeneration in auditory hair cells. *PLoS Biol.* 11:e1001583. doi: 10.1371/journal.pbio.1001583

Karasawa, T., Wang, Q., Fu, Y., Cohen, D. M., and Steyger, P. S. (2008). TRPV4 enhances the cellular uptake of aminoglycoside antibiotics. *J. Cell Sci.* 121, 2871–2879. doi: 10.1242/jcs.023705

Karashima, Y., Prenen, J., Talavera, K., Janssens, A., Voets, T., and Nilius, B. (2010). Agonist-induced changes in Ca(2+) permeation through the nociceptor cation channel TRPA1. *Biophys. J.* 98, 773–783. doi: 10.1016/j.bpj.2009.11.007

Kawashima, Y., Géléoc, G. S., Kurima, K., Labay, V., Lelli, A., Asai, Y., et al. (2011). Mechanotransduction in mouse inner ear hair cells requires transmembrane channel-like genes. *J. Clin. Invest.* 121, 4796–4809. doi: 10.1172/JCI60405

Kazmierczak, P., Sakaguchi, H., Tokita, J., Wilson-Kubalek, E. M., Milligan, R. A., Müller, U., et al. (2007). Cadherin 23 and protocadherin 15 interact to form tip-link filaments in sensory hair cells. *Nature* 449, 87–91. doi: 10.1038/nature06091

Kim, K. X., Beurg, M., Hackney, C. M., Furness, D. N., Mahendrasingam, S., and Fettiplace, R. (2013). The role of transmembrane channel-like proteins in the operation of hair cell mechanotransducer channels. *J. Gen. Physiol.* 142, 493–505. doi: 10.1085/jgp.201311068

Kurian, R., Krupp, N. L., and Saunders, J. C. (2003). Tip link loss and recovery on chick short hair cells following intense exposure to sound. *Hear. Res.* 181, 40–50. doi: 10.1016/s0378-5955(03)00165-5

Kwan, K. Y., Allchorne, A. J., Vollrath, M. A., Christensen, A. P., Zhang, D. S., Woolf, C. J., et al. (2006). TRPA1 contributes to cold, mechanical and chemical nociception but is not essential for hair-cell transduction. *Neuron* 50, 277–289. doi: 10.1016/j.neuron.2006.03.042

Legan, P. K., Lukashkina, V. A., Goodyear, R. J., Lukashkin, A. N., Verhoeven, K., Van Camp, G., et al. (2005). A deafness mutation isolates a second role for the tectorial membrane in hearing. *Nat. Neurosci.* 8, 1035–1042. doi: 10.1038/nn1496

Li, H., and Steyger, P. S. (2009). Synergistic ototoxicity due to noise exposure and aminoglycoside antibiotics. *Noise Health* 11, 26–32. doi: 10.4103/1463-1741.45310

Li, H., and Steyger, P. S. (2011). Systemic aminoglycosides are trafficked via endolymph into cochlear hair cells. *Sci. Rep.* 1:159. doi: 10.1038/srep00159

Li, H., Wang, Q., and Steyger, P. S. (2011). Acoustic trauma increases cochlear and hair cell uptake of gentamicin. *PLoS One* 6:e19130. doi: 10.1371/journal.pone.0019130

Lipovsek, M., Im, G. J., Franchini, L. F., Pisciottano, F., Katz, E., Fuchs, P. A., et al. (2012). Phylogenetic differences in calcium permeability of the auditory hair cell cholinergic nicotinic receptor. *Proc. Natl. Acad. Sci. U S A* 109, 4308–4313. doi: 10.1073/pnas.1115488109

Liu, K., Jiang, X., Shi, C., Shi, L., Yang, B., Xu, Y., et al. (2013). Cochlear inner hair cell ribbon synapse is the primary target of ototoxic aminoglycoside stimuli. *Mol. Neurobiol.* 48, 647–654. doi: 10.1007/s12035-013-8454-2

Luk, L., Vetter, D. E., Steyger, P. S., and Li, H. (2014). "Acetylcholine enhances aminoglycoside uptake in neonatal hair cells, via putative activation of nicotinic acetylcholine receptors", in *Association for Research in Otolaryngology: Midwinter Meeting Abstracts* (San Diego, CA), 37.

Marcotti, W., Corns, L. F., Desmonds, T., Kirkwood, N. K., Richardson, G. P., and Kros, C. J. (2014). Transduction without tip links in cochlear hair cells is mediated by ion channels with permeation properties distinct from those of the mechano-electrical transducer channel. *J. Neurosci.* 34, 5505–5514. doi: 10.1523/JNEUROSCI.4086-13.2014

Marcotti, W., Van Netten, S. M., and Kros, C. J. (2005). The aminoglycoside antibiotic dihydrostreptomycin rapidly enters mouse outer hair cells through the mechano-electrical transducer channels. *J. Physiol.* 567, 505–521. doi: 10.1113/jphysiol.2005.085951

Meyer, J., Furness, D. N., Zenner, H. P., Hackney, C. M., and Gummer, A. W. (1998). Evidence for opening of hair-cell transducer channels after tip-link loss. *J. Neurosci.* 18, 6748–6756.

Mitchell, C., Kempton, J. B., Creedon, T., and Trune, D. (1996). Rapid acquisition of auditory brainstem responses with multiple frequency and intensity tone-bursts. *Hear. Res.* 99, 38–46. doi: 10.1016/s0378-5955(96)00081-0

Müller, M., Von Hünerbein, K., Hoidis, S., and Smolders, J. W. (2005). A physiological place-frequency map of the cochlea in the CBA/J mouse. *Hear. Res.* 202, 63–73. doi: 10.1016/j.heares.2004.08.011

Murthy, V., Maison, S. F., Taranda, J., Haque, N., Bond, C. T., Elgoyhen, A. B., et al. (2009). SK2 channels are required for function and long-term survival of efferent synapses on mammalian outer hair cells. *Mol. Cell. Neurosci.* 40, 39–49. doi: 10.1016/j.mcn.2008.08.011

Myrdal, S. E., Johnson, K. C., and Steyger, P. S. (2005). Cytoplasmic and intra-nuclear binding of gentamicin does not require endocytosis. *Hear. Res.* 204, 156–169. doi: 10.1016/j.heares.2005.02.002

Ohlemiller, K. K., and Gagnon, P. M. (2007). Genetic dependence of cochlear cells and structures injured by noise. *Hear. Res.* 224, 34–50. doi: 10.1016/j.heares.2006.11.005

Ou, H. C., Harding, G. W., and Bohne, B. A. (2000). An anatomically based frequency-place map for the mouse cochlea. *Hear. Res.* 145, 123–129. doi: 10.1016/s0378-5955(00)00082-4

Pan, B., Géléoc, G. S., Asai, Y., Horwitz, G. C., Kurima, K., Ishikawa, K., et al. (2013). TMC1 and TMC2 are components of the mechanotransduction channel in hair cells of the mammalian inner ear. *Neuron* 79, 504–515. doi: 10.1016/j.neuron.2013.06.019

Pan, B., Waguespack, J., Schnee, M. E., LeBlanc, C., and Ricci, A. J. (2012). Permeation properties of the hair cell mechanotransducer channel provide insight into its molecular structure. *J. Neurophysiol.* 107, 2408–2420. doi: 10.1152/jn.01178.2011

Ryan, A. F., and Bone, R. C. (1982). Non-simultaneous interaction of exposure to noise and kanamycin intoxication in the chinchilla. *Am. J. Otolaryngol.* 3, 264–272. doi: 10.1016/s0196-0709(82)80065-3

Seiler, C., and Nicolson, T. (1999). Defective calmodulin-dependent rapid apical endocytosis in zebrafish sensory hair cell mutants. *J. Neurobiol.* 41, 424–434. doi: 10.1002/(sici)1097-4695(19991115)41:3<424::aid-neu10>3.3.co;2-7

Sellick, P. M. (2007). Long term effects of BAPTA in scala media on cochlear function. *Hear. Res.* 231, 13–22. doi: 10.1016/j.heares.2007.04.001

Sellick, P. M., Kirk, D. L., Patuzzi, R., and Robertson, D. (2007). Does BAPTA leave outer hair cell transduction channels closed? *Hear. Res.* 224, 84–92. doi: 10.1016/j.heares.2006.11.011

Seluakumaran, K., Mulders, W. H., and Robertson, D. (2008). Effects of medial olivocochlear efferent stimulation on the activity of neurons in the auditory midbrain. *Exp. Brain Res.* 186, 161–174. doi: 10.1007/s00221-007-1219-2

Stepanyan, R., Indzhykulian, A. A., Vélez-Ortega, A. C., Boger, E. T., Steyger, P. S., Friedman, T. B., et al. (2011). TRPA1-mediated accumulation of aminoglycosides in mouse cochlear outer hair cells. *J. Assoc. Res. Otolaryngol.* 12, 729–740. doi: 10.1007/s10162-011-0288-x

Syka, J., Melichar, I., and Ulehlova, L. (1981). Longitudinal distribution of cochlear potentials and the K^+ concentration in the endolymph after acoustic trauma. *Hear. Res.* 4, 287–298. doi: 10.1016/0378-5955(81)90013-7

Tran Ba Huy, P., Bernard, P., and Schacht, J. (1986). Kinetics of gentamicin uptake and release in the rat. Comparison of inner ear tissues and fluids with other organs. *J. Clin. Invest.* 77, 1492–1500. doi: 10.1172/jci112463

Vu, A. A., Nadaraja, G. S., Huth, M. E., Luk, L., Kim, J., Chai, R., et al. (2013). Integrity and regeneration of mechanotransduction machinery regulate aminoglycoside entry and sensory cell death. *PLoS One* 8:e54794. doi: 10.1371/journal.pone.0054794

Wang, Q., and Steyger, P. S. (2009). Trafficking of systemic fluorescent gentamicin into the cochlea and hair cells. *J. Assoc. Res. Otolaryngol.* 10, 205–219. doi: 10.1007/s10162-009-0160-4

Yamashita, D., Jiang, H. Y., Le Prell, C. G., Schacht, J., and Miller, J. M. (2005). Post-exposure treatment attenuates noise-induced hearing loss. *Neuroscience* 134, 633–642. doi: 10.1016/j.neuroscience.2005.04.015

Yu, H., Guo, C. K., Wang, Y., Zhou, T., and Kong, W. J. (2014). Gentamicin blocks the ACh-induced BK current in guinea pig type II vestibular hair cells by competing with Ca(2)(+) at the L-type calcium channel. *Int. J. Mol. Sci.* 15, 6757–6771. doi: 10.3390/ijms15046757

Zhao, Y., Yamoah, E. N., and Gillespie, P. G. (1996). Regeneration of broken tip links and restoration of mechanical transduction in hair cells. *Proc. Natl. Acad. Sci. U S A* 93, 15469–15474. doi: 10.1073/pnas.93.26.15469

3

Sensory hair cell death and regeneration in fishes

Jerry D. Monroe[1], *Gopinath Rajadinakaran*[2] *and Michael E. Smith*[1]*

[1] *Department of Biology, Western Kentucky University, Bowling Green, KY, USA,* [2] *Department of Genetics and Genome Sciences, University of Connecticut Health Center, Farmington, CT, USA*

Edited by:
Francesco Moccia, University of Pavia, Italy

Reviewed by:
Hernan Lopez-Schier, Helmholtz Zentrum Munchen, Germany
Jonathan I. Matsui, Harvard University, USA

***Correspondence:**
Michael E. Smith, Department of Biology, Western Kentucky University, 1906 College Heights Blvd., Bowling Green, KY 42101, USA
michael.smith1@wku.edu

Sensory hair cells are specialized mechanotransductive receptors required for hearing and vestibular function. Loss of hair cells in humans and other mammals is permanent and causes reduced hearing and balance. In the early 1980's, it was shown that hair cells continue to be added to the inner ear sensory epithelia in cartilaginous and bony fishes. Soon thereafter, hair cell regeneration was documented in the chick cochlea following acoustic trauma. Since then, research using chick and other avian models has led to great insights into hair cell death and regeneration. However, with the rise of the zebrafish as a model organism for studying disease and developmental processes, there has been an increased interest in studying sensory hair cell death and regeneration in its lateral line and inner ears. Advances derived from studies in zebrafish and other fish species include understanding the effect of ototoxins on hair cells and finding otoprotectants to mitigate ototoxin damage, the role of cellular proliferation vs. direct transdifferentiation during hair cell regeneration, and elucidating cellular pathways involved in the regeneration process. This review will summarize research on hair cell death and regeneration using fish models, indicate the potential strengths and weaknesses of these models, and discuss several emerging areas of future studies.

Keywords: hair cell, regeneration, ototoxicity, zebrafish, cell death, teleost, acoustic trauma, lateral line

Introduction

Hair cells are specialized mechanosensory receptors which convert external vibratory stimuli into neural signals (Hudspeth et al., 2000; Hackney and Furness, 2013). These cells are present in vertebrate auditory and vestibular organs and the lateral line system of aquatic vertebrates (Hudspeth, 1989; Corwin and Warchol, 1991; Nicolson, 2005). Hair cells can be damaged or destroyed by acoustic or chemical exposure, but non-mammalian hair cells, unlike their mammalian counterparts, can regenerate after they are damaged or lost (Corwin and Oberholtzer, 1997; Brignull et al., 2009; Rubel et al., 2013). This regenerative ability has sparked interest in studying hair cell death and restoration in fish in order to find means of promoting sensory hair cell regeneration in humans.

Ototoxic chemicals such as heavy metals, aminoglycoside antibiotics and platinum containing drugs like cisplatin that damage mammalian hair cells also target fish lateral line and inner ear hair cells (Lombarte et al., 1993; Ton and Parng, 2005; Hernández et al., 2006; Olivari et al., 2008; Giari et al., 2012; Uribe et al., 2013a). As in other vertebrates, auditory hair cells in fishes can also be damaged by intense acoustic stimuli (Smith et al., 2006; Schuck and Smith, 2009; Casper et al., 2013). Hair cell loss in fishes causes hearing and vestibular deficits (Corwin and Oberholtzer, 1997; Matsui and Ryals, 2005; Rubel et al., 2013) which can be assessed via behavioral and electrophysiological methods (Smith et al., 2006; Suli et al., 2012; Ladich and Schulz-Mirbach, 2013).

As mammalian and fish hair cells are damaged by similar chemical and acoustic insults, many researchers are interested in studying the mechanisms of hair cell death and otoprotection in fish with the objective of developing therapeutics that may treat or prevent human hair cell loss. A majority of this research has been done in zebrafish (*Danio rerio*), which has become an important vertebrate model for examining embryogenesis, organ development, disease, and genetic defects (Kimmel, 1989; Driever et al., 1996; Haddon and Lewis, 1996; Zon, 1999) and is also a valuable model in hearing research. For example, the zebrafish mutants mariner and sputnik, which do not respond to vibrational stimuli, have hair cell bundle defects where the stereociliary bundles are detached from the kinocilia and are splayed (Nicolson et al., 1998). Genetic screens using zebrafish inner ear mutants have identified alteration of ear morphology, including expansion of the ear lumen, and aberrant formation and shape of the otolith (Malicki et al., 1996; Schibler and Malicki, 2007). Further, zebrafish mutants can exhibit morphological and functional defects similar to those of mouse mutants (Ernest et al., 2000). Considerable genetic and organ system homology exists between zebrafish and humans (Barbazuk et al., 2000; Goldsmith and Jobin, 2012). Many of the genes expressed in the embryonic zebrafish inner ear during the onset of hair cell differentiation and innervation are also expressed in other vertebrates (Coimbra et al., 2002). These include members of the Notch signaling pathway which regulate sensory cell commitment in mammalian models as well as numerous other orthologs with human genes. Thus, zebrafish models can provide insight into human hearing diseases and their mechanisms and have some advantages over mammalian models (**Table 1**).

Both hair cell damage and regeneration research in fishes have primarily focused on the lateral line because of its accessibility and visibility, which greatly facilitates the study of cellular and molecular mechanisms of development and differentiation (Brignull et al., 2009; Groves, 2010; Esterberg et al., 2013; Lush and Piotrowski, 2014a; Thomas et al., 2015a), although, recent efforts have begun to characterize these processes in the teleost inner ear as well (Schuck and Smith, 2009; Millimaki et al., 2010; Tanimoto et al., 2011). Researchers are also beginning to elucidate the genetic and molecular signaling mechanisms that regulate fish auditory sensory hair cell loss and restoration (Brignull et al., 2009; Ma and Raible, 2009; Schuck et al., 2011; Namdaran et al., 2012). This article reviews the current knowledge regarding hair cell death and regeneration in fishes, the advantages and disadvantages of using fish in these studies, and concludes by suggesting several future avenues for study.

Anatomy and Physiology of Teleost Hair Cells

The Teleost Lateral Line

The fish lateral line contains hair cells in sensory patches known as neuromasts (**Figures 1A–D**). These patches are arrayed either on the surface (superficial neuromasts) or in a fluid-filled channel with pores connecting to the outside (canal neuromasts) (Coombs et al., 2001; McHenry and van Netten, 2007). Neuromasts ultimately develop 15–20 hair cells surrounded by two accessory cell types, supporting and mantle cells (Villegas et al., 2012). They are classified as being either part of the anterior lateral line (ALL), which are located on the head, or the posterior lateral line (PLL), which are found along the trunk and tail (Ghysen and Dambly-Chaudière, 2004). Lateral line hair cells detect hydrodynamic pressure variations providing crucial sensory information required for fundamental behaviors including rheotaxis, schooling, prey detection, and predator avoidance (Coombs et al., 2001; Liao, 2006; Suli et al., 2012). Neuromast cellular layers and nervous connections are similar to those of the inner ear sensory macula (Nicolson, 2005; Haehnel et al., 2012). However, the ciliary bundles of lateral line hair cells project into a gelatinous compartment, the cupula, where vibrational forces are transduced by the gel's motion against the ciliary bundles (Nicolson, 2005; McHenry and van Netten, 2007). Morphological observations show that newly differentiating or functionally immature hair cells mainly originate from the edge of the neuromast and migrate toward the center (Williams and Holder, 2000; López-Schier and Hudspeth, 2006; Kindt et al., 2012).

Most of what is known about hair cell death, regeneration and ototoxicity in fishes come from studies of zebrafish lateral line neuromasts (Williams and Holder, 2000; Harris et al., 2003; Hernández et al., 2006; López-Schier and Hudspeth, 2006; Ma et al., 2008). While the lateral line system has led to some remarkable discoveries, it has some potential weaknesses. First, the physical arrangement of neuromast hair cells and supporting cells is quite different from the auditory sensory epithelia in vertebrate inner ears. Secondly, most of the zebrafish lateral line studies are done within the first 5 days following fertilization. Thus, it is unclear whether the observed effects are influenced by developmental plasticity or distinct hair cell death and regenerative pathways. For these reasons, researchers are beginning to perform these studies in the inner ear of adult fishes (Smith et al., 2006; Schuck and Smith, 2009; Uribe et al., 2013b).

The Teleost Inner Ear

Unlike mammals, fishes have no external or middle ears. Instead, they possess two inner ears located adjacent to the brain enclosed in a pair of capsules in the cranium. The auditory system of teleost fishes consists of three sensory otolithic end organs, the saccule, lagena and utricle (Bever and Fekete, 2002; Nicolson, 2005; Inoue et al., 2013; **Figures 1E,F**). These end organ compartments are filled with endolymphatic fluid and are interconnected by vestibular semicircular canals (Nicolson, 2005; Cruz et al., 2009). In many ostariophysan fish, like zebrafish, these fluid-filled compartments are attached at their posterior end to a set of four small bones, the Weberian ossicles, which are interconnected by ligaments, and form a connection to the air-filled swim bladder (Bang et al., 2001). The Weberian ossicles function as an accessory hearing structure to transmit sound vibrations from the swim bladder to the inner ear sensory end organs. Fishes do not have a dedicated

TABLE 1 | Comparison of some advantages and disadvantages of zebrafish and rodent models of sensory hair cell death and regeneration.

Zebrafish		Rodent	
Low husbandry cost/space per animal	+	Higher husbandry cost/space per animal	–
Large # of synchronous developing embryos per mating	+	Production of 3–14 pups/litter	–
Embryos and larvae translucent for ex utero visualization	+	Embryos opaque and *in utero*	–
Easier access of sensory hair cells	+	Hair cells embedded in bony capsule	–
Hearing range lower frequency than humans	–	Hearing range comparable to humans	+
Large-scale mutagenesis	+	Several years to develop knockout mice	–
High-throughput genetic/drug screening	+	Lower-throughput genetic/drug screening	–
In vivo model using neuromast hair cells	+	Inner ear must be dissected out	–
Transgenic models available	+	Transgenic models available	+
70% homology with human genome*	–	90% homology with human genome*	+

*+/– Relative advantage/disadvantage. *Percentages are approximations.*

auditory organ like the mammalian cochlea, and while the otolithic organs have both vestibular and auditory functions it is generally thought that the utricle is primarily a vestibular organ, the saccule is thought to be primarily responsible for sound detection in most fish species, and the lagena supplements the functions of the saccule with roles in both orientation and hearing (Popper et al., 2003; Kwak et al., 2006; Khorevin, 2008). These pouch-like organs contain an area lined with sensory epithelia, referred to as a macula. The macula consists of a basal lamina which underlies a layer of non-sensory supporting cells with interspersed hair cells (Oesterle and Stone, 2008; Inoue et al., 2013). Neurons extend between the supporting cells forming synaptic connections with hair cells (Szabo et al., 2007; Tanimoto et al., 2009). Ciliary bundles consisting of one kinocilium and multiple stereocilia project from the hair cell body into the lumen where they contact an otolith, a

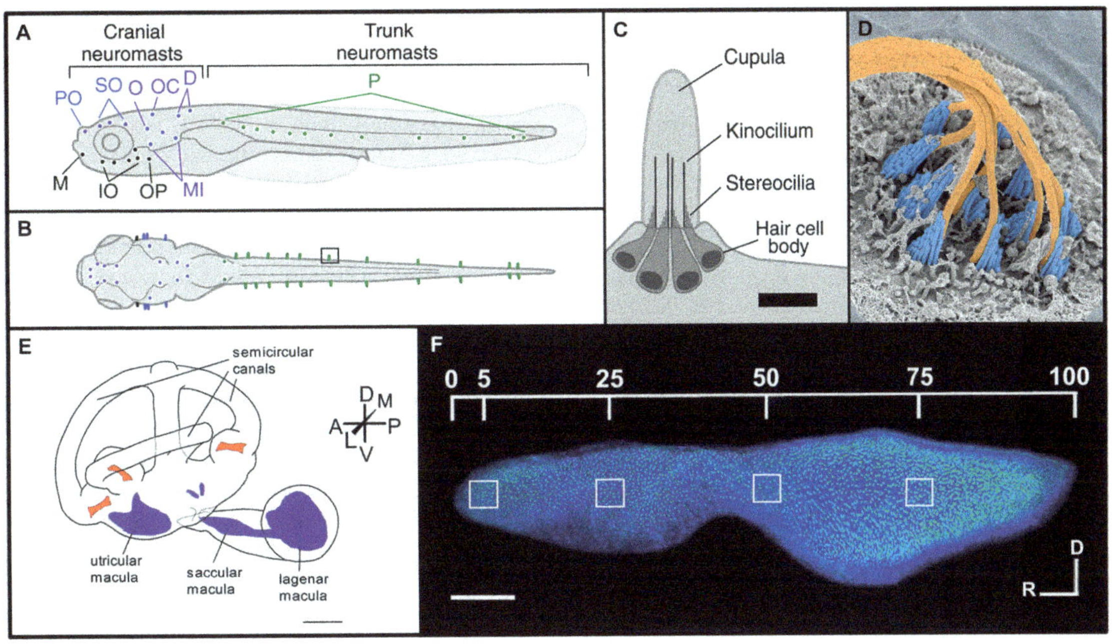

FIGURE 1 | Morphology of the lateral line and inner ear systems of zebrafish. (A) Lateral and **(B)** dorsal views of zebrafish larvae illustrate the distribution of neuromasts along the body. The supraorbital region (blue) includes the preoptic (PO) and supraorbital (SO) neuromasts. The infraorbital region (black) includes the mandibular (M), infraorbital (IO) and opercular (OP) neuromasts. The caudal–cranial region (purple) includes the otic (O), occipital (OC), dorsal (D) and middle (MI) neuromasts. Finally, the posterior (P) neuromasts are located in the trunk region (green). **(C)** The morphology of an individual neuromast illustrates its major anatomical features. Scale bar, 10 μm. Reproduced with permission from Van Trump and McHenry (2008) **(D)** False-colored SEM image of a zebrafish neuromast. The cupula has been removed to see the kinocilia (orange) and the stereocilia (blue). Reprinted from cover image of Developmental Cell, Vol. 23, (2), K.S. Kindt, G. Finch, T. Nicolson, Kinocilia mediate mechanosensitivity in developing zebrafish hair cells, 2012, with permission from Elsevier. **(E)** Morphology of the zebrafish inner ear, showing the relative positions of the sensory maculae (blue) and cristae (red). Scale bar, 500 μm. Adapted with permission from Hammond et al. (2010). **(F)** Phalloidin- and DAPI-labeled zebrafish saccule, showing locations used for quantifying hair cell bundle densities along the rostral-caudal axis. Scale bar, 100 μm. Reprinted from Hearing Research, Vol. 253, J.B. Schuck, M.E. Smith, Cell proliferation follows acoustically-induced hair cell bundle loss in the zebrafish saccule, 2009, with permission from Elsevier.

calcium carbonate structure found inside the lumen of each end organ (Bever and Fekete, 2002; Nicolson, 2005; Cruz et al., 2009; Inoue et al., 2013). Stereocilia are connected by elastic tip links and when deflected by the denser otolith, transduce either excitatory or inhibitory stimuli depending upon their directional movement (Nicolson, 2005). Newly formed hair cells may arise throughout the teleost inner ear maculae (Popper and Hoxter, 1990; Lombarte and Popper, 1994; Higgs et al., 2001).

Similarities and Differences Between Teleost and Mammalian Hair Cells

Since fishes are the common ancestor of all tetrapods (Clack, 2012), it is not surprising that teleost and mammalian hair cells share many fundamental features (Coffin et al., 2004). All sensory hair cells are elongate epithelial cells. On their apical surface there is a ciliary bundle composed of multiple actin-rich stereocilia and a single, eccentrically-placed kinocilium (a true cilium with 9 + 2 microtubule pattern; Popper, 1983). The stereocilia are graded in size, with the longest ones lying closest to the kinocilium, and shorter stereocilia positioned in rows in steplike positions away from the kinocilium. Filamentous tip links connect each stereocilia to its nearest neighbor (Pickles et al., 1988). These tip links are composed of two cadherin molecules- protocadherin 15 (PCDH15) and cadherin 23 (CDH23; Siemens et al., 2004; Ahmed et al., 2006), but it is likely that other proteins are also involved. It is hypothesized that the tip links interact with myosin motors that move along actin filaments in the stereocilia (Howard and Hudspeth, 1987; Holt and Corey, 2000; Furness et al., 2010).

Mechanotransduction occurs when hair cell stereociliary bundles are deflected toward the kinocilium, stretching the tip links, opening cation-selective channels, and thus depolarizing the cell, while deflection away from the kinocilium hyperpolarizes the cell (reviewed in Strassmaier and Gillespie, 2002). The precise structure of the mechanotransductive channel is currently not known but may incorporate transmembrane channel-like (TMC) 1 and 2 and TMIE proteins (Pan et al., 2013; Zhao et al., 2014). As this research has only been done using mammalian hair cells, there is no data available on the mechanotransduction channel structures in fishes.

There are obvious morphological differences between the hair cells of the inner ear and lateral line of teleosts and those of the mammalian cochlea. For example, cochlear hair cells are arranged in precise rows while the hair cells of teleost maculae are found as patches of fairly equally-spaced hair cells surrounded by supporting cells, similar to those of the mammalian utricle and saccule (Corwin and Warchol, 1991). Also, while auditory, vestibular, and lateral line teleost hair bundles are generally conical in shape with a kinocilium and many rows of stereocilia, mammalian cochlear hair bundles lose the kinocilium upon maturation and have stereocilia organized in fewer rows (3–4) arranged in a more or less pronounced W-shape (reviewed in Furness and Hackney, 2006).

Another morphological difference between teleost and mammalian hair cells that may represent a structural barrier to hair cell regeneration in mammals is cytoskeletal organization. A comparative study of six vertebrates, including zebrafish and dogfish sharks, showed that mammalian supporting cells have very large circumferential F-actin belts and intercellular junctions that express E-cadherin (Burns et al., 2013). However, supporting cells in zebrafish and adult sharks have thin F-actin belts and zebrafish have little E-cadherin. This suggests that fish supporting cells are able to divide and form new hair cells at least partially due to their unique cytoskeletal and cell adhesion characteristics.

Teleost hair cells exhibit considerable heterogeneity, but there are two basic types: Type I-like and Type II hair cells. Type I-like hair cells are located near the macular striola and have both afferent and efferent innervation (Popper, 2000). They are characterized by large, subnuclear bodies of endoplasmic reticulum, large mitochondria, and smaller synaptic bodies associated with synapses (Chang et al., 1992). Type II hair cells are extrastriolar with mostly afferent innervation. Studies suggest that the lateral line canal neuromasts are probably Type I-like cells and free neuromasts may be Type II hair cells (Song et al., 1995), although these identifications have been questioned (Van Trump et al., 2010; Brown et al., 2011). The mammalian cochlea also has two distinct hair cell types. There are inner hair cells (IHCs), the primary auditory receptors, which send afferent signals to the auditory processing centers of the brain, and outer hair cells (OHCs), which receive efferent signals from the brain and act as a cochlear amplifier which sharpens the frequency tuning curves along the length of the cochlea (Vater et al., 2004). It is thought that IHCs and OHCs are homologous to Type I-like and Type II hair cells, respectively. Mammalian vestibular Type I hair cells are amphora or cylindrically shaped but with a constricted neck and Type II hair cells are cylindrically shaped (Kevetter and Correia, 1996). A large nerve calyx surrounds the mammalian IHC hair cell, while this is usually not found in teleost hair cells (Popper, 2000).

Recently, whole-cell patch clamp analysis of zebrafish hair cells has allowed comparison of the physiological properties between hair cells from different locations (lateral line vs. inner ear) and with mammals (Olt et al., 2014). This study showed that all zebrafish hair cells exhibit a delayed rectifier K^+ current, but mature lateral line hair cells located in the center of neuromasts have large A-type K^+ currents (I_A) while immature hair cells at the neuromast edge expressed a large conductance Ca^{2+} -activated K^+ current ($I_{K,Ca}$) and a small I_A. Further, mature zebrafish hair cells physiologically resembled those of other lower vertebrates, and to some extent, the hair cells from immature mammalian vestibular and auditory systems (Olt et al., 2014). However, it is not certain whether zebrafish hair cell physiology resembles that of clinically relevant mature mammalian hair cells.

Causes and Mechanisms of Hair Cell Damage

Ototoxins

Fish inner ear and lateral line hair cells may be damaged by many of the same ototoxic chemicals that cause impaired auditory and vestibular function in mammals. These substances include heavy metals, platinum-based drugs, aminoglycoside antibiotics and alkaloids (Yan et al., 1991; Lombarte et al., 1993; Song et al., 1995; Harris et al., 2003; Ton and Parng, 2005; Hernández et al., 2006, 2007; Santos et al., 2006; Chiu et al., 2008; Ma et al., 2008; Olivari et al., 2008; Van Trump et al., 2010; Buck et al., 2012). Fish species tested with ototoxins include goldfish (*Carassius auratus*, Ramcharitar and Brack, 2010), Atlantic cod (*Gadus morhua*, Faucher et al., 2009), Mexican blind cavefish (*Astyanax mexicanus*, Van Trump et al., 2010), oscar (*Astronotus ocellatus*, Lombarte et al., 1993; Song et al., 1995), and zebrafish (*Danio rerio*, Hernández et al., 2006, 2007; Santos et al., 2006; Olivari et al., 2008; Van Trump et al., 2010; Uribe et al., 2013a). Ototoxic exposure of the lateral line can be accomplished by dissolving chemicals in the growth media of fish larvae (Harris et al., 2003; Ton and Parng, 2005; Hernández et al., 2006, 2007; Santos et al., 2006; Ma et al., 2008; Olivari et al., 2008; Van Trump et al., 2010), while exposure of the inner ear can be done via systemic or inner ear injection (Yan et al., 1991; Lombarte et al., 1993; Faucher et al., 2009; Uribe et al., 2013b). The degree of hair cell damage depends on ototoxin concentration (Yan et al., 1991; Ton and Parng, 2005; Hernández et al., 2006; Olivari et al., 2008) and exposure time (Song et al., 1995).

One heavy metal that is ototoxic to fish hair cells is copper. Treatment with 1 μM copper sulfate for 2 h did not cause morphological damage to larval zebrafish neuromasts, but hair cells were completely damaged at 50 μM (Hernández et al., 2006). Copper can also damage supporting cells. At 10 μM exposure, mantle and interneuromastic cells are moderately damaged, while at 50 μM, mantle, but not interneuromastic cells, are completely destroyed (Hernández et al., 2007). Mammalian studies have shown that copper transporters and pumps are responsible for cisplatin influx, sequestration and efflux (Ding et al., 2011). However, copper sulfate, an inhibitor of the copper transporter, CTR1, which modulates cisplatin influx in rodent models, can cause ototoxicity or otoprotection against cisplatin depending on dosage (More et al., 2010; Ding et al., 2011). In fact, CTR1 mRNA is expressed in zebrafish lateral line hair cells (McDermott et al., 2007), although, the level of CTR1 protein expression and its functionality has not yet been studied in either zebrafish lateral line or inner ear hair cells. Further, mRNA tissue expression of copper transporter genes can vary significantly between mammals, zebrafish and other fish species after copper exposure (Leung et al., 2014). Therefore, mammalian hair cells may respond differently than fish to copper-based compounds.

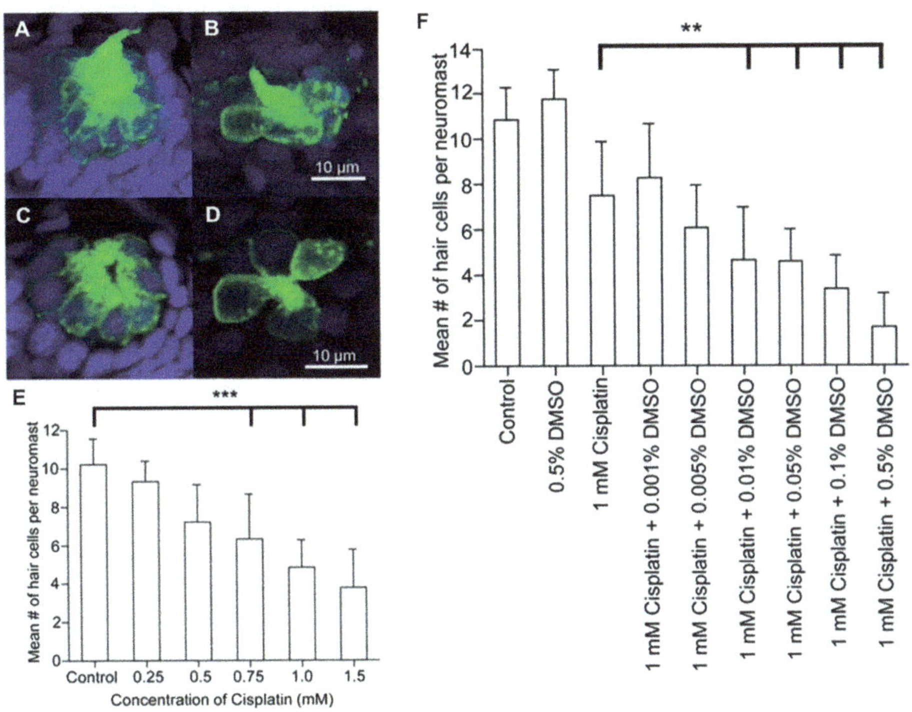

FIGURE 2 | Dose response curves following cisplatin and DMSO treatment. Brn3c-green fluorescent protein (GFP) transgenic zebrafish were exposed to varying doses of cisplatin for 4 h, then fixed and co-labeled with TO-PRO-3 (blue), and the GFP-tagged hair cells (green). Neuromasts were imaged using confocal microscopy. **(A,B)** *Z*-stack projections of two neuromasts under different treatment conditions showing the entire neuromast structure. **(C,D)** Slices from the same neuromasts as in A, B demonstrating the membrane-bound GFP label surrounding the nuclear dye. Neuromasts of untreated controls **(A,C)** and 1 mM cisplatin-treated fish **(B,D)**. **(E)** Dose-response curve for the effect of cisplatin on neuromast hair cell number. $^{***}p < 0.001$ when individual treatments are compared to untreated controls. **(F)** Dose-response curve showing the synergistic effects of cisplatin and DMSO on neuromast hair cell number. $^{**}p < 0.01$ when individual treatments are compared to untreated controls (modified from Uribe et al., 2013a).

Zebrafish hair cells can also be damaged by the anticancer platinum-based compound, cisplatin, which is also ototoxic in mammals (Ton and Parng, 2005; Ou et al., 2007; Chiu et al., 2008; Owens et al., 2008; Giari et al., 2012). Transmission and scanning electron microscopy shows that cisplatin damages inner ear more than lateral line hair cells with greater numbers of damaged mitochondria in the inner ear cells than in the lateral line (Giari et al., 2012). The mechanism responsible for increased inner ear sensitivity is not known, although lateral line hair cells require mechanotransduction for cisplatin influx (Thomas et al., 2013). However, rodent studies suggest that cisplatin uptake in mammals may depend upon membranous transporters (Ciarimboli et al., 2010; More et al., 2010; Ding et al., 2011; Ciarimboli, 2012). It is unknown whether cisplatin uptake in zebrafish inner ear hair cells is mechanotransduction or transporter dependent. Cisplatin-mediated hair cell damage may be modulated by other chemicals. For example, ototoxicity increases in zebrafish lateral line hair cells treated with cisplatin when they are also exposed to the pharmaceutical solvent, DMSO, although DMSO treatment alone does not cause hair cell death (Uribe et al., 2013a; **Figure 2**). Cisplatin and other anti-cancer drugs can produce synergistic ototoxic effects in the zebrafish lateral line (Hirose et al., 2011). Experiments investigating DMSO and synergistic effects have not been performed in zebrafish inner ear hair cells, however, in rats, DMSO can cause hair cell death by activating apoptotic pathways (Qi et al., 2008). Studies in guinea pigs have also found that DMSO has an otoprotective effect which can be enhanced by co-application of a synergistic agent (Momin et al., 2011). These results suggest that platinum-based compounds and synergistic agents may cause different ototoxic effects in mammalian vs. zebrafish hair cell models.

Aminoglycoside antibiotics that are ototoxic in mammals can also cause hair cell death in fish (Ton and Parng, 2005; Chiu et al., 2008). For example, gentamicin and neomycin cause ototoxicity in the zebrafish lateral line (Ton and Parng, 2005), and streptomycin damages the superficial and canal neuromasts of goldfish (Higgs and Radford, 2013). Although different levels of gentamicin-induced damage in superficial vs. canal neuromasts have been reported (Song et al., 1995), another study showed that zebrafish superficial and canal neuromasts were damaged to a similar extent when exposed to gentamicin (Van Trump et al., 2010). Therefore, results obtained with aminoglycosides may be species specific and warrant careful consideration regarding choice of a particular fish model. Zebrafish inner ear studies show that gentamicin injection also damages hair cells in the saccular and utricular sensory epithelium and causes auditory functional deficits (Uribe et al., 2013b).

Rodent models of aminoglycoside ototoxicity can present disadvantages. Induction of aminoglycoside-mediated ototoxicity in mice often requires drug treatments that cause significant mortality and complex delivery methods (Murillo-Cuesta et al., 2010). Furthermore, gentamicin studies in guinea pigs demonstrate that this drug is more vestibulotoxic than ototoxic (Zhai et al., 2010). Aminoglycoside studies in mice have also exhibited distributed hair cell damage patterns where outer hair cells are mostly destroyed but many inner hair cells are left intact (Taylor et al., 2008). Thus, the ototoxic effects of aminoglycosides on fish models may be different than that of their mammalian counterparts.

Developmental factors may play a significant and complicating role in zebrafish models of aminoglycoside ototoxicity. For example, in larval lateral line studies, hair cell susceptibility to neomycin increases during later stages of development (Murakami et al., 2003; Santos et al., 2006). Specifically, zebrafish treated four days post-fertilization exhibit little hair cell damage while older fish have many more damaged hair cells. This is generally the opposite of mammalian organisms where greater sensitivity to ototoxins is observed during early developmental stages and greater resistance is found in adult specimens (Henley and Rybak, 1995). Further, maturation-related sensitivity in the zebrafish lateral line has been associated with hair cell type as immature Type I-like hair cells are less susceptible to neomycin but are more strongly affected as they approach maturity (Harris et al., 2003). No studies to date have studied the role of developmental drug sensitivity in fish inner ear hair cells. Therefore, studies of aminoglycosides, and potentially other ototoxic drugs in fish models, should carefully consider how development might affect experimental outcomes.

Transgenic zebrafish expressing fluorescent protein reporters can exhibit impaired hearing. Zebrafish expressing green fluorescent protein (GFP) under the control of the *brn3c* promoter *Tg(Brn3c:GFP)* have elevated hearing threshold shifts compared to wild-type controls (Uribe et al., 2013b). This is similar to transgenic mouse models where GFP expression in hair cells is correlated with hearing deficits (Wenzel et al., 2007), while lower levels of GFP in these cells causes no hearing loss (Wang et al., 2013a). It is not certain whether GFP acts as an ototoxin. However, long-term GFP expression in transgenic mice has been linked to aberrant physiology (Huang et al., 2000). Future work will be required to determine whether the expression of fluorescent reporters causes ototoxic effects in zebrafish as well as in mammalian models.

Acoustic Damage

The hair cells of fishes, like mammals, can be damaged by a variety of sound stimuli. For example, 48 h of white noise at 180 dB re: 1 μPa produces hair cell damage in the lagena and saccule of goldfish with saccular damage being particularly localized in the central and caudal regions (Smith et al., 2006). Hair cell loss was also correlated with increased auditory threshold shifts over a range of frequencies (0.2–2 kHz). The goldfish saccule is tonotopically organized, and hair cells in discrete saccular locations are susceptible to stimuli of different frequencies, with low and high frequency sounds damaging hair cells of the caudal and rostral portions of the saccule, respectively (Smith et al., 2011). Similarly, low frequency sound exposure in zebrafish causes distributed hair cell damage in the caudal portion of the saccule (Schuck and Smith, 2009; Sun et al., 2011; **Figure 3**). Distributed damage patterns in the rostral and caudal portions of the saccule have also been identified

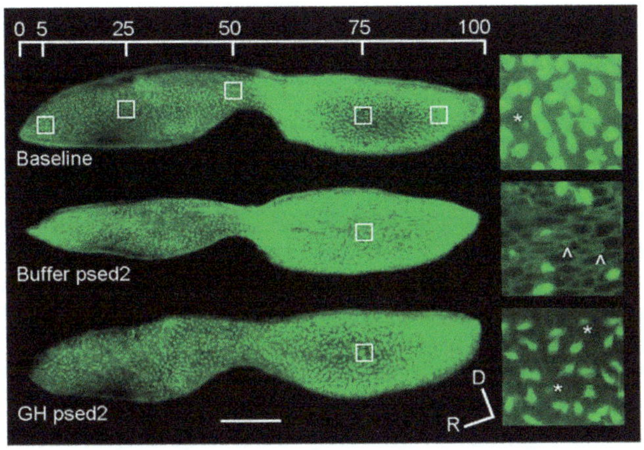

FIGURE 3 | Effect of acoustic exposure on zebrafish saccular hair cell bundle density. Phalloidin-labeled saccular epithelia of baseline, buffer-injected, and GH-injected zebrafish at post-sound exposure day 2 (psed2). The upper image shows the five locations of hair cell counts along the rostral-caudal axis of the saccule. The enlarged images to the right of the saccules are representative 100X images of saccules at 75% along the rostral-caudal axis. Scale bar, 100 μm, D = dorsal, R = rostral, * = presumed newly formed hair cell bundles, ^= scar formation characteristic of hair cell loss (modified from Sun et al., 2011).

in hybrid striped bass (white bass, *Morone chrysops* × striped bass, *Morone saxatilis*) and tilapia (*Oreochromis mossambicus*) exposed to pile driver noise (Casper et al., 2013). Similarly, studies conducted in mammalian models show that acoustic damage is often concentrated in different areas of the cochlea with lower frequencies typically damaging mainly outer hair cells and higher frequencies are required to damage inner hair cells (Stockwell et al., 1969; Lim, 1976; Park et al., 2013). As in fish, the mammalian auditory epithelia is tonotopically organized, although, mammalian organization is much more sophisticated (Mann and Kelley, 2011). However, it is unknown whether fish auditory sensory epithelia undergo tonotopic reorganization in response to acoustic damage, which in mammalian models includes changes in electrophysiological response, e.g., threshold response shifts and altered frequency detection, in different regions of the sensory epithelia (Wang et al., 2013b). In general, the cellular damage exhibited by fish and mammals after acoustic over-stimulation is similar. Immediately after zebrafish are sound exposed, hair cell stereociliary numbers are reduced, there are shorter and thinner ciliary bundles, and epithelial lesions where hair cells have been removed (Schuck and Smith, 2009). In mammalian models, after noise exposure, stereocilia are disarrayed or collapsed, and there is scarring where hair cells were located (Stockwell et al., 1969; Lim, 1976; Wang et al., 2002). Thus, fish and mammalian hair cells may be affected similarly by damaging noise stimuli, but there is still limited data on the effects of acoustic trauma on teleost hair cells.

Hair Cell Damage Mechanisms

Researchers have begun to characterize the mechanisms involved in fish hair cell death and how they relate to mammalian models. The terminal deoxynucleotidyl transferase dUTP nick end labeling (TUNEL) assay shows that noise exposure and ototoxins modulate apoptosis in zebrafish lateral line and inner ear hair cells (Sun et al., 2011; Chang et al., 2013; Hong et al., 2013; Song et al., 2013; Uribe et al., 2013b). Various indicators of apoptosis, e.g., nuclear condensation and fragmentation, can appear rapidly (30 min) in larval zebrafish neuromasts after cisplatin treatment (Ou et al., 2007). These results are consistent with noise-induced damage and ototoxicity studies conducted using TUNEL in mammalian organisms (Ahn et al., 2005; Chung et al., 2007; Taylor et al., 2008; Fu et al., 2012).

Non-apoptotic mechanisms can also be activated during fish hair cell death. For example, administration of low concentrations of copper causes apoptosis in zebrafish lateral line hair cells but higher concentrations modulate both apoptotic and necrotic mechanisms (Olivari et al., 2008). Non-apoptotic pathways are also activated in mammalian hair cell death. Mice exposed to the aminoglycoside, kanamycin, undergo hair cell death without activation of markers integral to the apoptotic pathway (Jiang et al., 2006). Further, hair cell death in noise-exposed mice can be due to activation of both apoptotic and necrotic pathways (Zheng et al., 2014).

Different pathways in fish hair cells may be targeted by specific ototoxins. Mutational studies show that multiple genes modulate aminoglycoside susceptibility in the larval zebrafish lateral line (Owens et al., 2008). It is likely that these genes function in different pathways, because they provide differential resistance to neomycin. Also, in zebrafish larvae, neomycin and gentamicin ototoxicity follows different time courses suggesting that different cell death mechanisms are targeted (Owens et al., 2009). Screens in larval zebrafish using signal transduction inhibitors targeting the molecules, Bax, Bcl2 and p53, suggest that specific pathways are associated with different otoprotective effects against various aminoglycosides and cisplatin (Coffin et al., 2013a). Studies conducted in mouse models also suggest that different ototoxins can signal through different hair cell death pathways (Jiang et al., 2006; Zheng et al., 2014). However, no studies have yet compared whether specific ototoxic drugs modulate the same apoptotic or necrotic pathways in zebrafish or mammalian models. Recent studies suggest that zebrafish auditory cell apoptosis and necrosis may signal through markers found in rodent models, e.g., Bax, Bcl2, p38, p53 and cytochrome c (Coffin et al., 2013a,b; Shin et al., 2014).

The role of mechanotransducive mechanisms in hair cell death is a potential point of divergence between fish and mammals. A study in the zebrafish lateral line shows that mechanotransduction is required to modulate the ototoxic effects of cisplatin (Thomas et al., 2013). The alkaloid, quinine, an ototoxic mechanotransduction blocker in mammals (Alharazneh et al., 2011), reduces mechanotransduction in the zebrafish lateral line and prevented cisplatin uptake (Thomas et al., 2013). However, work conducted with rodent models indicates that cisplatin uptake in mammals depends upon a variety of membranous transporters, e.g., CTR1, and, therefore, may not require mechanotransduction (Ciarimboli et al., 2010; More et al., 2010; Ding et al., 2011; Ciarimboli, 2012). These findings suggest that cisplatin influx in fish proceeds through a different mechanism than in mammals. An additional complicating factor is that hair cell development may intersect with mechanotransduction-modulated ototoxicity and affect the susceptibility of zebrafish to aminoglycosides. As zebrafish hair cells age they become more susceptible to neomycin, and age-related effects are not dependent upon the onset of functional mechanotransduction (Santos et al., 2006). Much additional work is needed before conclusions can be drawn as to whether zebrafish hair cell death mechanisms are largely equivalent to their mammalian counterparts and if the same pathways are involved in the response to specific ototoxins.

Hair Cell Regeneration

Cellular Differentiation and Proliferation

Hair cells can regenerate after damage through transdifferentiation or proliferation of supporting cells (Corwin and Oberholtzer, 1997; Warchol, 2010; Burns and Corwin, 2013; Rubel et al., 2013). Studies conducted using tritium and bromodeoxyuridine (BrdU) labeling show that hair cells in the teleost lateral line and inner ear can undergo continuous proliferation (Jørgensen, 1991; Lanford et al., 1996; Sun et al., 2011). Following acoustic trauma, fish can regenerate hair cells to control levels within one to two weeks, and functional recovery of hearing results (Smith et al., 2006; Faucher et al., 2009). However, regeneration may not proceed, at least in the lateral line, if a certain level of damage is reached. The regenerative potential of neuromasts can be dose-dependent and as damage increases, other cell types from which new hair cells are derived may be permanently destroyed (Hernández et al., 2006).

Several studies have shown that hair cells can regenerate from mitotic and proliferating supporting cells. In the oscar and goldfish inner ear saccule, supporting cells can enter mitotic S-phase and become hair cell precursors (Presson et al., 1995, 1996). In the zebrafish lateral line, hair cells normally undergo programmed cell death during development but are restored from mantle supporting cells at the periphery of the neuromast after S-phase has occurred (Williams and Holder, 2000; Harris et al., 2003). Proliferating supporting cells may either stay in the periphery or migrate inwards and their numbers increase after drug-induced hair cell death. Another zebrafish lateral line study found that most new hair cells are from proliferating supporting cells and that there are two sets of these cells within neuromasts (Ma et al., 2008). One group functions as the progenitors of hair cells and is centrally located. The other is peripheral and of uncertain function. This suggests that there may be functional specializations among neuromast supporting cell populations. These findings are similar to those of transgenic neonatal mouse models where new hairs cells can also proliferate from supporting cells (Shi et al., 2013). In contrast, hair cell regeneration does not occur in adult guinea pigs following damage to both hair and supporting cells suggesting that supporting cells are critical for regeneration (Izumikawa et al., 2008).

Fish hair cells can also regenerate from transdifferentiation of supporting cells. Inflicting high levels of damage to neuromasts causes replacement of hair cells from dividing surrounding supporting cells (Hernández et al., 2007). However, lower levels of damage can cause non-dividing precursor cells to differentiate into hair cells. In developing zebrafish embryos, laser-ablated inner ear hair cells were replaced by supporting cells that underwent transdifferentiation into new hair cells without mitotic proliferation (Millimaki et al., 2010). Transdifferentiation of supporting cells has also been observed in genetically-manipulated mammalian models (Izumikawa et al., 2005).

One potential complication involved in studying cellular differentiation and proliferation in zebrafish is that their lateral line and inner ear hair cells are continually replaced during life (Popper and Hoxter, 1984; Lombarte and Popper, 1994; Higgs et al., 2001, 2003). This could make it difficult to discriminate hair cell regeneration stemming from transdifferentiation as opposed to supporting cell division. However, the application of new technologies, such as laser-scanning confocal microscopy coupled with selective plane illumination microscopy, could facilitate study of these processes by allowing continuous videomicroscopy of different cell types labeled with unique fluorescent markers (Pinto-Teixeira et al., 2013). Thus, this technique could allow investigators to determine which cell types are involved in regeneration and whether new hair cells are produced by transdifferentiation or supporting cell division.

Hair cells in the fish inner ear may exhibit differential spatial patterns of regeneration. In noise-exposed goldfish, hair cell bundle density recovered in the central but not in the caudal portion of the saccule during the study time interval (Smith et al., 2006). After acoustic exposure, hair cells largely regenerated in the caudal region of the saccule, where higher hair cell loss and subsequent mitotic activity was greater than that found in the rostral region (Schuck and Smith, 2009; **Figure 4**). This was a result of the low frequency sound stimuli used and the tonotopic organization of the teleost saccule (Smith et al., 2011).

Regenerative Mechanisms

The ability of fish hair cells to regenerate has provoked great interest in identifying the genes and molecular mechanisms that control their differentiation and proliferation. Recent studies have used microarrays and next generation sequencing to identify genes that are activated after hair cell destruction. A microarray performed on zebrafish exposed to noise showed that many gene transcripts were either up- or down-regulated in the inner ear (Schuck et al., 2011; **Figure 5**). Growth hormone is particularly upregulated while myosin light chain, myosin heavy chain, and major histocompatibility complex I genes were significantly down-regulated. A subsequent study demonstrated that growth hormone can promote regeneration of acoustically- damaged inner ear hair cells in the saccule, utricle and lagena (Sun et al., 2011). Studies in mammalian models suggest that hormones and growth factors can modulate hair cell regeneration. For example, transforming growth factor α and insulin supplemented with epidermal growth factor induced cellular regeneration in mouse vestibular sensory epithelia (Yamashita and Oesterle, 1995). Although, the action of some growth factors, e.g., insulin-like growth factor-1, in mammals

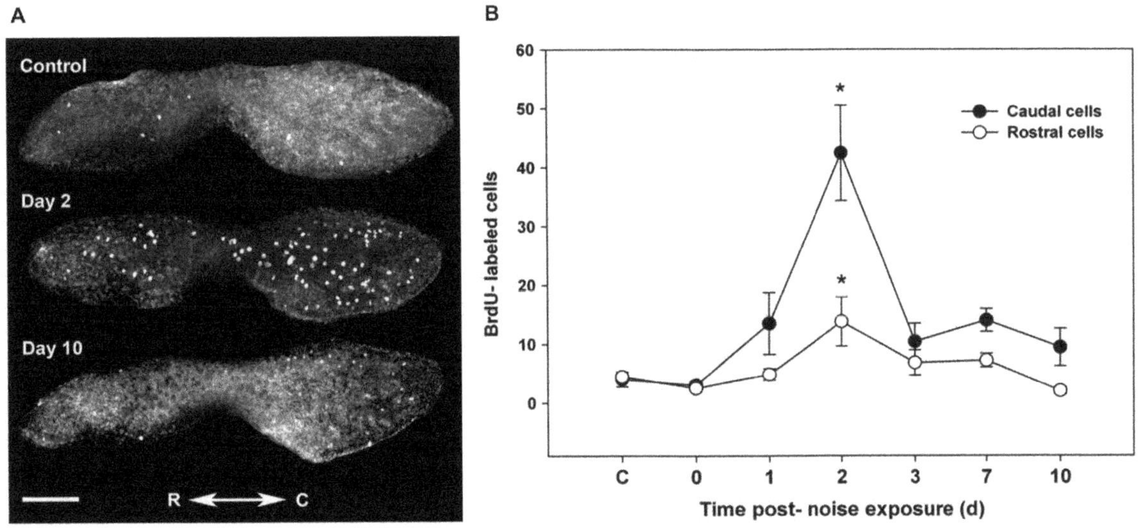

FIGURE 4 | Proliferation follows acoustic trauma to the zebrafish inner ear. (A) BrdU-labeled proliferating cells in a control zebrafish saccule and in saccules dissected for 2 and 10 days post-noise exposure. C = caudal, R = rostral; scale bar = 100 μm. **(B)** Mean (±SE) BrdU-labeled zebrafish saccular cells as a function of time following sound exposure (*$p < 0.001$; $n = 6$). Adapted from Hearing Research, Vol. 253, J.B. Schuck, M.E. Smith, Cell proliferation follows acoustically-induced hair cell bundle loss in the zebrafish saccule, 2009, with permission from Elsevier.

may be confined to protective and not regenerative effects (Yamamoto et al., 2014).

Digital gene expression, a form of next generation sequencing, has also been used to identify genes that modulate hair cell regeneration in adult and larval zebrafish (Liang et al., 2012). This showed that the *stat3/socs3* pathway can modulate hair cell production in the lateral line during development and the adult inner ear during hair cell regeneration, and its expression and activity is associated with supporting cells, differentiating hair cells, and cell division. In mouse models, upstream effectors of Stat3 may be involved in hair cell survival (Hertzano et al., 2004), but no role for Stat3 in hair cell regeneration has yet been reported in mammals.

While microarrays and digital gene expression studies typically use tissue preparations, gene expression can also be studied by collecting samples from individual progenitor cells. For example, lateral line mantle cells can be fluorescently-labeled, isolated by flow cytometry and then subjected to whole-transcriptome microarray analysis (Steiner et al., 2014). This approach revealed that after hair cell ablation, transcripts coding for transmembrane receptors and cell-adhesion molecules increased. Some of these transcripts were confined to particular mantle cell subsets in specific neuromast regions. Further, transcriptional levels followed a temporal course with maximal changes occurring within 3–5 h following ablation. Using this methodology, it may possible to further elaborate the mechanistic differences between mammalian and non-mammalian hair cell progenitors.

Chemical screens have also been used to identify compounds that enhance or inhibit hair cell regeneration in the zebrafish lateral line. For example, a chemical screen has been used to identify synthetic glucocorticoid enhancers that promote hair cell regeneration by increasing mitotic activity (Namdaran et al., 2012). This study also identified inhibitors that either reduced hair cell regeneration or prevented supporting cell proliferation, and some of these drugs targeted cell division mechanisms.

Zebrafish studies show that Wnt signaling is involved in hair cell regeneration. In neuromasts, inhibition of Wnt/β-catenin signaling reduces proliferation and hair cell differentiation while activation of Wnt increases hair cell numbers and promotes supporting cells to reenter the cell cycle and proliferate (Head et al., 2013; Jacques et al., 2013). Further, Wnt/β-catenin activation causes increased hair cell regeneration (Jacques et al., 2013). Neuromast size is also regulated by a negative feedback loop that incorporates Wnt signaling activity (Wada et al., 2013). This promotes surrounding cells to proliferate and is inhibited by Dkk activity from differentiated sensory cells. An analysis of RNA transcripts expressed in the zebrafish lateral line following neomycin-induced damage showed that Wnt/β-catenin signaling is down-regulated during earlier time points but becomes up-regulated later (Jiang et al., 2014). This suggests that Wnt is necessary for hair cell proliferation but not immediately after hair cell damage.

Studies of Wnt signaling in zebrafish indicate that the transcription factor Sox2 is involved in hair cell proliferation and transdifferentiation. In one study, new hair cells were derived from proliferating Sox2-positive cells in the prosensory domain (Jacques et al., 2013), and Sox2 is highly expressed in most proliferating neuromast progenitor cells (Hernández et al., 2007). Sox2 is also required for transdifferentiation of supporting cells (Millimaki et al., 2010). Another important regulator of Wnt/β-catenin signaling is ErbB/Neuregulin, which can act upstream to regulate the proliferation of zebrafish lateral line interneuromast cells and the development of intercalary

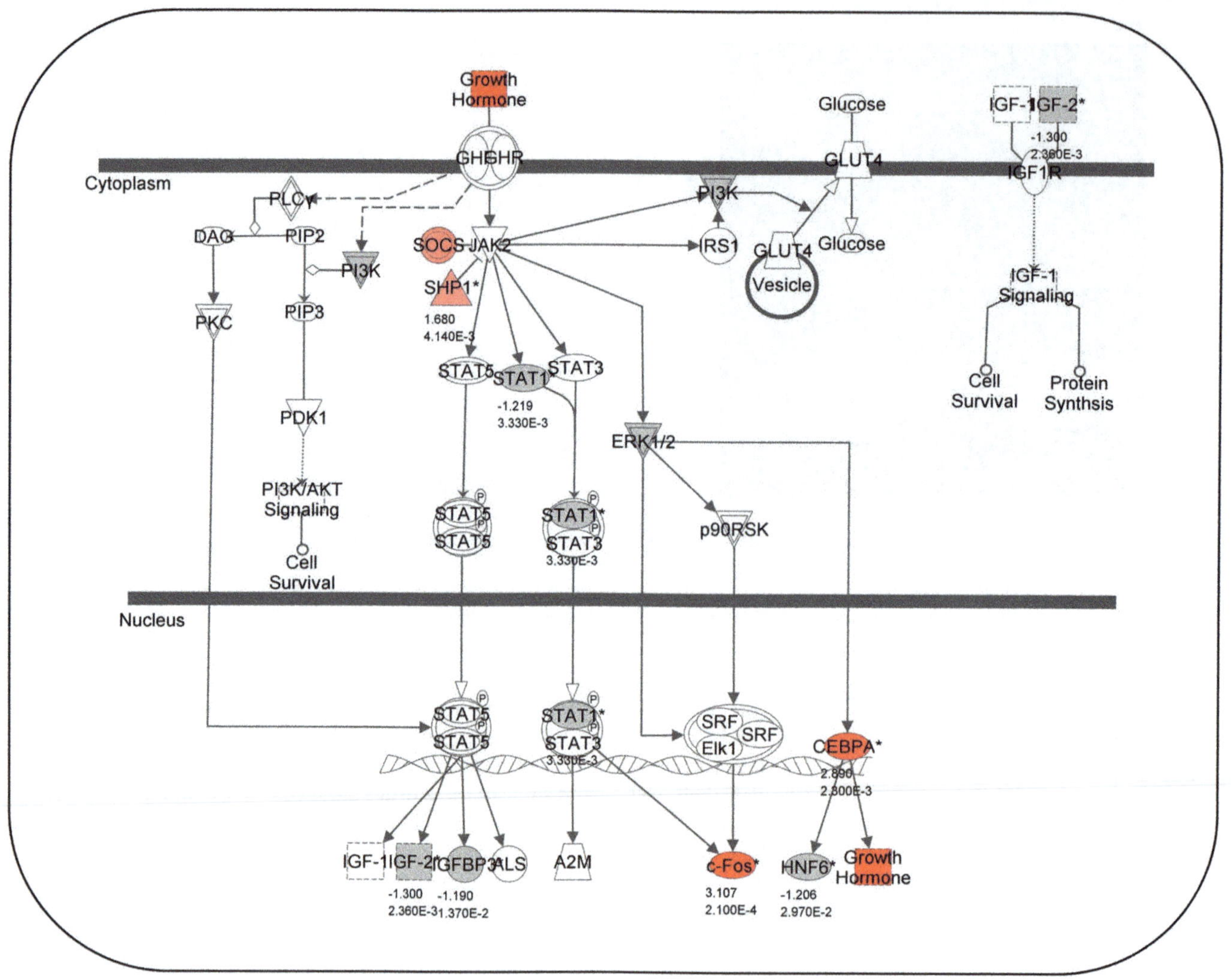

FIGURE 5 | Growth hormone-related gene expression. Canonical pathway analysis showing known growth-hormone related pathways. Red colored genes are up-regulated and gray-colored genes are down-regulated 2 days following acoustical trauma. Numbers below genes represent fold changes and *P*-values (Modified from Schuck et al., 2011).

neuromasts (Lush and Piotrowski, 2014b). ErbB signaling is required for the migration of Schwann cells and in the absence of ErbB signaling or Schwann cells, Wnt/β-catenin and Fgf (fibroblast growth factor) signaling is increased. Further, Wnt/β-catenin signaling is required for interneuromast proliferation, while protoneuromast formation and cellular differentiation requires Fgf signaling (Lush and Piotrowski, 2014b). When ErbB/Neuregulin signaling is reduced, Notch signaling is induced many hours after activation of Wnt/β-catenin but before Fgf signaling begins.

The Notch signaling pathway is also a key modulator of hair cell regeneration in the zebrafish lateral line. When supporting cell proliferation and formation of hair cell progenitors is maximal, transcript levels of the Notch pathway components, *notch3*, *deltaA*, and *atoh1a*, increase (Ma et al., 2008). However, inhibiting Notch signaling can also cause hair cell regeneration (Moon et al., 2011). These studies suggest that the Notch pathway modulates regeneration as part of a complex interplay of signaling elements. In the zebrafish *mind bomb* mutant, Delta-Notch signaling was responsible for controlling supporting cell differentiation into inner ear hair cells (Haddon et al., 1998). A time course analysis of lateral line hair cell regeneration in zebrafish found that Notch signaling is inhibited immediately following hair cell damage (Jiang et al., 2014). The Notch target genes, *her4.1*, *notch3*, and *sox2*, were down-regulated at 1 h, but were up-regulated between 3 and 5 h after damage. *Atoh1a*, a Notch target gene, was up-regulated at 1 h and *deltaD*, a target of Atoh1a, was up-regulated between 3 and 5 h following damage. The inhibition of Notch, and the up-regulation of *atoh1a* and *deltaD*, suggests that during hair cell regeneration, Notch inhibition needs to be relieved so that supporting cells can leave a quiescent state and begin proliferation. Constitutively expressing Notch can prevent hair cell proliferation from supporting cell progenitors, while eliminating Notch activity produces increased numbers of hair cell progenitors and ectopic hair cells (Wibowo et al., 2011). Further, Notch3 activity prevents supporting cells from becoming hair cell progenitors outside of the polar compartments where hair cells regenerate and establish directional symmetry. Thus, when Notch activity is low and Atoh1a expression is higher within the polar compartment, hair cell progenitor division and immature hair cell formation increases.

Differentiation of hair cell progenitors requires expression of the transcription factor, Atoh1 (Ma and Raible, 2009; Groves et al., 2013). Gain and loss-of-function techniques have been used to characterize the role of Atoh1 in hair cell regeneration. Knockdown of Atoh1a reduced hair cell formation in the zebrafish inner ear, while rescuing expression restored hair cells (Millimaki et al., 2007). However, excess Atoh1a expression did not produce ectopic or excess hair cells, as found in rodent models (Zheng and Gao, 2000). Interestingly, adjacent to the lateral line, excess Atoh1a increased ectopic hair cell placement (Millimaki et al., 2007). These results suggest that Atoh1 signaling may modulate inner ear and lateral line hair cell regeneration differently and may promote different effects in zebrafish and mammalian models. Knockdown of Atoh1 can also reduce zebrafish neuromast development; whereas, rescue or over-expression induces the activity of NeuroD, which is required for hair cell differentiation (Sarrazin et al., 2006). However, mantle and interneuromastic cells are not affected by reduction of Atoh1 protein. Activating Atoh1a signaling in the zebrafish inner ear at different time intervals can cause hair cell formation in distinct spatial regions (Sweet et al., 2011). For example, activation at 18 h post fertilization (hpf) causes formation of ectopic hair cells in the region normally occupied by the utricular and saccular maculae. At 36 hpf, activation caused two discrete and enlarged maculae to appear with an intervening region devoid of hair cells, while at 48 hpf, few hair cells develop and no ectopic cells were observed. Although increasing Atoh1 expression in mammalian models can cause hair cell regeneration, these cells typically exhibit aberrant placement and morphology (Sweet et al., 2011). Thus, future research is required to determine whether results obtained with zebrafish models can be applied to mammalian organisms.

Atoh1a can also regulate hair cell regeneration by modulating ion transport (Go et al., 2010). Specifically, knockdown and inhibition of the plasma membrane calcium transporter ATPase, Atp2b1a (Pmca1), which is controlled by Atoh1a, can affect hair cell regeneration. Knockdown of Atp2b1a blocks calcium export and increases hair cell progenitors. Thus, Atp2b1a might, under control of Atoh1a, affect progenitor cell proliferation and hair cell differentiation via a calcium signaling mechanism. Another ATPase gene, *atp1b2b*, which regulates Na^+/K^+ transport, can affect hair cell regeneration (Wang et al., 2008). Knockdown of Eya4, a transcriptional co-activator of Atp1b2b, decreased the number of hair cells in the zebrafish inner ear compartment and lateral line during development. Atp1b2b has a similar spatial and temporal expression as Eya4 and is reduced during Eya4 knockdown. Specific knockdown of Atp1b2b also reduced hair cell numbers in the inner ear compartment and lateral line while over-expression restored the normal phenotype, suggesting that Eya4 may regulate hair cell regeneration by modulating the Na^+/K^+-ATPase transporter.

As in zebrafish, Wnt, Notch and related signaling is involved in mammalian hair cell proliferation and transdifferentiation during development. For example, inhibition of Notch signaling causes proliferation of supporting cells in mouse cochlea by acting through the Wnt signaling pathway, however, transdifferentiation was Wnt-independent (Li et al., 2015). In the mouse utricle, inhibition of Notch signaling caused transdifferentiation of supporting cells with little mitotic proliferation (Lin et al., 2011). Transdifferentiation of supporting cells is also promoted by over-expressing Atoh1 in the guinea pig inner ear (Izumikawa et al., 2005). Over-expression in supporting cells of the downstream Wnt signaling molecule, β-catenin, caused proliferation in some cells and reduced expression of p27, a cell cycle inhibitor (Shi et al., 2013). Similarly, reducing p27 expression in mouse cochlea causes proliferation of hair and supporting cells (Chen and Segil, 1999; Ono et al., 2009). Interestingly, functional assays show no differences in hearing ability between wild type and p27 mutant animals (Walters et al., 2014). In the zebrafish lateral line, when histone deacetylases are inhibited, the numbers of hair and supporting cells decrease, neuromast cellular proliferation is reduced, and p27 mRNA levels increase (He et al., 2013). These studies suggest that p27 may regulate cellular proliferation in both zebrafish and mammalian models.

Caspase signaling may also play a role in hair cell regeneration. For example, caspase inhibition reduced hair cell death and supporting cell proliferation in zebrafish peripheral neuromasts (Williams and Holder, 2000). This suggests that caspases could be an integral part of a feedback mechanism that controls supporting cell division and entry into mitosis in response to hair cell death. Caspase activity in zebrafish may function similarly to mammalian models where caspases can modulate apoptosis (Zheng et al., 2014). However, hair cells could be continually renewed from supporting cells in the absence of cell death signaling. A study of hair cell regeneration in the oscar saccule and chicken utricle suggests that supporting cells may not require a cell death signal in the oscar in order to proliferate (Wilkins et al., 1999). In an avian study, caspase inhibition caused reduction of hair cell death and supporting cell proliferation (Matsui et al., 2002) similar to findings in the zebrafish lateral line (Williams and Holder, 2000). Teleosts could have a population of supporting cells that undergo continual renewal without a cell death signal requirement or require such a signal for some or all supporting cells. Alternatively, new hair cells might trigger the death of older cells. Further, as the oscar saccule continues to enlarge during adult life, developmental mechanisms may also be implicated in hair cell regeneration (Wilkins et al., 1999). Future research is needed to characterize the roles played by developmental and intracellular cell death signaling mechanisms in teleosts and their effects on hair cell regeneration.

Other mechanisms have been identified that can modulate teleost hair cell regeneration. The phoenix gene (*pho*), which is strongly expressed in supporting cells, affects zebrafish hair cell proliferation and regeneration (Behra et al., 2009). Pho mutants exhibit normal neuromast and hair cell development. However, when progenitor cells are destroyed in the mutants, supporting cell proliferation and hair cell regeneration is greatly reduced. This suggests that Pho may regulate entry into mitosis. Another mechanism involves histone methylation by lysine specific demethylase 1 (LSD1), which can regulate hair and supporting cell proliferation during development (He et al., 2013). Inhibition of LSD1 reduces the number of hair and supporting cells and suppressed neuromast cellular proliferation. Increased inhibition caused apoptosis within neuromasts. While investigating the origin of new hair cells in the zebrafish lateral line, Lin et al. (2013), found that Rb (retinoblastoma protein) and Raf-1 kinase were involved in asymmetric cell division in neuromasts. Blocking the interaction between Rb and Raf-1, and Rb phosphorylation, prevented hair cell regeneration from supporting cells. In a rat model, inhibition of phosphorylated Rb promoted proliferation of supporting cells which transdifferentiated into hair cells by activating the sonic hedgehog pathway (Lu et al., 2013).

While most of the research on hair cell regeneration has focused on protein expression at the gene level, microRNAs (miRNAs), which are small, non-coding RNAs that regulate gene expression by translation repression or mRNA destabilization (Friedman et al., 2009), have been shown to play an important role in hair cell development. For example, miRNAs can regulate hair cell proliferation in embryonic zebrafish inner ears (Wienholds et al., 2005; Li et al., 2010). Knockdown of miR-96, -182 and -183 causes a reduction in the numbers of inner ear hair cells. Conversely, over-expressing miR-96 and -182 promotes hair cell production. These miRNAs are also expressed in the mouse inner ear (Weston et al., 2006), and they have been shown to have roles in inner ear development (Sacheli et al., 2009; Soukup, 2009). Further, miR-96 can regulate differentiation of cochlear hair cells (Kuhn et al., 2011). A more in depth review of miRNAs regulated in vertebrate hair cells is provided elsewhere (Smith and Rajadinakaran, 2013).

Future Directions

Otoprotectants

One strategy for preventing damage to hair cells is to administer otoprotective drugs that counteract cellular injury from otherwise beneficial drugs (Coffin et al., 2010; Ou et al., 2010; Esterberg et al., 2013). Otoprotectants mainly work by interfering with antibiotic uptake (Hailey et al., 2012; Ou et al., 2012) or inhibiting generation of reactive oxygen species (Le Prell et al., 2007; Wu et al., 2014). The antioxidant epicatechin protects both mammalian and zebrafish hair cells against cisplatin damage and decreases reactive oxygen species generation (Kim et al., 2008). Similarly, Shin et al. (2013), demonstrated that the drug 3-amino-3-(4-fluoro-phenyl)-1H-quinoline-2, 4-dione (KR-22332) provided otoprotective benefits against cisplatin damage in zebrafish and a rat model. The utility of the zebrafish model for discovering potentially otoprotective drugs is well documented. Owens et al. (2008), investigated a library of 10,960 compounds for otoprotective effects in zebrafish larvae and found that two benzothiophene carboximides, PROTO-1 and PROTO-2, acted as otoprotectants. A recent screen in the zebrafish lateral line of 10,000 small molecule inhibitors of cisplatin-mediated hair cell death showed that two compounds, cisplatin hair cell protectant 1 and 2 (CHCP1 and 2), may respectively reduce uptake of a cisplatin analog and affect an intracellular mechanism (Thomas et al., 2015b). Quinoline drugs protective against neomycin and gentamicin mediated damage have also been identified (Ou et al., 2012). Vlasits et al. (2012), discovered 10 compounds that prevent several aminoglycosides and cisplatin from damaging hair cells in the larval zebrafish lateral line. Evidently, fish models could provide a very productive framework in the future for screening drug molecules that could offer protection against ototoxic damage, but these drugs still need to be tested in mammalian models.

Cell Cycle Mechanisms

Studies in zebrafish and mouse models demonstrate that they share key components of several hair cell proliferation pathways, e.g., Wnt, Notch and Rb (Hernández et al., 2007; Liu and Zuo, 2008; Ma et al., 2008; Moon et al., 2011; Head et al., 2013; Jacques et al., 2013; Lin et al., 2013; Mizutari et al., 2013; Wada et al., 2013). Despite this fact, hair cell proliferation does not normally occur in mammals after cells become post-mitotic (Burns and Corwin, 2013). One potential nexus for this divergent cellular behavior could involve regulation of the cell cycle (Liu and Zuo, 2008). Mammalian studies have identified a number of molecules that regulate hair cell entry into mitosis. One of these, the cell cycle inhibitor p27kip, can modulate mammalian hair cell regeneration (Chen and Segil, 1999; Löwenheim et al., 1999; Kanzaki et al., 2006; Ono et al., 2009; Oesterle et al., 2011; Liu et al., 2012; Walters et al., 2014). However, to this date, there is little information available on how cell cycle regulatory mechanisms function in fish hair cell regeneration or what environmental cues modulate them. Studies on this topic, and related signal transduction pathways, would be beneficial not only for our understanding of hair cell regenerative phenomena in fish, but could also have translational applications towards human health.

Reinnervation

Reinnervation, the reestablishing of functional nervous system connections with target cells, is a necessary concomitant of hair cell regeneration. If neurons are unable to establish appropriate communication with new hair cells, then auditory and vestibular signaling to the brain will not occur. The neuromasts and associated neurons of the embryonic zebrafish lateral line can be stained facilitating the study of neural innervation of the neuromasts using mutant models (Raible and Kruse, 2000). Hair cell polarity in the zebrafish lateral line is important for establishing an appropriate sense of equilibrium (López-Schier et al., 2004). Mutant fish lacking a planar-polarity protein (Vangl2) have improperly oriented hair cells (López-Schier and Hudspeth, 2006). Nagiel et al. (2008), and Faucherre et al. (2009), have shown that PLL afferent neurons establish synaptic connections with regenerated hair cells with a particular orientation suggesting that they target a polarity guidance cue.

Zebrafish unable to transduce mechanical stimuli have afferent neurons that exhibit increased arborization, less stability and more pathfinding errors (Faucherre et al., 2010). Intact lateral line hair cells are not required for neuronal regeneration, but in their absence deviation in pathfinding occurs (Villegas et al., 2012). Also, the synaptic ribbon protein, Ribeye, is required for synaptogenesis and afferent innervation in zebrafish (Sheets et al., 2011). Mo and Nicolson (2011), have investigated the role of N-ethylmaleimide-sensitive factor (Nsf) protein in hair cell synapse maintenance. Afferent neurons retract when Nsf decreases. Reduction of Nsf also caused brain-derived neurotrophic factor, BDNF, to accumulate suggesting that Nsf is required for BDNF release. Injection of BDNF only partially restores afferent synapses indicating that other signaling molecules may be involved in promoting hair cell synaptogenesis. Studies performed in mammalian models show that various stem cell populations can develop the features of spiral ganglion neurons and that their transplantation into the inner ear can restore some auditory function (Diensthuber et al., 2014; Géléoc and Holt, 2014). Another study transplanted spiral ganglion neurons into mice where these neurons had been destroyed and found that the replaced neurons reinnervated and formed new synaptic connections with hair cells (Martinez-Monedero et al., 2006). Additional studies in zebrafish will be needed to elucidate the mechanisms that modulate neuronal reinnervation with hair cells and their relatedness to mammalian organisms.

Conclusion

Much has been learned in the last decade about hair cell death and regeneration in teleost fishes. Advances derived from studies in zebrafish and other fish species include understanding how ototoxins affect hair cells and discovering new otoprotectants that mitigate ototoxin damage, the role played by cellular proliferation and transdifferentiation during hair cell regeneration, and characterization of the cellular pathways involved in regeneration. Although the zebrafish model has the advantage of higher throughput and easier access to sensory hair cells than mammalian models, because of the different cellular and molecular characteristics of teleost and mammalian auditory cells, data obtained in zebrafish models may not apply to mammalian models. Thus, additional comparative studies involving zebrafish and mammal-based models will be needed to determine whether results obtained in teleosts can be translated into therapeutics to prevent or treat human hearing loss.

Acknowledgments

This work was supported by an Institutional Development Award (IDeA) from NIH (8 P20 GM103436-12), the Kentucky Science and Engineering Foundation (KSEF-149-502-14-325), and a Western Kentucky University Research and Creative Activities Program Grant to MES.

References

Ahmed, Z. M., Goodyear, R., Riazuddin, S., Lagziel, A., Leagan, P. K., Behra, M., et al. (2006). The tip-link antigen, a protein associated with the transduction complex of sensory hair cells, is Protocadherin-15. *J. Neurosci.* 26, 7022–7034. doi: 10.1523/jneurosci.1163-06.2006

Ahn, J. H., Kang, H. H., Kim, Y. J., and Chung, J. W. (2005). Anti-apoptotic role of retinoic acid in the inner ear of noise-exposed mice. *Biochem. Biophys. Res. Commun.* 335, 485–490. doi: 10.1016/j.bbrc.2005.07.114

Alharazneh, A., Luk, L., Huth, M., Monfared, A., Steyger, P. S., Cheng, A. G., et al. (2011). Functional hair cell mechanotransducer channels are required for aminoglycoside ototoxicity. *PLoS One* 6:e22347. doi: 10.1371/journal.pone.0022347

Bang, P. I., Sewell, W. F., and Malicki, J. J. (2001). Morphology and cell type heterogeneities of the inner ear epithelia in adult and juvenile zebrafish (*Danio rerio*). *J. Comp. Neurol.* 438, 173–190. doi: 10.1002/cne.1308

Barbazuk, W. B., Korf, I., Kadavi, C., Heyen, J., Tate, S., Wun, E., et al. (2000). The syntenic relationship of the zebrafish and human genomes. *Genome Res.* 10, 1351–1358. doi: 10.1101/gr.144700

Behra, M., Bradsher, J., Sougrat, R., Gallardo, V., Allende, M. L., and Burgess, S. M. (2009). *Phoenix* is required for mechanosensory hair cell regeneration in the zebrafish lateral line. *PLoS Genet.* 5:e1000455. doi: 10.1371/journal.pgen.1000455

Bever, M. M., and Fekete, D. M. (2002). Atlas of the developing inner ear in zebrafish. *Dev. Dyn.* 223, 536–543. doi: 10.1002/dvdy.10062

Brignull, H. R., Raible, D. W., and Stone, J. S. (2009). Feathers and fins: non-mammalian models for hair cell regeneration. *Brain Res.* 1277, 12–23. doi: 10.1016/j.brainres.2009.02.028

Brown, A. D., Mussen, T. D., Sisneros, J. A., and Coffin, A. B. (2011). Reevaluating the use of aminoglycoside antibiotics in behavioral studies of the lateral line. *Hear. Res.* 272, 1–4. doi: 10.1016/j.heares.2010.10.014

Buck, L. M., Winter, M. J., Redfern, W. S., and Whitfield, T. T. (2012). Ototoxin-induced cellular damage in neuromasts disrupts lateral line function in larval zebrafish. *Hear. Res.* 284, 67–81. doi: 10.1016/j.heares.2011.12.001

Burns, J. C., Collado, M. S., Oliver, E. R., and Corwin, J. T. (2013). Specializations of intercellular junctions are associated with the presence and absence of hair cell regeneration in ears from six vertebrate classes. *J. Comp. Neurol.* 521, 1430–1448. doi: 10.1002/cne.23250

Burns, J. C., and Corwin, J. T. (2013). A historical to present-day account of efforts to answer the question: "what puts the brakes on mammalian hair cell regeneration?" *Hear. Res.* 297, 52–67. doi: 10.1016/j.heares.2013.01.005

Casper, B. M., Smith, M. E., Halvorsen, M. B., Sun, H., Carlson, T. J., and Popper, A. N. (2013). Effects of exposure to pile driving sounds on fish inner ear tissues. *Comp. Biochem. Physiol. A Mol. Integr. Physiol.* 166, 352–360. doi: 10.1016/j.cbpa.2013.07.008

Chang, J., Im, G. J., Chae, S. W., Lee, S. H., Kwon, S. Y., Jung, H. H., et al. (2013). Protective role of trimetazidine against neomycin-induced hair cell damage in zebrafish. *Clin. Exp. Otorhinolaryngol.* 6, 219–225. doi: 10.3342/ceo.2013.6.4.219

Chang, J. S. Y., Popper, A. N., and Saidel, W. M. (1992). Heterogeneity of sensory hair cells in a fish ear. *J. Comp. Neurol.* 324, 621–640. doi: 10.1002/cne.903240413

Chen, P., and Segil, N. (1999). p27^{Kip1} links cell proliferation to morphogenesis in the developing organ of Corti. *Development* 126, 1581–1590.

Chiu, L. L., Cunningham, L. L., Raible, D. W., Rubel, E. W., and Ou, H. C. (2008). Using the zebrafish lateral line to screen for ototoxicity. *J. Assoc. Res. Otolaryngol.* 9, 178–190. doi: 10.1007/s10162-008-0118-y

Chung, J. W., Ahn, J. H., Kim, J. Y., Lee, H. J., Kang, H. H., Lee, Y. K., et al. (2007). The effect of isoflurane, halothane and pentobarbital on noise-induced hearing loss in mice. *Anesth. Analg.* 104, 1404–1408. doi: 10.1213/01.ane.0000261508.24083.6c

Ciarimboli, G. (2012). Membrane transporters as mediators of cisplatin effects and side effects. *Scientifica (Cairo)* 2012:473829. doi: 10.6064/2012/473829

Ciarimboli, G., Deuster, D., Knief, A., Sperling, M., Holtkamp, M., Edemir, B., et al. (2010). Organic cation transporter 2 mediates cisplatin-induced oto- and nephrotoxicity and is a target for protective interventions. *Am. J. Pathol.* 176, 1169–1180. doi: 10.2353/ajpath.2010.090610

Clack, J. A. (2012). *Gaining Ground: The Origin and Evolution of Tetrapods.* Bloomington, Indiana, USA: Indiana University Press.

Coffin, A., Kelley, M. W., Manley, G. A., and Popper, A. N. (2004). "Evolution of sensory hair cells," in *Evolution of the Vertebrate Auditory System*, eds G. A. Manley, A. N. Popper, R. R. Fay (New York, NY: Springer Science and Business Media), 55–94.

Coffin, A. B., Ou, H., Owens, K. N., Santos, F., Simon, J. A., Rubel, E. W., et al. (2010). Chemical screening for hair cell loss and protection in the zebrafish lateral line. *Zebrafish* 7, 3–11. doi: 10.1089/zeb.2009.0639

Coffin, A. B., Rubel, E. W., and Raible, D. W. (2013a). Bax, Bcl2 and p53 differentially regulate neomycin- and gentamicin-induced hair cell death in the zebrafish lateral line. *J. Assoc. Res. Otolaryngol.* 14, 645–659. doi: 10.1007/s10162-013-0404-1

Coffin, A. B., Williamson, K. L., Mamiya, A., Raible, D. W., and Rubel, E. W. (2013b). Profiling drug-induced cell death pathways in the zebrafish lateral line. *Apoptosis* 18, 393–408. doi: 10.1007/s10495-013-0816-8

Coimbra, R. S., Weil, D., Brottier, P., Blanchard, S., Levi, M., Hardelin, J. P., et al. (2002). A subtracted cDNA library from the zebrafish (*Danio rerio*) embryonic inner ear. *Genome Res.* 12, 1007–1011. doi: 10.1101/gr.227502

Coombs, S., Braun, C. B., and Donovan, B. (2001). The orienting response of Lake Michigan mottled sculpin is mediated by canal neuromasts. *J. Exp. Biol.* 204, 337–348.

Corwin, J. T., and Oberholtzer, J. C. (1997). Fish n' chicks: model recipes for hair-cell regeneration? *Neuron* 9, 951–954. doi: 10.1016/s0896-6273(00)80386-4

Corwin, J. T., and Warchol, M. E. (1991). Auditory hair cells: structure, function, development and regeneration. *Annu. Rev. Neurosci.* 14, 301–333. doi: 10.1146/annurev.neuro.14.1.301

Cruz, S., Shiao, J. C., Liao, B. K., Huang, C. J., and Hwang, P. P. (2009). Plasma membrane calcium ATPase required for semicircular canal formation and otolith growth in the zebrafish inner ear. *J. Exp. Biol.* 212, 639–647. doi: 10.1242/jeb.022798

Diensthuber, M., Zecha, V., Wagenblast, J., Arnhold, S., Edge, A. S., and Stöver, T. (2014). Spiral ganglion stem cells can be propagated and differentiated into neurons and glia. *Biores. Open Access* 3, 88–97. doi: 10.1089/biores.2014.0016

Ding, D., He, J., Allman, B. L., Yu, D., Jiang, H., Seigel, G. M., et al. (2011). Cisplatin ototoxicity in rat cochlear organotypic cultures. *Hear. Res.* 282, 196–203. doi: 10.1016/j.heares.2011.08.002

Driever, W., Solnica-Krezel, L., Schier, A. F., Neuhauss, S. C., Malicki, J., Stemple, D. L., et al. (1996). A genetic screen for mutations affecting embryogenesis in zebrafish. *Development* 123, 37–46.

Ernest, S., Rauch, G. J., Haffter, P., Geisler, R., Petit, C., and Nicolson, T. (2000). *Mariner*is defective in *myosin VIIA*: a zebrafish model for human hereditary deafness. *Hum. Mol. Genet.* 9, 2189–2196. doi: 10.1093/hmg/9.14.2189

Esterberg, R., Coffin, A. B., Ou, H., Simon, J. A., Raible, D. W., and Rubel, E. W. (2013). Fish in a dish: drug discovery for hearing habilitation. *Drug Discov. Today Dis. Models* 10, e23–e29. doi: 10.1016/j.ddmod.2012.02.001

Faucher, K., Aas-Hansen, Ø., Damsgård, B., Laukli, E., and Stenklev, N. C. (2009). Damage and functional recovery of the Atlantic cod (*Gadus morhua*) inner ear hair cells following local injection of gentamicin. *Int. J. Audiol.* 48, 456–464. doi: 10.1080/14992020902738029

Faucherre, A., Baudoin, J. P., Pujol-Martí, J., and López-Schier, H. (2010). Multispectral four-dimensional imaging reveals that evoked activity modulates peripheral arborization and the selection of plane-polarized targets by sensory neurons. *Development* 137, 1635–1643. doi: 10.1242/dev.047316

Faucherre, A., Pujol-Martí, J., Kawakami, K., and López-Schier, H. (2009). Afferent neurons of the zebrafish lateral line are strict selectors of hair-cell orientation. *PLoS One* 4:e4477. doi: 10.1371/journal.pone.0004477

Friedman, R. C., Farh, K. K.-H., Burge, C. B., and Bartel, D. P. (2009). Most mammalian mRNAs are conserved targets of microRNAs. *Genome Res.* 19, 92–105. doi: 10.1101/gr.082701.108

Fu, Y., Ding, D., Jiang, H., and Salvi, R. (2012). Ouabain-induced cochlear degeneration in rat. *Neurotox. Res.* 22, 158–169. doi: 10.1007/s12640-012-9320-0

Furness, D. N., and Hackney, C. M. (2006). "The structure and composition of the stereociliary bundle of vertebrate hair cells," in *Vertebrate Hair Cells*, eds R. A. Eatock, R. R. Fay, A. N. Popper (New York, NY: Springer Science + Business Media, Inc.), 95–153.

Furness, D. N., Hackney, C. M., and Evans, M. G. (2010). Localisation of the mechanotransducer channels in mammalian cochlear hair cells provides clues to their gating. *J. Physiol.* 588, 765–772. doi: 10.1113/jphysiol.2009.179614

Géléoc, G. S., and Holt, J. R. (2014). Sound strategies for hearing restoration. *Science* 344:1241062. doi: 10.1126/science.1241062

Ghysen, A., and Dambly-Chaudière, C. (2004). Development of the zebrafish lateral line. *Curr. Opin. Neurobiol.* 14, 67–73. doi: 10.1016/j.conb.2004.01.012

Giari, L., Dezfuli, B. S., Astolfi, L., and Martini, A. (2012). Ultrastructural effects of cisplatin on the inner ear and lateral line system of zebrafish (*Danio rerio*) larvae. *J. Appl. Toxicol.* 32, 293–299. doi: 10.1002/jat.1691

Go, W., Bessarab, D., and Korzh, V. (2010). *atp2b1a*regulates Ca^{2+} export during differentiation and regeneration of mechanosensory hair cells in zebrafish. *Cell Calcium* 48, 302–313. doi: 10.1016/j.ceca.2010.09.012

Goldsmith, J. R., and Jobin, C. (2012). Think small: zebrafish as a model system of human pathology. *J. Biomed. Biotechnol.* 2012:817341. doi: 10.1155/2012/817341

Groves, A. K. (2010). The challenge of hair cell regeneration. *Exp. Biol. Med. (Maywood)* 235, 434–446. doi: 10.1258/ebm.2009.009281

Groves, A. K., Zhang, K. D., and Fekete, D. M. (2013). The genetics of hair cell development and regeneration. *Annu. Rev. Neurosci.* 36, 361–381. doi: 10.1146/annurev-neuro-062012-170309

Hackney, C. M., and Furness, D. N. (2013). The composition and role of cross links in mechanoelectrical transduction in vertebrate sensory hair cells. *J. Cell Sci.* 126, 1721–1731. doi: 10.1242/jcs.106120

Haddon, C., Jiang, Y. J., Smithers, L., and Lewis, J. (1998). Delta-Notch signaling and the patterning of sensory cell differentiation in the zebrafish ear: evidence from the *mind bomb* mutant. *Development* 125, 4637–4644.

Haddon, C., and Lewis, J. (1996). Early ear development in the embryo of the zebrafish, *Danio rerio*. *J. Comp. Neurol.* 365, 113–128. doi: 10.1002/(sici)1096-9861(19960129)365:1<113::aid-cne9>3.0.co;2-6

Haehnel, M., Taguchi, M., and Liao, J. C. (2012). Heterogeneity and dynamics of lateral line afferent innervation during development in zebrafish (*Danio rerio*). *J. Comp. Neurol.* 520, 1376–1386. doi: 10.1002/cne.22798

Hailey, D. W., Roberts, B., Owens, K. N., Stewart, A. K., Linbo, T., Pujol, R., et al. (2012). Loss of Slc4a1b chloride/bicarbonate exchanger function protects mechanosensory hair cells from aminoglycoside damage in the zebrafish mutant *persephone*. *PLoS Genet.* 8:e1002971. doi: 10.1371/journal.pgen.1002971

Hammond, K. L., van Eeden, F. J. M., and Whitfield, T. T. (2010). Repression of hedgehog signaling is required for the acquisition of dorsolateral cell fates in the zebrafish otic vesicle. *Development* 137, 1361–1371. doi: 10.1242/dev.045666

Harris, J. A., Cheng, A. G., Cunningham, L. L., MacDonald, G., Raible, D. W., and Rubel, E. W. (2003). Neomycin-induced hair cell death and rapid regeneration in the lateral line of zebrafish (*Danio rerio*). *J. Assoc. Res. Otolaryngol.* 4, 219–234. doi: 10.1007/s10162-002-3022-x

He, Y., Wu, J., Mei, H., Yu, H., Sun, S., Shou, J., et al. (2013). Histone deacetylase activity is required for embryonic posterior lateral line development. *Cell Prolif.* 47, 91–104. doi: 10.1111/cpr.12081

Head, J. R., Gacioch, L., Pennisi, M., and Meyers, J. R. (2013). Activation of canonical Wnt/β-catenin signaling stimulates proliferation in neuromasts in the zebrafish posterior lateral line. *Dev. Dyn.* 242, 832–846. doi: 10.1002/dvdy.23973

Henley, C. M., and Rybak, L. P. (1995). Ototoxicity in developing mammals. *Brain Res. Brain Res. Rev.* 20, 68–90. doi: 10.1016/0165-0173(94)00006-b

Hernández, P. P., Moreno, V., Olivari, F. A., and Allende, M. L. (2006). Sub-lethal concentrations of waterborne copper are toxic to lateral line neuromasts in zebrafish (*Danio rerio*). *Hear. Res.* 213, 1–10. doi: 10.1016/j.heares.2005.10.015

Hernández, P. P., Olivari, F. A., Sarrazin, A. F., Sandoval, P. C., and Allende, M. L. (2007). Regeneration in zebrafish lateral line neuromasts: expression of the neural progenitor cell marker Sox2 and proliferation-dependent and-independent mechanisms of hair cell renewal. *Dev. Neurobiol.* 67, 637–654. doi: 10.1002/dneu.20386

Hertzano, R., Montcouquiol, M., Rashi-Elkeles, S., Elkon, R., Yücel, R., Frankel, W. N., et al. (2004). Transcription profiling of inner ears from *Pou4f3* $^{ddl/ddl}$ identifies Gfi1 as a target of the Pou4f3 deafness gene. *Hum. Mol. Genet.* 13, 2143–2153. doi: 10.1093/hmg/ddh218

Higgs, D. M., and Radford, C. A. (2013). The contribution of the lateral line to 'hearing' in fish. *J. Exp. Biol.* 216, 1484–1490. doi: 10.1242/jeb.078816

Higgs, D. M., Rollo, A. K., Souza, M. J., and Popper, A. N. (2003). Development of form and function in peripheral auditory structures of the zebrafish (*Danio rerio*). *J. Acoust. Soc. Am.* 113, 1145–1154. doi: 10.1121/1.1536185

Higgs, D. M., Souza, M. J., Wilkins, H. R., Presson, J. C., and Popper, A. N. (2001). Age- and size-related changes in the inner ear and hearing ability of the adult zebrafish (*Danio rerio*). *J. Assoc. Res. Otolaryngol.* 3, 174–184. doi: 10.1007/s101620020035

Hirose, Y., Simon, J. A., and Ou, H. C. (2011). Hair cell toxicity in anti-cancer drugs: evaluating an anti-cancer drug library for independent and synergistic toxic effects on hair cells using the zebrafish lateral line. *J. Assoc. Res. Otolaryngol.* 12, 719–728. doi: 10.1007/s10162-011-0278-z

Holt, J. R., and Corey, D. P. (2000). Two mechanisms for transducer adaptation in vertebrate hair cells. *Proc. Natl. Acad. Sci. U S A* 97, 11730–11735. doi: 10.1073/pnas.97.22.11730

Hong, S. J., Im, G. J., Chang, J., Chae, S. W., Lee, S. H., Kwon, S. Y., et al. (2013). Protective effects of edaravone against cisplatin-induced hair cell damage in zebrafish. *Int. J. Pediatr. Otorhinolaryngol.* 77, 1025–1031. doi: 10.1016/j.ijporl.2013.04.003

Howard, J., and Hudspeth, A. J. (1987). Mechanical relaxation of the hair bundle mediates adaptation in mechanoelectrical transduction by the bullfrog's saccular hair cell. *Proc. Natl. Acad. Sci. U S A* 84, 3064–3068. doi: 10.1073/pnas.84.9.3064

Huang, W. Y., Aramburu, J., Douglas, P. S., and Izumo, S. (2000). Transgenic expression of green fluorescence protein can cause dilated cardiomyopathy. *Nat. Med.* 6, 482–483. doi: 10.1038/74914

Hudspeth, A. J. (1989). How the ear's works work. *Nature* 341, 397–404. doi: 10.1038/341397a0

Hudspeth, A. J., Choe, Y., Mehta, A. D., and Martin, P. (2000). Putting ion channels to work: mechanoelectrical transduction, adaptation and amplification by hair cells. *Proc. Natl. Acad. Sci. U S A* 97, 11765–11772. doi: 10.1073/pnas.97.22.11765

Inoue, M., Tanimoto, M., and Oda, Y. (2013). The role of ear stone size in hair cell acoustic sensory transduction. *Sci. Rep.* 3:2114. doi: 10.1038/srep02114

Izumikawa, M., Batts, S. A., Miyazawa, T., Swiderski, D. L., and Raphael, Y. (2008). Response of the flat cochlear epithelium to forced expression of *Atoh1*. *Hear Res.* 240, 52–56. doi: 10.1016/j.heares.2008.02.007

Izumikawa, M., Minoda, R., Kawamoto, K., Abrashkin, K. A., Swiderski, D. L., Dolan, D. F., et al. (2005). Auditory hair cell replacement and hearing improvement by *Atoh1* gene therapy in deaf mammals. *Nat. Med.* 11, 271–276. doi: 10.1038/nm1193

Jacques, B. E., Montgomery, W. H. 4th, Uribe, P. M., Yatteau, A., Asuncion, J. D., Resendiz, G., et al. (2013). The role of Wnt/β-catenin signaling in proliferation and regeneration of the developing basilar papilla and lateral line. *Dev. Neurobiol.* 74, 438–456. doi: 10.1002/dneu.22134

Jiang, L., Romero-Carvajal, A., Haug, J. S., Seidel, C. W., and Piotrowski, T. (2014). Gene-expression analysis of hair cell regeneration in the zebrafish lateral line. *Proc. Natl. Acad. Sci. U S A* 111, E1383–E1392. doi: 10.1073/pnas.1402898111

Jiang, H., Sha, S. H., Forge, A., and Schacht, J. (2006). Caspase-independent pathways of hair cell death induced by kanamycin *in vivo*. *Cell Death Differ.* 13, 20–30. doi: 10.1038/sj.cdd.4401706

Jørgensen, J. M. (1991). Regeneration of lateral line and inner ear vestibular cells. *Ciba Found. Symp.* 160, 151–163; discussion 163–170.

Kanzaki, S., Beyer, L. A., Swiderski, D. L., Izumikawa, M., Stöver, T., Kawamoto, K., et al. (2006). $p27^{Kip1}$ deficiency causes organ of Corti pathology and hearing loss. *Hear. Res.* 214, 28–36. doi: 10.1016/j.heares.2006.01.014

Kevetter, G. A., and Correia, M. J. (1996). "Vestibular system," in *Hearing Loss*, eds P. S. Roland, B. F. Marple and W. L. Meyerhoff (New York, NY: Theime Medical Publishers, Inc.), 54–70.

Khorevin, V. I. (2008). The lagena (the third otolithic endorgan in vertebrates). *Neurophysiology* 40, 142–159. doi: 10.1007/s11062-008-9021-8

Kim, C. H., Kang, S. U., Pyun, J., Lee, M. H., Hwang, H. S., and Lee, H. (2008). Epicatechin protects auditory cells against cisplatin-induced death. *Apoptosis* 13, 1184–1194. doi: 10.1007/s10495-008-0242-5

Kimmel, C. B. (1989). Genetics and early development of zebrafish. *Trends Genet.* 5, 283–288. doi: 10.1016/0168-9525(89)90103-0

Kindt, K. S., Finch, G., and Nicolson, T. (2012). Kinocilia mediate mechanosensitivity in developing zebrafish hair cells. *Dev. Cell* 23, 329–341. doi: 10.1016/j.devcel.2012.05.022

Kuhn, S., Johnson, S. L., Furness, D. N., Chen, J., Ingham, N., Hilton, J. M., et al. (2011). miR-96 regulates the progression of differentiation in mammalian cochlear inner and outer hair cells. *Proc. Natl. Acad. Sci. U S A* 108, 2355–2360. doi: 10.1073/pnas.1016646108

Kwak, S. J., Vemaraju, S., Moorman, S. J., Zeddies, D., Popper, A. N., and Riley, B. B. (2006). Zebrafish *pax5* regulates development of the utricular macula and vestibular function. *Dev. Dyn.* 235, 3026–3038. doi: 10.1002/dvdy.20961

Ladich, F., and Schulz-Mirbach, T. (2013). Hearing in cichlid fishes under noise conditions. *PLoS One* 8:e57588. doi: 10.1371/journal.pone.0057588

Lanford, P. J., Presson, J. C., and Popper, A. N. (1996). Cell proliferation and hair cell addition in the ear of goldfish, *Carassius auratus*. *Hear. Res.* 100, 1–9. doi: 10.1016/0378-5955(96)00110-4

Le Prell, C. G., Hughes, L. F., and Miller, J. M. (2007). Free radical scavengers vitamins A, C, and E plus magnesium reduce noise trauma. *Free Radic. Biol. Med.* 42, 1454–1463. doi: 10.1016/j.freeradbiomed.2007.02.008

Leung, K. P., Chen, D., and Chan, K. M. (2014). Understanding copper sensitivity in zebrafish (*Danio rerio*) through the intracellular localization of copper transporters in a hepatocyte cell-line ZFL and the tissue expression profiles of copper transporters. *Metallomics* 6, 1057–1067. doi: 10.1039/c3mt00366c

Li, H., Kloosterman, W., and Fekete, D. M. (2010). MicroRNA-183 family members regulate sensorineural fates in the inner ear. *J. Neurosci.* 30, 3254–3263. doi: 10.1523/JNEUROSCI.4948-09.2010

Li, W., Wu, J., Yang, J., Sun, S., Chai, R., Chen, Z. Y., et al. (2015). Notch inhibition induces mitotically generated hair cells in mammalian cochleae via activating the Wnt pathway. *Proc. Natl. Acad. Sci. U S A* 112, 166–171. doi: 10.1073/pnas.1415901112

Liang, J., Wang, D., Renaud, G., Wolfsberg, T. G., Wilson, A. F., and Burgess, S. M. (2012). The *stat3/socs3a* pathway is a key regulator of hair cell regeneration in zebrafish *stat3/socs3a* pathway: regulator of hair cell regeneration. *J. Neurosci.* 32, 10662–10673. doi: 10.1523/JNEUROSCI.5785-10.2012

Liao, J. C. (2006). The role of the lateral line and vision on body kinematics and hydrodynamic preference of rainbow trout in turbulent flow. *J. Exp. Biol.* 209, 4077–4090. doi: 10.1242/jeb.02487

Lim, D. J. (1976). Ultrastructural cochlear changes following acoustic hyperstimulation and ototoxicity. *Ann. Otol. Rhinol. Laryngol.* 85, 740–751. doi: 10.1177/000348947608500604

Lin, V., Golub, J. S., Nguyen, T. B., Hume, C. R., Oesterle, E. C., and Stone, J. S. (2011). Inhibition of notch activity promotes nonmitotic regeneration of hair cells in the adult mouse utricles. *J. Neurosci.* 31, 15329–15339. doi: 10.1523/JNEUROSCI.2057-11.2011

Lin, Q., Li, W., Chen, Y., Sun, S., and Li, H. (2013). Disrupting Rb-Raf-1 interaction inhibits hair cell regeneration in zebrafish lateral line neuromasts. *Neuroreport* 24, 190–195. doi: 10.1097/WNR.0b013e32835e3279

Liu, Z., Walters, B. J., Owen, T., Brimble, M. A., Steigelman, K. A., Zhang, L., et al. (2012). Regulation of $p27^{Kip1}$ by Sox2 maintains quiescence of inner pillar cells in the murine auditory sensory epithelium. *J. Neurosci.* 32, 10530–10540. doi: 10.1523/JNEUROSCI.0686-12.2012

Liu, Z., and Zuo, J. (2008). Cell cycle regulation in hair cell development and regeneration in the mouse cochlea. *Cell Cycle* 7, 2129–2133. doi: 10.4161/cc.7.14.6423

Lombarte, A., and Popper, A. N. (1994). Quantitative analyses of postembryonic hair cell addition in the otolithic end organs of the inner ear of the European hake, *Merluccius merluccius* (Gadiformes, Teleostei). *J. Comp. Neurol.* 345, 419–428. doi: 10.1002/cne.903450308

Lombarte, A., Yan, H. Y., Popper, A. N., Chang, J. S., and Platt, C. (1993). Damage and regeneration of hair cell ciliary bundles in a fish ear following treatment with gentamicin. *Hear. Res.* 64, 166–174. doi: 10.1016/0378-5955(93)90002-i

López-Schier, H., and Hudspeth, A. J. (2006). A two-step mechanism underlies the planar polarization of regenerating sensory hair cells. *Proc. Natl. Acad. Sci. U S A* 103, 18615–18620. doi: 10.1073/pnas.0608536103

López-Schier, H., Starr, C. J., Kappler, J. A., Kollmar, R., and Hudspeth, A. J. (2004). Directional cell migration establishes the axes of planar polarity in the posterior lateral-line organ of the zebrafish. *Dev. Cell.* 7, 401–412. doi: 10.1016/j.devcel.2004.07.018

Löwenheim, H., Furness, D. N., Kil, J., Zinn, C., Gültig, K., Fero, M. L., et al. (1999). Gene disruption of $p27^{Kip1}$ allows cell proliferation in the postnatal and adult organ of Corti. *Proc. Natl. Acad. Sci. U S A* 96, 4084–4088. doi: 10.1073/pnas.96.7.4084

Lu, N., Chen, Y., Wang, Z., Chen, G., Lin, Q., Chen, Z. Y., et al. (2013). Sonic hedgehog initiates cochlear hair cell regeneration through downregulation of retinoblastoma protein. *Biochem. Biophys. Res. Commun.* 430, 700–705. doi: 10.1016/j.bbrc.2012.11.088

Lush, M. E., and Piotrowski, T. (2014a). Sensory hair cell regeneration in the zebrafish lateral line. *Dev. Dyn.* 10, 1187–1202. doi: 10.1002/dvdy.24167

Lush, M. E., and Piotrowski, T. (2014b). ErbB expressing Schwann cells control lateral line progenitor cells via non-cell-autonomous regulation of Wnt/β-catenin. *Elife* 3:e01832. doi: 10.7554/eLife.01832

Ma, E. Y., and Raible, D. W. (2009). Signaling pathways regulating zebrafish lateral line development. *Curr. Biol.* 19, R381–R386. doi: 10.1016/j.cub.2009.03.057

Ma, E. Y., Rubel, E. W., and Raible, D. W. (2008). Notch signaling regulates the extent of hair cell regeneration in the zebrafish lateral line. *J. Neurosci.* 28, 2261–2273. doi: 10.1523/JNEUROSCI.4372-07.2008

Malicki, J., Schier, A. F., Solnica-Krezel, L., Stemple, D. L., Neuhauss, S. C., Stainier, D. Y., et al. (1996). Mutations affecting development of the zebrafish ear. *Development* 123, 275–283.

Mann, Z. F., and Kelley, M. W. (2011). Development of tonotopy in the auditory periphery. *Hear. Res.* 276, 2–15. doi: 10.1016/j.heares.2011.01.011

Martinez-Monedero, R., Corrales, C. E., Cuajungco, M. P., Heller, S., and Edge, A. S. (2006). Reinnervation of hair cells by auditory neurons after selective removal of spiral ganglion neurons. *J. Neurobiol.* 66, 319–331. doi: 10.1002/neu.20232

Matsui, J. I., Ogilvie, J. M., and Warchol, M. E. (2002). Inhibition of caspases prevents ototoxic and ongoing hair cell death. *J. Neurosci.* 22, 1218–1227.

Matsui, J. I., and Ryals, B. M. (2005). Hair cell regeneration: an exciting phenomenon. . .but will restoring hearing and balance be possible? *J. Rehabil. Res. Dev.* 42, 187–198. doi: 10.1682/jrrd.2005.01.0008

McDermott, B. M. Jr., Baucom, J. M., and Hudspeth, A. J. (2007). Analysis and functional evaluation of the hair-cell transcriptome. *Proc. Natl. Acad. Sci. U S A* 104, 11820–11825. doi: 10.1073/pnas.0704476104

McHenry, M. J., and van Netten, S. M. (2007). The flexural stiffness of superficial neuromasts in the zebrafish (*Danio rerio*) lateral line. *J. Exp. Biol.* 210, 4244–4253. doi: 10.1242/jeb.009290

Millimaki, B. B., Sweet, E. M., Dhason, M. S., and Riley, B. B. (2007). Zebrafish *atoh1* genes: classic proneural activity in the inner ear and regulation by Fgf and Notch. *Development* 134, 295–305. doi: 10.1242/dev.02734

Millimaki, B. B., Sweet, E. M., and Riley, B. B. (2010). Sox2 is required for maintenance and regeneration, but not initial development, of hair cells in the zebrafish inner ear. *Dev. Biol.* 338, 262–269. doi: 10.1016/j.ydbio.2009.12.011

Mizutari, K., Fujioka, M., Hosoya, M., Bramhall, N., Okano, H. J., Okano, H., et al. (2013). Notch inhibition induces cochlear hair cell regeneration and recovery of hearing after acoustic trauma. *Neuron* 77, 58–69. doi: 10.1016/j.neuron.2012.10.032

Mo, W., and Nicolson, T. (2011). Both pre- and postsynaptic activity of Nsf prevents degeneration of hair-cell synapses. *PLoS One* 6:e27146. doi: 10.1371/journal.pone.0027146

Momin, S. R., Melki, S. J., Obokhare, J. O., Fares, S. A., Semaan, M. T., and Megerian, C. A. (2011). Hearing preservation in Guinea pigs with long-standing endolymphatic hydrops. *Otol. Neurotol.* 32, 1583–1589. doi: 10.1097/MAO.0b013e3182382a64

Moon, I. S., So, J. H., Jung, Y. M., Lee, W. S., Kim, E. Y., Choi, J. H., et al. (2011). Fucoidan promotes mechanosensory hair cell regeneration following amino glycoside-induced cell death. *Hear. Res.* 282, 236–242. doi: 10.1016/j.heares.2011.07.007

More, S. S., Akil, O., Ianculescu, A. G., Geier, E. G., Lustig, L. R., and Giacomini, K. M. (2010). Role of the copper transporter, CTR1, in platinum-induced ototoxicity. *J. Neurosci.* 30, 9500–9509. doi: 10.1523/JNEUROSCI.1544-10.2010

Murakami, S. L., Cunningham, L. L., Werner, L. A., Bauer, E., Pujol, R., Raible, D. W., et al. (2003). Developmental differences in susceptibility to neomycin-induced hair cell death in the lateral line neuromasts of zebrafish (*Danio rerio*). *Hear. Res.* 186, 47–56. doi: 10.1016/s0378-5955(03)00259-4

Murillo-Cuesta, S., Contreras, J., Cediel, R., and Varela-Nieto, I. (2010). Comparison of different aminoglycoside antibiotic treatments to refine ototoxicity studies in adult mice. *Lab. Anim.* 44, 124–131. doi: 10.1258/la.2009.009046

Nagiel, A., Andor-Ardó, D., and Hudspeth, A. J. (2008). Specificity of afferent synapses onto plane-polarized hair cells in the posterior lateral line of the zebrafish. *J. Neurosci.* 28, 8442–8453. doi: 10.1523/JNEUROSCI.2425-08.2008

Namdaran, P., Reinhart, K. E., Owens, K. N., Raible, D. W., and Rubel, E. W. (2012). Identification of modulators of hair cell regeneration in the zebrafish lateral line. *J. Neurosci.* 32, 3516–3528. doi: 10.1523/JNEUROSCI.3905-11.2012

Nicolson, T. (2005). The genetics of hearing and balance in zebrafish. *Annu. Rev. Genet.* 39, 9–22. doi: 10.1146/annurev.genet.39.073003.105049

Nicolson, T., Rüsch, A., Friedrich, R. W., Granato, M., Ruppersberg, J. P., and Nüsslein-Volhard, C. (1998). Genetic analysis of vertebrate sensory hair cell mechanosensation: the zebrafish circler mutants. *Neuron* 20, 271–283. doi: 10.1016/s0896-6273(00)80455-9

Oesterle, E. C., Chien, W. M., Campbell, S., Nellimarla, P., and Fero, M. L. (2011). $p27^{Kip1}$ is required to maintain proliferative quiescence in the adult cochlea and pituitary. *Cell Cycle* 10, 1237–1248. doi: 10.4161/cc.10.8.15301

Oesterle, E. C., and Stone, J. S. (2008). "Hair cell regeneration: mechanisms guiding cellular proliferation and differentiation," in *Hair Cell Regeneration, Repair and Protection*, eds R. J. Salvi, A. N. Popper and R. R. Fay (New York: Springer), 141–198.

Olivari, F. A., Hernández, P. P., and Allende, M. L. (2008). Acute copper exposure induces oxidative stress and cell death in lateral line hair cells of zebrafish larvae. *Brain Res.* 1244, 1–12. doi: 10.1016/j.brainres.2008.09.050

Olt, J., Johnson, S. L., and Marcotti, W. (2014). *In vivo* and *in vitro* biophysical properties of hair cells from the lateral line and inner ear of developing and adult zebrafish. *J. Physiol.* 592, 2041–2058. doi: 10.1113/jphysiol.2013.265108

Ono, K., Nakagawa, T., Kojima, K., Matsumoto, M., Kawauchi, T., Hoshino, M., et al. (2009). Silencing p27 reverses post-mitotic state of supporting cells in neonatal mouse cochleae. *Mol. Cell. Neurosci.* 42, 391–398. doi: 10.1016/j.mcn.2009.08.011

Ou, H. C., Raible, D. W., and Rubel, E. W. (2007). Cisplatin-induced hair cell loss in zebrafish (*Danio rerio*) lateral line. *Hear. Res.* 233, 46–53. doi: 10.1016/j.heares.2007.07.003

Ou, H. C., Santos, F., Raible, D. W., Simon, J. A., and Rubel, E. W. (2010). Drug screening for hearing loss: using the zebrafish lateral line to screen for drugs that prevent and cause hearing loss. *Drug Discov. Today* 15, 265–271. doi: 10.1016/j.drudis.2010.01.001

Ou, H., Simon, J. A., Rubel, E. W., and Raible, D. W. (2012). Screening for chemicals that affect hair cell death and survival in the zebrafish lateral line. *Hear. Res.* 288, 58–66. doi: 10.1016/j.heares.2012.01.009

Owens, K. N., Coffin, A. B., Hong, L. S., Bennett, K. O., Rubel, E. W., and Raible, D. W. (2009). Response of mechanosensory hair cells of the zebrafish lateral line to aminoglycosides reveals distinct cell death pathways. *Hear. Res.* 253, 32–41. doi: 10.1016/j.heares.2009.03.001

Owens, K. N., Santos, F., Roberts, B., Linbo, T., Coffin, A. B., Knisely, A. J., et al. (2008). Identification of genetic and chemical modulators of zebrafish mechanosensory hair cell death. *PLoS Genet.* 4:e1000020. doi: 10.1371/journal.pgen.1000020

Pan, B., Géléoc, G. S., Asai, Y., Horwitz, G. C., Kurima, K., Ishikawa, K., et al. (2013). TMC1 and TMC2 are components of the mechanotransduction channel in hair cells of the mammalian inner ear. *Neuron* 79, 504–515. doi: 10.1016/j.neuron.2013.06.019

Park, S. N., Back, S. A., Park, K. H., Seo, J. H., Noh, H. I., Akil, O., et al. (2013). Comparison of functional and morphologic characteristics of mice models of noise-induced hearing loss. *Auris Nasus Larynx* 40, 11–17. doi: 10.1016/j.anl.2011.11.008

Pickles, J. O., Brix, J., Gleich, O., Köppl, C., Manley, G. A., Osborne, M. P., et al. (1988). "The fine structure and organization of tip links on hair cell stereovilli," in *Basic Issues in Hearing*, eds H. Duifhuis, J. W. Horst and H. P. Wit (London: Academic Press), 56–63.

Pinto-Teixeira, F., Muzzopappa, M., Swoger, J., Mineo, A., Sharpe, J., and López-Schier, H. (2013). Intravital imaging of hair-cell development and regeneration in the zebrafish. *Front. Neuroanat.* 7:33. doi: 10.3389/fnana.2013.00033

Popper, A. N. (1983). "Organization of the inner ear and processing of acoustic information," in *Fish Neurobiology and Behavior*, eds R. G. Northcutt and R. E. Davis (Ann Arbor, MI: University of Michigan Press), 125–178.

Popper, A. N. (2000). Hair cell heterogeneity and ultrasonic hearing: recent advances in understanding fish hearing. *Philos. Trans. R. Soc. Lond. B Biol. Sci.* 355, 1277–1280. doi: 10.1098/rstb.2000.0683

Popper, A. N., Fay, R. R., Platt, C., and Sand, O. (2003). "Sound detection mechanisms and capabilities of teleost fishes," in *Sensory Processing in Aquatic Environments*, eds S. P. Collin and N. J. Marshall (New York, NY: Springer-Verlag New York, Inc.), 3–38.

Popper, A. N., and Hoxter, B. (1984). Growth of a fish ear: 1. Quantitative analysis of hair cell and ganglion cell proliferation. *Hear. Res.* 15, 133–142. doi: 10.1016/0378-5955(84)90044-3

Popper, A. N., and Hoxter, B. (1990). Growth of a fish ear. II. Locations of newly proliferated sensory hair cells in the saccular epithelium of *Astronotus ocellatus*. *Hear. Res.* 45, 33–40. doi: 10.1016/0378-5955(90)90180-w

Presson, J. C., Lanford, P. J., and Popper, A. N. (1996). Hair cell precursors are ultrastructurally indistinguishable from mature support cells in the ear of a postembryonic fish. *Hear. Res.* 100, 10–20. doi: 10.1016/0378-5955(96)00109-8

Presson, J. C., Smith, T., and Mentz, L. (1995). Proliferating hair cell precursors in the ear of a postembryonic fish are replaced after elimination by cytosine arabinoside. *J. Neurobiol.* 26, 579–584. doi: 10.1002/neu.480260410

Qi, W., Ding, D., and Salvi, R. J. (2008). Cytotoxic effects of dimethyl sulphoxide (DMSO) on cochlear organotypic cultures. *Hear. Res.* 236, 52–60. doi: 10.1016/j.heares.2007.12.002

Raible, D. W., and Kruse, G. J. (2000). Organization of the lateral line system in embryonic zebrafish. *J. Comp. Neurol.* 421, 189–198. doi: 10.1002/(sici)1096-9861(20000529)421:2<189::aid-cne5>3.3.co;2-b

Ramcharitar, J. U., and Brack, C. L. (2010). Physiological dimensions of ototoxic responses in a model fish species. *J. Clin. Neurosci.* 17, 103–106. doi: 10.1016/j.jocn.2009.08.003

Rubel, E. W., Furrer, S. A., and Stone, J. S. (2013). A brief history of hair cell regeneration research and speculations on the future. *Hear. Res.* 297, 42–51. doi: 10.1016/j.heares.2012.12.014

Sacheli, R., Nguyen, L., Borgs, L., Vandenbosch, R., Bodson, M., Lefebvre, P., et al. (2009). Expression patterns of miR-96, miR-182 and miR-183 in the development inner ear. *Gene Expr. Patterns* 9, 364–370. doi: 10.1016/j.gep.2009.01.003

Santos, F., MacDonald, G., Rubel, E. W., and Raible, D. W. (2006). Lateral line hair cell maturation is a determinant of aminoglycoside susceptibility in zebrafish (*Danio rerio*). *Hear. Res.* 213, 25–33. doi: 10.1016/j.heares.2005.12.009

Sarrazin, A. F., Villablanca, E. J., Nuñez, V. A., Sandoval, P. C., Ghysen, A., and Allende, M. L. (2006). Proneural gene requirement for hair cell differentiation in the zebrafish lateral line. *Dev. Biol.* 295, 534–545. doi: 10.1016/j.ydbio.2006.03.037

Schibler, A., and Malicki, J. (2007). A screen for genetic defects of the zebrafish ear. *Mech. Dev.* 124, 592–604. doi: 10.1016/j.mod.2007.04.005

Schuck, J. B., and Smith, M. E. (2009). Cell proliferation follows acoustically-induced hair cell bundle loss in the zebrafish saccule. *Hear. Res.* 253, 67–76. doi: 10.1016/j.heares.2009.03.008

Schuck, J. B., Sun, H., Penberthy, W. T., Cooper, N. G., Li, X., and Smith, M. E. (2011). Transcriptomic analysis of the zebrafish inner ear points to growth hormone mediated regeneration following acoustic trauma. *BMC Neurosci.* 12:88. doi: 10.1186/1471-2202-12-88

Sheets, L., Trapani, J. G., Mo, W., Obholzer, N., and Nicolson, T. (2011). Ribeye is required for presynaptic Ca_V1.3a channel localization and afferent innervation of sensory hair cells. *Development* 138, 1309–1319. doi: 10.1242/dev.059451

Shi, F., Hu, L., and Edge, A. S. (2013). Generation of hair cells in neonatal mice by β-catenin overexpression in Lgr5-positive cochlear progenitors. *Proc. Natl. Acad. Sci. U S A* 110, 13851–13856. doi: 10.1073/pnas.1219952110

Shin, Y. S., Hwang, H. S., Kang, S. U., Chang, J. W., Oh, Y. T., and Kim, C. H. (2014). Inhibition of p38 mitogen-activated protein kinase ameliorates radiation-induced ototoxicity in zebrafish and cochlea-derived cell lines. *Neurotoxicology* 40, 111–122. doi: 10.1016/j.neuro.2013.12.006

Shin, Y. S., Song, S. J., Kang, S. U., Hwang, H. S., Choi, J. W., Lee, B. H., et al. (2013). A novel synthetic compound, 3-amino-3-(4-fluoro-phenyl)-1H-quinoline-2,4-dione, inhibits cisplatin-induced hearing loss by the suppression of reactive oxygen species: *In vitro* and *in vivo* study. *Neuroscience* 232, 1–12. doi: 10.1016/j.neuroscience.2012.12.008

Siemens, J., Lillo, C., Dumont, R. A., Reynolds, A., Williams, D. S., Gillespie, P. G., et al. (2004). Cadherin 23 is a component of the tip link in hair-cell stereocilia. *Nature* 428, 950–955. doi: 10.1038/nature02483

Smith, M. E., Coffin, A. B., Miller, D. L., and Popper, A. N. (2006). Anatomical and functional recovery of the goldfish (*Carassius auratus*) ear following noise exposure. *J. Exp. Biol.* 209, 4193–4202. doi: 10.1242/jeb.02490

Smith, M. E., and Rajadinakaran, G. (2013). The transcriptomics to proteomics of hair cell regeneration: looking for a hair cell in a haystack. *Microarrays (Basel)* 2, 186–207. doi: 10.3390/microarrays2030186

Smith, M. E., Schuck, J. B., Gilley, R. R., and Rogers, B. D. (2011). Structural and functional effects of acoustic exposure in goldfish: evidence for tonotopy in the teleost saccule. *BMC Neurosci.* 12:19. doi: 10.1186/1471-2202-12-19

Song, J. J., Chang, J., Choi, J., Im, G. J., Chae, S. W., Lee, S. H., et al. (2013). Protective role of NecroX-5 against neomycin-induced hair cell damage in zebrafish. *Arch. Toxicol.* 88, 435–441. doi: 10.1007/s00204-013-1124-3

Song, J., Yan, H. Y., and Popper, A. N. (1995). Damage and recovery of hair cells in fish canal (but not superficial) neuromasts after gentamicin exposure. *Hear. Res.* 91, 63–71. doi: 10.1016/0378-5955(95)00170-0

Soukup, G. A. (2009). Little but loud: small RNAs have a resounding affect on ear development. *Brain Res.* 1277, 104–114. doi: 10.1016/j.brainres.2009.02.027

Steiner, A. B., Kim, T., Cabot, V., and Hudspeth, A. J. (2014). Dynamic gene expression by putative hair-cell progenitors during regeneration in the zebrafish lateral line. *Proc. Natl. Acad. Sci. U S A* 111, E1393–E1401. doi: 10.1073/pnas.1318692111

Stockwell, C. W., Ades, H. W., and Engström, H. (1969). Patterns of hair cell damage after intense auditory stimulation. *Ann. Otol. Rhinol. Laryngol.* 78, 1144–1168. doi: 10.1177/000348946907800602

Strassmaier, M., and Gillespie, P. G. (2002). The hair cell's transduction channel. *Curr. Opin. Neurobiol.* 12, 380–386. doi: 10.1016/S0959-4388(02)00344-6

Suli, A., Watson, G. M., Rubel, E. W., and Raible, D. W. (2012). Rheotaxis in larval zebrafish is mediated by lateral line mechanosensory hair cells. *PLoS One* 7:e29727. doi: 10.1371/journal.pone.0029727

Sun, H., Lin, C. H., and Smith, M. E. (2011). Growth hormone promotes hair cell regeneration in the zebrafish (*Danio rerio*) inner ear following acoustic trauma. *PLoS One* 6:e28372. doi: 10.1371/journal.pone.0028372

Sweet, E. M., Vemaraju, S., and Riley, B. B. (2011). Sox2 and Fgf interact with Atoh1 to promote sensory competence throughout the zebrafish inner ear. *Dev. Biol.* 358, 113–121. doi: 10.1016/j.ydbio.2011.07.019

Szabo, T. M., McCormick, C. A., and Faber, D. S. (2007). Otolith endorgan input to the Mauthner neuron in the goldfish. *J. Comp. Neurol.* 505, 511–525. doi: 10.1002/cne.21499

Tanimoto, M., Ota, Y., Horikawa, K., and Oda, Y. (2009). Auditory input to CNS is acquired coincidentally with development of inner ear after formation of functional afferent pathway in zebrafish. *J. Neurosci.* 29, 2762–2767. doi: 10.1523/JNEUROSCI.5530-08.2009

Tanimoto, M., Ota, Y., Inoue, M., and Oda, Y. (2011). Origin of inner ear hair cells: morphological and functional differentiation from ciliary cells into hair cells in zebrafish inner ear. *J. Neurosci.* 31, 3784–3794. doi: 10.1523/jneurosci.5554-10.2011

Taylor, R. R., Nevill, G., and Forge, A. (2008). Rapid hair cell loss: a mouse model for cochlear lesions. *J. Assoc. Res. Otolaryngol.* 9, 44–64. doi: 10.1007/s10162-007-0105-8

Thomas, E. D., Cruz, I. A., Hailey, D. W., and Raible, D. W. (2015b). There and back again: development and regeneration of the zebrafish lateral line system. *Wiley Interdiscip. Rev. Dev. Biol.* 4, 1–16. doi: 10.1002/wdev.160

Thomas, A. J., Hailey, D. W., Stawicki, T. M., Wu, P., Coffin, A. B., Rubel, E. W., et al. (2013). Functional mechanotransduction is required for cisplatin-induced hair cell death in the zebrafish lateral line. *J. Neurosci.* 33, 4405–4414. doi: 10.1523/jneurosci.3940-12.2013

Thomas, A. J., Wu, P., Raible, D. W., Rubel, E. W., Simon, J. A., and Ou, H. C. (2015a). Identification of small molecule inhibitors of Cisplatin-induced hair cell death: results of a 10,000 compound screen in the zebrafish lateral line. *Otol. Neurotol.* 36, 519–525. doi: 10.1097/mao.0000000000000487

Ton, C., and Parng, C. (2005). The use of zebrafish for assessing ototoxic and otoprotective agents. *Hear. Res.* 208, 79–88. doi: 10.1016/j.heares.2005.05.005

Uribe, P. M., Mueller, M. A., Gleichman, J. S., Kramer, M. D., Wang, Q., Sibrian-Vazquez, M., et al. (2013a). Dimethyl sulfoxide (DMSO) exacerbates cisplatin-induced sensory hair cell death in zebrafish (*Danio rerio*). *PLoS One* 8:e55359. doi: 10.1371/journal.pone.0055359

Uribe, P. M., Sun, H., Wang, K., Asuncion, J. D., Wang, Q., Chen, C. W., et al. (2013b). Aminoglycoside-induced hair cell death of inner ear organs causes functional deficits in adult zebrafish (*Danio rerio*). *PLoS One* 8:e58755. doi: 10.1371/journal.pone.0058755

Van Trump, W. J., Coombs, S., Duncan, K., and McHenry, M. J. (2010). Gentamicin is ototoxic to all hair cells in the fish lateral line system. *Hear. Res.* 261, 42–50. doi: 10.1016/j.heares.2010.01.001

Van Trump, W. J., and McHenry, M. J. (2008). The morphology and mechanical sensitivity of lateral line receptors in zebrafish larvae (*Danio rerio*). *J. Exp. Biol.* 211, 2105–2115. doi: 10.1242/jeb.016204

Vater, M., Meng, J., and Fox, R. C. (2004). "Hearing organ evolution and specialization: early and later mammals," in *Evolution of the Vertebrate Auditory System*, eds G. A. Manley, A. N. Popper and R. R. Fay (New York: Springer-Verlag), 256–288.

Villegas, R., Martin, S. M., O'Donnell, K. C., Carrillo, S. A., Sagasti, A., and Allende, M. L. (2012). Dynamics of degeneration and regeneration in developing zebrafish peripheral axons reveals a requirement for extrinsic cell types. *Neural Dev.* 7:19. doi: 10.1186/1749-8104-7-19

Vlasits, A. L., Simon, J. A., Raible, D. W., Rubel, E. W., and Owens, K. N. (2012). Screen of FDA-approved drug library reveals compounds that protect hair cells from aminoglycosides and cisplatin. *Hear. Res.* 294, 153–165. doi: 10.1016/j.heares.2012.08.002

Wada, H., Ghysen, A., Asakawa, K., Abe, G., Ishitani, T., and Kawakami, K. (2013). Wnt/Dkk negative feedback regulates sensory organ size in zebrafish. *Curr. Biol.* 23, 1559–1565. doi: 10.1016/j.cub.2013.06.035

Walters, B. J., Liu, Z., Crabtree, M., Coak, E., Cox, B. C., and Zuo, J. (2014). Auditory hair cell-specific deletion of $p27^{Kip1}$ in postnatal mice promotes cell-autonomous generation of new hair cells and normal hearing. *J. Neurosci.* 34, 15751–15763. doi: 10.1523/jneurosci.3200-14.2014

Wang, Y., Hirose, K., and Liberman, M. C. (2002). Dynamics of noise-induced cellular injury and repair in the mouse cochlea. *J. Assoc. Res. Otolaryngol.* 3, 248–268. doi: 10.1007/s101620020028

Wang, L., Sewell, W. F., Kim, S. D., Shin, J. T., MacRae, C. A., Zon, L. I., et al. (2008). Eya4 regulation of Na^+/K^+-ATPase is required for sensory system development in zebrafish. *Development* 135, 3425–3434. doi: 10.1242/dev.012237

Wang, Y., Sun, Y., Chang, Q., Ahmad, S., Zhou, B., Kim, Y., et al. (2013a). Early postnatal virus inoculation into the scala media achieved extensive expression of exogenous green fluorescent protein in the inner ear and preserved auditory brainstem response thresholds. *J. Gene Med.* 15, 123–133. doi: 10.1002/jgm.2701

Wang, F., Zuo, L., Hong, B., Han, D., Range, E. M., Zhao, L., et al. (2013b). Tonotopic reorganization and spontaneous firing in inferior colliculus during both short and long recovery periods after noise overexposure. *J. Biomed. Sci.* 20:91. doi: 10.1186/1423-0127-20-91

Warchol, M. E. (2010). Cellular mechanisms of aminoglycoside ototoxicity. *Curr. Opin. Otolaryngol. Head Neck Surg.* 18, 454–458. doi: 10.1097/moo.0b013e32833e05ec

Wenzel, G. I., Xia, A., Funk, E., Evans, M. B., Palmer, D. J., Ng, P., et al. (2007). Helper-dependent adenovirus-mediated gene transfer into the adult mouse cochlea. *Otol. Neurotol.* 28, 1100–1108. doi: 10.1097/mao.0b013e318158973f

Weston, M. D., Pierce, M. L., Rocha-Sanchez, S., Beisel, K. W., and Soukup, G. A. (2006). MicroRNA gene expression in the mouse inner ear. *Brain Res.* 1111, 95–104. doi: 10.1016/j.brainres.2006.07.006

Wibowo, I., Pinto-Teixeira, F., Satou, C., Higashijima, S., and López-Schier, H. (2011). Compartmentalized Notch signaling sustains epithelial mirror symmetry. *Development* 138, 1143–1152. doi: 10.1242/dev.060566

Wienholds, E., Kloosterman, W. P., Miska, E., Alvarez-Saavedra, E., Berezikov, E., de Bruijn, E., et al. (2005). MicroRNA expression in zebrafish embryonic development. *Science* 309, 310–311. doi: 10.1126/science.1114519

Wilkins, H. R., Presson, J. C., and Popper, A. N. (1999). Proliferation of vertebrate inner ear supporting cells. *J. Neurobiol.* 39, 527–535. doi: 10.1002/(sici)1097-4695(19990615)39:4<527::aid-neu6>3.0.co;2-k

Williams, J. A., and Holder, N. (2000). Cell turnover in neuromasts of zebrafish larvae. *Hear. Res.* 143, 171–181. doi: 10.1016/s0378-5955(00)00039-3

Wu, C. Y., Lee, H. J., Liu, C. F., Korivi, M., Chen, H. H., and Chan, M. H. (2014). Protective role of L-ascorbic acid, N-acetylcysteine and apocynin on neomycin-induced hair cell loss in Zebrafish. *J. Appl. Toxicol.* 35, 273–279. doi: 10.1002/jat.3043

Yamamoto, N., Nakagawa, T., and Ito, J. (2014). Application of insulin-like growth factor-1 in the treatment of inner ear disorders. *Front. Pharmacol.* 5:208. doi: 10.3389/fphar.2014.00208

Yamashita, H., and Oesterle, E. C. (1995). Induction of cell proliferation in mammalian inner-ear sensory epithelia by transforming growth factor α and epidermal growth factor. *Proc. Natl. Acad. Sci. U S A* 92, 3152–3155. doi: 10.1073/pnas.92.8.3152

Yan, H. Y., Saidel, W. M., Chang, J. S., Presson, J. C., and Popper, A. N. (1991). Sensory hair cells of a fish ear: evidence of multiple types based on ototoxicity sensitivity. *Proc. Biol. Sci.* 245, 133–138. doi: 10.1098/rspb.1991.0099

Zhai, F., Liu, J. P., Dai, C. F., Wang, Q., and Steyger, P. S. (2010). Evidence-based modification of intratympanic gentamicin injections in patients with intractable vertigo. *Otol. Neurotol.* 31, 642–648. doi: 10.1097/mao.0b013e3181dbb30e

Zhao, B., Wu, Z., Grillet, N., Yan, L., Xiong, W., Harkins-Perry, S., et al. (2014). TMIE is an essential component of the mechanotransduction machinery of cochlear hair cells. *Neuron* 84, 954–967. doi: 10.1016/j.neuron.2014.10.041

Zheng, H. W., Chen, J., and Sha, S. H. (2014). Receptor-interacting protein kinases modulate noise-induced sensory hair cell death. *Cell Death Dis.* 5:e1262. doi: 10.1038/cddis.2014.177

Zheng, J. L., and Gao, W.-Q. (2000). Overexpression of *Math1* induces robust production of extra hair cells in postnatal rat inner ears. *Nat. Neurosci.* 3, 580–586. doi: 10.1038/75753

Zon, L. I. (1999). Zebrafish: a new model for human disease. *Genome Res.* 9, 99–100. doi: 10.1101/gr.9.2.99

4

Epidermal stem cells in hair follicle cycling and skin regeneration: a view from the perspective of inflammation

Elena I. Morgun and Ekaterina A. Vorotelyak*

Laboratory of Cell Biology, Koltzov Institute of Developmental Biology of Russian Academy of Sciences, Moscow, Russia

Edited by:
Mingxing Lei,
Chongqing University, China

Reviewed by:
Zhili Deng,
Central South University, China
Stéphanie Claudinot,
Centre Hospitalier Universitaire Vaudois (CHUV), Switzerland

***Correspondence:**
Elena I. Morgun
lady.morgun2016@yandex.ru

There are many studies devoted to the role of hair follicle stem cells in wound healing as well as in follicle self-restoration. At the same time, the influence of the inflammatory cells on the hair follicle cycling in both injured and intact skin is well established. Immune cells of all wound healing stages, including macrophages, $\gamma\delta$T cells, and T_{regs}, may activate epidermal stem cells to provide re-epithelization and wound-induced hair follicle neogenesis. In addition to the ability of epidermal cells to maintain epidermal morphogenesis through differentiation program, they can undergo de-differentiation and acquire stem features under the influence of inflammatory milieu. Simultaneously, a stem cell compartment may undergo re-programming to adopt another fate. The proportion of skin resident immune cells and wound-attracted inflammatory cells (e.g., neutrophils and macrophages) in wound-induced hair follicle anagen and plucking-induced anagen is still under discussion to date. Experimental data suggesting the role of reactive oxygen species and prostaglandins, which are uncharacteristic of the intact skin, in the hair follicle cycling indicates the role of neutrophils in injury-induced conditions. In this review, we discuss some of the hair follicles stem cell activities, such as wound-induced hair follicle neogenesis, hair follicle cycling, and re-epithelization, through the prism of inflammation. The plasticity of epidermal stem cells under the influence of inflammatory microenvironment is considered. The relationship between inflammation, scarring, and follicle neogenesis as an indicator of complete wound healing is also highlighted. Taking into consideration the available data, we also conclude that there may exist a presumptive interlink between the stem cell activation, inflammation and the components of programmed cell death pathways.

Keywords: hair follicle, stem cells, regeneration, wound, skin, inflammation

INTRODUCTION

As an outmost barrier of the organism, the skin has multiple functions, including a vitally important protective mission. Being exposed to an aggressive environment, it has developed a complex system of mutually dependent stem cell populations as well as immune response. Stem cells replenish regular tissue losses and are ready to upregulate their activity in case of injury. Immune system supports regenerative processes via direct interactions with invaders and clearance of wound debris.

Also, it has the ability to intensify stem cell activity for production of differentiated progeny and restoration of lesions (Rahmani et al., 2020).

Epidermal homeostasis is maintained by stem cells that either self-renew or undergo differentiation forming the spinous, granular and cornified layers of the interfollicular epidermis (IFE) or multiple types of keratinocytes in the hair follicle (HF) generating the hair shaft (Gonzales and Fuchs, 2017).

The concept of epidermal stem cells (EpiSC) evolved from the assumption of equipotent basal cells of IFE toward the scheme of complicated hierarchy, kinetics, and behavior. Several approaches were proposed to determine stem cells in IFE and epithelial part of appendages. Among the most prominent characteristics is their ability to retain DNA label (for review see: Terskikh et al., 2012). Another widely accepted property of EpiSC is to form large clones (holoclones) *in vitro* in contrast to small abortive clones produced by their progeny as it was shown by pioneering experiments performed by Barrandon and Green (Barrandon and Green, 1987). Potten proposed the concept of proliferating epidermal unit containing slow-cycling stem cell in the center (Potten, 1974) for murine IFE where columnar structures could be observed at certain sites (Mackenzie, 1970). Labeling of EpiSC progeny in mouse epidermis confirmed the clonal organization of IFE (Ghazizadeh and Taichman, 2001). At the same time, the hypothesis of a single population of progenitor cells in homeostatic IFE of mouse tail with no role for stem cells was proposed (Clayton et al., 2007). The authors pointed out that the stem cell population undetectable in steady-state conditions might be recruited in wound healing. To identify interfollicular EpiSC, β1- and α6-integrins as well as keratin 15 (Krt15), LRIG1, and MCSP were utilized as markers (Solanas and Benitah, 2013).

The most potent EpiSC reside in a specialized niche of HF named the bulge, where label-retaining cells were found by landmark paper of Cotsarelis with colleagues (Cotsarelis et al., 1990). They provide continuous cycling of HF and its regeneration (Jahoda et al., 1996) as well as the source of epithelial cells in the course of skin regeneration. The bulge zone of HF contains several subsets of EpiSC with diverse functions and regenerative potential. Pioneering experiments by Cotsarelis and his group revealed Krt15 as a putative marker of bulge cells (Lyle et al., 1998; Liu et al., 2003). *In vitro* lineage tracing showed that the progeny of Krt15 + cells contribute to all HF epithelial cell lines (Morris et al., 2004). Later on, the list of bulge markers was supplemented with CD34, Keratin 19, Lgr5, Gli1, Hopx, Lhx2, Nfatc1, Sox9, Tcf3/4, integrin α6, and Lhx2 (Rompolas and Greco, 2014; Gonzales and Fuchs, 2017). Another region of HF, the isthmus, contains cells with stem-like properties. They are expressing Lrig1, Gli1, MTS24, and Lgr6. Lrig1 + cells of the isthmus are involved in the infundibulum regeneration, at the top of which there is a population of cells expressing Sca-1 (Rompolas and Greco, 2014). The secondary germ is believed to be another source of HF renewal (Panteleyev et al., 2001).

Healthy human and mouse skin is populated by several types of immune cells such as dendritic cells, innate lymphoid cells (ILCs), T lymphocytes and macrophages (Mansfield and Naik, 2020), as well as mast cells and neutrophils (Nakamizo et al., 2020). Immune cells that are located above the basement membrane include CD8 + resident memory T cells (T_{RM}), Langerhans cells, ILCs, and dendritic epidermal DT cells (DETCs). The dermal immune cells are represented by macrophages located near blood vessels, and T cells, which include near-follicular effector and regulatory CD4 + T cells (T_{regs}), and γδT cells. Thus, each type of immune cell is situated in a specific compartment of the skin, and this is achieved by the homing to the corresponding microenvironment – different fractions of the HF and IFE keratinocytes have diverse chemokine signatures (Mansfield and Naik, 2020). It was shown *in vivo* and *in vitro* experiments that T_{regs}, which express CCR6 on their surface, migrate to CCL20 ligand, derived from infundibulum cells (Scharschmidt et al., 2017). A similar mechanism of homing is implemented in the case of ILCs migration toward the upper part of HF. However, in addition to the CCR6-CCL20 interaction, ILCs are attracted to the epidermis by cytokines IL-7 and TSLP (Kobayashi et al., 2019). CD10-expressing DETCs, as well as T_{RM} are recruited to IFE cells due to the expression of CCL27 (Morales et al., 1999; Jin et al., 2010). Thus, the steady skin state is immunologically active, and there is an interplay between keratinocytes and inflammatory cells. Subsequently, EpiSC is in close interaction with cells of the immune system and are able to recruit them when the tissue is damaged (Naik et al., 2018).

Wound healing begins with an inflammatory phase involving cells of the immune system. Macrophages and neutrophils are the first and foremost, which secrete inflammatory mediators and phagocytize debris disinfecting the wound bed and enabling its further successful closure (Eming et al., 2007). Wound regeneration is incomplete without wound resurfacing, i.e., re-epithelization (Santoro and Gaudino, 2005). Dermal part of the skin is subjected to active regeneration and reorganization during wound healing and affects its outcome (Rippa et al., 2019). Blood and lymphatic vessels which supply the skin with nutrients and replenish immune cell pool in steady-state are extensively reorganized during wound healing providing proper regulation and structural reconstruction of damaged tissue. The effectiveness of wound healing correlates with the phase of HF cycle. It was found that skin containing anagen HF regenerates more effectively than that with HF in telogen. Wounds of mice anagen skin showed improved angiogenesis, increased proliferation of keratinocytes, accelerated transition to terminal differentiation, and ameliorated matrix synthesis, while telogen skin demonstrated an increase in the number of neutrophils and macrophages in the granulation tissue, as well as a high expression of macrophage migration inhibitory factor (Ansell et al., 2011).

During wound healing, epithelial HF stem cells (HFSCs) provide both HF neogenesis and wound re-epithelialization (Rompolas and Greco, 2014). HF regeneration in the middle of a full-thickness wound in mice is similar to embryonic hair morphogenesis. It is called wound-induced hair neogenesis (WIHN) (Wang et al., 2017; Gong et al., 2018). Formation of new HFs in adult skin may also be induced in experimental conditions by ectopic activation of specific signaling pathways (Sun et al., 2020). However, WIHN is appropriate only for mouse wound healing, while most mammals, including humans, do not regenerate skin appendages (Lim et al., 2018).

Activation of EpiSC is important condition for restoration of the structure and functions of the skin after injury. We will overview the characteristics of EpiSC, immune cells and inflammatory-related agents in the context of their interactions and functioning during wound healing and HF morphogenesis. As wound healing and inflammation are tightly connected with cell death, we tried to make brief references to possible interlinks with stem cell activation, where data are available.

EPISC PLASTICITY DURING WOUND HEALING UNDER THE INFLUENCE OF IMMUNE REACTION

Since the skin delimits the body with the environment, it often undergoes damage and healing, and keratinocytes meet a first thrust (Proksch et al., 2008). The inflammatory milieu in the wound gets cells ready for re-epithelialization affecting their migratory and proliferation activities. Inflammation-induced cell dedifferentiation and can modulate cell stemness. However, the details of cellular behavior in the course of re-epithelization are not known at the moment. There is experimental evidence in favor of at least two models. According to the first, the cells of the basal layer migrate to the wound bed and then differentiate into suprabasal, and according to the second, suprabasal cells move from wound edges to the wound bed due to "leapfrog" mechanism and become basal (Rognoni and Watt, 2018). Thereby, epidermal cells possess certain plasticity: they can undergo de-differentiation as well as differentiation under the influence of accompanying wound healing inflammatory agents (Haensel et al., 2020). Noteworthy, similar transitions are known in inflammatory diseases. For example, exposure to IL-17 and IL-22, interleukins, which are elevated in psoriasis (Kim and Krueger, 2015), caused the expression of stem markers p63, CD44, CD29, and CD49f in keratinocytes *in vitro* due to activation of the RAC1/MEC/ERK/NF-κB pathway (Ekman et al., 2019). Nelson and colleagues found that activation of TLR3 by polyriboinosinic-polyribocytidylic acid (polyI: C), simulating the viral dsRNA in keratinocyte cell culture (Takada et al., 2017), causes a loss of Keratin1 and filaggrin (markers of differentiated keratinocytes) and an increase in the expression of Lgr5 and Lgr6 HF progenitor markers as well as Krt15 (Nelson et al., 2015). Besides, the participation of IL-6/STAT3 pathway in the acquisition of stem status is indirectly confirmed by the fact that STAT3 phosphorylation under the influence of IL-6 family members IL-11 and Oncostatin M (OSM) contributes to WIHN (Nelson et al., 2016b_B). There is experimental evidence that TA isoforms of stem/progenitor marker p63, which expression is affected by IL-6/STAT3, are involved both in the inhibition of keratinocytes ability to differentiate and in the stimulation of WIHN (Nelson et al., 2016a_A).

In addition to the acquisition of a stem marker profile by mature keratinocytes, other data are confirming the ability of epidermal cells to de-differentiate under the influence of the wound environment. Haensel and colleagues using RNA velocity analysis showed a significant proportion of *col17a1*^{Hi} basal cells and spinous cells of the SP1 population of wounded mice to demonstrate faster RNA dynamics than those from non-wounded skin. This indicated increased plasticity of cell fate in the skin sample of wounded mice with bidirectional transitions in several cell states between basal and spinous cells, which was not observed in the non-wounded animals. Thus, the wound inflammatory milieu stimulates epidermal cell plasticity and enfeebles restrictions on cell differentiation compared to their non-wounded counterparts (Haensel et al., 2020).

The implication of bulge HFSCs in re-epithelization has been established for a long time. However, different strategies for HFSCs labeling and a variety of markers employed led to a conclusion about different inputs of HFSCs subpopulations into the process (Garcin and Ansell, 2017). Some HF cells have been shown to play a dual role. In mice, Lgr6 + cells of the isthmus area provide ongoing skin restoration, including WIHN (Snippert et al., 2010). However, it seems now that both Lgr6 + and Lgr5 + stem cells are involved in IFE regeneration. Infundibulum Sca-1 + cells and Gli + stem cells are also involved (Brownell et al., 2011; Rompolas and Greco, 2014). HFSCs move downward for the regeneration and neogenesis of HF, while their upward migration contributes to re-epithelization. In spite of intuitive imagination of EpiSC as attached tightly to the niche, they probably may be highly motile making input into morphogenesis far from their original location. Nanba and co-authors showed *in vitro* that human EpiSC could be identified by their motility: the faster the cells move, the higher "stemness" they possess (Nanba et al., 2015). Another activity of HFSCs is linked to the barrier maintenance directly in the bulge niche where they are interacting with recruited immune cells to overcome telogen cell cycle inhibitory signals (Lay et al., 2018).

To accomplish regeneration, EpiSC can undergo reprogramming. Experimental data of Joost et al. suggest that inflammatory environment affects the expression of "follicular" (*Lgr5, Cd34, Cxcl14, and Sparc*) and "interfollicular" (*Krt14, Ifitm3, Eef1b2, Ly6e*) markers. Wound healing experiment with subsequent single-cell analysis showed that after wounding, the Lgr5 + progeny, while still in the bulge, begin to express both interfollicular and HF markers. However, interfollicular markers are upregulated; meanwhile, bulge markers are downregulated. Besides, Lgr6 + progeny in the intact skin expresses numerous receptors for interaction with wound ligands, and when the skin is damaged, their number slightly changes. Lgr5 + progeny expresses a few such receptors; however, when wounded, their number increases. This suggests that Lgr5 + progeny may become competent to interact with the wound environment at the level of Lgr6 + descendants. Moreover, this early upregulation of genes makes Lgr5 + progeny motile, as the number of genes (*Cd44, Cd9, Itgb1, Itga3,* and *Itga6*) that begin to be expressed are associated with cell migration (Joost et al., 2018), which indicates acquisition of the ability to re-epithelization. Thus, epidermal cells, beyond classical differentiation of basal cells to suprabasal ones, may change their status by loss of their maturity or reprogramming. from follicular to interfollicular state. Whether interfollicular cells can be reprogrammed into follicular cells under the influence of inflammation and what conditions determine the direction of differentiation/dedifferentiation/reprogramming, remains unknown and requires further research. Intriguingly, cells stemness was induced by inflammatory pathways, which intersected with programmed cell death pathways to some extent. It was mentioned above that de-differentiation of mature keratinocytes, and their acquisition of stem features may be associated with the influence of such an inflammatory agent as dsRNA, as well as upregulation of cytokines IL-17 and IL-22, which occurs during wound healing (Sasaki et al., 2011; Zhu et al., 2017). At the same time, the effect of dsRNA on TLR3 is a proven trigger of apoptosis and necroptosis (Seya et al., 2012) and upregulation of IL-17 and IL-22 in the psoriasis model is associated with a decrease in the expression of a RIPK-1, traditionally considered as a necroptosis component (Saito et al., 2018). Therefore, the stem status of epidermal cells may be affected not only by inflammation but also by the components of programmed cell death occurring during wound healing.

However, the relationship of epidermal cells with the immune system is two-component. On the one hand, inflammatory agents can affect epidermal cell activity; on the other hand, keratinocytes possess their own intrinsic immune activity. The basis of this phenomenon is the necessity to respond adequately to the inflammatory milieu that occurs as a result of injury or infection and to transmit a signal to surrounding cells. Epidermal cells are able to release IL-1, IL-6, IL -7, IL -8, IL -10, IL -12, IL -15, IL -18, IL -20, and tumor necrosis factor-alpha (TNF-α), which causes proliferation and differentiation of keratinocytes, production of cytokines by them, and migration of immune cells into the wound (Gröne, 2002). Innate immunity is a well-known characteristic of epidermal keratinocytes, presumably including those located in the basal layer. It was shown that interfolicular EpiSC could "remember" episodes of acute inflammation. Wound healing in mice previously exposed to imiquimod, which induced skin inflammation via TLR7-NALP3 axis, was more effective than in the control group. Moreover, this process was experimentally proven not to depend on macrophages or T cells. "Inflammatory memory" was based both on a transcription of the inflammasome pathway component *Aim2* in interfollicular EpiSC and the expression of its downstream effector *caspase-1* in post-inflamed skin. Caspase-1, in turn, is involved in the maturation and secretion of IL-18 and IL-1β, which were also increased in skin of the experimental animals (Naik et al., 2017). Therefore, previous "inflammation experience" could augment cutaneous wound healing due to EpiSC activity. Interestingly, all of the above agents are participants of the pyroptosis, the type of programmed cell death with morphological signs of necrosis (Vande Walle and Lamkanfi, 2016). However, Naik with colleagues did not show cell death in the experiment (Naik et al., 2017).

To summarize, immunocompetence of stem cells and changes in their stem status under the influence of inflammation are the two facets of the interaction of immunity and stem cells providing re-epithelialization after skin damage. As we can see, these processes involve various members of the TLR family. Activation of TLR7 is responsible for the "inflammatory memory" of interfollicular EpiSC, the influence of dsRNA on TLR3 causes the loss of differentiation markers by mature keratinocytes and the expression of stem cell markers Lgr5 and Lgr6 and Krt15. Therefore, immunoreactivity and the mechanism of dedifferentiation can also be interlinked. Furthermore, activation of pyroptosis and necroptosis also occurs through the TLR receptors. Consequently, various members of TLR family may be the "hubs" through which the pathways of immunity activation, stemness, and cell death can intersect.

Facets of EpiSC plastsicity under the influence of inflammatory agents is summarized in **Figure 1**.

THE HF CYCLE AND IMMUNITY IN PHYSIOLOGICAL AND INJURY-INDUCED CONDITIONS

Cyclic changes in HF, namely, a continuity of successive phases of telogen, anagen, and catagen, partly occur owing to HFSC activity. Immune cell dynamics is associated with the transition of HF through the cycle and, in some degree, provides regulatory keys for it. We will discuss some striking features of this interconnection (for review see: Wang and Higgins, 2020) along with specific stage characteristics.

After the regression, HF passes into telogen, the phase of relative rest in terms of proliferation and biochemical activity (Paus and Cotsarelis, 1999; Krause and Foitzik, 2006). HF stays dormant until it is reactivated by intrafollicular and extrafollicular signals (Paus and Cotsarelis, 1999). Inactivity of HFSCs at this stage is provided mainly by bulge expression of BMP6 and FGF18 (Hsu et al., 2014). At the same time, telogen is supposed to be a stage of "progressive molecular activity". In late telogen, the activity aimed at inhibiting quiescence predominates, whereas, in early and middle telogen, inhibition of cellular activity prevails. Also, there is a proliferative activity of several cell types: while bulge and secondary hair germ HFSCs are quiescent, keratinocytes from upper HF proliferate (Geyfman et al., 2015).

Anagen begins with the proliferation of Lgr5 + HFSCs, which are activated in late telogen. Hair germ HFSCs give rise to transit-amplifying cells that populate the germinative layer of the matrix. Outer root sheath (ORS) is formed by cells of the lower bulge (Welle and Wiener, 2016). It is well known that the key factors that induce anagen are the Wnt proteins, while the level of BMP signaling is downregulated by expression of its antagonist noggin (Botchkarev and Sharov, 2004). Sonic hedgehog, HGF, and FGF7, among others, support this process and stimulate the subsequent HF entry into anagen (Krause and Foitzik, 2006). In mice, anagen induction in response to exogenous stimuli and entry into the second anagen differ by underlying mechanisms, at least in terms of STAT3 signaling (Sano et al., 2000).

Upon completion of anagen, a controlled involution of HF occurs denoting onset of catagen, when most follicular keratinocytes undergo apoptosis (Paus and Cotsarelis, 1999; Krause and Foitzik, 2006; Welle and Wiener, 2016). At this stage, poorly dividing ORS cells create a new bulge, while slightly faster dividing cells form the secondary hair germ (Welle and Wiener, 2016). Unlike ORS and the hair matrix, the cells of DP do not die, though they express the suppressor of apoptosis bcl-2 (Krause and Foitzik, 2006). Toward the end of catagen, DP condenses and moves upward transiting into a resting stage to reside under the bulge (Paus and Cotsarelis, 1999).

Spontaneous HF cycle is mediated by different types of skin resident immune cells, which were listed above. Among multiple signals and niche components, stay of HF in telogen is regulated by FoxP3-expressing CD4 + T cells (also known as regulatory T cells, T_{regs}) (Ali et al., 2017) and macrophages (Castellana et al., 2014). T_{regs} are associated with telogen. The abundance of these cells in telogen is threefold higher as compared to anagen. Moreover, their proliferative index correlates with the phase of the HF cycle: they are more active in telogen. Ali and colleagues found the bulge-associated subpopulation of T_{regs} (Ali et al., 2017). Disruption of adherence of the cell-cell junctions in bulge HFSC niche by E-cadherin removal activated proliferation program in telogen bulge HFSC repurposing new daughters to restore the breached integrity of the niche. In addition to cell cycle genes activation necessary during normal anagen, this proliferation activity needed elevation of the immune-signaling transcriptome. Notably, no transition to anagen was observed. Thus, proliferating stem cells were activated to restore the niche rather than to launch a new hair cycle. Proliferating HFSCs attracted immune cells, including

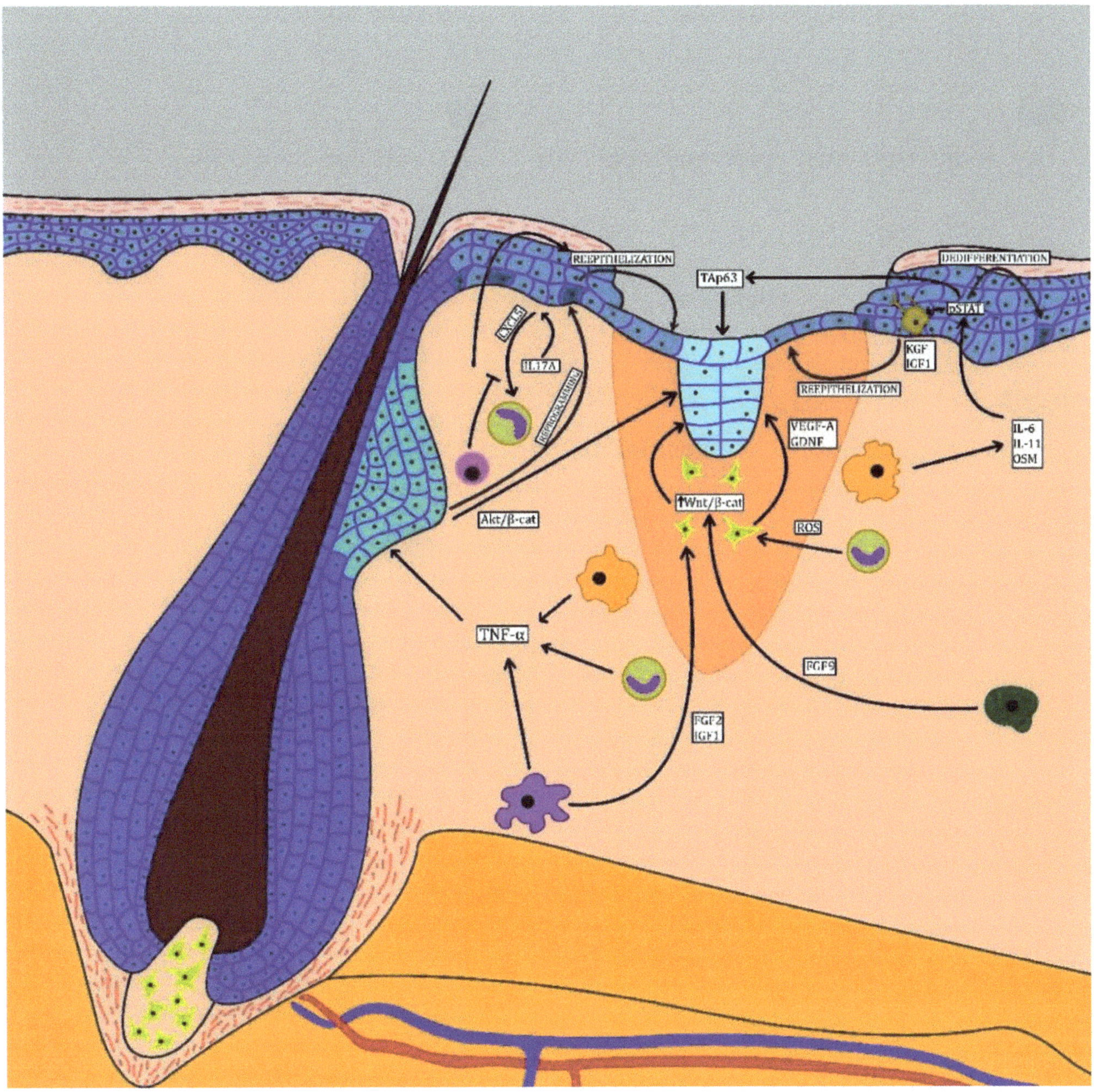

FIGURE 1 | Continued

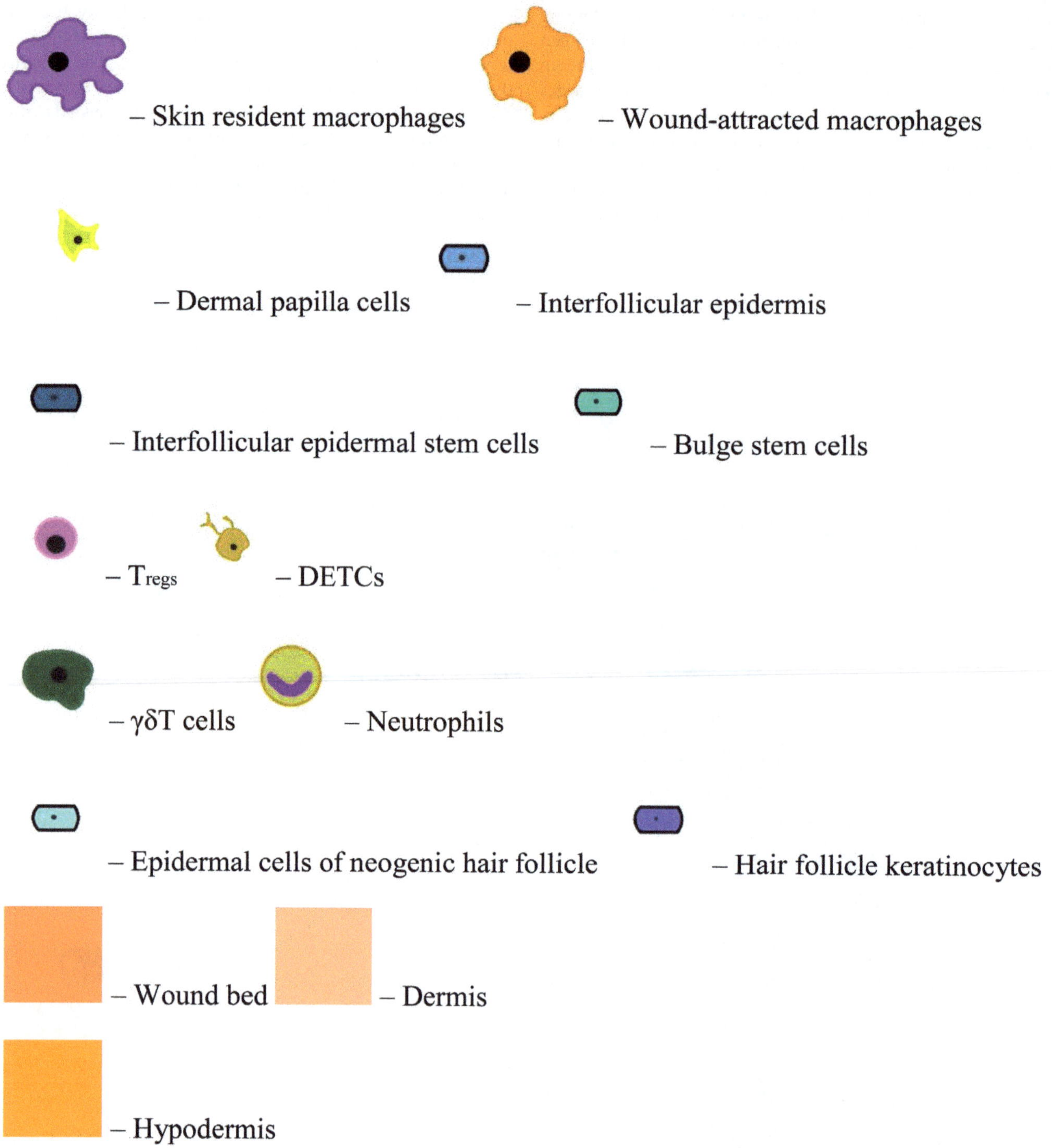

FIGURE 1 | Facets of EpiSC plasticity under the influence of inflammatory agents.

T_{regs}, increasing their numbers as compared to the resident skin population in a steady state.

Interestingly, this effect was independent of microbial presence. Moreover, immune cells, in turn, were necessary for activation of HFSC proliferation as the regular telogen proliferation-inhibitory cues were still active in the disrupted niche (Lay et al., 2018). Thus, telogen bulge cells are capable of proliferation independent of HF activation, and immune cells regulate this activity. The role of macrophages in telogen regulation is controversial. Not only they activate anagen but also prolong telogen: TREM2 + macrophages maintain the dormancy of HFSCs through OSM (Wang et al., 2019). Castellana and the colleagues showed that macrophage apoptosis promoted the entry of HFSCs into the anagen phase. As soon as the number of macrophages decreased due to liposome-induced apoptosis, HF of the experimental mice entered anagen, while the control group remained in telogen (Castellana et al., 2014).

As mentioned above, the telogen-to-anagen transition (TAT) is associated with macrophage apoptosis. Expression of *Wnt7b* and *Wnt10a* responsible for HFSC activation was elevated in skin resident macrophages during TAT. Moreover, experiments in the culture of mouse macrophages showed that their apoptosis occurs in parallel with the release of Wnts and that apoptotic macrophages stimulate the expression of Wnts by neighboring macrophages (Castellana et al., 2014). Interestingly, macrophages seem to produce extracellular vesicles containing Wnt3a and Wnt7b (Rajendran et al., 2020). Thus, the apoptotic reduction of macrophages during TAT is associated with the activation of the Wnt/β-catenin cascade (Castellana et al., 2014). Therefore, TAT and the Wnt/β-catenin cascade are related both to the activity of inflammatory cells and their apoptosis. Consequently, the activation mechanisms of HFSCs can be coupled with the pathways of programmed cell death.

Tissue-resident T_{regs} localized in close contact with HF sustain the bulge stem cells functions. Ali and colleagues demonstrated the role of T_{regs} in the activation of bulge HFSCs (Ali et al., 2017). In mice with T_{regs} depletion, a proliferative defect of the HFSC bulge zone during depilation-induced TAT was observed. In addition, lineage tracing showed a decrease in genes associated with the proliferation and differentiation of HFSCs (e.g., *Bgn, Bncl, Cks2, Hmgn3, Gdf10,* and *Sox4*) in CD34 + integrin α6 $(ITGA6)^{high}$ basal bulge HFSCs from depilated mice lacking T_{regs}. When comparing the transcriptome of skin T_{regs} with those of skin draining lymph nodes (SDLN), it was shown that skin T_{regs} express Notch signaling ligand Jagged 1 (Jagl) 150 times higher than SDLN T_{regs} do (Ali et al., 2017). During anagen, the switching on Notch cascade activates Kit signaling and suppresses TGF-β establishing an optimal environment for the proliferation of matrix cells (Rishikaysh et al., 2014). Exogenous administration of Jagl restores the proliferative function of stem cells in mice lacking T_{regs}. Deletion of *Jagl* in T_{regs} reduces the expression of epidermal differentiation genes *Bgn, Ccnd1, Gdf10, Sox4, Sox7,* and *Timp3* as well as provokes anagen deterioration (Ali et al., 2017).

At the end of anagen, some significant changes occur in HF, in particular, downregulation of IGF1 (Krause and Foitzik, 2006). This growth factor is well known for its anagen-stimulating effect, as it decreases the expression of the negative regulator of anagen TGF-β1 and also promotes the proliferation of HF keratinocytes (Li et al., 2014). One of the sources of IGF1 is DETCs, the subpopulation of γδT cells that prevented epidermal apoptosis in a model *in vitro* (Sharp et al., 2005). Presumably, DETCs support anagen through secretion of IGF1 in three ways: through inhibition of TGF-β1, stimulation of keratinocytes proliferation, and downregulation of apoptosis, which is a key catagen pathway. Anagen ends with downregulation not only of IGF1 but also of other factors (including HGF, and FGF5) supporting anagen phase and with upregulation of hair growth inhibitors, such as TGF-β1, TGF-β2, FGF5 (Krause and Foitzik, 2006).

Catagen is induced by growth factors and cytokines, including FGF5 secreted by perifollicular macrophages and IFN-γ (Wang and Higgins, 2020). *Fgf5* mutations cause catagen retention in humans (Higgins et al., 2014). In certain pathological conditions, for example, in case of stress, mast cells were also shown to stimulate the onset of catagen in mice. In this situation, mast cell-deficient mice demonstrated catagen delay, as did knockout mice, which were not able to respond to the substance P produced by nerve fibers in stress conditions (Arck et al., 2005). Mature mast cells release a lot of significant inflammatory mediators and are involved in wound healing (Komi et al., 2020).

Interestingly, mouse vibrissal HF contains precursors capable of differentiation into competent mast cells *in vitro* and probably provide a niche for their differentiation *in vivo* (Kumamoto et al., 2003). Inflammation and HF cells in catagen are interconnected through cell death processes: apoptotic keratinocytes are cleared by macrophages in the mouse, whereas in humans, the macrophages themselves undergo apoptosis. In the experiment by Hardman with colleagues, a cyclic change in the number of perifollicular macrophages in a freshly isolated HF was shown with a minimal rate in late catagen (Hardman et al., 2019). The close interdependence between inflammatory cytokine TNF-α, Keratin 17 and apoptosis in keratinocytes was shown in the next study (Tong and Coulombe, 2006). In *Krt17* $^{-/-}$ mice, alopecia developed in the first week after birth due to increased apoptosis. *Tnf* ablation led to catagen delay. It is thought that apoptosis in *Krt17* $^{-/-}$ keratinocytes occurs due to accelerated sensitivity to TNF-α. In turn, apoptosis in *Krt17*-null keratinocytes led to premature onset of catagen. Consequently, cytoskeletal protein Keratin 17 is responsible for HF detention in anagen, meanwhile TNF-α leads to anagen-catagen transition. Tong and Coulombe suggest that Keratin 17 interacts with the TRADD adapter necessary to transmit a signal from TNFR1 (Tong and Coulombe, 2006).

Thus, HF stays in a specific phase is regulated by various types of skin resident inflammatory cells. Macrophages and T_{regs} play a significant role in telogen and anagen and by mast cells and macrophages in catagen. It is believed that during TAT, the induction of Wnt/β-catenin is associated with the apoptosis of macrophages, and activation of bulge HFSCs is associated with their induction by the T_{reg} cluster. However, it is possible that in certain conditions, inflammatory cells that are absent in normal skin contribute to the HF cycling.

In addition to the physiological conditions, TAT may be induced by injury. In the case of hair plucking, CCL2 is released, which leads to the recruitment of inflammatory macrophages and, as a result, the stimulation of anagen by TNF-α (Chen et al., 2015). Macrophages are also involved in another type of injury-induced TAT, which is called wound-induced hair anagen re-entry/growth (WIH-A), when, under the influence of a wound milieu, HF located at the edges of the wound switch to anagen (Abbasi and Biernaskie, 2019). It was shown that macrophage production of TNF-α invoked an activation of HF Lgr5 + stem cells being important for WIH-A. Suppression of these inflammatory cell infiltration resulted in the loss of WIH-A ability in HFs. To assess the role of macrophages in WIH-A, Wang, and co-authors eliminated these cells with clodronate liposomes (Wang et al., 2017). It led to an inability of the HF to proceed to WIH-A. Furthermore, an *in vivo* experiment performed to assess the role of TNF-α in these processes showed that $Tnf^{-/-}$ mice did not develop HF anagen on post wound day (PWD) 15. In this study, $Lysm^{cre}/:Tnf^{flox/flox}$ mice with macrophages and neutrophils unable to express *Tnfa* were used. Skin regeneration in these mice occurred with a significantly reduced number of anagen HF, but an injection of lipopolysaccharide stimulated macrophages induced anagen. There is experimental evidence that activation of RAC-alpha serine/threonine-protein kinase (AKT) in Lgr5 + cells plays an essential role in the induction of TAT of HF. Knockdown of *Tnfr1* in Lgr5 + cells caused a decrease in TNF-induced p-AKT activity in cell culture. It is assumed that TNF-α activates β-catenin through the PI3K/AKT/mTOR cascade, and phosphorylation of β-catenin, in turn, is induced by AKT in Lgr5 + HFSC (Wang et al., 2017). There is also another way in which macrophages could cause anagen during skin damage. These cells secrete growth factors (Werner and Grose, 2003) that lead to activation of the PI3K-Akt-mTOR pathway involved in cell growth and survival (Fang et al., 2013) in epithelial cells during wound healing (Squarize et al., 2010). Activation of the mammalian target of rapamycin complex 1 (mTORC1) was observed in the bulge and hair germ cells in a growth phase-dependent manner suggesting its role in anagen activation (Kellenberger and Tauchi, 2013). Thus, macrophages are involved in both physiological TAT, plucking-induced anagen, and WIH-A in the described experiment; therefore, the contribution ratio of skin resident macrophages and those arrived at the wound bed is unknown (Rahmani et al., 2020).

However, there are indirect signs that, in addition to skin resident immune cells, wound cells that are completely unusual for intact skin can be involved in WIH-A. It can be supposed that the persistence of HFSC in anagen is regulated by polymorphonuclear leukocytes, as they can secrete reactive oxygen species (ROS) (Dunnill et al., 2017), and prostaglandins (PG) (Higgs et al., 1975), which are also involved in HF cycling (Valente Duarte de Sousa and Tosti, 2013; Zhao et al., 2015). PGE_2, acting synergistically with PGF_2, prolongs anagen and induces hair growth (Valente Duarte de Sousa and Tosti, 2013). PGE_2 does not induce TAT but has a stimulating effect on early anagen HF manifested by increased hair length. PGF_{2a} promotes protein kinase C (PKC) activation via phosphorylase C-associated receptors. Furthermore, PKC is upregulated in anagen, which indicates its significance for HF activity (Sasaki et al., 2005). ROS is an important mediator of inflammation being secreted during wound healing and contributing to wound disinfection (Dunnill et al., 2017). It was shown that adipose-derived stem cells are also able to secrete ROS this way promoting DP-induced hair growth and thus, may cause TAT (Choi et al., 2019). However, in an *in vivo* study during the transition from anagen to catagen, Zhao and colleagues showed elevation of ROS level by the Foxp1 protein via suppression of ROS scavenger Thioredoxin-1. This is also supported by the fact that administration of NAC antioxidant to *Foxp1* cKO mice led to the arrest of the HF cycle in anagen and increased HFSCs proliferation (Zhao et al., 2015). Thus, it is possible that in certain conditions, not only skin resident but wound-specific immune cells are also involved in the regulation of the HF cycle and morphogenesis. The relationship of the activation mechanisms of EpiSC with molecular cascades of wound healing will be considered in the next section.

HF NEOGENESIS AND RE-EPITHELIALIZATION IN THE COURSE OF WOUND HEALING

Widely recognized course of wound regeneration includes phases of inflammation, proliferation, and remodeling (Gurtner et al., 2008). Below we will consider these phases with critical elements of inflammatory reactions affecting epidermal cell activity, regeneration, and morphogenesis. Surprisingly, some of these elements demonstrate delayed effects in this respect. For example, macrophages acting in the inflammation phase (Eming et al., 2007) contribute to WIHN, which occurs during the time of the scar remodeling phase (Gay et al., 2020), and re-epithelialization begins in the proliferation phase under the influence of T_{regs}.

Inflammation Phase

TNF alpha. Platelets, leukocytes, macrophages, and mast cells are involved in the inflammation phase replacing each other. First of all, after a wound, platelets and polymorphonuclear leukocytes create a blood clot, and thus the tissue reaches hemostasis (Eming et al., 2007). Platelets form a clot interacting by GpIIb-IIIa receptors and adhering to the collagen of the disrupted subendothelium. Fibrin polymerization promotes the formation of a mature clot, which serves as a scaffold for infiltrating leukocytes and fibroblasts playing a sequential role in healing. Platelets also contribute to the subsequent stages of healing, for example, secreting catecholamines and serotonin, which act through receptors on the endothelium and cause vasoconstriction surrounding the wound (Gantwerker and Hom, 2011). In addition, platelets and polymorphonuclear leukocytes secrete TNF-α and IL-1 (Werner and Grose, 2003; Mussano et al., 2016) activating capillary endothelial cells and contributing to leukocyte transmigration (Bevilacqua et al., 1987). Neutrophils disinfect the wound eliminating debris and bacteria and provide antimicrobial protection by releasing H_2O_2, which produce ROS into the surrounding space.

Meanwhile, ROS not only protect the wound from infection, but they are also engaged in normal wound healing. ROS are involved in the proliferation of fibroblasts and vascular endothelial cells, promote proliferation and migration of keratinocytes, stimulate angiogenesis, and act as a chemoattractant for neutrophils, mononuclear phagocytes, eosinophils, basophils, and lymphocytes by stimulating the production of macrophage inflammatory protein (MIP)-1α (Dunnill et al., 2017). The importance of ROS for wound healing was confirmed in a study by Carrasco and colleagues, who showed the beneficial effects of ROS on wound healing and on HFSCs. The researchers induced transient ROS generation via the photodynamic effect as a result of the application of a photosensitizer (5-aminolevulinic acid (ALA) or its methyl derivative (mALA) cream) to mice in combination with red rays.

This effect is used in clinical practice for induction of cell death in tumors. Generation of transient ROS in such a way led to the proliferation of bulge HFSC, as well as epidermal and dermal skin layers (Carrasco et al., 2015). ROS can also affect HF neogenesis through DP. Zheng et al. showed proliferation of DP cells and increased mRNA expression levels of vascular endothelial growth factor (VEGF)-A and glial cell line-derived neurotrophic factor (GDNF), leading to WIHN under ROS-induced hypoxia (Zheng et al., 2019). Also, one of the most critical cellular events mediated by ROS is mitochondrial apoptosis. When the mitochondrial membrane is permeabilized with ROS, apoptosis agents (cytochrome c, AIF, or Smac/Diablo) enter the cytosol (Circu and Aw, 2010), implementing relationship between HFSCs activity and wound healing through ROS as an inflammatory mediator and an apoptotic agent.

However, the role of neutrophils, ROS, and other inflammatory mediators produced by them is controversial. Dysregulation of neutrophils can lead to skin lesions. Abundant neutrophil infiltration into the wound bed is a key factor in the development of chronic inflammation, which underlies non-healing wounds. Excess of neutrophils causes overproduction of ROS, which provokes cell membrane and extracellular matrix (ECM) damage with subsequent premature cell aging (Zhao et al., 2016).

Neutrophils are also capable of recruiting macrophages leading to a transition from the neutrophilic stage of wound healing to the stage of macrophage infiltration (Eming et al., 2007).

Macrophages appear in the wounded skin after neutrophils and phagocytize them (Gurtner et al., 2008; Greenlee-Wacker, 2016). Macrophage infiltration is regulated by fibrin clot platelets, fibroblasts, leukocytes, a gradient of growth factors, pro-inflammatory cytokines and chemokines released by hyperproliferative keratinocytes along the margins of the wound (Werner and Grose, 2003). Macrophages express many receptors on their surface, for example, the TLRs of different types (Karin et al., 2006). In addition to phagocytic and antigen-presenting functions, they produce various growth factors, such as TGF-β, TGF-α, and VEGF, which regulate fibroplasia and angiogenesis (Werner and Grose, 2003). Macrophage ablation during the inflammatory phase in an experimental model of wound regeneration in mice was shown to delay wound healing.

In addition, macrophages are known to play an essential role in angiogenesis. There is a hypothesis, that they form "tunnels" in the ECM which are colonized by capillary sprouts, circulating progenitor endothelial cells or transdifferentiated endothelial cells during later stages of wound healing (Moldovan, 2002). Also, there are experimental data in favor of the fact that macrophages can also participate in lymphangiogenesis during wound healing: the number of macrophages reaches a peak during the period of migration and organization of lymphatic endothelial cells (Rutkowski et al., 2006).

It is well known that macrophages are polarized into two subtypes, M1 and M2, with different phenotypes (Xu et al., 2013) though continuum of intermediate states exists. M1 macrophages are CCR2 + cells (Fadini et al., 2013). They secrete pro-inflammatory cytokines and phagocyte dead cells and pathogens. They can acquire this phenotype under the influence of bacterial metabolites, IFN-γ, and a granulocyte-macrophage colony-stimulating factor (GM-CSF) (Xu et al., 2013). Anti-inflammatory M2 macrophages, which activation is regulated by IL-13 and/or IL-4 (Qing, 2017), secrete angiogenic factors and anti-inflammatory cytokines and stimulate wound closure (Xu et al., 2013). They express CX3CR1 (Fadini et al., 2013). In M2-deficient mice, a delay in healing is observed, which is most prominent in the late stages of regeneration (Minutti et al., 2017).

Macrophage ablation using diphtheria toxin (DT) leads to WIHN inhibition in mouse experiments. M2 macrophages produce follicle-stimulating growth factors, such as FGF2 and IGF1. These factors are thought to take part in WIHN, since they participate in the Wnt pathway (Kasuya et al., 2018). The study of Wang and colleagues, which was mentioned in the previous section, in contrast, showed the valuable role of M1 macrophages in WIHN. It was found that in Lgr5 + HFSCs, TNF-α released by M1 macrophages induced not only TAT and WIH-A but also WIHN through activation of AKT/β-catenin (Wang et al., 2017).

TNF-α is a critical player in the inflammatory response (Efimov et al., 2009). It is upregulated during the inflammatory phase of wound healing (Barrientos et al., 2008). In response to skin damage, TNF-α is secreted by polymorphonuclear leukocytes, then by macrophages over a period from 12 to 24 hours after skin injury (Xu et al., 2013). In keratinocyte culture, TNF-α and IFN-γ stimulate the secretion of growth factors (e.g., TGF- α), HLA-DR, interleukins (IL-1, IL-6 and IL-8), ICAM-1, and monocyte chemotactic and activating factor (MCAF) (Barker et al., 1991). During regeneration, TNF-α is expressed in proliferating keratinocytes along the wound margins (Xu et al., 2013). Exposure of a culture of keratinocytes to TNF-α led to the expression of chemokines, cytokines, growth factors, and cell surface receptors, which can *in vivo* attract hematopoietic cells, monocytes, macrophages, and neutrophils, as well as memory T-cells that provide an innate immune response (Banno et al., 2004).

Îiwever, the upregulation of TNF-α is a noticeable factor in the transition of the acute wound to non-healing status, including diabetic wound development (Siqueira et al., 2010; Xu et al., 2013; Zhang et al., 2017). In *in vivo* and *in vitro* experiments, TNF-α exhibits a pro-inflammatory and pro-apoptotic effect, as well as prevents scar formation, fibroblast migration, re-epithelialization and, as a result, prolongs the period of wound closure.

Overexpression of TNF-α leads to an increase in the number of neutrophils and macrophages in the wound bed through NF-κB signaling. Anti-TNF-α therapy helps to reduce the activity of NF-κB, to normalize the number of inflammatory cells, and to decrease the size of the wound bed. Experiments with mice knockout for the gene of TNF-α inhibitor, a secretory leukocyte protease inhibitor (SLPI), showed that upregulation of TNF-α induces matrix metalloprotease 9 (MMP9), which leads to collagen destruction and, as a result, abnormal healing (Ashcroft et al., 2012). In an *in vivo* experiment, application of recombinant TNF-α to a wound reduced the expression of genes associated with collagen synthesis (Salomon et al., 1991), while TNF-α induced the expression of collagenase in dermal fibroblast culture in several studies (Dayer et al., 1985; Brenner et al., 1989). In human keratinocyte culture, TNF-α induces the expression of gelatinase capable of degrading type IV collagen (Banno et al., 2004). Secretion of TNF-α in high doses for a long period harms healing because it suppresses the expression of TIMPs and ECM proteins and induces the expression of MMP-1, -2, -3, -9, -13 and MT1-MMP, thus leading to the degradation of ECM, the decline of cell migration, and collagen deposition. TNF-α contributes to non-healing wounds by increasing gelatinases, collagenases, and stromelysins levels (Barrientos et al., 2008). The result of therapy aimed at inhibiting TNF- α is not only a decrease in the inflammatory response but also the normalization of ECM synthesis (Ashcroft et al., 2012).

There is some evidence that TNF-α inhibits normal scar formation not only due to enzyme activity. It was shown in an *in vitro* contacting wound model that TNF-α suppresses TGF-β-induced expression of myofibroblast genes, such as *α-SMA, fibronectin type 1A*, and *collagen*. The authors confirmed that the effect of TNF-α is in the inhibition of TGF-β1-induced differentiation of myofibroblasts, which leads to the formation of a more fragile matrix with reduced contractile properties. It is thought that the high level of TNF-α in a non-healing wound prevents the differentiation of myofibroblasts and changes in the cytoskeleton configuration, which leads to the impairment in normal matrix contraction during wound healing (Goldberg et al., 2007). TNF-α also suppresses re-epithelialization during wound healing (Barrientos et al., 2008). The *in vitro* study showed that administration of TNF-α led to an elevation of the mRNA expression of IL-8, ICAM-1, and MCP-1 in HaCaT through PKCζ; however, TNF-α-induced decline in the proliferative and migratory activity of HaCaT cells did not depend on PKCζ (Zhang et al., 2017). In another study, exposure of human keratinocyte culture to TNF-α stimulated the expression of pro-apoptotic genes *BIK, BID*, and *TNFSF10* (Banno et al., 2004).

As one can see, TNF-α is not just an activator of the pro-survival and inflammatory pathways as well as the trigger of apoptosis and necroptosis, itis also involved in wound healing, stem cell activation, and in the HF cycling. Multiple complementary data are indicating that delicate balance of TNF-α expression and related signaling is required for proper skin restoration, including WIHN.

In addition to TNF-α, important mediators of inflammation during wound healing are PG secreted by damaged tissues under the influence of leukocytes and other immune cells (Higgs et al., 1975). The role of PG in wound healing is controversial. They activate apoptotic cascades and thus prevent excessive scarring because impaired apoptosis does not give fibroblasts and myofibroblasts disappear during the later stages of skin regeneration (Su et al., 2010). Dysregulation of PG levels causes both WIHN and wound healing abnormalities. Thus, in a model of a non-healing diabetic wound in *ob/ob* mice, a decrease in PGE_2/PGD_2 levels was shown, and leptin injections retained normal wound healing and proper levels of PGE_2/PGD_2 (Kampfer et al., 2005). However, not only their abnormal decrease but also increase can lead to aberrations in wound healing and HFSCs activation. It was shown that the expression levels of the prostaglandin D_2 synthase enzyme (PTGDS) and its product PGD_2 correlated with WIHN: high levels of PTGDS and PGD_2 were interlinked with impaired neogenesis of HFs (Nelson et al., 2013). Despite the harmful effect of PGD_2 on WIHN, there is a suggestion that another type of prostaglandin, PGE_2, may induce WIHN through Wnt activation, as it was demonstrated in hematopoietic stem cells (Goessling et al., 2009; Gong et al., 2018).

Besides neutrophils and macrophages mast cells also take part in an inflammatory phase. They are a source of pro-inflammatory mediators and cytokines and modulate the number of neutrophils in the wound bed. The number of mast cells in the wound bed returns to its standard value within the first 48 hours after injury and then increases in the course of regeneration (Eming et al., 2007; Gurtner et al., 2008). As mentioned above, mast cells contribute to the regulation of the HF activity, namely, its entry into catagen (Arck et al., 2005).

To summarize, the inflammatory cells, which take part in wound healing, are mainly polymorphonuclear leukocytes (namely, neutrophil compartment) and macrophages. They and their mediators (TNF-α, ROS and PG) are involved not only in the regulation of the HF cycling but also in other activities of EpiSC including WIHN. Excessive inflammation alters HF homeostasis and wound healing process. It is expected that WIHN failure in this respect makes an additional indirect contribution to wound chronicity because of the importance of HF neogenesis in skin regeneration.

Proliferation Phase

T$_{regs}$. This stage of wound healing is characterized by proliferation and migration of cells, mainly keratinocytes and fibroblasts (Gurtner et al., 2008). The transition from the phase of inflammation to the stages of proliferation and remodeling is controlled by immunomegulatory mechanisms. In particular, T_{regs} are accumulated at inflammatory sites and are involved in modulating the immune response. These cells secrete Amphiregulin, an epidermal growth factor-like growth factor that is associated with maintaining tissue homeostasis, inflammation, and immunity. Amphiregulin via PCLγ induces "inside-out" activation of the integrin-αν-containing complex, which causes the transition of TGF-β from an inactive form to an active one. Active TGF-β has a dual role: it suppresses excessive inflammation and makes mesenchymal vascular progenitor cells, pericytes, differentiate into myofibroblasts, thus contributing to angiogenesis (Zaiss et al., 2019). Also, during angiogenesis, endothelial progenitor cells arrive from the bone marrow to the healing tissue to form new vessels (Gurtner et al., 2008). Xu et al. (2013) and Qing (2017).

T_{regs} contribute to re-epithelialization, which occurs due to differentiation of HFSCs into IFE keratinocytes, their proliferation, migration to the center of the wound, and synthesis of a new basement membrane (Gurtner et al., 2008; Gantwerker and Hom, 2011; Mathur et al., 2019). Re-epithelialization is activated by growth factors of the HGF, FGF, and EGF families (Martin and Nunan, 2015).

Mathur and co-authors showed in *in vivo* experiments that T_{regs} stimulated differentiation of HFSCs into IFE through the control of the IL-17-CXCL5-neutrophil inflammatory cascade. In a model of subacute skin injury inflicted by tape stripping, T_{reg} depleted mice demonstrated thinner epidermis upon regeneration and downregulation of genes related to keratinocyte differentiation and stratum corneum formation. T_{regs} suppress the keratinocyte expression of *Cxcl5*, which is induced by the neutrophil regulator IL-17A. In the T_{reg}-cell-lacking mice, neutralization of CXCL5 by antibodies restored differentiation, while IL-17A neutralization or co-depletion of neutrophils saved the migratory defect of Lgr5-derived cells in IFE during healing (Mathur et al., 2019). Thus, T_{regs} contribute to wound healing affecting a wide range of cells. In addition to initiating re-epithelialization, the fibrin matrix is replaced by granulation tissue consisting of fibroblasts, germinating vessels, and immature type III collagen in the proliferation phase (Gantwerker and Hom, 2011). Either T_{regs} can stimulate bulge cells and cause HF cycle changes in normal conditions or promote re-epithelization during wound healing due to immunomodulating properties.

Fibroblasts are the key players in this phase of wound healing. It is well-known that fibroblasts and myofibroblasts secrete procollagen molecules, as well as fibronectin, thus providing ECM development. Fibroblasts migrating from the edges of the wound under the influence of TGF-β, cell fibronectin, and endothelin-1 differentiate into myofibroblasts contributing to wound contraction (Xu et al., 2013). Nevertheless, there is another surprising way, in which fibroblasts contribute to wound healing: they can produce nitric oxide (NO), an inflammatory mediator, which is also involved in skin regeneration. Several facts are indicating that NO is associated with collagen production. First, *in vitro* wound fibroblasts produce NO, and inhibition of NO synthases (NOS) leads to a decrease in collagen production (Schaffer et al., 1997). Second, transfection of tissues of wounded rats with a plasmid containing murine inducible NOS (iNOS) increased collagen deposition (Thornton et al., 1998). Third, ablation of endothelial NOS (eNOS) in mice leads to prolonged wound healing (Lee et al., 1999). Besides, there is some evidence that NO can affect EpiSC activation. Zhu and colleagues treated burn wounds in rats with NO-gel with sodium nitrite and showed that this treatment improved both wound healing and follicular neogenesis. Application of the gel contributed to re-epithelialization of the wound, caused an increase in the number of procollagen-expressing fibroblasts by 40%. Also, blood vessels number augmentation and neutrophils and monocytes infiltration was observed in the wound bed. In the wound bed of the treated group, more HFs and CD34 + stem cells were observed (Zhu et al., 2008). Wolf et al. in an *in vitro* experiment showed basal production of NO by human DP cells. The authors suggest that NO secretion promotes hair growth by mediating the proliferation and differentiation of matrix keratinocytes surrounding the DP (Wolf et al., 2003).

However, we should note that excessive exposure of the wound to NO can have the opposite outcome. There are some data on the harmful effect of NO on wound healing, for example, the delay in wound healing under its influence in an aged rat model (Bauer et al., 1998).

Scar Remodeling and Re-epithelialization Phase

During this stage, most endothelial cells, macrophages, and myofibroblasts undergo apoptosis or migrate from the wound bed, which consists of collagen and other ECM proteins. Type III collagen is replaced by type I collagen with the assistance of MMPs secreted by fibroblasts, macrophages, and endothelial cells (Gurtner et al., 2008). In this phase, HF neogenesis begins (Gay et al., 2020).

The mechanism of apoptosis that inflammatory cells undergo during healing remains under discussion. There is some evidence that the death receptor pathway mediates it due to TNFR activation, but some data indicate that the mitochondrial pathway via the anti-proliferative protein p53 is also possible. Fibroblasts die after they have synthesized a sufficient amount of fibers. And then, excessive endothelial cells are discarded (Greenhalgh, 1998). Thus, an involution of granulation tissue and retraction of blood vessels are observed (Gantwerker and Hom, 2011).

At the stage of remodeling, T cells are acting (Eming et al., 2007). Lee et al. showed that γδT cells are activated by IL-1α and IL-7, which are secreted by keratinocytes after injury (Lee P. et al., 2017_A). DETCs play diverse roles in wound healing. They contribute to the proliferation of keratinocytes by secretion of IGF1. In the mouse wound healing model, IGF1 secreted by DETCs caused a proliferation of keratin 14 + mouse epidermal cells and inhibited their terminal differentiation. IL-17A secreted by another subtype of γδT cells, Vγ4 T cells, can promote proliferation and terminal differentiation of mouse keratin 14 + epidermal cells (Zhu et al., 2019). There is also evidence of a stimulatory effect of KGF secreted by activated DETCs on keratinocyte proliferation. In addition to participating in the survival and proliferation of keratinocytes, activated DETCs affect inflammatory cells. They produce CCL3 and CCL4, which regulate the recruitment of inflammatory cells. DETC-derived KGF stimulates hyaluronan deposition by keratinocytes attracting macrophages (Ramirez et al., 2015).

γδT cells are the source of FGF9, which is involved in neofolliculogenesis in wounds (Gay et al., 2013). Gay with colleagues showed that *Fgf9* was upregulated in the dermis, just before the development of the hair placode during wound healing begins. The administration of antibodies against FGF9 into wound dermis decreased the number of newly formed HF. The number of γδT cells in the wound increased just before the raise of FGF9. The researchers showed that on PWD 12 Vγ4 + γδT population was the predominant source of FGF9, while DETCs was inactive in this respect. The study on $Tcrd^{-/-}$ mice lacking γδT cells showed a significant decrease in the number of newly formed HF in the wound bed compared with control. An analysis of the timeline of *Fgf9* expression and *in situ* hybridization of wound skin at different time points allowed the authors to conclude that γδT cells are the primary source of FGF9 at PWD 10–12, which caused the expression of Wnt2a in dermal fibroblasts and thus led to the activation of Wnt pathway as well as to the expression of FGF9 in fibroblasts later on, and, consequently, increased Wnt activation in the dermis. Researchers found a small number of resident γδT cells in the human dermis with low density per area compared with the mouse dermis. Also, there were differences in the localization of γδT cells. In mice, cells were scattered throughout the dermis, usually at a distance from αβT cells and blood vessels. Human cells formed clusters with αβ T cells in vascularized dermal "pockets," indicating that they rarely migrate between skin and blood. A small number of γδT cells in the human skin, as compared to mice, may explain the lower regeneration ability of human skin when injured (Gay et al., 2013).

The Wnt pathway makes an important contribution to *de novo* HF formation (Gong et al., 2018). Myung and co-authors used K14-CreER;*Wls*$^{fl/fl}$ (WlsK14cKO) mice with knockout of *Wintless*, the gene, corresponding to Wnt secretion in the basal cells of IFE and HF. In the mouse model of wound healing, the absence of DP formation in the dermis of mutant animals was shown using alkaline phosphatase (AP) whole-mount staining (Myung et al., 2013). Transfection of human HFDP cells by negative Wnt regulator *CXXC5* led to downregulation of β-catenin, AP and PCNA, and knockdown of CXXC5 had the opposite effect. Lee and colleagues assume that Wnt3a activates CXXC5. Exposure of human DP cells to Wnt3a increased CXXC5 via a negative feedback mechanism. It is suggested that interruption of Wnt inhibitory signaling may stimulate WIHN, especially in humans (Lee S.H. et al., 2017_B). As it was mentioned above, in addition to γδT cells, the Wnt pathway can be activated by macrophages.

Lee and colleagues showed that γδT cells affect HFSCs not only indirectly through Wnt-mediated contributions to WIHN. These cells are an excellent example of the direct relationship between wound healing and HFSCs activation, as they stimulate the proliferation of bulge CD34 + HFSCs. The authors used the conditional knockout model for the *caspase-8* gene in epidermal cells for simulating wound healing to investigate the role of IL-1 in EpiSC activation during this process (Lee P. et al., 2017_A). Previously it was shown that *caspase-8* loss led to upregulation of IL-1α secretion because of an influence on caspase-1, which take part in the conversion of IL-1 precursor into an active form (Lee et al., 2009). Caspase-8 is widely known for its participation in the process of death receptor apoptosis, but besides, it has other functions. For example, it is involved in the processing of IL-1β, which contributes to inflammation (Gurung and Kanneganti, 2015).

Furthermore, IL-1β can indirectly influence HF: transplantation of IL-1β-stimulated bone marrow-derived macrophages into mice induced hair growth (Osaka et al., 2007). Lee and colleagues proposed the following HFSCs activation scheme: after wounding, the expression of caspase-8 decreases and, as a result, IL-1α is released from keratinocytes, which, together with IL-7, increases the population of γδT-cells (Lee P. et al., 2017_A). The latter stimulates the proliferation of bulge stem cells and mobilize them for wound healing. In inflammatory conditions keratinocytes also secrete CCL2 (Behfar et al., 2018), which attracts macrophages secreting IL-1β inducing hair growth. This mechanism potentiates the effect of IL-1 and IL-7/γδT cells on HFSCs proliferation (Lee P. et al., 2017_A). The above data once again proves the complicated interconnections between HFSCs activation pathways, inflammation participants, and cell death.

The scarring, which accomplishes the regeneration, much depends on the inflammatory process features, as well as on the expression of the cytokine profile (Liechty et al., 2000). However, scar development precludes restoration of the structure and functions of the wounded skin amply, not to mention severe complications such as keloids (Lim et al., 2018). Therefore, studies focusing on the possibility of regulating scar development via modulating the inflammation are of great practical importance. For example, in mice lacking T-lymphocytes, wounds heal without scars; however, in mice that do not develop both T- and B-lymphocytes, skin regeneration ends with scarring (Gawronska-Kozak et al., 2006). In the fetus, the skin regenerates without scars, since fetal wound healing occurs with a reduced inflammatory reaction, in part because macrophages, neutrophils, and mast cells of the fetus differ in size and maturity from those in adult tissues (Takeo et al., 2015). Martin et al. (2003) argue that inflammation is not prerequisite for effective wound healing if antibiotics stop the development of a bacterial infection. In the *pu.1* $^{-/-}$ mouse model, which does not develop functioning neutrophils and macrophages, skin regeneration is similar to fetal healing without the development of an inflammatory response and, as a result, under conditions of lower levels of TGF-β and IL-6. Thus, at the moment, information about the possibility of a direct influence on the scar through inflammation modulation is contradictory.

Nevertheless, studies are pointing out the possibility of indirect eliminating the effects of excess inflammation manifested by fibrotic scarring via agents produced by dermal cells. Lim and colleagues showed in their work that activation of Sonic hedgehog pathway leads to the formation of DP, which is a necessary condition for follicular neogenesis, which, in turn, leads to the restoration of skin functions at the site of injury and prevents the formation of scars (Lim et al., 2018).

Consequently, inflammation, scarring, and WIHN are interlinked. This is confirmed by fibrotic healing in WIHN^{-} mice wounds. In this type of wounds, unlike WIHN^{+} ones, late macrophages phagocytized a Wnt inhibitor SFRP4. In the late stages of wound healing, Wnt ligands paradoxically induced fibrotic healing, and these ligands are decreased in WIHN^{+} wounds. A similar process occurs in humans (Gay et al., 2020), where wounds lack WIHN and commonly heal with a cosmetic defect. Thereby, the role of Wnt ligands in wound healing is controversial: on the one hand, they can promote WIHN, which prevents scar formation and causes skin restoration; on the other hand, chronic expression of such ligands can cause wound fibrosis. Since macrophages phagocytize Wnt-inhibitor, it can be assumed that the chronic presence of Wnt ligands in the wound may be a consequence of prolonged inflammation, causing impaired regeneration and abnormal scarring.

At the moment, the involvement of different types of stem cells in HF neogenesis is under discussion (Plikus et al., 2015).

There is evidence that first telogen Lgr6 + stem cells transplanted onto the backs of nude mice are capable of reconstructing HF (Snippert et al., 2010). Another study gives a key role in follicular neogenesis to bulge Lgr5 + stem cells. Depletion of Lgr5 + cells in Lgr5-Cre:R26^{DTR}/ + mice resulted in WIH-A arrest on PWD 15 as well as a decrease in the number of neogenic HF by PWD 21-23 (Wang et al., 2017). However, another type of bulge stem cells, Krt15-expressing cells, are not involved in WIHN (Plikus et al., 2015).

Proper WIHN requires dermal papilla (DP) formation likely occurring by condensation of dermal fibroblasts or pre-existing progenitors. Experiments on *Blimp-1* knock-out mice demonstrated a violation of WIHN, suggesting an essential function of fibroblasts expressing Blimp-1 in DP neogenesis (Telerman et al., 2017). On the other hand, DP cells themselves take part in wound healing. Being one of the main components of the wound environment, TGF-β1 upregulates the expression of fibroblast-specific protein 1 (FSP1) and vimentin in DP cells and downregulated α-SMA expression suggesting that DP cells can differentiate into fibroblasts during wound healing (Bin et al., 2013). DP can also contribute to wound healing by secreting the anagen-inducing hormone leptin (Jimenez et al., 2015), which was shown to improve the migration and proliferation of keratinocytes as well as to accelerate angiogenesis (Tadokoro et al., 2015).

Thus, to sum up, inflammation during wound healing is like a double-edged sword. On the one hand, excessive inflammation leads to the establishment of long-term non-healing wounds. The optionality of inflammation for wound healing was shown by a series of experiments, for example, with the ablation of functioning neutrophils and macrophages. On the other hand, the release of the inflammatory cytokine TNF-α is a significant factor in WIHN, which is a prerequisite for scar formation without a cosmetic defect. Also, we can make one more conclusion about the potential intersection of wound healing and activation of HFSCs not only through wound healing cascades but also in other ways, for example, through programmed cell death. These considerations are prompted by data on the role of the upstream activator of apoptosis and necroptosis TNF-α and the downstream participant of apoptosis Caspase-8 (Varfolomeev and Vucic, 2018) in the activation of HFSCs as well as in normal and pathological wound healing.

DISCUSSION

Undoubtedly, there is a close interplay between the activation of EpiSC, specifically, HFSCs, as a whole and WIHN as its particular manifestation with the participation of wound healing via inflammatory cells, mediators, and dsRNA. Inflammation is involved in the regulation of HF cycling in intact skin and into the activation of HFSCs during wound healing. However, there is a reason to believe that the relationship between HFSCs functioning and wound healing has a much more complex regulation. We want to take a chance here and suppose that this regulation may comprise not only inflammatory agents but also components of the signaling pathways of cell death, including apoptosis and necroptosis. As it was discussed above, ROS, activators of pro-apoptotic and inflammatory cascades, together with the "external" apoptosis and necroptosis activators TNF-α and dsRNA, and the downstream mediator of apoptosis caspase-8 influence wound healing and HFSC activation. These findings are particularly interesting since apoptosis is classically considered to be a non-inflammatory way of cell death (Nagata, 2018). There are also new data suggesting that apoptotic cells are not inert: they may trigger genes associated with wound healing, proliferation, and a decrease in inflammation in adjacent cells (Medina et al., 2020). It is known that the signaling pathways of inflammation and cell death are interconnected through RIPK-1 and RIPK-3, including the situation of wound healing, as shown in several studies (Takahashi et al., 2014; Godwin et al., 2015; Moriwaki et al., 2015; Gupta et al., 2018). Such intersections can also occur in the HF. Moreover, it can be speculated that RIPK-1 and RIPK-3 play an unexpected role in HF dynamics. We found the cycle-related expression of RIPK-1 and RIPK-3 in mouse and human HF cells: It was found in the anagen HFs and absent in telogen ones (Morgun et al., 2020). As it was described above, hair growth may be promoted via dsRNA/TLR3/IL-6/STAT3 pathway (Nelson et al., 2015, 2016a_A; Nelson et al., 2016b_B). Based on Moriwaki data obtained in a mouse model of colitis, as well as in an experiment on bone-marrow-derived dendritic cells, it can be concluded that after LPS-induced stimulation of TLR4, RIPK-3 participates in the activation of the NF-κβ pathway, which leads to interleukin expression and STAT3 phosphorylation (Moriwaki et al., 2014). It may be speculated that RIPK-3-induced activation of NF-κβ is an additional intermediate link between the stimulation of the TLR3 and IL-6/STAT3-induced hair growth.

The regulation of inflammation and other processes that occur during wound healing is very complex and multidirectional. Excessive scarring can cause a cosmetic defect, while a delay in the formation of a scar (like in a non-healing wound) can cause severe complications during the wound healing process. The functions of HF in wound healing are also a two-way street: it is a source of stem cells both for re-epithelialization and for self-regeneration, while its neogenesis in the wound bed is essential for the functional recovery of the skin after injury. However, humans are unable to accomplish WIHN. Likewise, there is no adequate model for studying the damaged human HF. There are several *in vivo* and *in vitro* models admitting studies of human HF life activities. For example, researchers offer a humanized scalp model (Yamao et al., 2015), a SCID mouse xenotransplantation model (Oh et al., 2016), and *in vitro* culture model of a single human HF (Ma et al., 2016), and DP organoid model (Gupta et al., 2018). It is believed that the use of HF or their cellular components can significantly affect the course of wound healing, while *in situ* induction of hair growth during wound healing can stimulate epimorphic regeneration instead of scarring (Rippa et al., 2019). Attempts to transplant or "grow" HF in the wound bed have a long history. There is a classic work of the Jahoda with co-authors, where the induction of hair growth by transplantation of cultured DP cells in the lower part-amputated HF, was shown (Jahoda et al., 1984). Kageyama and colleagues showed HF development after the transplantation of bead-based HF germs, which were prepared with mouse embryonic mesenchymal cells or human DP cells and epithelial cells, into the back of nude mice (Kageyama et al., 2019). Lei and co-workers accomplish *in vivo* hair growth after transplantation of organoids, which were developed from mice neonatal epidermal and dermal cells (Lei et al., 2017). Lee and co-authors generated the artificial HF using mouse pluripotent stem cells in an *in vitro* study (Lee et al., 2018). Using skin epidermal keratinocytes and human DP cells we fabricated an artificial hair germ-like structures expressing a number markers, such as Lef1, EpCAM, and P cadherin attributed to folliculogenesis (Kalabusheva et al., 2017). Abaci and colleagues managed to compose a factitious human HF inside bioengineered skin constructs (HSCs) using 3D-printed molds. Transfection of DP cells with *Lef-1* restored the intact transcription signature of the DP and significantly increased expression of markers of the inner and outer root sheath, as well as the medulla, which indicated the efficiency of cell differentiation within the HSCs toward the HF. Moreover, human umbilical vein endothelial cells (HUVECs) were encapsulated into HSCs, and this resulted in HF vascularization and in the hair growth stimulation in immunodeficient mice (Abaci et al., 2018). Returning to the subject of our review, we suggest that engagement of inflammatory cells during HF-like structure fabrication may improve the outcome of transplantation. Notably, there could be used not only distinctive for skin in steady state immune cells, such as T_{regs} or γδT cells but also polymorphonuclear leukocytes (in particular, neutrophils) and macrophages. Thus, partial simulation of wound milieu may be helpful to reproduce WIH-A and WIHN microenvironment during hair transplantation into the scar, which is a promising method of its amelioration (Jung et al., 2013), or into the balding scalp. It may be proposed, that macrophages within the hair-bearing graft could improve hair growth by three ways: trough AKT/β-catenin activation (Wang et al., 2017); via induction of Wnt-signaling by dint of growth factors release (Kasuya et al., 2018), or production of Wnt-ligands upon their apoptosis activation (Castellana et al., 2014). Neutrophils, releasing ROS, could stimulate secretion of growth factors by DP cells and, thus, cause hair growth, maintain DP identity and support correct epithelial-mesenchymal interactions through the restoration of native DP signature (Zheng et al., 2019).

Thereby, the study of the components of inflammatory cascades as general targets for the treatment of wound healing and pathologies assumes a new significance. According to EpiSC plasticity, it may be proposed, that inflammation milieu can promote HF development from cultured cells transplanted into the wound. However, inflammation- induced effect on stemness can not only ameliorate wound healing but also cause diseases associated with pathological cell proliferation and differentiation failure, for example, psoriasis. Likewise, several germinative epidermal cells have an "inflammatory memory", which in the experiment leads to better healing, though the long-term outcome of this approach in humans is unknown. In addition, it is known, that skin pathologies characterized by excessive inflammation such as epidermolysis bullosa (Mallipeddi, 2002) and burns (Koh et al., 2014) improve the risk of squamous cell carcinoma. It can be assumed that inflammation so radically affects the homeostasis of the epidermis that differentiated epidermal cells acquire stem features, and epidermal SC overreact, resulting in malignant skin degeneration. This is another indirect evidence of the ambiguity of the effect of inflammation on the differentiation status of epidermal cells. Consequently, using TNF-α, ROS, and NO, as well as cells, which release these inflammatory agents, can be problematic, as they can cause quite severe skin pathologies. Thus, it is necessary to find a delicate regulation of inflammatory cascades.

AUTHOR CONTRIBUTIONS

EM analyzed the literature and wrote the manuscript. EV edited the text and proposed ideas. Both authors contributed to the article and approved the submitted version.

FUNDING

The work was funded by the Russian Science Foundation (Project No. 16-14-00204).

ACKNOWLEDGMENTS

The authors would like to thank Ekaterina P. Kalabusheva, Elina S. Chermnykh, and Alexandra A. Rippa for valuable consultations, Evgeny I. Kiselev for assisting with the figure.

REFERENCES

Abaci, H. E., Coffman, A., Doucet, Y., Chen, J., Jacków, J., Wang, E., et al. (2018). Tissue engineering of human hair follicles using a biomimetic developmental approach. *Nat. Commun.* 9:5301. doi: 10.1038/s41467-018-07579-y

Abbasi, S., and Biernaskie, J. (2019). Injury modifies the fate of hair follicle dermal stem cell progeny in a hair cycle-dependent manner. *Exp. Dermatol.* 28, 419–424. doi: 10.1111/exd.13924

Ali, N., Zirak, B., Rodriguez, R. S., Pauli, M. L., Truong, M. A., Lai, K., et al. (2017). Regulatory T cells in skin facilitate epithelial stem cell differentiation. *Cell* 169, 1119–1129.e11. doi: 10.1016/j.cell.2017.05.002

Ansell, D. M., Kloepper, J. E., Thomason, H. A., Paus, R., and Hardman, M. J. (2011). Exploring the "hair growth–wound healing connection": anagen phase promotes wound re-epithelialization. *J. Invest. Dermatol.* 131, 518–528. doi: 10.1038/jid.2010.291

Arck, P. C., Handjiski, B., Kuhlmei, A., Peters, E. M. J., Knackstedt, M., Peter, A., et al. (2005). Mast cell deficient and neurokinin-1 receptor knockout mice are protected from stress-induced hair growth inhibition. *J. Mol. Med.* 83, 386–396. doi: 10.1007/s00109-004-0627-z

Ashcroft, G. S., Jeong, M. J., Ashworth, J. J., Hardman, M., Jin, W., Moutsopoulos, N., et al. (2012). Tumor necrosis factor-alpha (TNF-α) is a therapeutic target for impaired cutaneous wound healing. *Wound Repair Regen.* 20, 38–49. doi: 10.1111/j.1524-475x.2011.00748.x

Banno, T., Gazel, A., and Blumenberg, M. (2004). Effects of tumor necrosis factor-α (TNFα) in epidermal keratinocytes revealed using global transcriptional profiling. *J. Biol. Chem.* 279, 32633–32642. doi: 10.1074/jbc.m400642200

Barker, J. N. W. N., Mitra, R. S., Griffiths, C. E. M., Dixit, V. M., and Nickoloff, B. J. (1991). Keratinocytes as initiators of inflammation. *Lancet* 337, 211–214. doi: 10.1016/0140-6736(91)92168-2

Barrandon, Y., and Green, H. (1987). Three clonal types of keratinocyte with different capacities for multiplication. *Proc. Natl. Acad. Sci. U.S.A.* 84, 2302–2306. doi: 10.1073/pnas.84.8.2302

Barrientos, S., Stojadinovic, O., Golinko, M. S., Brem, H., and Tomic-Canic, M. (2008). Perspective article: growth factors and cytokines in wound healing. *Wound Repair Regen.* 16, 585–601. doi: 10.1111/j.1524-475x.2008.00410.x

Bauer, J. A., Rao, W., and Smith, D. (1998). Evaluation of linear polyethyleneimine/nitric oxide adduct on wound repair: therapy versus toxicity. *Wound Repair Regen.* 6, 569–577. doi: 10.1046/j.1524-475x.1998.60609.x

Behfar, S., Hassanshahi, G., Nazari, A., and Khorramdelazad, H. (2018). A brief look at the role of monocyte chemoattractant protein-1 (CCL2) in the pathophysiology of psoriasis. *Cytokine* 110, 226–231. doi: 10.1016/j.cyto.2017.12.010

Bevilacqua, M. P., Pober, J. S., Mendrick, D. L., Cotran, R. S., and Gimbrone, M. A. (1987). Identification of an inducible endothelial-leukocyte adhesion molecule. *Proc. Natl. Acad. Sci. U.S.A.* 84, 9238–9242. doi: 10.1073/pnas.84.24.9238

Bin, S., Li, H. D., Xu, Y. B., Qi, S. H., Li, T. Z., Liu, X. S., et al. (2013). BMP-7 attenuates TGF-β1-induced fibroblast-like differentiation of rat dermal papilla cells. *Wound Repair Regen.* 21, 275–281. doi: 10.1111/wrr.12015

Botchkarev, V. A., and Sharov, A. A. (2004). BMP signaling in the control of skin development and hair follicle growth. *Differentiation* 72, 512–526. doi: 10.1111/j.1432-0436.2004.07209005.x

Brenner, D. A., O'Hara, M., Angel, P., Chojkier, M., and Karin, M. (1989). Prolonged activation of jun and collagenase genes by tumour necrosis factor-α. *Nature* 337, 661–663. doi: 10.1038/337661a0

Brownell, I., Guevara, E., Bai, C. B., Loomis, C. A., and Joyner, A. L. (2011). Nerve-derived sonic hedgehog defines a niche for hair follicle stem cells capable of becoming epidermal stem cells. *Cell Stem Cell* 8, 552–565. doi: 10.1016/j.stem.2011.02.021

Carrasco, E., Calvo, M., Blázquez-Castro, A., Vecchio, D., Zamarrón, A., Dias de Almeida, I. J., et al. (2015). Photoactivation of ROS production *in situ* transiently activates cell proliferation in mouse skin and in the hair follicle stem cell niche promoting hair growth and wound healing. *J. Invest. Dermatol.* 135, 2611–2622. doi: 10.1038/jid.2015.248

Castellana, D., Paus, R., and Perez-Moreno, M. (2014). Macrophages contribute to the cyclic activation of adult hair follicle stem cells. *PLoS Biol.* 12:e1002002. doi: 10.1371/journal.pbio.1002002

Chen, C. C., Wang, L., Plikus, M. V., Jiang, T. X., Murray, P. J., Ramos, R., et al. (2015). Organ-level quorum sensing directs regeneration in hair stem cell populations. *Cell* 161, 277–290. doi: 10.1016/j.cell.2015.02.016

Choi, N., Kim, W. S., Oh, S. H., and Sung, J. H. (2019). HB-EGF improves the hair regenerative potential of adipose-derived stem cells via ros generation and Hck phosphorylation. *Int. J. Mol. Sci.* 21:122. doi: 10.3390/ijms21010122

Circu, M. L., and Aw, T. Y. (2010). Reactive oxygen species, cellular redox systems, and apoptosis. *Free Radic. Biol. Med.* 48, 749–762. doi: 10.1016/j.freeradbiomed.2009.12.022

Clayton, E., Doupé, D. P., Klein, A. M., Winton, D. J., Simons, B. D., and Jones, P. H. (2007). A single type of progenitor cell maintains normal epidermis. *Nature* 446, 185–189. doi: 10.1038/nature05574

Cotsarelis, G., Sun, T. T., and Lavker, R. M. (1990). Label-retaining cells reside in the bulge area of pilosebaceous unit: implications for follicular stem cells, hair cycle, and skin carcinogenesis. *Cell* 61, 1329–1337. doi: 10.1016/0092-8674(90)90696-c

Dayer, J. M., Beutler, B., and Cerami, A. (1985). Cachectin/tumor necrosis factor stimulates collagenase and prostaglandin E2 production by human synovial cells and dermal fibroblasts. *J. Exp. Med.* 162, 2163–2168. doi: 10.1084/jem.162.6.2163

Dunnill, C., Patton, T., Brennan, J., Barrett, J., Dryden, M., Cooke, J., et al. (2017). Reactive oxygen species (ROS) and wound healing: the functional role of ROS and emerging ROS-modulating technologies for augmentation of the healing process. *Int. Wound J.* 14, 89–96. doi: 10.1111/iwj.12557

Efimov, G. A., Kruglov, A. A., Tillib, S. V., Kuprash, D. V., and Nedospasov, S. A. (2009). Tumor necrosis factor and the consequences of its ablation *in vivo*. *Mol. Immunol.* 47, 19–27. doi: 10.1016/j.molimm.2009.01.007

Ekman, A.-K., Bivik Eding, C., Rundquist, I., and Enerback, C. (2019). IL-17 and IL-22 promote keratinocyte stemness in the germinative compartment in psoriasis. *J. Invest. Dermatol.* 139, 1564–1573.e8. doi: 10.1016/j.jid.2019.03.368

Eming, S. A., Krieg, T., and Davidson, J. M. (2007). Inflammation in wound repair: molecular and cellular mechanisms. *J. Invest. Dermatol.* 127, 514–525. doi: 10.1038/sj.jid.5700701

Fadini, G. P., Cappellari, R., Mazzucato, M., Agostini, C., Vigili de Kreutzenberg, S., and Avogaro, A. (2013). Monocyte–macrophage polarization balance in pre-diabetic individuals. *Acta Diabetol.* 50, 977–982. doi: 10.1007/s00592-013-0517-3

Fang, X., Zhou, X., and Wang, X. (2013). Clinical development of phosphatidylinositol 3-kinase inhibitors for non-Hodgkin lymphoma. *Biomark. Res.* 1:30. doi: 10.1186/2050-7771-1-30

Gantwerker, E. A., and Hom, D. B. (2011). Skin: histology and physiology of wound healing. facial plast surg clin. *North Am.* 19, 441–453. doi: 10.1016/j.fsc.2011.06.009

Garcin, C. L., and Ansell, D. M. (2017). The battle of the bulge: re-evaluating hair follicle stem cells in wound repair. *Exp. Dermatol.* 26, 101–104. doi: 10.1111/exd.13184

Gawronska-Kozak, B., Bogacki, M., Rim, J. S., Monroe, W. T., and Manuel, J. A. (2006). Scarless skin repair in immunode cient mice. *Wound Repair Regen.* 14, 265–276. doi: 10.1111/j.1743-6109.2006.00121.x

Gay, D., Ghinatti, G., Guerrero-Juarez, C. F., Ferrer, R. A., Ferri, F., Lim, C. H., et al. (2020). Phagocytosis of Wnt inhibitor SFRP4 by late wound macrophages drives chronic Wnt activity for fibrotic skin healing. *Sci. Adv.* 6:eaay3704. doi: 10.1126/sciadv.aay3704

Gay, D., Kwon, O., Zhang, Z., Spata, M., Plikus, M. V., Holler, P. D., et al. (2013). Fgf9 from dermal γδ T cells induces hair follicle neogenesis after wounding. *Nat. Med.* 19, 916–923. doi: 10.1038/nm.3181

Geyfman, M., Plikus, M., Treffeisen, E., Andersen, B., and Paus, R. (2015). Resting no more: re-defining telogen, the maintenance stage of the hair growth cycle. *Biol. Rev.* 90, 1179–1196. doi: 10.1111/brv.12151

Ghazizadeh, S., and Taichman, L. B. (2001). Multiple classes of stem cells in cutaneous epithelium: a lineage analysis of adult mouse skin. *EMBO J.* 20, 1215–1222. doi: 10.1093/emboj/20.6.1215

Godwin, A., Sharma, A., Yang, W.-L., Wang, Z., Nicastro, J., Coppa, G. F., et al. (2015). Receptor-interacting protein kinase 3 deficiency delays cutaneous wound healing. *PLoS One* 10:e0140514. doi: 10.1371/journal.pone.0140514

Goessling, W., North, T. E., Loewer, S., Lord, A. M., Lee, S., Stoick-Cooper, C. L., et al. (2009). Genetic interaction of PGE2 and Wnt signaling regulates developmental specification of stem cells and regeneration. *Cell* 136, 1136–1147. doi: 10.1016/j.cell.2009.01.015

Goldberg, M. T., Han, Y. P., Yan, C., Shaw, M. C., and Garner, W. L. (2007). TNF-α suppresses α-Smooth Muscle Actin expression in human dermal fibroblasts: an implication for abnormal wound healing. *J. Invest. Dermatol.* 127, 2645–2655. doi: 10.1038/sj.jid.5700890

Gong, L., Xu, X. G., and Li, Y. H. (2018). Embryonic-like regenerative phenomenon: wound-induced hair follicle neogenesis. *Regen. Med.* 13, 729–739. doi: 10.2217/rme-2018-0028

Gonzales, K. A. U., and Fuchs, E. (2017). Skin and its regenerative powers: an alliance between stem cells and their niche. *Dev. Cell* 43, 387–401. doi: 10.1016/j.devcel.2017.10.001

Greenhalgh, D. G. (1998). The role of apoptosis in wound healing. *Int. J. Biochem. Cell Biol.* 30, 1019–1030. doi: 10.1016/s1357-2725(98)00058-2

Greenlee-Wacker, M. C. (2016). Clearance of apoptotic neutrophils and resolution of inflammation. *Immunol. Rev.* 273, 357–370. doi: 10.1111/imr.12453

Gröne, A. (2002). Keratinocytes and cytokines. *Vet. Immunol. Immunopathol.* 88, 1–12. doi: 10.1016/s0165-2427(02)00136-8

Gupta, A. C., Chawla, S., Hegde, A., Singh, D., Bandyopadhyay, B., Lakshmanan, C. C., et al. (2018). Establishment of an *in vitro* organoid model of dermal papilla of human hair follicle. *J. Cell. Physiol.* 233, 9015–9030. doi: 10.1002/jcp.26853

Gurtner, G. C., Werner, S., Barrandon, Y., and Longaker, M. T. (2008). Wound repair and regeneration. *Nature* 453, 314–321. doi: 10.1038/nature07039

Gurung, P., and Kanneganti, T. D. (2015). Novel roles for caspase- 8 in IL-1beta and inflammasome regulation. *Am. J. Pathol.* 185, 17–25.

Haensel, D., Jin, S., Sun, P., Cinco, R., Dragan, M., Nguyen, Q., et al. (2020). Defining epidermal basal cell states during skin homeostasis and wound healing using single-cell transcriptomics. *Cell Rep.* 30, 3932–3947.e6. doi: 10.1016/j.celrep.2020.02.091

Hardman, J. A., Muneeb, F., Pople, J., Bhogal, R., Shahmalak, A., and Paus, R. (2019). Human perifollicular macrophages undergo apoptosis, express wnt ligands, and switch their polarization during catagen. *J. Invest. Dermatol.* 139, 2543–2546.e9. doi: 10.1016/j.jid.2019.04.026

Higgins, C. A., Petukhova, L., Harel, S., Ho, Y. Y., Drill, E., Shapiro, L., et al. (2014). FGF5 is a crucial regulator of hair length in humans. *Proc. Natl. Acad. Sci. U.S.A.* 111, 10648–10653. doi: 10.1073/pnas.1402862111

Higgs, G. A., McCall, E., and Youlten, L. G. F. (1975). A chemotactic role for prostaglandins released from polymorphonuclear leucocytes during phagocytosis. *Br. J. Pharmacol.* 53, 539–546. doi: 10.1111/j.1476-5381.1975.tb07392.x

Hsu, Y., Li, L., and Fuchs, E. (2014). Emerging interactions between skin stem cells and their niches. *Nat. Med.* 20, 847–856. doi: 10.1038/nm.3643

Jahoda, C. A., Horne, K. A., and Oliver, R. F. (1984). Induction of hair growth by implantation of cultured dermal papilla cells. *Nature* 311, 560–562. doi: 10.1038/311560a0

Jahoda, C. A., Oliver, R. F., Reynolds, A., Forrester, J., and Horne, K. (1996). Human hair follicle regeneration following amputation and grafting into the nude mouse. *J. Invest. Dermatol.* 107, 804–807. doi: 10.1111/1523-1747.ep12330565

Jimenez, F., Poblet, E., and Izeta, A. (2015). Reflections on how wound healing-promoting effects of the hair follicle can be translated into clinical practice. *Exp. Dermatol.* 24, 91–94. doi: 10.1111/exd.12521

Jin, Y., Xia, M., Sun, A., Saylor, C. M., and Xiong, N. (2010). CCR10 is important for the development of skin-specific γδT cells by regulating their migration and location. *J. Immunol.* 185, 5723–5731. doi: 10.4049/jimmunol.1001612

Joost, S., Jacob, T., Sun, X., Annusver, K., La Manno, G., Sur, I., et al. (2018). Single-cell transcriptomics of traced epidermal and hair follicle stem cells reveals rapid adaptations during wound healing. *Cell Rep.* 25, 585–597.e7. doi: 10.1016/j.celrep.2018.09.059

Jung, S., Oh, S. J., and Hoon Koh, S. (2013). Hair follicle transplantation on scar tissue. *J. Craniofac. Surg.* 24, 1239–1241. doi: 10.1097/scs.0b013e31828a78ad

Kageyama, T., Yan, L., Shimizu, A., Maruo, S., and Fukuda, J. (2019). Preparation of hair beads and hair follicle germs for regenerative medicine. *Biomaterials* 212, 55–63. doi: 10.1016/j.biomaterials.2019.05.003

Kalabusheva, E. P., Terskikh, V. V., and Vorotelyak, E. A. (2017). Hair germ model in vitro via human postnatal keratinocyte-dermal papilla interactions: impact of hyaluronic acid. *Stem Cells Int.* 2017:9271869. doi: 10.1155/2017/9271869

Kampfer, H., Schmidt, R., Geisslinger, G., Pfeilschifter, J., and Frank, S. (2005). Wound inflammation in diabetic *ob/ob* mice: functional coupling of prostaglandin biosynthesis to cyclooxygenase-1 activity in diabetes-impaired wound healing. *Diabetes Metab. Res. Rev.* 54, 1543–1551. doi: 10.2337/diabetes.54.5.1543

Karin, M., Lawrence, T., and Nizet, V. (2006). Innate immunity gone awry: linking microbial infections to chronic inflammation and cancer. *Cell* 124, 823–835. doi: 10.1016/j.cell.2006.02.016

Kasuya, A., Ito, T., and Tokura, Y. (2018). M2 macrophages promote wound-induced hair neogenesis. *J. Dermatol. Sci.* 91, 250–255. doi: 10.1016/j.jdermsci.2018.05.004

Kellenberger, A., and Tauchi, M. (2013). Mammalian target of rapamycin complex 1 (mTORC1) may modulate the timing of anagen entry in mouse hair follicles. *Exp. Dermatol.* 22, 77–80. doi: 10.1111/exd.12062

Kim, J., and Krueger, J. (2015). The immunopathogenesis of psoriasis. *Dermatol. Clin.* 33, 13–23. doi: 10.1016/j.det.2014.09.002

Kobayashi, T., Voisin, B., Kim, D. Y., Kennedy, E. A., Jo, J., Shih, H. Y., et al. (2019). Homeostatic control of sebaceous glands by innate lymphoid cells regulates commensal bacteria equilibrium. *Cell* 176, 982–997.e16. doi: 10.1016/j.cell.2018.12.031

Koh, S. H., Oh, S. J., Chun, H., and Kim, S. J. (2014). Pseudoangiosarcomatous squamous cell carcinoma developing on a burn scar: a case report and review of the literature. *Burns* 40, e47–e52. doi: 10.1016/j.burns.2014.02.019

Komi, D. E. A., Khomtchouk, K., and Santa Maria, P. L. (2020). A review of the contribution of mast cells in wound healing: involved molecular and cellular mechanisms. *Clin. Rev. Allergy Immunol.* 58, 298–312. doi: 10.1007/s12016-019-08729-w

Krause, K., and Foitzik, K. (2006). Biology of the hair follicle: the basics. *Semin. Cutan. Med. Surg.* 25, 2–10. doi: 10.1016/j.sder.2006.01.002

Kumamoto, T., Shalhevet, D., Matsue, H., Mummert, M. E., Ward, B. R., Jester, J. V., et al. (2003). Hair follicles serve as local reservoirs of skin mast cell precursors. *Blood* 102, 1654–1660. doi: 10.1182/blood-2003-02-0449

Lay, K., Yuan, S., Gur-Cohen, S., Miao, Y., Han, T., Naik, S., et al. (2018). Stem cells repurpose proliferation to contain a breach in their niche barrier. *eLife* 7:e41661. doi: 10.7554/elife.41661

Lee, J., Böscke, R., Tang, P. C., Hartman, B. H., Heller, S., and Koehler, K. R. (2018). Hair follicle development in mouse pluripotent stem cell-derived skin organoids. *Cell Rep.* 22, 242–254. doi: 10.1016/j.celrep.2017.12.007

Lee, P., Gund, R., Dutta, A., Pincha, N., Rana, I., Ghosh, S., et al. (2017). Stimulation of hair follicle stem cell proliferation through an IL-1α dependent activation of γδT-cells. *J. Invest. Dermatol.* 138:S229. doi: 10.1016/j.jid.2018.03.1366_A

Lee, P., Lee, D. J., Chan, C., Chen, S. W., Ch'en, I., and Jamora, C. (2009). Dynamic expression of epidermal caspase 8 simulates a wound healing response. *Nature* 458, 519–523. doi: 10.1038/nature07687

Lee, P. C., Salyponsge, N., Bragdon, G. A., Shears, L. L., Watkins, S. C., Endington, H. D., et al. (1999). Impaired wound healing and angiogenesis in eNOS deficient mice. *Am. J. Physiol.* 46, 1600–1608. doi: 10.1152/ajpheart.1999.277.4.H1600

Lee, S. H., Seo, S. H., Lee, D. H., Pi, L. Q., Lee, W. S., and Choi, K. Y. (2017). Targeting of CXXC5 by a competing peptide stimulates hair regrowth and wound-induced hair neogenesis. *J. Invest. Dermat.* 137, 2260–2269. doi: 10.1016/j.jid.2017.04.038_B

Lei, M., Schumacher, L. J., Lai, Y. C., Juan, W. T., Yeh, C. Y., Wu, P., et al. (2017). Self-organization process in newborn skin organoid formation inspires strategy to restore hair regeneration of adult cells. *Proc. Natl. Acad. Sci. U.S.A.* 114, E7101–E7110. doi: 10.1073/pnas.1700475114

Li, J., Yang, Z., Li, Z., Gu, L., Wang, Y., and Sung, C. (2014). Exogenous IGF-1 promotes hair growth by stimulating cell proliferation and down regulating TGF-β1 in C57BL/6 mice in vivo. *Growth Horm. IGF Res.* 24, 89–94. doi: 10.1016/j.ghir.2014.03.004

Liechty, K. W., Kim, H. B., Adzick, N. S., and Crombleholme, T. M. (2000). Fetal wound repair results in scar formation in interleukin-10–deficient mice in a syngeneic murine model of scarless fetal wound repair. *J. Pediatr. Surg.* 35, 866–873. doi: 10.1053/jpsu.2000.6868

Lim, C. H., Sun, Q., Ratti, K., Lee, S.-H., Zheng, Y. I., Takeo, M., et al. (2018). Hedgehog stimulates hair follicle neogenesis by creating inductive dermis during murine skin wound healing. *Nat. Commun.* 9:4903. doi: 10.1038/s41467-018-07142-9

Liu, Y., Lyle, S., Yang, Z., and Cotsarelis, G. (2003). Keratin 15 promoter targets putative epithelial stem cells in the hair follicle bulge. *J. Invest. Dermat.* 121, 963–968. doi: 10.1046/j.1523-1747.2003.12600.x

Lyle, S., Christofidou-Solomidou, M., Liu, Y., Elder, D. E., Albelda, S., and Cotsarelis, G. (1998). The C8/144b monoclonal antibody recognizes cytokeratin 15 and defines the location of human hair follicle stem cells. *J. Cell Sci.* 111, 3179–3188.

Ma, L., Wang, J., Feng, S., Li, Y., Zhao, K., and Lei, M. (2016). Establishment of an *in vitro* culture model of single human hair follicle. *Zhonghua Zheng Xing Wai Ke Za Zhi* 32, 55–59.

Mackenzie, I. C. (1970). Relationship between mitosis and the ordered structure of the stratum corneum in mouse epidermis. *Nature* 226, 653–655. doi: 10.1038/226653a0

Mallipeddi, R. (2002). Epidermolysis bullosa and cancer. *Clin. Exp. Dermatol.* 27, 616–623. doi: 10.1046/j.1365-2230.2002.01130.x

Mansfield, K., and Naik, S. (2020). Unraveling immune-epithelial interactions in skin homeostasis and injury. *Yale J. Biol. Med.* 93, 133–143.

Martin, P., D'Souza, D., Martin, J., Grose, R., Cooper, L., Maki, R., et al. (2003). Wound healing in the PU.1 null mouse—tissue repair is not dependent on inflammatory cells. *Curr. Biol.* 13, 1122–1128. doi: 10.1016/s0960-9822(03)00396-8

Martin, P., and Nunan, R. (2015). Cellular and molecular mechanisms of repair in acute and chronic wound healing. *Br. J. Dermatol.* 173, 370–378. doi: 10.1111/bjd.13954

Mathur, A. N., Zirak, B., Boothby, I. C., Tan, M., Cohen, J. N., Mauro, T. N., et al. (2019). Treg-cell control of a CXCL5-IL-17 inflammatory axis promotes hair-follicle-stem-cell differentiation During Skin-Barrier Repair. *Immunity* 50, 655–667.e4. doi: 10.1016/j.immuni.2019.02.013

Medina, C. B., Mehrotra, P., Arandjelovic, S., Perry, J. S. A., Guo, Y., Morioka, S., et al. (2020). Metabolites released from apoptotic cells act as tissue messengers. *Nature* 580, 130–135. doi: 10.1038/s41586-020-2121-3

Minutti, C. M., Knipper, J. A., Allen, J. E., and Zaiss, D. M. W. (2017). Tissue-specific contribution of macrophages to wound healing. *Semin. Cell Dev. Biol.* 61, 3–11. doi: 10.1016/j.semcdb.2016.08.006

Moldovan, N. I. (2002). Role of monocytes and macrophages in adult angiogenesis: a light at the Tunnel's End. *J. Hematother. Stem Cell Res.* 11, 179–194. doi: 10.1089/152581602753658394

Morales, J., Homey, B., Vicari, A. P., Hudak, S., Oldham, E., Hedrick, J., et al. (1999). CTACK, a skin-associated chemokine that preferentially attracts skin-homing memory T cells. *Proc. Natl. Acad. Sci. U.S.A.* 96, 14470–14475. doi: 10.1073/pnas.96.25.14470

Morgun, E. I., Pozdniakova, E. D., and Vorotelyak, E. A. (2020). Expression of protein kinases RIPK-1 and RIPK-3 in mousee and human hair follicle. Doklady Rossiiskoi Akademii Nauk. *Nauki o Zhizni* 494, 500–503. doi: 10.1134/S1607672920050105 [in English - Doklady Biochemistry and Biophysics (in press)].

Moriwaki, K., Balaji, S., McQuade, T., Malhotra, N., Kang, J., and Chan, F. (2014). The necroptosis adaptor RIPK3 promotes injury-induced cytokine expression and tissue repair. *Immunity* 41, 567–578. doi: 10.1016/j.immuni.2014.09.016

Moriwaki, K., Bertin, J., Gough, P., and Chan, F. K.-M. (2015). A RIPK3–Caspase 8 complex mediates atypical Pro–IL-1β Processing. *J. Immunol.* 194, 1938–1944. doi: 10.4049/jimmunol.1402167

Morris, R. J., Liu, Y., Marles, L., Yang, Z., Tremous, C., Li, S., et al. (2004). Capturing and profiling adult hair follicle stem cells. *Nat. Biotechnol.* 22, 411–417. doi: 10.1038/nbt950

Mussano, F., Genova, T., Munaron, L., Petrillo, S., Erovigni, F., and Carossa, S. (2016). Cytokine, chemokine, and growth factor profile of platelet-rich plasma. *Platelets* 27, 467–471. doi: 10.3109/09537104.2016.1143922

Myung, P. S., Takeo, M., Ito, M., and Atit, R. P. (2013). Epithelial Wnt ligand secretion is required for adult hair follicle growth and regeneration. *J. Invest. Dermatol.* 133, 31–41. doi: 10.1038/jid.2012.230

Nagata, S. (2018). Apoptosis and clearance of apoptotic cells. *Annu. Rev. Immunol.* 36, 489–517. doi: 10.1146/annurev-immunol-042617-053010

Naik, S., Larsen, S. B., Cowley, C. J., and Fuchs, E. (2018). Two to tango: dialog between immunity and stem cells in health and dsease. *Cell* 175, 908–920. doi: 10.1016/j.cell.2018.08.071

Naik, S., Larsen, S. B., Gomez, N. C., Alaverdyan, K., Sendoel, A., Yuan, S., et al. (2017). Inflammatory memory sensitizes skin epithelial stem cells to tissue damage. *Nature* 550, 475–480. doi: 10.1038/nature24271

Nakamizo, S., Egawa, G., Tan, J. T. K., and Kabashima, K. (2020). Intravital imaging of cutaneous immune responses. *Cell. Immunol.* 350:103813. doi: 10.1016/j.cellimm.2018.05.006

Nanba, D., Toki, F., Tate, S., Imai, M., Matsushita, N., Shiraishi, K., et al. (2015). Cell motion predicts human epidermal stemness. *J. Exp. Med.* 212:2125OIA31. doi: 10.1084/jem.2125oia31

Nelson, A. M., Katseff, A. S., Ratliff, T. S., and Garza, L. A. (2016a). Interleukin 6 and STAT3 regulate p63 isoform expression in keratinocytes during regeneration. *Exp. Dermatol.* 25, 155–157. doi: 10.1111/exd.12896_A

Nelson, A. M., Katseff, A. S., Resnik, S. R., Ratliff, T. S., Zhu, A. S., and Garza, L. A. (2016b). Interleukin-6 null mice paradoxically display increased STAT3 activity and wound-induced hair neogenesis. *J. Invest. Dermatol.* 136, 1051–1053. doi: 10.1016/j.jid.2015.12.043_B

Nelson, A. M., Loy, D. E., Lawson, J. A., Katseff, A. S., FitzGerald, G. A., and Garza, L. A. (2013). Prostaglandin D2 inhibits wound-induced hair follicle neogenesis through the receptor, Gpr44. *J. Invest. Dermatol.* 133, 881–889. doi: 10.1038/jid.2012.398

Nelson, A. M., Reddy, S. K., Ratliff, T. S., Hossain, M. Z., Katseff, A. S., Zhu, A. S., et al. (2015). dsRNA released by tissue damage activates TLR3 to drive skin regeneration. *Cell Stem Cell* 17, 139–151. doi: 10.1016/j.stem.2015.07.008

Oh, J. W., Kloepper, J., Langan, E. A., Kim, Y., Yeo, J., Kim, M. J., et al. (2016). A guide to studying human hair follicle cycling *in vivo*. *J. Invest. Dermat.* 136, 34–44. doi: 10.1038/JID.2015.354

Osaka, N., Takahashi, T., Murakami, S., Matsuzawa, A., Noguchi, T., Fujiwara, T., et al. (2007). ASK1-dependent recruitment and activation of macrophages induce hair growth in skin wounds. *J. Exp. Med.* 204:i9. doi: 10.1084/jem2044oia9

Panteleyev, A. A., Jahoda, C. A. B., and Christiano, A. M. (2001). Hair follicle predetermination. *J. Cell Sci.* 114, 3419–3431.

Paus, R., and Cotsarelis, G. (1999). The biology of hair follicles. *N. Engl. J. Med.* 341, 491–497.

Plikus, M. V., Guerrero-Juarez, C. F., Treffeisen, E., and Gay, D. V. (2015). Epigenetic control of skin and hair regeneration after wounding. *Exp. Dermatol.* 24, 167–170. doi: 10.1111/exd.12488

Potten, C. S. (1974). The epidermal proliferative unit: the possible role of the central basal cell. *Cell Prolif.* 7, 77–88. doi: 10.1111/j.1365-2184.1974.tb00401.x

Proksch, E., Brandner, J. M., and Jensen, J.-M. (2008). The skin: an indispensable barrier. *Exp. Dermatol.* 17, 1063–1072. doi: 10.1111/j.1600-0625.2008.00786.x

Qing, C. (2017). The molecular biology in wound healing & non-healing wound. *Chin. J. Traumatol.* 20, 189–193. doi: 10.1016/j.cjtee.2017.06.001

Rahmani, W., Sinha, S., and Biernaskie, J. (2020). Immune modulation of hair follicle regeneration. *NPJ Regen. Med.* 5:9. doi: 10.1038/s41536-020-0095-2

Rajendran, R. L., Gangadaran, P., Seo, C. H., Kwack, M. H., Oh, J. M., Lee, H. W., et al. (2020). Macrophage-derived extracellular vesicle promotes hair growth. *Cells* 9:856. doi: 10.3390/cells9040856

Ramirez, K., Witherden, D. A., and Havran, W. L. (2015). All hands on DE(T)C: epithelial-resident γδ T cells respond to tissue injury. *Cell. Immunol.* 296, 57–61. doi: 10.1016/j.cellimm.2015.04.003

Rippa, A. L., Kalabusheva, E. P., and Vorotelyak, E. A. (2019). Regeneration of dermis: scarring and cells involved. *Cells* 8:607. doi: 10.3390/cells8060607

Rishikaysh, P., Dev, K., Diaz, D., Qureshi, W. M. S., Filip, S., and Mokry, J. (2014). Signaling involved in hair follicle morphogenesis and development. *Int. J. Mol. Sci.* 15, 1647–1670. doi: 10.3390/ijms15011647

Rognoni, E., and Watt, F. M. (2018). Skin cell heterogeneity in development, wound healing, and cancer. *Trends Cell Biol.* 28, 709–722. doi: 10.1016/j.tcb.2018.05.002

Rompolas, P., and Greco, V. (2014). Stem cell dynamics in the hair follicle niche. *Semin. Cell Dev. Biol.* 2, 34–42. doi: 10.1016/j.semcdb.2013.12.005

Rutkowski, J. M., Boardman, K. C., and Swartz, M. A. (2006). Characterization of lymphangiogenesis in a model of adult skin regeneration. *Am. J. Physiol. Heart Circ. Physiol.* 291, H1402–H1410. doi: 10.1152/ajpheart.00038.2006

Saito, N., Honma, M., Shibuya, T., Iinuma, S., Igawa, S., Kishibe, M., et al. (2018). RIPK1 downregulation in keratinocyte enhances TRAIL signaling in psoriasis. *J. Dermatol. Sci.* 91, 79–86. doi: 10.1016/j.jdermsci.2018.04.007

Salomon, G. D., Kasid, A., Cromack, D. T., Director, E., Talbot, T. L., Sank, A., et al. (1991). The local effects of cachectin/tumor necrosis factor on wound healing. *Ann. Surg.* 214, 175–180. doi: 10.1097/00000658-199108000-00012

Sano, S., Kira, M., Takagi, S., Yoshikawa, K., Takeda, J., and Itami, S. (2000). Two distinct signaling pathways in hair cycle induction: Stat3-dependent and -independent pathways. *Proc. Natl. Acad. Sci. U.S.A.* 97, 13824–13829. doi: 10.1073/pnas.240303097

Santoro, M. M., and Gaudino, G. (2005). Cellular and molecular facets of keratinocyte reepithelization during wound healing. *Exp. Cell Res.* 304, 274–286. doi: 10.1016/j.yexcr.2004.10.033

Sasaki, J. R., Zhang, Q., and Schwacha, M. G. (2011). Burn induces a Th-17 inflammatory response at the injury site. *Burns* 37, 646–651. doi: 10.1016/j.burns.2011.01.028

Sasaki, S., Hozumi, Y., and Kondo, S. (2005). Influence of prostaglandin F2alpha and its analogues on hair regrowth and follicular melanogenesis in a murine model. *Exp. Dermatol.* 14, 323–328. doi: 10.1111/j.0906-6705.2005.00270.x

Schaffer, M. R., Efron, P. A., Thorton, F. J., Klingel, K., Gross, S., and Barbul, A. (1997). Nitric oxide, an autocrine regulator of wound fibroblast synthetic function. *J. Immunol.* 158, 2275–2381.

Scharschmidt, T. C., Vasquez, K. S., Pauli, M., Leitner, E., Chu, K., Truong, H., et al. (2017). Commensal microbes and hair follicle morphogenesis coordinately drive treg migration into neonatal skin. *Cell Host Microbe* 21, 467–477.e5. doi: 10.1016/j.chom.2017.03.001

Seya, T., Shime, H., Takaki, H., Azuma, M., Oshiumi, H., and Matsumoto, M. (2012). TLR3/TICAM-1 signaling in tumor cell RIP3-dependent necroptosis. *Oncoimmunology* 1, 917–923. doi: 10.4161/onci.21244

Sharp, L. L., Jameson, J. M., Cauvi, G., and Havran, W. L. (2005). Dendritic epidermal T cells regulate skin homeostasis through local production of insulin-like growth factor 1. *Nat. Immunol.* 6, 73–79. doi: 10.1038/ni1152

Siqueira, M. F., Li, J., Chehab, L., Desta, T., Chino, T., Krothpali, N., et al. (2010). Impaired wound healing in mouse models of diabetes is mediated by TNF-α dysregulation and associated with enhanced activation of forkhead box O1 (FOXO1). *Diabetologia* 53, 378–388. doi: 10.1007/s00125-009-1529-y

Snippert, H. J., Haegebarth, A., Kasper, M., Jaks, V., van Es, J. H., Barker, N., et al. (2010). Lgr6 marks stem cells in the hair follicle that generate all cell lineages of the skin. *Science* 327, 1385–1389. doi: 10.1126/science.1184733

Solanas, G., and Benitah, S. A. (2013). Regenerating the skin: a task for the heterogeneous stem cell pool and surrounding niche. *Nat. Rev. Mol. Cell Biol.* 14, 737–748. doi: 10.1038/nrm3675

Squarize, C. H., Castilho, R. M., Bugge, T. H., and Gutkind, J. S. (2010). Accelerated wound healing by mTOR activation in genetically defined mouse models. *PLoS One* 5:e10643. doi: 10.1371/journal.pone.0010643

Su, W. H., Cheng, M. H., Lee, W. L., Tsou, T. S., Chang, W. H., Chen, C. S., et al. (2010). Nonsteroidal anti-inflammatory drugs for wounds: pain relief or excessive scar formation? *Mediators Inflamm.* 2010:413238. doi: 10.1155/2010/413238

Sun, X., Are, A., Annusver, K., Sivan, U., Jacob, T., Dalessandri, T., et al. (2020). Coordinated hedgehog signaling induces new hair follicles in adult skin. *eLife* 9:e46756. doi: 10.7554/elife.46756

Tadokoro, S., Ide, S., Tokuyama, R., Umeki, H., Tatehara, S., Kataoka, S., et al. (2015). Leptin promotes wound healing in the skin. *PLoS One* 10:e0121242. doi: 10.1371/journal.pone.0121242

Takada, K., Komine-Aizawa, S., Hirohata, N., Trinh, Q. D., Nishina, A., Kimura, H., et al. (2017). Poly I:C induces collective migration of HaCaT keratinocytes via IL-8. *BMC Immunol.* 18:19. doi: 10.1186/s12865-017-0202-3

Takahashi, N., Vereecke, L., Bertrand, M. J. M., Duprez, L., Berger, S. B., Divert, T., et al. (2014). RIPK1 ensures intestinal homeostasis by protecting the epithelium against apoptosis. *Nature* 513, 95–99. doi: 10.1038/nature13706

Takeo, M., Lee, W., and Ito, M. (2015). Wound healing and skin regeneration. *Cold Spring Harb. Perspect. Med.* 5, a023267. doi: 10.1101/cshperspect.a023267

Telerman, S. B., Rognoni, E., Sequeira, I., Pisco, A. O., Lichtenberger, B. M., Culley, O. J., et al. (2017). Dermal Blimp1 acts downstream of epidermal TGFβ and Wnt/β-catenin to regulate hair follicle formation and growth. *J. Invest. Dermatol.* 137, 2270–2281. doi: 10.1016/j.jid.2017.06.015

Terskikh, V. V., Vasiliev, A. V., and Vorotelyak, E. A. (2012). Label retaining cells and cutaneous stem cells. *Stem Cell Rev. Rep.* 8, 414–425. doi: 10.1007/s12015-011-9299-6

Thornton, F. J., Schaffer, M. R., Witte, M. B., Moldawer, L. L., MacKay, S. L., Abouhamze, A., et al. (1998). Enhanced collagen accumulation following direct transfection of the inducible nitric oxide synthase gene in cutaneous wounds. *Biochem. Biophys. Res. Commun.* 246, 654–659. doi: 10.1006/bbrc.1998.8681

Tong, X., and Coulombe, P. A. (2006). Keratin 17 modulates hair follicle cycling in a TNF-dependent fashion. *Genes Dev.* 20, 1353–1364. doi: 10.1101/gad.1387406

Valente Duarte de Sousa, I. C., and Tosti, A. (2013). New investigational drugs for androgenetic alopecia. *Expert Opin. Investig. Drugs* 22, 573–589. doi: 10.1517/13543784.2013.784743

Vande Walle, L., and Lamkanfi, M. (2016). Pyroptosis. *Curr. Biol.* 26, R568–R572. doi: 10.1016/j.cub.2016.02.019

Varfolomeev, E., and Vucic, D. (2018). Intracellular regulation of TNF activity in health and disease. *Cytokine* 101, 26–32. doi: 10.1016/j.cyto.2016.08.035

Wang, E. C. E., Dai, Z., Ferrante, A. W., Drake, C. G., and Christiano, A. M. (2019). A subset of TREM2+ dermal macrophages secretes oncostatin M to maintain hair follicle stem cell quiescence and Inhibit Hair Growth. *Cell Stem Cell* 24, 654–669.e6. doi: 10.1016/j.stem.2019.01.011

Wang, E. C. E., and Higgins, C. A. (2020). Immune cell regulation of the hair cycle. *Exp. Dermatol.* 29, 322–333. doi: 10.1111/exd.14070

Wang, X., Chen, H., Tian, R., Zhang, Y., Drutskaya, M. S., Wang, C., et al. (2017). Macrophages induce AKT/β-catenin-dependent Lgr5+ stem cell activation and hair follicle regeneration through TNF. *Nat. Commun.* 8:14091. doi: 10.1038/ncomms14091

Welle, M. M., and Wiener, D. J. (2016). The hair follicle. *Toxicol. Pathol.* 44, 564–574. doi: 10.1177/0192623316631843

Werner, S., and Grose, R. (2003). Regulation of wound healing by growth factors and cytokines. *Physiol. Rev.* 83, 835–870. doi: 10.1152/physrev.2003.83.3.835

Wolf, R., Schönfelder, G., Paul, M., and Blume-Peytavi, U. (2003). Nitric oxide in the human hair follicle: constitutive and dihydrotestosterone-induced nitric oxide synthase expression and NO production in dermal papilla cells. *J. Mol. Med.* 81, 110–117. doi: 10.1007/s00109-002-0402-y

Xu, F., Zhang, C., and Graves, D. T. (2013). Abnormal cell responses and role of TNF-α in impaired diabetic wound healing. *Biomed Res. Int.* 2013:754802. doi: 10.1155/2013/754802

Yamao, M., Inamatsu, M., Okada, T., Ogawa, Y., Ishida, Y., Tateno, C., et al. (2015). Restorative effect of hair follicular dermal cells on injured human hair follicles in a mouse model. *Exp. Dermatol.* 24, 225–227. doi: 10.1111/exd.12625

Zaiss, D. M., Minutti, C. M., and Knipper, J. A. (2019). Immune- and non-immune-mediated roles of regulatory T-cells during wound healing. *Immunology* 157, 190–197. doi: 10.1111/imm.13057

Zhang, J., Yang, X., Wang, H., Zhao, B., Wu, X., Su, L., et al. (2017). PKCζ as a promising therapeutic target for TNFα-induced inflammatory disorders in chronic cutaneous wounds. *Int. J. Mol. Med.* 40, 1335–1346. doi: 10.3892/ijmm.2017.3144

Zhao, J., Li, H., Zhou, R., Ma, G., Dekker, J. D., Tucker, H. O., et al. (2015). Foxp1 regulates the proliferation of hair follicle stem cells in response to oxidative stress during hair cycling. *PLoS One* 10:e0131674. doi: 10.1371/journal.pone.0131674

Zhao, R., Liang, H., Clarke, E., Jackson, C., and Xue, M. (2016). Inflammation in chronic wounds. *Int. J. Mol. Sci.* 17:2085. doi: 10.3390/ijms17122085

Zheng, M., Jang, Y., Choi, N., Kim, D. Y., Han, T. W., Yeo, J. H., et al. (2019). Hypoxia improves hair inductivity of dermal papilla cells via nuclear NADPH oxidase 4-mediated reactive oxygen species generation'. *Br. J. Dermatol.* 181, 523–534. doi: 10.1111/bjd.17706

Zhu, A. S., Li, A., Ratliff, T. S., Melsom, M., and Garza, L. A. (2017). After skin wounding, Noncoding dsRNA coordinates prostaglandins and wnts to promote regeneration. *J. Invest. Dermatol.* 137, 1562–1568. doi: 10.1016/j.jid.2017.03.023

Zhu, H., Wei, X., Bian, K., and Murad, F. (2008). Effects of nitric oxide on skin burn wound healing. *J. Burn Care Res.* 29, 804–814. doi: 10.1097/bcr.0b013e3181848119

Zhu, H. J., Li, Y. S., Wang, Y. P., Hu, X. H., Zhang, X. R., Qiu, L., et al. (2019). Effects of skin γδ T lymphocytes on wound healing of mice through regulating proliferation and differentiation of mice epidermal cells. *Zhonghua Shao Shang Za Zhi* 35, 298–307. doi: 10.3760/cma.j.issn.1009-2587.2019.04.010

Conflict of Interest: The authors declare that the research was conducted in the absence of any commercial or financial relationships that could be construed as a potential conflict of interest.

5

Molecular regulation of auditory hair cell death and approaches to protect sensory receptor cells and/or stimulate repair following acoustic trauma

Christine T. Dinh[1], *Stefania Goncalves*[1], *Esperanza Bas*[1], *Thomas R. Van De Water*[1] and *Azel Zine*[2,3]*

[1] University of Miami Ear Institute, University of Miami Miller School of Medicine, Miami, FL, USA, [2] Integrative and Adaptive Neurosciences, Aix-Marseille Université, CNRS, UMR 7260, Marseille, France, [3] Faculty of Pharmacy, Biophysics Department, University of Montpellier, Montpellier, France

Edited by:
Allison B. Coffin,
Washington State University, USA

Reviewed by:
Richardson N. Leão,
Brain Institute, Brazil
Dale Warren Hailey,
University or Washington, USA

***Correspondence:**
Azel Zine,
Integrative and Adaptive Neurosciences, Aix-Marseille Université, CNRS, UMR 7260, 3 Place Victor Hugo, 13331 Marseille Cedex 03, France
azel.zine@univ-amu.fr

Loss of auditory sensory hair cells (HCs) is the most common cause of hearing loss. This review addresses the signaling pathways that are involved in the programmed and necrotic cell death of auditory HCs that occur in response to ototoxic and traumatic stressor events. The roles of inflammatory processes, oxidative stress, mitochondrial damage, cell death receptors, members of the mitogen-activated protein kinase (MAPK) signal pathway and pro- and anti-cell death members of the Bcl-2 family are explored. The molecular interaction of these signal pathways that initiates the loss of auditory HCs following acoustic trauma is covered and possible therapeutic interventions that may protect these sensory HCs from loss via apoptotic or non-apoptotic cell death are explored.

Keywords: trauma, cochlea, auditory hair cells, apoptosis, inflammation, necrosis, otoprotection, repair

Introduction

Auditory hair cells (HCs) are important for the conversion of acoustic sound energy into electrical impulses that travel to the auditory centers of the brain for hearing. Sensorineural hearing loss (SNHL) is a form of hearing impairment that occurs most commonly from damagedHCs within the cochlea; it is a prevalent disability, affecting one in five people and more than 48 million Americans (Lin et al., 2011). There are numerous causes of acquired SNHL. Some of these etiologies include viral infections, platinum-based chemotherapeutic agents, aminoglycoside antibiotics, acoustic trauma, labyrinthine concussion, cochlear hypoxia, radiation exposure, cochlear implant electrode insertion trauma, and meningitis (Kuhn et al., 2011). Genetic mutations can also cause structural or physiologic abnormalities within the cochlea and impair cochlear homeostasis. These insults to the inner ear can promote cell death of auditory HCs and hearing loss.

Several signaling cascades are activated following an insult to the cochlea; these pathways can be pro-inflammatory, pro-death, and even pro-survival. The signaling cascades that occur on a cellular and a molecular level are highly complex and in many ways entwine; there is significant cross communication between pathways and it is the culmination of all of these activities that tilt the pendulum of cell survival and cell death in one direction or the other.

Although there has been great progress in understanding the pathways of cell death in auditory HCs, several pro-death concepts are still speculative and extrapolated from studies of other cell types. As research in necrobiology of the inner ear progresses, these pathways specific to auditory HC death will be more stream-lined and refined. This review will discuss general concepts and pathways in apoptosis and necrosis that contribute to the understanding of key events in acoustic trauma. Several drug therapies take advantage of key events that occur following acoustic injury by targeting, promoting, or inhibiting different pathways that favor cell survival.

Cell Death

Auditory HCs undergo cell death through apoptosis and necrosis, in response to different insults to the inner ear. Apoptosis is an organized form of programmed cell death that is characterized by blebbing of the cell membrane, shrinkage of the cell body, fragmentation of the nucleus, condensation of the chromatin, and cleavage of chromosomal DNA. The cell is then divided into numerous fragments called apoptotic bodies that are disposed by phagocytosis (**Figure 1**). Particular to HCs undergoing apoptotic cell death, mitochondria swell, stereocilia are disrupted and lost, cuticular plates shrink, and chromatin condensation occurs in the nucleus, prior to disruption of junctional complexes and extrusion of auditory HCs (Hirose et al., 2004). Necrosis, originally thought to be an uncontrolled process, is another form of cell death that appears to be highly regulated. During necrotic cell death, the cell volume increases, the organelles swell, and the plasma membrane ruptures. There is spillage of intracellular contents in the extracellular space and postlytic DNA fragmentation occurs (**Figure 1**). Necrosis of auditory HCs can occur in concert with mechanisms of apoptosis. Most of the molecular and cellular mechanisms responsible for apoptosis and necrosis in auditory HCs originate in studies of other cell types. A review of general concepts in apoptosis and necrosis and stress signaling is offered below.

Apoptosis

Apoptosis can occur through two different signaling cascades, called the intrinsic [mitochondrial death] and extrinsic [death receptor, DR] pathways. These two particular pathways can interweave and can promote synergism in cell death in many contexts (Roy and Nicholson, 2000).

Intrinsic Pathway

In the intrinsic pathway, a stress signal initiates a disturbance between the pro- and anti-apoptotic proteins of the Bcl-2 family that promote supramolecular openings or activation of mega-channels in the outer membrane of the mitochondria (Marzo et al., 1998; Kuwana et al., 2002). In particular, Bcl-2-like protein 4 (Bax) activation is a key regulator of this phenomenon. This results in the release of pro-death proteins from the intermembrane space of the mitochondria into the cytosol. These regulatory mitochondrial proteins that are liberated into the cytoplasm can activate both caspase-dependent and caspase-independent cell death pathways. These proteins include cytochrome *c* (cyt *c*), endonuclease G (EndoG), apoptosis inducing factor (AIF), second mitochondria-derived activator of caspases/direct inhibitor of apoptosis protein binding protein with low pI (Smac/DIABLO), and mammalian homolog of bacterial high temperature requirement protein A2 (Omi/HtrA2; **Figure 2**).

When released into the cytoplasm, cyt *c* binds with apoptotic protease-activating factor-1 (Apaf-1) and recruits pro-caspase-9 to form an apoptosome (Cain et al., 2000). This apoptosome can induce caspase-3 dependent apoptosis (Bratton et al., 2001). Subsequently, caspase-3 initiates apoptosis by promoting DNA fragmentation through caspase-activated DNase (CAD), chromatin condensation via apoptotic chromatin condensation inducer in the nucleus (ACINUS), and acceleration of DNA degradation through cleavage of cytosolic helicase with an N-terminal caspase-recruitment domain (HELI-CARD; Liu et al., 1997; Enari et al., 1998; Sahara et al., 1999; Kovacsovics et al., 2002).

EndoG is a mitochondrion-specific nuclease that translocates into the nucleus and works in concert with exonucleases and DNAse I to ensure efficient nucleosomal fragmentation of DNA, independent of caspase activation (Li et al., 2001; Widlak et al., 2001). Similar to EndoG, AIF is also a caspase-independent death effector; once released into the cytosol, AIF migrates into the nucleus to stimulate chromatin condensation and large scale DNA fragmentation (Lorenzo et al., 1999; Daugas et al., 2000).

Smac and Omi/HtrA2 are similar because both promote caspase-dependent apoptosis by binding and inhibiting X-linked inhibitor of apoptosis protein (XIAP). XIAP is a cytosolic protein that has three baculoviral inhibitory repeat (BIR) domains—BIR1 and BIR2 specifically bind and inhibit caspase-3 and -7, while BIR3 is a specific inhibitor of caspase-9 (Deveraux et al., 1999). Smac functions by neutralizing the caspase-inhibiting properties of XIAP, thereby promoting caspase-3, -7, and -9 activations (Chai et al., 2000, 2001). Similar to Smac, Omi/HtrA2 competes with caspase -3, -7, and -9 for XIAP binding and therefore promotes caspase-dependent cell death (Suzuki et al., 2001; Hegde et al., 2002). However, Omi/HtrA2 is a ubiquitously expressed mitochondrial serine protease that can also promote apoptosis through caspase-independent activity through alternate mechanisms that rely on its serine protease properties (Li et al., 2002).

Extrinsic Death Pathway

The extrinsic cell death pathway is intricate and involves several molecular interactions that occur in succession: (1) binding of a death ligand to its complementary receptor; (2) recruitment of adaptor molecules such as FAS-associated death domain protein (FADD) and tumor necrosis factor receptor type 1-associated death domain protein (TRADD); (3) binding, dimerizing, and activation of initiator caspase-8 and -10; and (4) formation of a death-inducing signaling complex (DISC; Itoh and Nagata, 1993; Tartaglia et al., 1993; Chinnaiyan et al., 1995; Hsu et al., 1995; Nagata, 1999; Fischer et al., 2006). DISC is a multi-protein

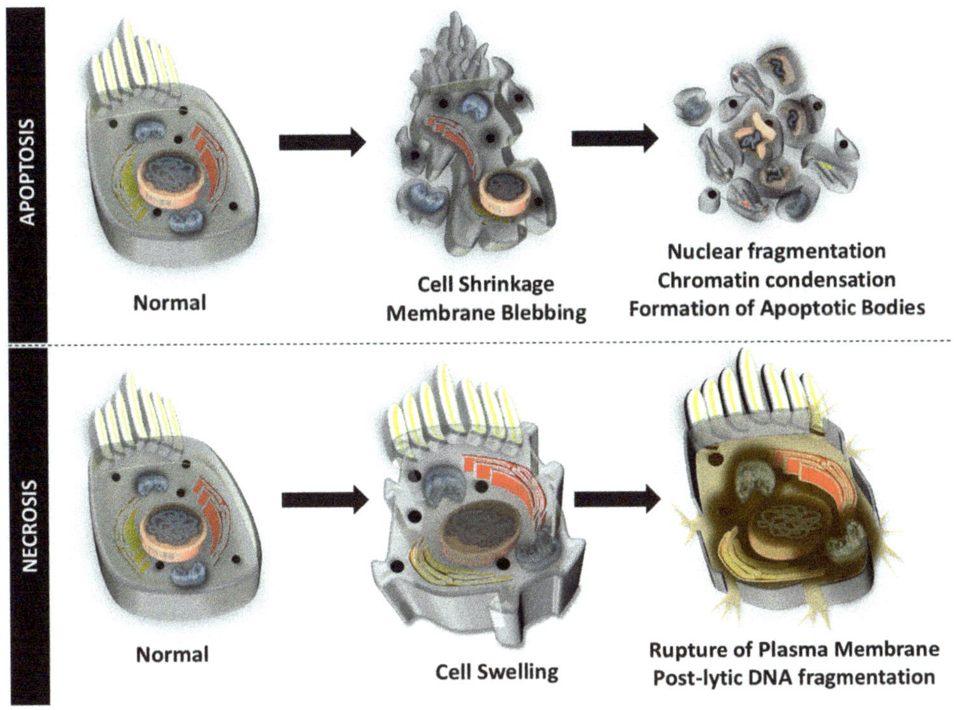

FIGURE 1 | Apoptotic and necrotic cell death. Apoptosis is an organized form of programmed cell death that is characterized by shrinkage of the cell body, blebbing of the cell membrane, chromatin condensation, fragmentation of the nucleus, cleavage of chromosomal DNA, and division into numerous cell fragments (apoptotic bodies).Necrosis occurs when the volume of the cell increases, organelles swell, the plasma membrane ruptures, intracellular contents spill into the extracellular matrix, and there is postlytic DNA fragmentation.

complex that subsequently cleaves and promotes executioner caspase-3 and -7 activities to promote programmed cell death (**Figure 2**).

The most well recognized and studied death ligands include TNFα and FasL or CD95L. Their complementary receptors are TNFR1, also known as p55 or CD120a and Fas receptor (FasR, also referred to as CD95 or apoptosis antigen 1, APO-1), respectively (Itoh and Nagata, 1993; Tartaglia et al., 1993). Other DRs that have been described include TNF-like receptor apoptosis mediating protein (TRAMP, also called DR3, APO-3), TNF-related apoptosis inducing ligand receptors-1 (TRAIL-R1 or DR4) and -2 (TRAIL-R2, also named DR5 and APO-2), and DR6 (Bodmer et al., 1997; Guicciardi and Gores, 2009).

Initiators caspase-8 and caspase-10 can cleave and activate effector caspase-3 to initiate programmed cell death (Ng et al., 1999; Wang et al., 2001; Fischer et al., 2006). Caspase-8 can also promote effector caspase-7 activity. In addition, both caspase-8 and caspase-10 can cleave Bcl-2 homology 3 interacting domain death agonist (BID) into truncated BID (tBID) that triggers mitochondrial cell death pathways mediated by Bax and Bcl-2 homologous antagonist killer (Bak) activation (Chandler et al., 1998; Li et al., 1998; Luo et al., 1998; Korsmeyer et al., 2000; Kandasamy et al., 2003; Milhas et al., 2005). Bax and Bak are pro-death proteins that belong to the Bcl-2 family of proteins that can stimulate mitochondrial release of pro-apoptotic proteins such as cyt *c* and Smac. There are likely other levels of modulation between the intrinsic and extrinsic pathways of apoptosis that have not yet been discovered.

Necrosis

Mechanisms of regulated necrosis include necroptosis and MPT. Parthanatos, ferroptosis and pyroptosis have also been described as mechanisms of non-apoptotic cell death; however, they may not represent distinct forms of necrosis (Galluzzi et al., 2012; Vanden Berghe et al., 2014; **Figure 2**).

Necroptosis

Receptor interacting protein kinases (RIPK) are important regulators of cell survival and cell death. Necroptosis refers to a RIPK3-dependent molecular cascade of events that promotes regulated necrotic cell death (Galluzzi et al., 2012). Necroptosis and apoptosis share similar upstream signaling elements and regulator molecules such as Fas-associated death domain-like interleukin-1β-converting enzyme-like inhibitory proteins (FLIP) and cellular inhibitors of apoptosis proteins 1 and 2 (cIAP1 and cIAP2; McComb et al., 2012; Silke and Strasser, 2013). When caspase-8 is inhibited by genetic manipulation or pharmacologic therapies, RIPK3 is recruited to RIPK1 to form a necrosis-inducing complex (necrosome) that phosphorylates pseudokinase mixed lineage kinase domain-like protein (MLKL) and engages in downstream activities that lead to RIPK1/RIPK3 dependent necroptosis (He et al., 2009; Zhang et al., 2009;

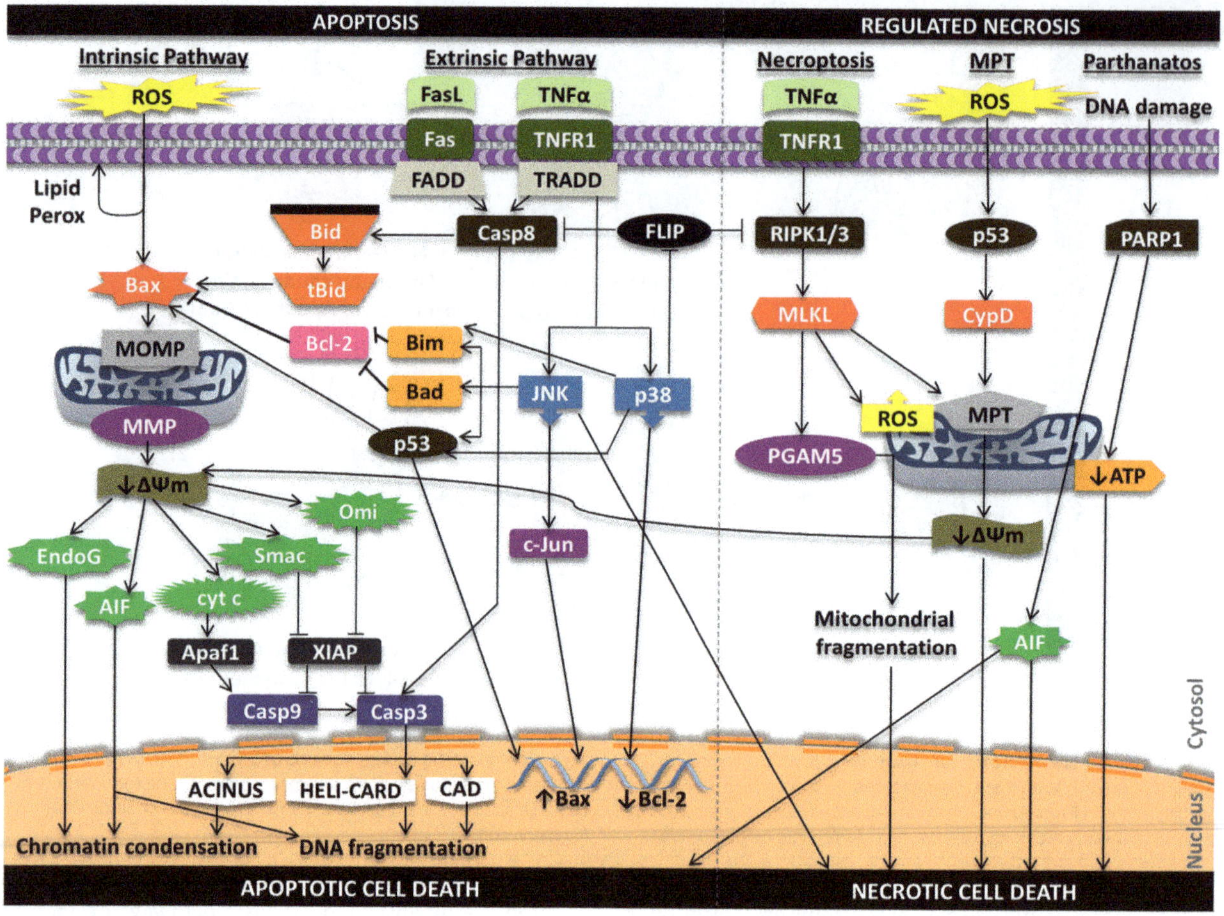

FIGURE 2 | Signaling in apoptosis and regulated necrosis. ROS can promote lipid peroxidation of the phosopholipid membrane, proteolytic degradation, and mitochondrial and cellular DNA damage that can propagate the apoptotic effects of oxidative stress. Oxidative stress can activate pro-apoptotic Bax protein that initiates damage to the outer mitochondrial membrane (i.e., pore formation) that results in release of pro-death proteins from the mitochondria into the cytosol that act in caspase-independent and caspase-dependent mechanisms to induce chromatin condensation, DNA fragmentation and intrinsic apoptotic cell death. Ligands such as Fas ligand (FasL) and tumor necrosis factor alpha (TNFα) can promote extrinsic programmed cell death through caspase-8 activation and downstream caspase-3 activity, while also triggering intrinsic apoptosis through truncation of Bid (tBid). Tumor necrosis factor receptor type 1 (TNFR1) signaling can induce phosphorylation and activation of p38 and JNK that can lead to Bax-mediated mitochondrial cell death and phosphorylation of transcription factors that increase pro-death and reduce pro-survival gene expression. Activation of TNFR1 can also initiate a RIPK1 and RIPK3-dependent form of regulated necrosis (necroptosis) through regulation of PGAM5, ROS, and the mitochondrial permeability transition (MPT). MPT-mediated regulated necrotic cell death can be triggered following oxidative stress; downstream signaling results in activation of cyclophilin D (CypD), increased permeability of the inner mitochondrial membrane, and mitochondrial swelling and rupture that promotes necrosis. Alterations in the transmembrane potential of the mitochondria can also induce intrinsic cell death. Lastly, hyper-activation of PARP1 from persistent DNA damage that can inhibit mitochondrial ATP synthesis and promote mitochondrial release of AIF to initiate necrotic form of cell death. AIF, in this situation, can promote both apoptosis and necrosis. $\Delta\Psi m$, mitochondrial membrane potential; Casp3, caspase-3; Casp8, caspase-8; Casp9, caspase-9; MMP, mitochondrial membrane permeability; MOMP, mitochondrial outer membrane permeability.

Vandenabeele et al., 2010). The events that occur downstream to promote necroptosis are controversial, convoluted, and poorly characterized, but may include production of mitochondrial reactive oxygen species (ROS), activation of mitochondrial phosphatase, i.e., PGAM5, and induction of MPT (Wang et al., 2012a,b; Marshall and Baines, 2014). PGAM5 is a mitochondrial protein phosphatase that can activate dynamin related protein 1 (Drp1) and its GTPase activity, which can stimulate fragmentation of mitochondria and execution of necrosis (Wang et al., 2012a,b).

Mitochondrial Permeability Transition

The MPT refers to an abrupt increase in the permeability of the inner mitochondrial membrane to small solutes that lead to osmotic influx of water into the mitochondrial matrix, mitochondrial swelling and rupture of the outer mitochondrial membrane (Tsujimoto and Shimizu, 2007). Although it is not well characterized, cyclophilin D (CypD; also known as peptidylprolyl isomerase F) is believed to be crucial in the formation of the permeability transition pore complex associated with MPT-dependent necrosis (Li et al., 2004; Baines et al.,

2005; Nakagawa et al., 2005). Interestingly, the shift in the transmembrane potential in MPT can also initiate intrinsic cell death by halting the bioenergetics and redox functions of the mitochondria and initiating release of pro-apoptotic mitochondrial proteins into the cytosol (Marchetti et al., 1996; Scarlett and Murphy, 1997; Brenner and Grimm, 2006; Kroemer et al., 2007).

Other Forms of Non-Apoptotic Cell Death

Parthanatos is a poly(ADP-ribose) polymerase 1 (PARP1) dependent form of non-apoptotic death. PARP1 is recruited to sites of DNA damage where it is able to catalyze ADP ribosylation of various proteins and histones and generate negative charges by overconsumption of nicotinamide adenine dinucleotide (NAD) during the ADP ribosylation process. Ultimately, other factors important for DNA repair are recruited. However, when PARP1 becomes hyper-activated in situations of persistent DNA damage, there is a depletion of NAD and inhibition of mitochondrial ATP synthesis, which is essential in ATP-dependent apoptosis pathways (Yu et al., 2006; Wang et al., 2011). Overactivation of PARP-1 can lead to unregulated synthesis of poly (ADP-ribose) (PAR) that can bind to and initiate release of AIF into the cytoplasm. PARP-1 mediated AIF expression can promote DNA condensation and widespread cell death that is independent of caspases and distinct from apoptosis (Andrabi et al., 2008). There is controversy whether parthanatos represents a form of regulated necrosis or is a distinct entity.

Ferroptosis refers to an iron-dependent form of non-apoptotic cell death that is morphologically, biochemically, and genetically different from both apoptosis and necrosis (Dixon et al., 2012). Pyroptosis refers to caspase-1 dependent cell death that exhibits a spectrum of morphotypes that range from necrosis to purely apoptosis (Kepp et al., 2010). Caspase-1 is activated through a supramolecular complex called a pyroptosome or inflammasome and is thought to cause pore formation in the plasma membrane that leads to osmotic cell lysis (necrosis) and activation of caspase-7 (apoptosis) (Fink and Cookson, 2006; Fernandes-Alnemri et al., 2007; Lamkanfi et al., 2008). The elements behind regulated necrosis are still unclear; however, research in this topic has become more and more prevalent especially in the context of cancer research.

Auditory Hair Cell Death

Depending on the cochlear insult, various elements of the apoptotic and necrotic cell death pathway are activated (Op de Beeck et al., 2011; **Figure 1**). In acoustic trauma, loss of auditory HCs occur through direct mechanical injury and activation of apoptosis and necrosis related pathways (Saunders et al., 1985; Pirvola et al., 2000; Yang et al., 2004). Intense noise exposure can displace the tympanic membrane, vibrate the ossicles, and create large displacements of the basilar membrane that can sheer and injure stereocilia, auditory HCs, and supporting cells of the organ of Corti important for hearing. Downstream stress signaling from acoustic trauma are activated, including expression of free radicals and pro-inflammatory factors that trigger both apoptotic and necrotic cell death (discussed in subsequent sections). Following intense noise exposure Bax activation promotes mitochondrial release of pro-apoptotic factors (i.e., cyt *c*, AIF, and EndoG), caspase-3 activation, and intrinsic cell death (Nicotera et al., 2003; Yamashita et al., 2004a,b; Han et al., 2006; Wang et al., 2007a,b). Acoustic trauma also stimulates TNFR1 and Fas DR signaling that activates downstream pathway leading to caspase-8 activity and extrinsic apoptotic cell death (Nicotera et al., 2003; Fujioka et al., 2006; Jamesdaniel et al., 2011). Although the molecular mechanisms are still unclear, necrosis of outer HCs occur early following acoustic trauma and persist weeks after acoustic trauma (Yang et al., 2004; Hu et al., 2006). Lastly, intense noise exposure can also promote loss of auditory HCs through HC extrusion (Cotanche et al., 1997).

Although there are several drugs that can injure auditory HCs, the most commonly encountered ototoxic drugs are aminoglycosides and cisplatin. In brief, aminoglycoside antibiotics, such as gentamicin, amikacin, kanamycin, and neomycin, can initiate apoptotic cell death in auditory HCs and vestibular HCs. In particular, the outer HCs of the basal turn are the most vulnerable to aminoglycoside ototoxicity. The most predominant form of cell death is apoptosis, however necrotic features are also seen following exposure to aminoglycosides (Jiang et al., 2006). Aminoglycosides can induce mitochondrial apoptotic cell death and DNA fragmentation through oxidative stress, Bax activation, mitochondrial release of cyt *c* and caspase-3 activity (Mangiardi et al., 2004; Matsui et al., 2004; Coffin et al., 2013). Evidence for the role of caspase-8 and extrinsic apoptosis is aminoglycoside ototoxicity is not strong (Tabuchi et al., 2007; Ding et al., 2010).

Cisplatin is a platinum-based chemotherapeutic drug used to treat cancer and can promote ototoxicity, nephrotoxicity, and even neurotoxicity. Cisplatin predominantly affects the outer HCs of the basal turn of the cochlea; spiral ganglion neurons are affected by this drug. Similar to aminoglycosides, cisplatin stimulates free radical production in the cochlea that leads to Bax activation, mitochondrial release of cyt *c*, caspase activation, and intrinsic apoptotic cell death (Rybak et al., 2007). Unfortunately, regulated necrosis and potential pathways associated with this form of cell death are still unclear in the field of cell biology. The contribution of pathways described in regulated necrosis is still speculative in cochlear injury. Progress in necrobiology research can improve our understanding of necrosis in auditory HCs.

Stress Signaling in Auditory Hair Cell Death

There are several signaling pathways that are involved in apoptosis and necrosis of auditory HCs, including (1) expression of extracellular pro-inflammatory cytokines such as tumor necrosis factor alpha (TNFα) and recruited of neutrophils and macrophages to the cochlea; and (2) generation of oxidative stress in the form of ROS and reactive nitrogen species (RNS) such as superoxide ($O_2^{\cdot-}$), peroxynitrite ($ONOO^-$), and hydroxyl ($OH^\cdot$) radicals (**Figure 2**). These stress signals can activate intrinsic and extrinsic apoptotic cell death of auditory HCs as well as initiate molecular mechanisms for necrosis. Although signaling mechanisms discussed are extrapolated from studies investigating the effects of various cochlear insults on apoptosis and necrosis in auditory HCs and studies of other cell types, many of these pathways are relevant and expressed following acoustic trauma. Studies pertaining to stress signaling in the cochlea are bolded in subsequent sections.

Inflammatory Cytokines and Chemokines

Several cytokines and chemokines are upregulated in the cochlea following an inner ear insult. TNFα is one of the most well studied and possibly most important cytokines as it possesses pro-inflammatory properties and can also initiated cell death of auditory HCs. TNFα is expressed within the cochlea during acoustic trauma, cisplatin ototoxicity, aminoglycoside exposure, electrode insertion trauma, autoimmune inner ear disease, as well as various other traumas to the inner ear (Ichimiya et al., 2000; Satoh et al., 2002, 2003; Aminpour et al., 2005; Zou et al., 2005; Fujioka et al., 2006; Van Wijk et al., 2006; So et al., 2007; Bas et al., 2009, 2012a,b).

Following a cochlear insult, the stria vascularis and spiral ligament express and release TNFα, which promotes leukocyte migration through the spiral modiolar vein and tributaries (Keithley et al., 2008). TNFα also stimulates expression of other cytokines, chemokines, and adhesion molecules such as interleukin (IL)-1β, IL-6, monocyte chemoattractant protein-1 (MCP-1), macrophage inflammatory protein-2 (MIP-2), soluble intercellular adhesion molecule-1 (siCAM-1), vascular cell adhesion molecule-1 (VCAM-1), intercellular adhesion molecule-1 (ICAM-1), and vascular endothelial growth factor (VEGF; Yoshida et al., 1999; Ichimiya et al., 2000, 2003; Maeda et al., 2005). These inflammatory mediators can promote migration and adhesion of inflammatory cells such as neutrophils, monocytes, macrophages, lymphocytes, eosinophils, basophils, and even natural killer cells. (Taub et al., 1995; Proost et al., 1996; Mutsaers et al., 1997; Deshmane et al., 2009). These inflammatory cells are themselves a major source of cytokines and chemokines, creating a positive feedback loop that propagates and intensifies the inflammatory process.

In particular, expression of TNFα can promote neutrophil migration, adhesion, and generation of superoxide free radicals in the cochlea (Tsujimoto et al., 1986; Figari et al., 1987). Neutrophils, one type of polymorphonuclear white blood cell, are among the first immune cells to arrive in response to inflammation. They relesase a number of pro-inflammatory cytokines that stimulate migration of other immune cells, such as monocytes (Mutsaers et al., 1997). In response to local cytokines, monocytes will differentiate into M1 and M2 macrophages. M1 macrophages are primarily involved in clearance of injured cells; they can secrete inflammatory factors, stimulate inducible nitrous oxide synthetase (iNOS) activity, and generate oxidative stress in the form of ROS and RNS that can diffuse into surrounding tissue. M2 macrophages are known to release several growth factors from the transforming growth factor-beta (TGF-β) family of proteins, which are important for initiation of a fibroproliferative response, wound healing, and tissue repair (Mahdavian Delavary et al., 2011).

Not only is TNFα a leukocyte attractant; extracellular TNFα can bind to tumor necrosis factor receptor 1 (TNFR1) on the cell surface of auditory HCs and initiate a signaling cascade that can lead to cell death (Dinh et al., 2008a,b, 2011, 2013; Haake et al., 2009; **Figure 2**). Adaptor protein TRADD, receptor interacting protein (RIP), and FADD are recruited along with caspase-8 to form a DISC that cleaves and activates caspase-3 and -7 and triggers extrinsic apoptosis. TNFα-mediated Bax activation and intrinsic programmed cell death also occurs, likely through truncation of Bid.

The binding of TNFα to TNFR1 can also promote formation of another signaling complex consisting of TNFR1, TRADD, RIP, and TNF receptor-associated factor 2 (TRAF2) that promotes mitogen-activated protein kinase (MAPK) and nuclear factor kappa B (NFkB) signaling (Shen and Pervaiz, 2006). NFkB is a transcription factor that can mediate cellular inflammation, proliferation, and apoptosis. When activated, NFkB can translocate into the nucleus of an affected cell and activate transcription of several genes that are pro-inflammatory, pro-survival and pro-death, depending on the cell type (Pahl, 1999). TNFα initiates NFkB signaling in an attempt to block cell death by up regulation of pro-survival genes Bcl-2 and Bcl-xL in auditory HCs (Haake et al., 2009; Dinh et al., 2011).

High levels of IL-1beta (β) have also been detected in OC and cochlea following various inner ear challenges such as exposure to gentamicin, electrode insertion trauma, and autoimmune responses mediated by inner ear tissues (Pathak et al., 2011; Bas et al., 2012a,b). This cytokine can promote formation of a pyroptosome or inflammasome that mediates caspase-1 dependent cell death via pyroptosis (Brough and Rothwell, 2007). As discussed earlier, caspase-1 activation can promote apoptosis by inducing caspase-7 activity or necrosis through pore formation in the cell membrane and cell lysis through an osmotic imbalance (Fink and Cookson, 2006; Fernandes-Alnemri et al., 2007; Lamkanfi et al., 2008). In summary, TNFα expression in the cochlea can promote a robust inflammatory response and activation of downstream pro-apoptotic cell signaling that can promote cell death of auditory HCs. Blocking TNFα expression and associated signaling cascades may mitigate the inflammatory and pro-death responses in the cochlea. In particular, glucocorticoids have been shown to reduce inflammatory cell trafficking as well as inhibit TNFα-mediated downstream pathways of cell death (Dinh et al., 2008a,b; Haake et al., 2009). Steroids can also activate NFkB signaling that promotes cell survival pathways following TNFα-induced death of auditory HCs (Dinh et al., 2011). Inhibition of Bax expression by short interfering RNA can also abrogate TNFα-mediated HC loss (Dinh et al., 2013).

MAPK Signaling

In response to TNFα, auditory HCs can initiate MAPK signaling pathways. There are several distinct groups of MAPKs; however, the most extensively studied MAPKs are extracellular signal-regulated kinases (ERK) 1 and 2 (ERK1/2), c-Jun N-terminal kinases (JNK 1, 2, and 3), and p38 kinases (Roux and Blenis, 2004). Growth factors are the primary initiators of ERK1/2 activation, while JNK and p38 activities are stimulated by a number of physical and chemical stressors such as oxidative stress, UV irradiation, hypoxia, and various inflammatory

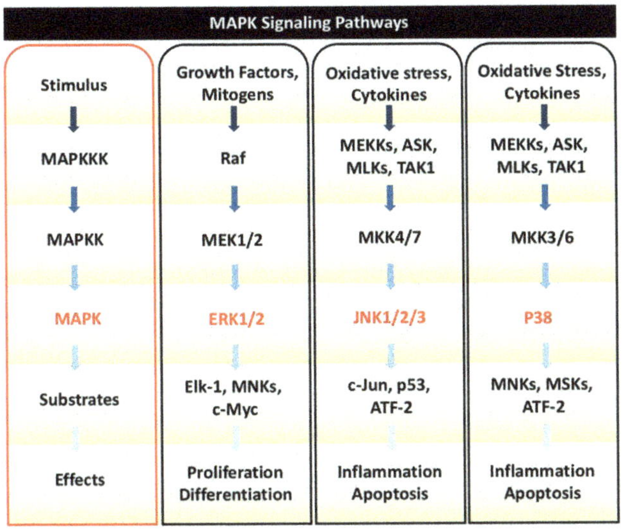

FIGURE 3 | MAPK Signaling. There are three tiers of protein kinases that comprise each family of MAPKs: (1) MAPK; (2) MAPK kinase (MAPKK); and (3) MAPKK kinase (MAPKKK). Following a specific stimulus, MAPKKK phosphorylates and activates MAPKK, which then phosphorylates and activates MAPK to then phosphorylate target substrates that can regulate cellular proliferation, survival, inflammation, and cell death. The three main classes of MAPK include ERK1/2, JNK1/2/3, and p38. Oxidative stress and cytokines such as TNFα can trigger JNK and p38 to phosphorylate downstream transcription factors that initiate pro-death and pro-inflammatory signaling and gene transcription.

cytokines including TNFα (Chen et al., 2001; Kyriakis and Avruch, 2001). There are three tiers of protein kinases that comprise each family of MAPKs: (1) MAPK; (2) MAPK kinase (MAPKK); and (3) MAPKK kinase (MAPKKK; **Figure 3**). MAPKKK phosphorylates and activates MAPKK, which then phosphorylates and activates MAPK to then phosphorylate target substrates (Keshet and Seger, 2010).

While ERK1/2 signaling has been implicated in cell proliferation and survival, TNFα activation of JNK and p38 signaling cascades promotes downstream events associated with cell death (Wajant et al., 2003). P38 is a mediator of apoptosis and it does so through several transcriptional and posttranscriptional molecular mechanisms. P38 activation can promote Bax mRNA and protein expression while phosphorylating and deactivating pro-survival Bcl-2 protein, thereby stimulating Bax-mediated mitochondrial apoptosis and cyt *c* release (Porras et al., 2004; Capano and Crompton, 2006; Markou et al., 2009; Owens et al., 2009). Pro-death factors such as Bcl-2-like protein 11 (Bim, a pro-apoptotic regulator), FasL, and FasR have also been positively regulated following p38 MAPK activation to stress stimuli (Hsu et al., 1999; Stephanou et al., 2001; Porras et al., 2004; Cai et al., 2006). Through inhibition of cellular FLIP (c-FLIP) in the DISC of the extrinsic apoptotic pathway, p38 may also trigger Fas-mediated caspase-8 dependent programmed cell death (Tourian et al., 2004). There is some evidence that p38 may also promote apoptosis by blocking ERK1/2 signaling cascades associated with cell survival (Porras et al., 2004). Blocking p38 MAPK activity has been associated with protection against noise trauma, aminoglycoside, cisplatin, radiation and TNFα-induced ototoxicity (Wei et al., 2005; Tabuchi et al., 2010; Bas et al., 2012a,b; Park et al., 2012; Wang et al., 2012a,b; Maeda et al., 2013; Kim et al., 2014; Kurioka et al., 2014; Shin et al., 2014).

JNK has three isoforms: JNK1, JNK2, and JNK3. JNK1 and JNK2 are expressed ubiquitously while JNK3 is primarily localized to cardiac and neuronal tissues. In response to an extracellular stimulus, JNK signaling can promote apoptosis through two distinct mechanisms: one targeting the nucleus and the other targeting the mitochondria. JNK can translocate to the nucleus and phosphorylate c-Jun and other transcription factors such as p53, subsequently promoting expression of pro-apoptotic genes (such as TNFα, FasL, Bak, Bim, and Bax) and blocking transcription of anti-apoptotic genes (such as Bcl-2) (Faris et al., 1998; Budhram-Mahadeo et al., 1999; Eichhorst et al., 2000; Fan et al., 2001; Whitfield et al., 2001; Liu and Lin, 2005; Oleinik et al., 2007; Dhanasekaran and Reddy, 2008; Amaral et al., 2010). The JNK-mediated upregulation of pro-inflammatory and pro-apoptotic proteins and downregulation of pro-survival proteins can provide the necessary substrates for fueling pro-death cellular events.

In addition, activated JNK can phosphorylate a number of proteins that are intimately involved in mitochondrial cell death. By phosphorylating the pro-death proteins Bim and Bad, activated JNK can neutralize Bcl-2 and Bcl-xL protein inhibition while promoting Bax activation of intrinsic apoptotic cell death (Ottilie et al., 1997; Puthalakath et al., 1999; Donovan et al., 2002; Lei et al., 2002; Lei and Davis, 2003; Wang et al., 2007a,b). Furthermore, phosphorylated JNK can indirectly trigger pro-apoptotic Bax-mediated mitochondrial death signaling through truncation of Bid. The constellation of these events results in release of cyt *c*, Smac, and other mitochondrial pro-death proteins into the cytoplasm that promote caspase-dependent and -independent mechanisms of programmed cell death (Tournier et al., 2000; Madesh et al., 2002; Deng et al., 2003; Dhanasekaran and Reddy, 2008).

Although JNK activity is primarily linked to apoptotic cell death, prolonged JNK activation is thought to divert TNFα-induced cell death from apoptosis to necrosis. Elevated levels of ROS can promote prolonged JNK activation, while prolonged JNK signaling can lead to increased mitochondrial production of ROS, creating a positive feedback loop that favors TNFα-induced necrotic cell death (Sakon et al., 2003; Wajant et al., 2003; Ventura et al., 2004).

Similar to p38, JNK signaling is implicated in noise, aminoglycoside, cisplatin, radiation and TNFα-initiated loss of auditory HCs and with a resultant hearing loss. The insertion of an electrode array of a cochlea implant into the cochlea also exhibits effects of JNK and downstream molecular events. Direct inhibition of JNK by either CEP-1347 or D-JNKI-1 (aka AM-111) have demonstrated protection against HC and hearing losses following aminoglycoside, acoustic, and electrode insertion injury to the cochlea (Ylikoski et al., 2002; Wang et al., 2003, 2007a,b; Eshraghi et al., 2006, 2010; Jiang et al., 2006; Suckfuell et al., 2007). Indirect modulation of JNK activity by various drug therapies have been associated with HC and hearing protection (Nakamagoe et al., 2010; Pyun et al., 2011; Shin et al., 2014).

Oxidative Stress

ROS are free radicals containing oxygen. They are very reactive and in high amounts can damage cells. Extracellular ROS can be generated by activated phagocytes such as neutrophils, monocytes, and macrophages, and play a vital role in host defense against pathogens (Evans and Halliwell, 1999). Intracellular ROS are primarily produced by the cell's mitochondria (Turrens, 2003). Oxygen-derived free radicals can induce apoptosis and necrosis by peroxidation of a cell's phospholipid membranes, proteolytic degradation, and DNA damage in mitochondria and in the nucleus (Beckman and Ames, 1997; Kohen and Nyska, 2002).

Oxygen (O_2) contains two unpaired electrons. Superoxide anion ($O_2^-\cdot$) is the product of one electron reduction of O_2 and is the precursor for several ROS. $O_2^-\cdot$ can react with nitric oxide and produce RNS, such as peroxynitrite, that are also detrimental to cell viability (Beckman and Koppenol, 1996).

The main enzymatic source of $O_2^-\cdot$ is NAD phosphate (NADPH) oxidases, which are located on the cellular membrane of phagocytes. NADPH oxidases can transfer electrons from NADPH to O_2 to produce $O_2^-\cdot$ (Dworakowski et al., 2006). The mitochondrial electron transport chain (ETC) is the predominant non-enzymatic supplier of $O_2^-\cdot$. The ETC involves several redox enzymes that act in sequence to couple electron transfer to proton translocation across the mitochondrial membrane, creating a transmembrane electrochemical proton gradient. This gradient is crucial for driving ATP synthesis and cellular events that depend on ATP as an energy source. The ETC can leak electrons to O_2, partially reducing this molecule to $O_2^-\cdot$ (Turrens, 2003). Overproduction of ROS can promote cell death following various stress signals.

Classically, ROS is not associated with the DR (death receptor)-mediated apoptosis; however there is some recent evidence that oxidative stress can turn on extrinsic cell death signaling. This again demonstrates the many levels of communication that occur both upstream and downstream in events of programmed cell death. ROS can activate apoptosis signal-regulating kinase-1 (ASK-1), which is a MAPKKK that can phosphorylate and activate mediators of the JNK and p38 pathways of extrinsic programmed cell death (Nagai et al., 2007). ROS may also promote JNK-mediated extrinsic apoptosis through oxidation and inhibition of MAPK phosphatases that normally suppress JNK activity (Kamata et al., 2005).

Intrinsic cell death can also be affected by oxidative stress. High levels of ROS can initiate nuclear accumulation of FOXO3 (O subclass of the forkhead family of transcription factors) that can trigger up regulation of genes important for cell death such as Bim and Bcl-6 (Hagenbuchner et al., 2012; Sinha et al., 2013). FOXO3 can promote Bim translocation to the mitochondria and knockdown of anti-apoptotic protein Bcl-xL, which can modulate Bax-mediated mitochondrial cell death (Sedlak et al., 1995; Khawaja et al., 2008). It is hypothesized that FOXO3 can regulate the expression and activation of various pro-apoptotic and pro-survival proteins of the Bcl-2 family that can lead to mitochondrial stress, transient opening of the MPT pore, collapse of the mitochondrial membrane potential, release of mitochondrial pro-death proteins into the cytoplasm, and transient increases in ROS from the ETC. This downstream mitochondrial production of ROS can promote a positive feedback loop that converges into apoptosis (Sinha et al., 2013). In this positive response, overproduction of ROS can then promote more oxidation of lipids, proteins, and nucleic acids, disruption of mitochondrial integrity and induction of apoptosis and possibly necrosis. In addition, these free radicals can also oxidize cardiolipin, which results in tBID binding of the voltage-dependent anion channel (VDAC) of the MPT pore and downstream events associated with intrinsic apoptosis (Kagan et al., 2005).

Cochlear tissues produce high levels of ROS in response to a variety of challenges, such as gentamicin, radiation, cisplatin, electrode insertion trauma, and noise exposure (Henderson et al., 2006; Rybak et al., 2007; Choung et al., 2009; Low et al., 2009; Bas et al., 2012a,b). Cells can counteract the effects of oxidative stress through an antioxidant defense system that comprises free radical scavengers and antioxidant enzymes such as reduced glutathione (GSH), superoxide dismutases, and catalase. Insufficient levels of antioxidants such as GSH and vitamins A, C, and E are also associated with oxidative stress. It is the imbalance produced by ROS and antioxidant activity that can help determine the fate of an affected cell. Antioxidants and free-radical scavengers that have demonstrated protection against cochlear injury include iron chelators, manipulation of dietary glutathione, D-Methionine, lipoic acid, N-acetylcysteine, alpha-tocopherol, and m40403 (a superoxide dismutase mimetic), resveratrol, nitro-L-arginine methyl ester (L-NAME) and co-enzyme (Evans and Halliwell, 1999; Ohlemiller et al., 1999, 2000; Huang et al., 2000; Teranishi et al., 2001; Seidman et al., 2003; Nicotera et al., 2004; Samson et al., 2008; Fetoni et al., 2009; Rewerska et al., 2013). Dexamethasone is a synthetic steroid that has demonstrated beneficial effects against several inner ear disorders; dexamethasone can block the expression of ROS as well as reduce the extracellular inflammatory response and block extrinsic cell death signaling through activation of NFkB (Bas et al., 2012a).

Acoustic Trauma and Auditory HC Death

Although a number of stressors can initiate pro-inflammatory and pro-cell death signaling within the cochlea, the most studied insult to the inner ear is acoustic trauma. Acoustic trauma initiates a sequence of events within the cochlea that can culminate in apoptosis and regulated necrosis of auditory HCs (**Figure 4**).

Loud noise exposures produce large displacements of the tympanic membrane and propagate waves of mechanical energy into the inner ear. These intense pulses can produce rapid displacement of cochlear fluid within the inner ear, causing shearing force damage to the OC and basilar membrane, injuring auditory HCs, and altering the endocochlear potential (EP). Acoustic trauma can also initiate inflammation and edema of the stria vascularis and compromise the blood supply to the

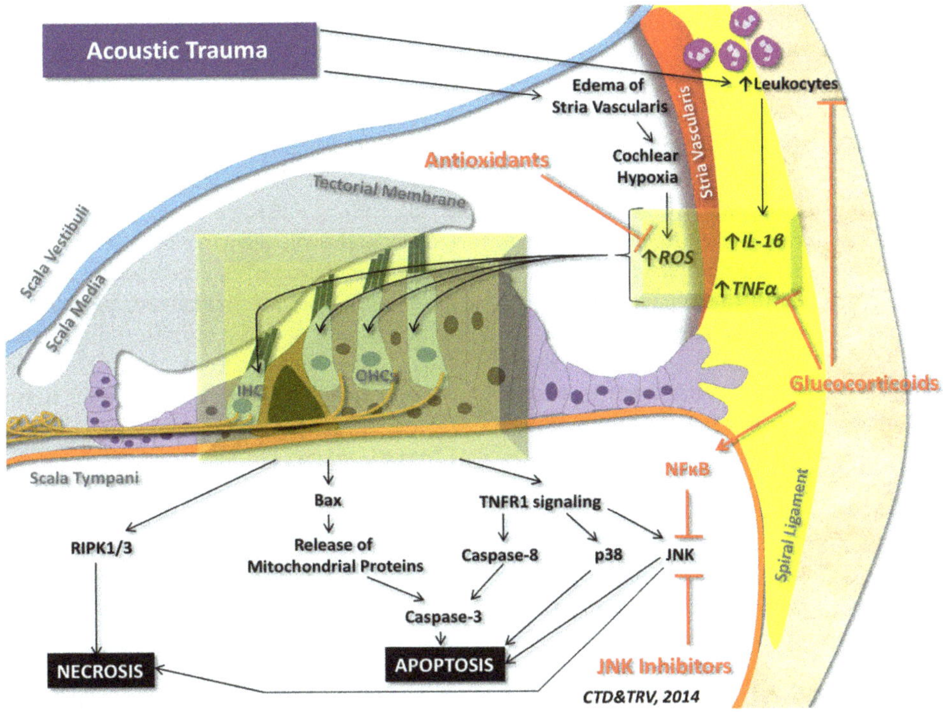

FIGURE 4 | Cell death signaling following acoustic trauma. Acoustic trauma can promote edema of the stria vascularis, resulting in cochlear hypoxia, formation of ROS, and oxidative stress. Noise trauma can also stimulate the spiral ligament to express cytokines (such as TNFα and IL-1β) and chemokines that initiate migration of leukocytes to the cochlea; leukocytes will then release a number of other pro-inflammatory factors and free radicals that propagate the inflammatory process. Oxidative stress and pro-inflammatory cytokines can travel to the inner hair cells (IHC) and outer hair cells (OHCs) of the organ of Corti and induce intrinsic and extrinsic apoptotic signaling cascades. Prolonged activation of JNK and induction of RIPK1/3 activity can promote necrotic cell death. Glucocorticoids have demonstrated protection against acoustic trauma, in part by reducing leukocyte migration, decreasing expression of pro-inflammatory factors, and activating NFκB inhibition of JNK signaling. Antioxidants and free radical scavengers can neutralize ROS and downstream effects of oxidative stress. Inhibitors of JNK can also mitigate noise-induced loss of auditory HCs by preventing downstream signaling cascades that lead to apoptosis and necrosis.

cochlea (Smith et al., 1985). Since there is minimal redundancy in cochlear blood flow, even transient reductions in cochlear blood flow can result in hypoxia and injury to auditory HCs. Injuries to the stria vascularis and spiral ligament occur following noise trauma, damaging type II and type IV fibrocytes that are important for maintenance of theEP) and lead to permanent hearing loss (Hirose and Liberman, 2003).

Acoustic trauma can lead to ROS release by the marginal cells of the stria vascularis as a result of reductions in cochlear blood flow and cochlear hypoxia (Yamane et al., 1995; Ohlemiller et al., 1999). It is controversial how hypoxia results in oxidative stress; however, it may be related to an increase in oxygen demand by auditory HCs followed by increased aerobic respiration by mitochondria to produce ATP and production of free radical byproducts via the ETC (Yamane et al., 1995; Taylor, 2008). The lateral wall structures of the cochlea also express cytokines (such as TNFα and IL-1β) and chemokines following acoustic trauma, which stimulate migration of leukocytes into the cochlea via the spiral modiolar vein (Keithley et al., 2008). These inflammatory cells will in turn release more cytokines and chemokines as well as produce ROS and RNS that will propagate the inflammatory process in the inner ear.

When TNFα binds to its complementary receptor TNFR1, TRADD and FADD are recruited along with caspase-8. Caspase-8 can activate executioner caspase-3 to promote extrinsic cell death through DNA fragmentation and chromatin condensation via CAD, ACINUS, and HELI-CARD or it can cleave BID into tBID, which can activate Bax-mediated intrinsic, mitochondrial cell death (Liu et al., 1997; Enari et al., 1998; Li et al., 1998; Kovacsovics et al., 2002; Nicotera et al., 2003; Wang et al., 2003; Murai et al., 2008; Jamesdaniel et al., 2011; Infante et al., 2012). Furthermore, loud noise exposure can upregulate TNFα-mediated p38 and JNK signaling in the sensory epithelium of the inner ear that promotes transcription of pro-death genes and Bax-mediated mitochondrial release of apoptotic proteins such as cyt *c* (Wang et al., 2007a,b; Dinh et al., 2008a,b; Infante et al., 2012; Jamesdaniel et al., 2011). Fas-mediated apoptosis also occurs following acoustic trauma (Jamesdaniel et al., 2011).

Oxidative stress from noise exposure can also initiate intrinsic apoptotic cell death in auditory HCs, resulting in mitochondrial release of cyt *c* into the cytoplasm, generation of apoptosomes, and activation of caspase-3 dependent cell death. AIF and EndoG are also released into the cytosol, translocate into the nucleus, and can initiate chromatin condensation and DNA fragmentation of auditory HCs (Nicotera et al., 2003; Yamashita et al., 2004a,b; Han et al., 2006; Henderson et al., 2006).

In addition to apoptosis, acoustic trauma can result in regulated necrosis through RIPK3/RIPK1 activation in rats, that was reversed with necrosis inhibitor necrostatin-1 (Zheng et al., 2014).

Acoustic trauma can also promote swelling and rupture of dendritic terminals of cochlear nerve afferent fibers (Spoendlin, 1971). Intense noise exposure can trigger inner HCs to release significant amounts of glutamate into the synapses with type I fibers of the cochlear nerve. The glutamate overwhelms the postsynaptic glutamate receptors and results in ion influx into dendritic terminals of the cochlear nerve that leads to loss of auditory nerve fibers (Pujol et al., 1990; Kujawa and Liberman, 2009).

Furthermore, intense noise exposure can increase intracellular calcium in auditory HCs and activate calcium-dependent calpains—cysteine proteases that promote proteolysis and breakdown of cytoskeletal and membrane proteins, kinases, phosphatases, and transcription factors (Wang et al., 1999). Subsequently, calpain cleaves and activates calcineurin that promotes Bad-mediated mitochondrial release of apoptotic factors that lead to intrinsic cell death (Le Prell et al., 2007).

Otoprotective drugs can target different levels in apoptosis and necrosis signaling pathways following acoustic trauma (**Figure 4**). Glucocorticoids can reduce extracellular inflammatory cell trafficking, reduce the level of TNFα expression in spiral ligament fibrocytes, and bind to its glucocorticoid receptors in auditory HCs to activate pro-survival NFkB signaling and inhibit JNK signaling. Additionally, they can reduce oxidative stress, and regulate pro-death and pro-survival gene transcription (Maeda et al., 2005; Tahera et al., 2006; Dinh et al., 2008a,b, 2011; Bas et al., 2012b). Regulation of MAPK signaling can also protect against noise-induced hearing loss by reducing p38 and JNK MAPKs (Tabuchi et al., 2010). In particular, direct and indirect inhibitors of JNK can block JNK phosphorylation of c-Jun and p53 and suppress downstream activation of intrinsic and extrinsic forms of apoptosis and potentially necrosis following acoustic trauma (Sakon et al., 2003; Wang et al., 2003, 2007a,b; Ventura et al., 2004; Coleman et al., 2007; Suckfuell et al., 2007). Lastly, antioxidants and free-radical scavengers can neutralize ROS that is responsible for lipid peroxidation of cell membranes, protein degradation, DNA injury and other mechanisms related to oxidative stress induced apoptosis and necrosis of noise-injured auditory HCs (Seidman et al., 2003; Nicotera et al., 2004; Nordang and Anniko, 2005; Samson et al., 2008; Fetoni et al., 2009; Rewerska et al., 2013).

Conclusion

Numerous diverse insults to the inner ear can cause auditory HC damage and hearing loss. The evolutionarily conserved apoptotic and necrotic cell death signaling that occurs in auditory HCs is shared among many ototoxic and traumatic stressor events. The most well studied molecular mechanisms behind cell death in auditory HCs involve TNFα signaling, JNK and p38 activation and the effect of high levels of oxidative stress. Although their effects on intrinsic and extrinsic pathways of apoptosis have been studied extensively, there are likely many levels of cross communication between signaling cascades that are still undiscovered. Research in this area is becoming more prevalent, as well as research into mechanisms of regulated necrosis in auditory HCs. A number of otoprotective drug therapies target different levels along this pro-inflammatory pro-death signaling cascade to block downstream events that lead to cell death and promote auditory HC viability and hearing protection.

References

Amaral, J. D., Xavier, J. M., Steer, C. J., and Rodrigues, C. M. (2010). The role of p53 in apoptosis. *Discov. Med.* 9, 145–152.

Aminpour, S., Tinling, S. P., and Brodie, H. A. (2005). Role of tumor necrosis factor-alpha in sensorineural hearing loss after bacterial meningitis. *Otol. Neurotol.* 26, 602–609. doi: 10.1097/01.mao.0000178121.28365.0d

Andrabi, S. A., Dawson, T. M., and Dawson, V. L. (2008). Mitochondrial and nuclear cross talk in cell death: parthanatos. *Ann. N Y Acad. Sci.* 1147, 233–241. doi: 10.1196/annals.1427.014

Baines, C. P., Kaiser, R. A., Purcell, N. H., Blair, N. S., Osinska, H., Hambleton, M. A., et al. (2005). Loss of cyclophilin D reveals a critical role for mitochondrial permeability transition in cell death. *Nature* 434, 658–662. doi: 10.1038/nature03434

Bas, E., Gupta, C., and Van De Water, T. R. (2012a). A novel organ of corti explant model for the study of cochlear implantation trauma. *Anat. Rec. (Hoboken)* 295, 1944–1956. doi: 10.1002/ar.22585

Bas, E., Martinez-Soriano, F., Láinez, J. M., and Marco, J. (2009). An experimental comparative study of dexamethasone, melatonin and tacrolimus in noise-induced hearing loss. *Acta. Otolaryngol.* 129, 385–389. doi: 10.1080/00016480802566279

Bas, E., Van De Water, T. R., Gupta, C., Dinh, J., Vu, L., Martínez-Soriano, F., et al. (2012b). Efficacy of three drugs for protecting against gentamicin-induced hair cell and hearing losses. *Br. J. Pharmacol.* 166, 1888–1904. doi: 10.1111/j.1476-5381.2012.01890.x

Beckman, K. B., and Ames, B. N. (1997). Oxidative decay of DNA. *J. Biol. Chem.* 272, 19633–19636. doi: 10.1074/jbc.272.32.19633

Beckman, J. S., and Koppenol, W. H. (1996). Nitric oxide, superoxide and peroxynitrite: the good, the bad and ugly. *Am. J. Physiol.* 271, C1424–C1437.

Bodmer, J. L., Burns, K., Schneider, P., Hofmann, K., Steiner, V., Thome, M., et al. (1997). TRAMP, a novel apoptosis-mediating receptor with sequence homology to tumor necrosis factor receptor 1 and Fas (Apo-1/CD95). *Immunity* 6, 79–88. doi: 10.1016/s1074-7613(00)80244-7

Bratton, S. B., Walker, G., Srinivasula, S. M., Sun, X. M., Butterworth, M., Alnemri, E. S., et al. (2001). Recruitment, activation and retention of caspases-9 and -3 by Apaf-1 apoptosome and associated XIAP complexes. *EMBO J.* 20, 998–1009. doi: 10.1093/emboj/20.5.998

Brenner, C., and Grimm, S. (2006). The permeability transition pore complex in cancer cell death. *Oncogene* 25, 4744–4756. doi: 10.1038/sj.onc.1209609

Brough, D., and Rothwell, N. J. (2007). Caspase-1-dependent processing of pro-interleukin-1beta is cytosolic and precedes cell death. *J. Cell Sci.* 120, 772–781. doi: 10.1242/jcs.03377

Budhram-Mahadeo, V., Morris, P. J., Smith, M. D., Midgley, C. A., Boxer, L. M., and Latchman, D. S. (1999). P53 suppresses the activation of the Bcl-2 promoter by the Brn-3a POU family transcription factor. *J. Biol. Chem.* 274, 15237–15244. doi: 10.1074/jbc.274.21.15237

Cai, B., Chang, S. H., Becker, E. B., Bonni, A., and Xia, Z. (2006). p38 MAP kinase mediates apoptosis through phosphorylation of BimEL at Ser-65. *J. Biol. Chem.* 281, 25215–25222. doi: 10.1074/jbc.m512627200

Cain, K., Bratton, S. B., Langlais, C., Walker, G., Brown, D. G., Sun, X. M., et al. (2000). Apaf-1 oligomerizes into biologically active approximately 700-kDa and inactive approximately 1.4-MDa apoptosome complexes. *J. Biol. Chem.* 275, 6067–6070. doi: 10.1074/jbc.275.9.6067

Capano, M., and Crompton, M. (2006). Bax translocates to mitochondria of heart cells during simulated ischaemia: involvement of AMP-activated and p38 mitogen-activated protein kinases. *Biochem. J.* 395, 57–64. doi: 10.1042/bj20051654

Chai, J., Du, C., Wu, J. W., Kyin, S., Wang, X., and Shi, Y. (2000). Structural and biochemical basis of apoptotic activation by Smac/DIABLO. *Nature* 406, 855–862. doi: 10.1038/35022514

Chai, J., Shiozaki, E., Srinivasula, S. M., Wu, Q., Datta, P., Alnemri, E. S., et al. (2001). Structural basis of caspase-7 inhibition by XIAP. *Cell* 104, 769–780. doi: 10.1016/s0092-8674(02)02034-2

Chandler, J. M., Cohen, G. M., and MacFarlane, M. (1998). Different subcellular distribution of caspase-3 and caspase-7 following Fas-induced apoptosis in mouse liver. *J. Biol. Chem.* 273, 10815–10818. doi: 10.1074/jbc.273.18.10815

Chen, Z., Gibson, T. B., Robinson, F., Silvestro, L., Pearson, G., Xu, B., et al. (2001). MAP kinases. *Chem. Rev.* 101, 2449–2476. doi: 10.1021/cr000241p

Chinnaiyan, A. M., O'Rourke, K., Tewari, M., and Dixit, V. M. (1995). FADD, a novel death domain-containing protein, interacts with the death domain of Fas and initiates apoptosis. *Cell* 81, 505–512. doi: 10.1016/0092-8674(95)90071-3

Choung, Y. H., Taura, A., Pak, K., Choi, S. J., Masuda, M., and Ryan, A. F. (2009). Generation of highly-reactive oxygen species is closely related to hair cell damage in rat organ of Corti treated with gentamicin. *Neuroscience* 161, 214–226. doi: 10.1016/j.neuroscience.2009.02.085

Coffin, A. B., Rubel, E. W., and Raible, D. W. (2013). Bax, Bcl2 and p53 differentially regulate neomycin- and gentamicin-induced hair cell death in the zebrafish lateral line. *J. Assoc. Res. Otolaryngol.* 14, 645–659. doi: 10.1007/s10162-013-0404-1

Coleman, J. N. K., Littlesunday, C., Jackson, R., and Meyer, T. (2007). AM-111 protects against permanent hearing loss from impulse noise trauma. *Hear. Res.* 226, 70–78. doi: 10.1016/j.heares.2006.05.006

Cotanche, D. A., Hennig, A. K., Riedl, A. E., and Messana, E. P. (1997). "Hair cell regeneration in the chick cochlea – were we stand after 10 years of work," in *Psychophysical and Physiological Advances in Hearing: Proceedings of the 11th International Symposium on Hearing*, eds A. R. Palmer, A. Rees, A. Q. Summerfield and A. Meddis (London: Whurr), 109–115.

Daugas, E., Susin, S. A., Zamzami, N., Ferri, K. F., Irinopoulou, T., Larochette, N., et al. (2000). Mitochondrio-nuclear translocation of AIF in apoptosis and necrosis. *FASEB J.* 14, 729–739.

Deng, Y., Ren, X., Yang, L., Lin, Y., and Wu, X. (2003). A JNK-dependent pathway is required for TNFalpha-induced apoptosis. *Cell* 115, 61–70. doi: 10.1016/s0092-8674(03)00757-8

Deshmane, S. L., Kremlev, S., Amini, S., and Sawaya, B. E. (2009). Monocyte chemoattractant protein-1 (MCP-1): an overview. *J. Interferon Cytokine Res.* 29, 313–326. doi: 10.1089/jir.2008.0027

Deveraux, Q. L., Leo, E., Stennicke, H. R., Welsh, K., Salvesen, G. S., and Reed, J. C. (1999). Cleavage of human inhibitor of apoptosis protein XIAP results in fragments with distinct specificities for caspases. *EMBO J.* 18, 5242–5251. doi: 10.1093/emboj/18.19.5242

Dhanasekaran, D. N., and Reddy, E. P. (2008). JNK signaling in apoptosis. *Oncogene* 27, 6245–6251. doi: 10.1038/onc.2008.301

Ding, D., Jiang, H., and Salvi, R. J. (2010). Mechanisms of rapid sensory hair-cell death following co-administration of gentamicin and ethacrynic acid. *Hear. Res.* 259, 16–23. doi: 10.1016/j.heares.2009.08.008

Dinh, C. T., Bas, E., Chan, S. S., Dinh, J. N., Vu, L., and Van De Water, T. R. (2011). Dexamethasone treatment of tumor necrosis factor-alpha challenged organ of Corti explants activates nuclear factor kappa B signaling that induces changes in gene expression that favor hair cell survival. *Neuroscience* 188, 157–167. doi: 10.1016/j.neuroscience.2011.04.061

Dinh, C., Bas, E., Dinh, J., Vu, L., Gupta, C., and Van De Water, T. R. (2013). Short interfering RNA against Bax attenuates TNFα-induced ototoxicity in rat organ of Corti explants. *Otolaryngol. Head Neck Surg.* 148, 834–840. doi: 10.1177/0194599813477631

Dinh, C. T., Haake, S., Chen, S., Hoang, K., Nong, E., Eshraghi, A. A., et al. (2008b). Dexamethasone protects organ of corti explants against tumor necrosis factor-alpha-induced loss of auditory hair cells and alters the expression levels of apoptosis-related genes. *Neuroscience* 157, 405–413. doi: 10.1016/j.neuroscience.2008.09.012

Dinh, C., Hoang, K., Haake, S., Chen, S., Angeli, S., Nong, E., et al. (2008a). Biopolymer-released dexamethasone prevents tumor necrosis factor alpha-induced loss of auditory hair cells in vitro: implications toward the development of a drug-eluting cochlear implant electrode array. *Otol. Neurotol.* 29, 1012–1019. doi: 10.1097/mao.0b013e3181859a1f

Dixon, S. J., Lemberg, K. M., Lamprecht, M. R., Skouta, R., Zaitsev, E. M., Gleason, C. E., et al. (2012). Ferroptosis: an iron-dependent form of nanopoptotic cell death. *Cell* 149, 1060–1072. doi: 10.1016/j.cell.2012.03.042

Donovan, N., Becker, E. B., Konishi, Y., and Bonni, A. (2002). JNK phosphorylation and activation of BAD couples the stress-activated signaling pathway to the cell death machinery. *J. Biol. Chem.* 277, 40944–40949. doi: 10.1074/jbc.m206113200

Dworakowski, R., Anilkumar, N., Zhang, M., and Shah, A. M. (2006). Redox signaling involving NADPH oxidase-derived reactive oxygen species. *Biochem. Soc. Trans.* 34, 960–964. doi: 10.1042/bst0340960

Eichhorst, S. T., Müller, M., Li-Weber, M., Schulze-Bergkamen, H., Angel, P., and Krammer, P. H. (2000). A novel AP-1 element in the CD95 ligand promoter is required for induction of apoptosis in hepatocellular carcinoma cells upon treatment with anticancer drugs. *Mol. Cell. Biol.* 20, 7826–7837. doi: 10.1128/mcb.20.20.7826-7837.2000

Enari, M., Sakahira, H., Yokoyama, H., Okawa, K., Iwamatsu, A., and Nagata, S. (1998). A caspase-activated DNase that degrades DNA during apoptosis and its inhibitos ICAD. *Nature* 391, 43–50. doi: 10.1038/34112

Eshraghi, A. A., He, J., Mou, C. H., Polak, M., Zine, A., Bonny, C., et al. (2006). D-JNKI-1 treatment prevents the progression of hearing loss in a model of cochlear implantation trauma. *Otol. Neurotol.* 27, 504–511. doi: 10.1097/00129492-200606000-00012

Eshraghi, A. A., Hoosien, G., Ramsay, S., Dinh, C. T., Bas, E., Balkany, T. J., et al. (2010). Inhibition of the JNK signal cascade conserves hearing against electrode insertion trauma-induced loss. *Cochlear Implants Int.* 11, 104–109. doi: 10.1179/146701010x12671177544104

Evans, P., and Halliwell, B. (1999). Free radicals and hearing. Cause, consequence and criteria. *Ann. N Y Acad. Sci.* 884, 19–40. doi: 10.1111/j.1749-6632.1999.tb08633.x

Fan, M., Goodwin, M. E., Birrer, M. J., and Chambers, T. C. (2001). The c-Jun NH(2)-terminal protein kinase/AP-1 pathway is required for efficient apoptosis induced by vinblastine. *Cancer Res.* 61, 4450–4458.

Faris, M., Kokot, N., Latinis, K., Kasibhatla, S., Green, D. R., Koretzky, G. A., et al. (1998). The c-Jun N-terminal kinase cascade plays a role in stress-induced apoptosis in Jurkat cells by up-regulating Fas ligand expression. *J. Immunol.* 160, 134–144.

Fernandes-Alnemri, T., Wu, J., Yu, J. W., Datta, P., Miller, B., Jankowski, W., et al. (2007). The pyroptosome: a supramolecular assembly of ASC dimers mediating inflammatory cell death via caspase-1 activation. *Cell Death Differ.* 14, 1590–1604. doi: 10.1038/sj.cdd.4402194

Fetoni, A. R., Piacentini, R., Fiorita, A., Paludetti, G., and Troiani, D. (2009). Water-solube Coenzyme Q10 formulation (Q-ter) promotes outer hair cell survival in a guinea pig model of noise-induced hearing loss (NIHL). *Brain Res.* 1257, 108–116. doi: 10.1016/j.brainres.2008.12.027

Figari, I. S., Mori, N. A., and Palladino, M. A. Jr. (1987). Regulation of neutrophil migration and superoxide production by recombinant tumor necrosis factors-alpha and -beta: comparison to recombinant interferon-gamma and interleukin-1 alpha. *Blood* 70, 979–984.

Fink, S. L., and Cookson, B. T. (2006). Caspase-1-dependent pore formation during pyroptosis leads to osmotic lysis of infected host macrophages. *Cell. Microbiol.* 8, 1812–1825. doi: 10.1111/j.1462-5822.2006.00751.x

Fischer, U., Stroh, C., and Schulze-Osthoff, K. (2006). Unique and overlapping substrate specificities of caspase-8 and caspase-10. *Oncogene* 25, 152–159. doi: 10.1038/sj.onc.1209015

Fujioka, M., Kanzaki, S., Okano, H. J., Masuda, M., Ogawa, K., and Okano, H. (2006). Proinflammatory cytokines expression in noise-induced damaged cochlea. *J. Neurosci. Res.* 83, 575–583. doi: 10.1002/jnr.20764

Galluzzi, L., Vitale, I., Abrams, J. M., Alnemri, E. S., Baehreck, E. H., Blagosklonny, M. V., et al. (2012). Molecular definitions of cell death subroutines: recommendations of the nomenclature committee on cell death 2012. *Cell Death Differ.* 19, 107–120. doi: 10.1038/cdd.2011.96

Guicciardi, M. E., and Gores, G. J. (2009). Life and death by death receptors. *FASEB J.* 23, 1625–1637. doi: 10.1096/fj.08-111005

Haake, S. M., Dinh, C. T., Chen, S., Eshraghi, A. A., and Van De Water, T. R. (2009). Dexamethasone protects auditory hair cells against TNFalpha-initiated apoptosis via activation of PI3K/Akt and NFkappaB signaling. *Hear. Res.* 255, 22–32. doi: 10.1016/j.heares.2009.05.003

Hagenbuchner, J., Kuznetsov, A., Hermann, M., Hausott, B., Obexer, P., and Ausserlechner, M. J. (2012). FOXO3-induced reactive oxygen species are regulated by BCL2L11 (Bim) and SESN3. *J. Cell Sci.* 125, 1191–1203. doi: 10.1242/jcs.092098

Han, W., Shi, X., and Nuttall, A. L. (2006). AIF and endoG translocation in noise exposure induced hair cell death. *Hear. Res.* 211, 85–95. doi: 10.1016/j.heares.2005.10.004

He, S., Wang, L., Miao, L., Wang, T., Du, F., Zhao, L., et al. (2009). Receptor interacting protein kinase-3 determines cellular necrotic response to TNF-alpha. *Cell* 137, 1100–1111. doi: 10.1016/j.cell.2009.05.021

Hegde, R., Srinivasula, S. M., Zhang, Z., Wassell, R., Mukattash, R., Cilenti, L., et al. (2002). Identification of Omi/HtrA2 as a mitochondrial apoptotic serine protease that disrupts inhibitor of apoptosis protein-caspase interaction. *J. Biol. Chem.* 277, 432–438. doi: 10.1074/jbc.M109721200

Henderson, D., Bielefeld, E. C., Harris, K. C., and Hu, B. H. (2006). The role of oxidative stress in noise-induced hearing loss. *Ear Hear.* 27, 1–19. doi: 10.1097/01.aud.0000191942.36672.f3

Hirose, K., and Liberman, M. C. (2003). Lateral wall histophatology and endoncochlear potential in the noise-damage mouse cochlea. *J. Assoc. Res. Otolaryngol.* 4, 339–352. doi: 10.1007/s10162-002-3036-4

Hirose, K., Westrum, L. E., Cunningham, D. E., and Rubel, E. W. (2004). Electron microscopy of degenerative changes in the chick basilar papilla after gentamicin exposure. *J. Comp. Neurol.* 470, 164–180. doi: 10.1002/cne.11046

Hsu, S. C., Gavrilin, M. A., Tsai, M. H., Han, J., and Lai, M. Z. (1999). p38 mitogen-activated protein kinase is involved in Fas ligand expression. *J. Biol. Chem.* 274, 25769–25776. doi: 10.1074/jbc.274.36.25769

Hsu, H., Xiong, J., and Goeddel, D. V. (1995). The TNF receptor 1-associated protein TRADD signals cell death and NF-kappa B activation. *Cell* 81, 495–504. doi: 10.1016/0092-8674(95)90070-5

Hu, B. H., Henderson, D., and Nicotera, T. M. (2006). Extremely rapid induction of outer hair cell apoptosis in the chinchilla cochlea following exposure to impulse noise. *Hear. Res.* 211, 16–25. doi: 10.1016/j.heares.2005.08.006

Huang, T., Cheng, A. G., Stupak, H., Liu, W., Kim, A., Staecker, H., et al. (2000). Oxidative stress-induced apoptosis of cochlear sensory cells: otoprotective strategies. *Int. J. Dev. Neurosci.* 18, 259–270. doi: 10.1016/s0736-5748(99)00094-5

Ichimiya, I., Yoshida, K., Hirano, T., Suzuki, M., and Mogi, G. (2000). Significance of spiral ligament fibrocytes with cochlear inflammation. *Int. J. Pediatr. Otorhinolaryngol.* 56, 45–51. doi: 10.1016/s0165-5876(00)00408-0

Ichimiya, I., Yoshida, K., Suzuki, M., and Mogi, G. (2003). Expression of adhesion molecules by cultured spiral ligament fibrocytes stimulated with proinflammatory cytokines. *Ann. Otol. Rhinol. Laryngol.* 112, 722–728. doi: 10.1177/000348940311200813

Infante, E. B., Channer, G. A., Telischi, F. F., Gupta, C., Dinh, J. T., Vu, L., et al. (2012). Mannitol protects hair cells against tumor necrosis factor α-induced loss. *Otol. Neurotol.* 33, 1656–1663. doi: 10.1097/mao.0b013e31826bedd9

Itoh, N., and Nagata, S. (1993). A novel protein domain required for apoptosis mutational analysis of human Fas antigen. *J. Biol. Chem.* 268, 10932–10937.

Jamesdaniel, S., Hu, B., Kermany, M. H., Jiang, H., Ding, D., Coling, D., et al. (2011). Noise induced changes in the expression of p38/MAPK signaling proteins in the sensory epithelium of the inner ear. *J. Proteomics* 75, 410–424. doi: 10.1016/j.jprot.2011.08.007

Jiang, H., Sha, S. H., Forge, A., and Schacht, J. (2006). Caspase-independent pathways of hair cell death induced by kanamycin in vivo. *Cell Death Differ.* 13, 20–30. doi: 10.1038/sj.cdd.4401706

Kagan, V. E., Tyurin, V. A., Jiang, J., Tyurina, Y. Y., Ritov, V. B., Amoscato, A. A., et al. (2005). Cytochrome c acts as a cardiolipin oxygenase required for release of proapoptotic factors. *Nat. Chem. Biol.* 1, 223–232. doi: 10.1038/nchembio727

Kamata, H., Honda, S., Maeda, S., Chang, L., Hirata, H., and Karin, M. (2005). Reactive oxygen species promotes TNFalpha-induced death and sustained JNK activation by inhibiting MAP kinase phosphatases. *Cell* 120, 649–661. doi: 10.1016/j.cell.2004.12.041

Kandasamy, K., Srinivasula, S. M., Alnemri, E. S., Thompson, C. B., Korsmeyer, S. J., Bryant, J. L., et al. (2003). Involvement of proapoptotic molecules Bax and Bak in tumor necrosis factor-related apoptosis-inducing ligand (TRAIL)-induced mitochondrial disruption and apoptosis: differential regulation of cytochrome c and Smac/DIABLo release. *Cancer Res.* 63, 1712–1721.

Keithley, E. M., Wang, X., and Barkdull, G. C. (2008). Tumor necrosis factor alpha can induce recruitment of inflammatory cells to the cochlea. *Otol. Neurotol.* 29, 854–859. doi: 10.1097/mao.0b013e31818256a9

Kepp, O., Galluzzi, L., Zitvogel, L., and Kroemer, G. (2010). Pyroptosis: a cell death modality of its kind. *Eur. J. Immunol.* 40, 627–630. doi: 10.1002/eji.200940160

Keshet, Y., and Seger, R. (2010). The MAP kinase signaling cascades: a system of hundreds of components regulates a diverse array of physiological functions. *Methods Mol. Biol.* 661, 3–38. doi: 10.1007/978-1-60761-795-2_1

Khawaja, N. R., Carré, M., Kovacic, H., Estève, M. A., and Braguer, D. (2008). Patupilone-induced apoptosis is mediated by mitochondrial reactive oxygen species through Bim relocalization to mitochondria. *Mol. Pharmacol.* 74, 1072–1083. doi: 10.1124/mol.108.048405

Kim, J., Cho, H. J., Sagong, B., Kim, S. J., Lee, J. T., So, H. S., et al. (2014). Alpha-lipoic acid protects against cisplatin-induced ototoxicity via the regulat of MAPKs and proinflammatory cytokines. *Biochem. Biophys. Res. Commun.* 449, 183–189. doi: 10.1016/j.bbrc.2014.04.118

Kohen, R., and Nyska, A. (2002). Oxidation of biological systems: oxidative stress phenomena, antioxidants, redox reactions and methods for their quantification. *Toxicol. Pathol.* 30, 620–650. doi: 10.1080/01926230290166724

Korsmeyer, S. J., Wei, M. C., Saito, M., Weiler, S., Oh, K. J., and Schlesinger, P. H. (2000). Pro-apoptotic cascade activates BID, which oligomerizes BAK or BAX into pores that result in the release of cytochrome c. *Cell Death Differ.* 7, 1166–1173. doi: 10.1038/sj.cdd.4400783

Kovacsovics, M., Martinon, F., Micheau, O., Bodmer, J. L., Hofmann, K., and Tschopp, J. (2002). Overexpression of Helicard, a CARD-containing helicase cleaved during apoptosis, accelerates DNA degradation. *Curr. Biol.* 12, 838–843. doi: 10.1016/s0960-9822(02)00842-4

Kroemer, G., Galluzzi, L., and Brenner, C. (2007). Mitochondrial membrane permeabilization in cell death. *Physiol. Rev.* 87, 99–163. doi: 10.1152/physrev.00013.2006

Kuhn, M., Heman-Ackah, S. E., Shaikh, J. A., and Roehm, P. C. (2011). Sudden sensorineural hearing loss: a review of diagnosis, treatment and prognosis. *Trends Amplif.* 15, 91–105. doi: 10.1177/1084713811408349

Kujawa, S. G., and Liberman, M. C. (2009). Adding insult to injury: cochlear nerve degeneration after "temporary" noise-induced hearing loss. *J. Neurosci.* 29, 14077–14085. doi: 10.1523/JNEUROSCI.2845-09.2009

Kurioka, T., Matsunobu, T., Niwa, K., Tamura, A., Satoh, Y., and Shiotani, A. (2014). Activated protein C rescues the cochlea from noise-induced hearing loss. *Brain Res.* 1583, 201–210. doi: 10.1016/j.brainres.2014.07.052

Kuwana, T., Mackey, M. R., Perkins, G., Ellisman, M. H., Latterich, M., Schneiter, R., et al. (2002). Bid, Bax and lipids cooperat to form supramolecula ropenings in the outer mitochondrial membrane. *Cell* 111, 331–342. doi: 10.1016/s0092-8674(02)01036-x

Kyriakis, J. M., and Avruch, J. (2001). Mammalian mitogen-activated protein kinase signal transcution pathways activated by stress and inflammation. *Physiol. Rev.* 81, 807–869.

Lamkanfi, M., Kanneganti, T. D., Van Damme, P., Vanden Berghe, T., Vanoverberghe, I., Vandekerckhove, J., et al. (2008). Targeted peptidecentic proteomics reveals caspase-7 as a substrate of the caspase-1 inflammasomes. *Mol. Cell. Proteomics* 7, 2350–2363. doi: 10.1074/mcp.m800132-mcp200

Lei, K., and Davis, R. J. (2003). JNK phosphorylation of Bim-related members of the Bcl2 family induces Bax-dependent apoptosis. *Proc. Natl. Acad. Sci. U S A* 100, 2432–2437. doi: 10.1073/pnas.0438011100

Lei, K., Nimnual, A., Zong, W. X., Kennedy, N. J., Flavell, R. A., Thompson, C. B., et al. (2002). The Bax subfamily of Bcl2-related proteins is essential for apoptotic signal transduction of c-Jun NH(2)-terminal kinase. *Mol. Cell. Biol.* 22, 4929–4942. doi: 10.1128/mcb.22.13.4929-4942.2002

Le Prell, C. G., Yamashita, D., Minami, S. B., Yamasoba, T., and Miller, J. M. (2007). Mechanisms of noise-induced hearing loss indicated multiple methods of prevention. *Hear. Res.* 226, 22–43. doi: 10.1016/j.heares.2006.10.006

Li, Y., Johnson, N., Capano, M., Edwards, M., and Crompton, M. (2004). Cyclophilin-D promotes the mitochondrial permeability transition but has opposite effects on apoptosis and necrosis. *Biochem. J.* 383, 101–109. doi: 10.1042/bj20040669

Li, L. Y., Luo, X., and Wang, X. (2001). Endonuclease G is an apoptotic DNase when released from mitochondria. *Nature* 412, 95–99. doi: 10.1038/35083620

Li, W., Srinivasula, S. M., Chai, J., Li, P., Wu, J. W., Zhang, Z., et al. (2002). Structural insights into the pro-apoptotic function of mitochondrial serine protease HtrA2/Omi. *Nat. Struct. Biol.* 9, 436–441. doi: 10.1038/nsb795

Li, H., Zhu, H., Xu, C. J., and Yuan, J. (1998). Cleavage of BID by caspase 8 mediates the mitochondrial damage in the Fas pathway of apoptosis. *Cell* 94, 491–501. doi: 10.1016/s0092-8674(00)81590-1

Lin, F. R., Niparko, J. K., and Ferrucci, L. (2011). Hearing loss prevalence in the United States. *Arch. Intern. Med.* 171, 1851–1852. doi: 10.1001/archinternmed.2011.506

Liu, J., and Lin, A. (2005). Role of JNK activation in apoptosis: a double-edged sword. *Cell Res.* 15, 36–42. doi: 10.1038/sj.cr.7290262

Liu, X., Zou, H., Slaughter, C., and Wang, X. (1997). DFF, a heterodimeric protein that functions downstream of caspase-3 to trigger DNA fragmentation during apoptosis. *Cell* 89, 175–184. doi: 10.1016/s0092-8674(00)80197-x

Lorenzo, H. K., Susin, S. A., Penninger, J., and Kroemer, G. (1999). Apoptosis inducing factor (AIF): a phylogenetically old caspase-independent effector of cell death. *Cell Death Differ.* 6, 516–524. doi: 10.1038/sj.cdd.4400527

Low, W. K., Tan, M. G., Chua, A. W., Sun, L., and Wang, D. Y. (2009). 12th Yahya Cohen memorial lecture: the cellular and molecular basis of radiation-induced sensorineural hearing loss. *Ann. Acad. Med. Singapore* 38, 91–94.

Luo, X., Budihardjo, I., Zou, H., Slaughter, C., and Wang, X. (1998). Bid, a Bcl-2 interacting protein, mediates cytochrome c release from mitochondria in response to activation of cell surface death receptors. *Cell* 94, 481–490. doi: 10.1016/s0092-8674(00)81589-5

Madesh, M., Antonsson, B., Srinivasula, S. M., Alnemri, E. S., and Hajnoczky, G. (2002). Rapid kinetics of tBid-induced cytochrome c and Smac/DIABLO release and mitochondrial depolarization. *J. Biol. Chem.* 277, 5651–5659. doi: 10.1074/jbc.m108171200

Maeda, Y., Fukushima, K., Omichi, R., Kariya, S., and Nishizaki, K. (2013). Time courses of changes in phospho- and total-MAP kinases in the cochlea after intense noise exposure. *PLoS One* 8:e58775. doi: 10.1371/journal.pone.0058775

Maeda, K., Yoshida, K., Ichimiya, I., and Suzuki, M. (2005). Dexamethasone inhibits tumor necrosis factor-alpha-induced cytokine secretion from spiral ligament fibrocytes. *Hear. Res.* 202, 154–160. doi: 10.1016/j.heares.2004.08.022

Mahdavian Delavary, B., van der Veer, W. M., van Egmond, M., Niessen, F. B., and Beelen, R. H. (2011). Macrophages in skin injury and repair. *Immunobiology* 216, 753–762. doi: 10.1016/j.imbio.2011.01.001

Mangiardi, D. A., McLaughlin-Williamson, K., May, K. E., Messana, E. P., Mountain, D. C., and Cotanche, D. A. (2004). Progression of hair cell ejection and molecular markers of apoptosis in the avian cochlea following gentamicin treatment. *J. Comp. Neurol.* 475, 1–8. doi: 10.1002/cne.20129

Marchetti, P., Castedo, M., Susin, S. A., Zamzami, N., Hirsch, T., Macho, A., et al. (1996). Mitochondrial permeability transition is a central coordinating event in apoptosis. *J. Exp. Med.* 184, 1155–1160. doi: 10.1084/jem.184.3.1155

Markou, T., Dowling, A. A., Kelly, T., and Lazou, A. (2009). Regulation of Bcl-2 phosphorylation in response to oxidative stress in cardiac myocytes. *Free Radic. Res.* 42, 809–816. doi: 10.1080/10715760903071649

Marshall, K. D., and Baines, C. P. (2014). Necroptosis: is there a role for mitochondria? *Front. Physiol.* 5:323. doi: 10.3389/fphys.2014.00323

Marzo, I., Brenner, C., and Kroemer, G. (1998). The central role of the mitochondrial megachannel in apoptosis: evidence obtained with intact cells, isolated mitochondria and purified protein complexes. *Biomed. Pharmacother.* 52, 248–251. doi: 10.1016/s0753-3322(98)80009-7

Matsui, J. I., Gale, J. E., and Warchol, M. E. (2004). Critical signaling events during the aminoglycoside-induced death of sensory hair cells in vitro. *J. Neurobiol.* 61, 250–266. doi: 10.1002/neu.20054

McComb, S., Cheung, H. H., Korneluk, R. G., Wang, S., Krishnan, L., and Sad, S. (2012). cIAP1 and cIAP2 limit macrophage necroptosis by inhibiting Rip1 and Rip3 activation. *Cell Death Differ.* 19, 1791–1801. doi: 10.1038/cdd.2012.59

Milhas, D., Cuvillier, O., Therville, N., Clavé, P., Thomsen, M., Levade, T., et al. (2005). Caspase-10 triggers Bid cleavage and caspase cascade activation in FasL-induced apoptosis. *J. Biol. Chem.* 280, 19836–19842. doi: 10.1074/jbc.m414358200

Murai, N., Kirkegaard, M., Järlebark, L., Risling, M., Suneson, A., and Ulfendahl, M. (2008). Activation of JNK in the inner ear following impulse noise exposure. *J. Neurotrauma* 25, 72–77. doi: 10.1089/neu.2007.0346

Mutsaers, S. E., Bishop, J. E., McGrouther, G., and Laurent, G. J. (1997). Mechanisms of tissue repair: from wound healing to fibrosis. *Int. J. Biochem. Cell Biol.* 29, 5–17. doi: 10.1016/s1357-2725(96)00115-x

Nagai, H., Noguchi, T., Takeda, K., and Ichijo, H. (2007). Pathophysiological roles of ASK1-MAP kinase signaling pathways. *J. Biochem. Mol. Biol.* 40, 1–6. doi: 10.5483/bmbrep.2007.40.1.001

Nagata, S. (1999). Fas ligand-induced apoptosis. *Annu. Rev. Genet.* 33, 29–55. doi: 10.1146/annurev.genet.33.1.29

Nakagawa, T., Shimizu, S., Watanabe, T., Yamaguchi, O., Otsu, K., Yamagata, H., et al. (2005). Cyclophilin D-dependent mitochondrial permeability transition regulates some necrotic but not apoptotic cell death. *Nature* 434, 652–658. doi: 10.1038/nature03317

Nakamagoe, M., Tabuchi, K., Uemaetomari, I., Nishimura, B., and Hara, A. (2010). Estradiol protects the cochlea against gentamicin ototoxicity through inhibition of the JNK pathway. *Hear. Res.* 261, 67–74. doi: 10.1016/j.heares.2010.01.004

Ng, P. W., Porter, A. G., and Jänicke, R. U. (1999). Molecular cloning and characterization of two novel pro-apoptotic isoforms of caspase-10. *J. Biol. Chem.* 274, 10301–10308. doi: 10.1074/jbc.274.15.10301

Nicotera, T. M., Ding, D., McFadden, S. L., Salvemini, D., and Salvi, R. (2004). Paraquat-induced hair cell damage and protection with the superoxide dismutase mimetic m40403. *Audiol. Neurootol.* 9, 353–362. doi: 10.1159/000081284

Nicotera, T. M., Hu, B. H., and Henderson, D. (2003). The caspase pathway in noise-induced apoptosis of the chinchilla cochlea. *J. Assoc. Res. Otolaryngol.* 4, 466–477. doi: 10.1007/s10162-002-3038-2

Nordang, L., and Anniko, M. (2005). Nitro-L-arginine methyl ester: a potential protector against gentamicin ototoxicity. *Acta Otolaryngol.* 125, 1033–1038. doi: 10.1080/00016480510038022

Ohlemiller, K. K., McFadden, S. L., Ding, D. L., Lear, P. M., and Ho, Y. S. (2000). Targeted mutation of the gene for cellular glutathione peroxidase (Gpx1) increases noise-induced hearing loss in mice. *J. Assoc. Res. Otolaryngol.* 1, 243–254. doi: 10.1007/s101620010043

Ohlemiller, K. K., Wright, J. S., and Dugan, L. L. (1999). Early elevation of cochlear reactive oxygen species following noise exposure. *Audiol. Neurootol.* 4, 229–236. doi: 10.1159/000013846

Oleinik, N. V., Krupenko, N. I., and Krupenko, S. A. (2007). Cooperation between JNK1 and JNK2 in activation of p53 apoptotic pathway. *Oncogene* 26, 7222–7230. doi: 10.1038/sj.onc.1210526

Op de Beeck, K., Schacht, J., and Van Camp, G. (2011). Apoptosis in acquired and genetic hearing impairment: the programmed death of the hair cell. *Hear. Res.* 281, 18–27. doi: 10.1016/j.heares.2011.07.002

Ottilie, S., Diaz, J. L., Horne, W., Chang, J., Wang, Y., Wilson, G., et al. (1997). Dimerization properties of human BAD. Identification of a BH-3 domain and analysis of its binding to mutant BCL-2 and BCL-XL proteins. *J. Biol. Chem.* 272, 30866–30872. doi: 10.1074/jbc.272.49.30866

Owens, T. W., Valentijn, A. J., Upton, J. P., Keeble, J., Zhang, L., Lindsay, J., et al. (2009). Apoptosis commitment and activation of mitochondrial Bax during anoikis is regulated by p38MAPK. *Cell Death Differ.* 16, 1551–1562. doi: 10.1038/cdd.2009.102

Pahl, H. L. (1999). Activators and target genes of Rel/NF-kappaB transcription factors. *Oncogene* 18, 6853–6866. doi: 10.1038/sj.onc.1203239

Park, H. Y., Lee, M. H., Kang, S. U., Hwang, H. S., Park, K., Choung, Y. H., et al. (2012). Nitric oxide mediates TNF-α-induced apoptosis in the auditory cell line. *Laryngoscope* 122, 2256–2264. doi: 10.1002/lary.23444

Pathak, S., Goldofsky, E., Vivas, E. X., Bonagura, V. R., and Vambutas, A. (2011). IL-1β is overexpressed and aberrantly regulated in corticosteroid nonresponders with autoimmune inner ear disease. *J. Immunol.* 186, 1870–1879. doi: 10.4049/jimmunol.1002275

Pirvola, U., XingQun, L., Virkkala, J., Saarma, M., Murakata, C., Camoratto, A. M., et al. (2000). Rescue of hearing, auditory hair cells and neurons by CEP1347/KT7515, an inhibitor of cJun Nterminal kinase activation. *J. Neurosci.* 20, 43–50.

Porras, A., Zuluaga, S., Black, E., Valladares, A., Alvarez, A. M., Ambrosino, C., et al. (2004). P38 alpha mitogen-activated protein kinase sensitizes cells to apoptosis induced by different stimuli. *Mol. Biol. Cell.* 15, 922–933. doi: 10. 1091/mbc.E03-08-0592

Proost, P., Wuyts, A., and van Damme, J. (1996). The role of chemokines in inflammation. *Int. J. Clin. Lab. Res.* 26, 211–223. doi: 10.1007/BF0260 2952

Pujol, R., Rebillard, G., Puel, J. L., Lenoir, M., Eybalin, M., and Recasens, M. (1990). Glutamate neurotoxicity in the cochlea: a possible consequence of ischaemic or anoxic conditions accurring in ageing. *Acta Otolaryngol. Suppl.* 476, 32–36. doi: 10.3109/00016489109127253

Puthalakath, H., Huang, D. C., O'Reilly, L. A., King, S. M., and Strasser, A. (1999). The proapoptotic activity of the Bcl-2 family member Bim is regulated by interation with the dynein motor complex. *Mol. Cell* 3, 287–296. doi: 10. 1016/s1097-2765(00)80456-6

Pyun, J. H., Kang, S. U., Hwang, H. S., Oh, Y. T., Kang, S. H., Lim, Y. A., et al. (2011). Epicatechin inhibits radiation-induced auditory cell death by suppression of reactive oxygen species generation. *Neuroscience* 199, 410–420. doi: 10.1016/j.neuroscience.2011.09.012

Rewerska, A., Pawelczyk, M., Rajkowska, E., Politanski, P., and Sliwinska-Kowalska, M. (2013). Evaluating D-methionine dose to attenuate oxidative stress-mediated hearing loss following overexposure to noise. *Eur. Arch. Otorhinolaryngol.* 270, 1513–1520. doi: 10.1007/s00405-012-2265-3

Roux, P. P., and Blenis, J. (2004). ERK and p38 MAPK-activated protein kinases: a family of protein kinases with diverse biological functions. *Microbiol. Mol. Biol. Rev.* 68, 320–344. doi: 10.1128/mmbr.68.2.320-344.2004

Roy, S., and Nicholson, D. W. (2000). Cross-talk in cell death signaling. *J. Exp. Med.* 192, f21–f26. doi: 10.1084/jem.192.8.f21

Rybak, L. P., Whitworth, C. A., Mukherjea, D., and Ramkumar, V. (2007). Mechanisms of cisplatin-induced ototoxicity and prevention. *Hear. Res.* 226, 157–167. doi: 10.1016/j.heares.2006.09.015

Sahara, A., Aoto, M., Eguchi, Y., Imamoto, N., Yoneda, Y., and Tsujimoto, Y. (1999). Acinus is a caspase-3-activated protein required for apoptotic chromatin condensation. *Nature* 401, 168–173. doi: 10.1038/ 43678

Sakon, S., Xue, X., Takekawa, M., Sasazuki, T., Okazaki, T., Kojima, Y., et al. (2003). NFkappaB inhibits TNF-induced accumulation of ROS that mediate prolonged MAPK activation and necrotic cell death. *EMBO J.* 22, 3898–3909. doi: 10. 1093/emboj/cdg379

Samson, J., Wiktorek-Smagur, A., Politanski, P., Rajkowska, E., Pawlaczyk-Luszczynska, M., Dudarewicz, A., et al. (2008). Noise-induced time-dependent changes in oxidative stress in the mouse cochlea and attenuation by D-methionine. *Neuroscience* 152, 146–150. doi: 10.1016/j.neuroscience.2007. 11.015

Satoh, H., Firestein, G. S., Billings, P. B., Harris, J. P., and Keithley, E. M. (2002). Tumor necrosis factor-alpha, an initiator and etanercept and inhibitor of cochlear inflammation. *Laryngoscope* 112, 1627–1634. doi: 10.1097/00005537-200209000-00019

Satoh, H., Firestein, G. S., Billings, P. B., Harris, J. P., and Keithley, E. M. (2003). Proinflammatory cytokine expression in the endolymphatic sac during inner ear inflammation. *J. Assoc. Res. Otolaryngol.* 4, 139–147. doi: 10.1007/s10162-002-3025-7

Saunders, J. C., Dear, S. P., and Schneider, M. E. (1985). The anatomical consequences of acoustic injury: a review and tutorial. *J. Acoust. Soc. Am.* 78, 833–860. doi: 10.1121/1.392915

Scarlett, J. L., and Murphy, M. P. (1997). Release of apoptogenic proteins form the mitochondrial intermembrane space during the mitochondrial permeability transition. *FEBS Lett.* 418, 282–286. doi: 10.1016/s0014-5793(97) 01391-4

Sedlak, T. W., Oltvai, Z. N., Yang, E., Wang, K., Boise, L. H., Thompson, C. B., et al. (1995). Multiple Bcl-2 family members demonstrate selective dimerizations with Bax. *Proc. Natl. Acad. Sci. U S A* 92, 7834–7838. doi: 10.1073/pnas.92.17. 7834

Seidman, M., Babu, S., Tang, W., Naem, E., and Quirk, W. S. (2003). Effects of resveratrol on acoustic trauma. *Otolaryngol. Head Neck Surg.* 129, 463–470. doi: 10.1016/s0194-5998(03)01586-9

Shen, H. M., and Pervaiz, S. (2006). TNF receptor superfamily-induced cell death: redox-dependent execution. *FASEB J.* 20, 1589–1598. doi: 10.1096/fj.05-5603rev

Shin, Y. S., Hwang, H. S., Kang, S. U., Chang, J. W., Oh, Y. T., and Kim, C. H. (2014). Inhibition of p38 mitogen-activated protein kinase ameliorates radiation-induced ototoxicity in zebrafish and cochlea-derived cell lines. *Neurotoxicology* 40, 111–122. doi: 10.1016/j.neuro.2013.12.006

Silke, J., and Strasser, A. (2013). The FLIP side of life. *Sci. Signal.* 6:pe2. doi: 10. 1126/scisignal.2003845

Sinha, K., Das, J., Pal, P. B., and Sil, P. C. (2013). Oxidative stress: the mitochondria-dependent and mitochondria-independent pathways of apoptosis. *Arch. Toxicol.* 87, 1157–1180. doi: 10.1007/s00204-013-1034-4

Smith, D. I., Lawrence, M., and Hawkins, J. E. Jr. (1985). Effects of noise and quinine on the vessels of the stria vascularis: an image analysis study. *Am. J. Otolaryngol.* 6, 280–289. doi: 10.1016/s0196-0709(85)80056-9

So, H., Kim, H., Lee, J. H., Park, C., Kim, Y., Kim, E., et al. (2007). Cisplatin cytotoxicity of auditory cells requires secretions of proinflammatory cytokines via activation of ERK and NF-kappaB. *J. Assoc. Res. Otolaryngol.* 8, 338–355. doi: 10.1007/s10162-007-0084-9

Spoendlin, H. (1971). Primary structural changes in the organ of Corti after acoustic overstimulation. *Acta Otolaryngol.* 71, 166–176. doi: 10. 3109/00016487109125346

Stephanou, A., Scarabelli, T. M., Brar, B. K., Nakanishi, Y., Matsumura, M., Knight, R. A., et al. (2001). Induction of apoptosis and Fas receptor/Fas ligand expression by ischemi/reperfusion in cardiac myocytes requires serine 727 of the STAT-1 trancription factor but not tyrosine 701. *J. Biol. Chem.* 276, 28340--28347. doi: 10.1074/jbc.m101177200

Suckfuell, M., Canis, M., Strieth, S., Scherer, H., and Haisch, A. (2007). Intratympanic treatment of acute acoustic trauma with a cell-permeable JNK ligand: a prospective randomized phase I/II study. *Acta Otolaryngol.* 127, 938–942. doi: 10.1080/00016480601110212

Suzuki, Y., Imai, Y., Nakayama, H., Takahashi, K., Takio, K., and Takahashi, R. (2001). A serine protease, HtrA2, is released from the mitochondria and interacts with XIAP, inducing cell death. *Mol. Cell* 8, 613–621. doi: 10. 1016/s1097-2765(01)00341-0

Tabuchi, K., Oikawa, K., Hoshino, T., Nishimura, B., Hayashi, K., Yanagawa, T., et al. (2010). Cochlear protection from acoustic injury by inhibitors of p38 mitogen-activated protein kinase and sequestosome 1 stress protein. *Neuroscience* 166, 665–670. doi: 10.1016/j.neuroscience.2009.12.038

Tabuchi, K., Pak, K., Chavez, E., and Ryan, A. F. (2007). Role of inhibitor of apoptosis protein in gentamicin-induced cohlear hair cell damage. *Neuroscience* 149, 213–222. doi: 10.1016/j.neuroscience.2007.06.061

Tahera, Y., Meltser, I., Johansson, P., Bian, Z., Stierna, P., Hansson, A. C., et al. (2006). NF-kappaB mediated glucocorticoid response in the inner ear after acoustic trauma. *J. Neurosci. Res.* 83, 1066–1076. doi: 10.1002/jnr.20795

Tartaglia, L. A., Ayres, T. M., Wong, G. H., and Goeddel, D. V. (1993). A novel domain within the 55 kd TNF receptor signals cell death. *Cell* 74, 845–853. doi: 10.1016/0092-8674(93)90464-2

Taub, D. D., Proost, P., Murphy, W. J., Anver, M., Longo, D. L., van Damme, J., et al. (1995). Monocyte chemotactic protein-1 (MCP-1), -2 and -3 are chemotactic for human T lymphocytes. *J. Clin. Invest.* 95, 1370–1376. doi: 10. 1172/jci117788

Taylor, C. T. (2008). Mitochondria and cellular oxygen sensing in the HIF pathway. *Biochem. J.* 409, 19–26. doi: 10.1042/bj20071249

Teranishi, M., Nakashima, T., and Wakabayashi, T. (2001). Effects of alpha-tocopherol on cisplatin-induced ototoxicity in guinea pigs. *Hear. Res.* 151, 61–70. doi: 10.1016/s0300-2977(00)00080-2

Tourian, L. Jr., Zhao, H., and Srikant, C. B. (2004). P38alpha, but not p38beta, inhibits the phosphorylation and presence of c-FLIPS in DISC to potentiate Fas-mediated caspase-8 activation and type I apoptotic signaling. *J. Cell Sci.* 117, 6459–6471. doi: 10.1242/jcs.01573

Tournier, C., Hess, P., Yang, D. D., Xu, J., Turner, T. K., Nimnual, A., et al. (2000). Requirement of JNK for stress-induced activation of the cytochrome c-mediated death pathway. *Science* 288, 870–874. doi: 10.1126/science.288.5467.870

Tsujimoto, Y., and Shimizu, S. (2007). Role of the mitochondrial membrane permeability transition in cell death. *Apoptosis* 12, 835–840. doi: 10.1007/s10495-006-0525-7

Tsujimoto, M., Yokota, S., Vilcek, J., and Weissmann, G. (1986). Tumor necrosis factor provokes superoxide anion generation from neutrophils. *Biochem. Biophys. Res. Commun.* 137, 1094–1100. doi: 10.1016/0006-291x(86)90337-2

Turrens, J. F. (2003). Mitochondrial formation of reactive oxygen species. *J. Physiol.* 552, 335–344. doi: 10.1111/j.1469-7793.2003.00335.x

Vandenabeele, P., Galluzzi, L., Vanden Berghe, T., and Kroemer, G. (2010). Molecular mechanisms of necroptosis: an ordered cellular explosion. *Nat. Rev. Mol. Cell Biol.* 11, 700–714. doi: 10.1038/nrm2970

Vanden Berghe, T., Linkermann, A., Jouan-Lanhouet, S., Walczak, H., and Vandenabeele, P. (2014). Regulated necrosis: the expanding network of non-apoptotic cell death pathways. *Nat Rev. Mol. Cell Biol.* 15, 135–147. doi: 10.1038/nrm3737

Van Wijk, F., Staecker, H., Keithley, E., and Lefebvre, P. P. (2006). Local perfusion of the tumor necrosis factor alpha blocker infliximab to the inner ear improves autoimmune neurosensory hearing loss. *Audiol. Neurootol.* 11, 357–365. doi: 10.1159/000095897

Ventura, J. J., Cogswell, P., Flavell, R. A., Baldwin, A. S. Jr., and Davis, R. J. (2004). JNK potentiates TNF-stimulated necrosis by increasing the production of cytotoxic reactive oxygen species. *Genes Dev.* 18, 2905–2915. doi: 10.1101/gad.1223004

Wajant, H., Pfizenmaier, K., and Scheurich, P. (2003). Tumor necrosis factor signaling. *Cell Death Differ.* 10, 45–65. doi: 10.1038/sj.cdd.4401189

Wang, J., Chun, H. J., Wong, W., Spencer, D. M., and Lenardo, M. J. (2001). Caspase-10 is an initiator caspase in death receptor signaling. *Proc. Natl. Acad. Sci. U S A* 98, 13884–13888. doi: 10.1073/pnas.241358198

Wang, J., Ding, D., Shulman, A., Stracher, A., and Salvi, R. J. (1999). Leupeptin protects sensory hair cells from acoustic trauma. *Neuroreport* 10, 811–816. doi: 10.1097/00001756-199903170-00027

Wang, A., Hou, N., Bao, D., Liu, S., and Xu, T. (2012a). Mechanism of alpha-lipoic acid in attenuating kanamycin-induced ototoxiciy. *Neural Regen. Res.* 7, 2793–2800. doi: 10.3969/j.issn.1673-5374.2012.35.007

Wang, Z., Jiang, H., Chen, S., Du, F., and Wang, X. (2012b). The mitochondrial phosphatase PGAM5 functions at the convergence point of multiple necrotic death pathways. *Cell* 148, 228–243. doi: 10.1016/j.cell.2011.11.030

Wang, Y., Kim, N. S., Haince, J. F., Kang, H. C., David, K. K., Andrabi, S. A., et al. (2011). Poly(ADP-ribose) (PAR) binding to apoptosis-inducing factor is critical for PAR polymerase-1 dependent cell death (parthanatos). *Sci. Signal.* 4:ra20. doi: 10.1126/scisignal.2000902

Wang, X. T., Pei, D. S., Xu, J., Guan, Q. H., Sun, Y. F., Liu, X. M., et al. (2007a). Opposing effects of Bad phosphorylation at two distinct sites by Akt1 and JNK1/2 on ischemic brain injury. *Cell. Signal.* 19, 1844–1856. doi: 10.1016/j.cellsig.2007.04.005

Wang, J., Ruel, J., Ladrech, S., Bonny, C., Van de Water, T. R., and Puel, J. L. (2007b). Inhibition of the c-Jun N-terminal kinase-mediated mitochondrial cell death pathway restores auditory function in sound-exposed animals. *Mol. Pharmacol.* 71, 654–666. doi: 10.1124/mol.106.028936

Wang, J., Van De Water, T. R., Bonny, C., de Ribaupierre, F., Puel, J. L., and Zine, A. (2003). A peptide inhibitor of c-Jun N-terminal kinase protects against both aminoglycoside and acoustic trauma-induced auditory hair cell death and hearing loss. *J. Neurosci.* 23, 8596–8607.

Wei, X., Zhao, L., Liu, J., Dodel, R. C., Farlow, M. R., and Du, Y. (2005). Minocycline prevents gentamicin-induced ototoxicity by inhibiting p38 MAP kinase phosphorylation and caspase 3 activation. *Neuroscience* 131, 513–521. doi: 10.1016/j.neuroscience.2004.11.014

Whitfield, J., Neame, S. J., Paquet, L., Bernard, O., and Ham, J. (2001). Dominant-negative c-Jun promotes neuronal survival by reducing BIM expression and inhibiting mitochondrial cytochrome c release. *Neuron* 29, 629–643. doi: 10.1016/s0896-6273(01)00239-2

Widlak, P., Li, L. Y., Wang, X., and Garrard, W. T. (2001). Action of recombinant human apoptotic endonuclease G on naked DNA and chromatin substrates: cooperation with exonuclease and DNase I. *J. Biol. Chem.* 276, 48404–48409.

Yamane, H., Nakai, Y., Takayama, M., Konishi, K., Iguchi, H., Nakagawa, T., et al. (1995). The emergence of free radicals after acoustic trauma and strial blood flow. *Acta Otolaryngol. Suppl.* 519, 87–92. doi: 10.3109/00016489509121877

Yamashita, D., Jiang, H. Y., Schacht, J., and Miller, J. M. (2004a). Delayed production of free radicals following noise exposure. *Brain Res.* 1019, 201–209. doi: 10.1016/j.brainres.2004.05.104

Yamashita, D., Miller, J. M., Jiang, H. Y., Minami, S. B., and Schacht, J. (2004b). AIF and EndoG in noise-induced hearing loss. *Neuroreport* 15, 2719–2722.

Yang, W. P., Henderson, D., Hu, B. H., and Nicotera, T. M. (2004). Quantitative analysis of apoptotic and necrotic outer hair cells after exposure to different levels of continuous noise. *Hear. Res.* 196, 69–76. doi: 10.1016/j.heares.2004.04.015

Ylikoski, J., Xing-Qun, L., Virkkala, J., and Pirvola, U. (2002). Blockade of c-Jun N-terminal kinase pathway attenuates gentamicin-induced cochlear and vestibular hair cell death. *Hear. Res.* 163, 71–81. doi: 10.1016/s0378-5955(01)00380-x

Yoshida, K., Ichimiya, I., Suzuki, M., and Mogi, G. (1999). Effect of proinflammatory cytokines on cultured spiral ligament fibrocytes. *Hear. Res.* 137, 155–159. doi: 10.1016/s0378-5955(99)00134-3

Yu, S. W., Andrabi, S. A., Wang, H., Kim, N. S., Poirier, G. G., Dawson, T. M., et al. (2006). Apoptosis-inducing factor mediates poly(ADP-ribose)(PAR) polymer-induced cell death. *Proc. Natl. Acad. Sci. U S A* 103, 18314–18319. doi: 10.1073/pnas.0606528103

Zhang, D. W., Shao, J., Lin, J., Zhang, N., Lu, B. J., Lin, S. C., et al. (2009). RIP3, an energy metabolism regulator that switches TNF-induced cell death from apoptosis to necrosis. *Science* 325, 332–336. doi: 10.1126/science.1172308

Zheng, H. W., Chen, J., and Sha, S. H. (2014). Receptor-interacting protein kinases modulate noise induced sensory hair cell death. *Cell Death Dis.* 5:e1262. doi: 10.1038/cddis.2014.177

Zou, J., Pyykkö, I., Sutinen, P., and Toppila, E. (2005). Vibration induced hearing loss in guinea pig cochlea: expression of TNF-alpha and VEGF. *Hear. Res.* 202, 13–20. doi: 10.1016/j.heares.2004.10.008

6

Dynamic expression of *Lgr6* in the developing and mature mouse cochlea

Yanping Zhang[1,2,3†], *Yan Chen*[1,2†], *Wenli Ni*[4], *Luo Guo*[1,2], *Xiaoling Lu*[4], *Liman Liu*[2], *Wen Li*[1,2], *Shan Sun*[1,2], *Lei Wang*[3] and *Huawei Li*[2,4,5*]

[1] Research Center, Affiliated Eye and ENT Hospital of Fudan University, Shanghai, China, [2] Key Laboratory of Hearing Medicine, Ministry of Health, Affiliated Eye and ENT Hospital of Fudan University, Shanghai, China, [3] Institutes of Biomedical Sciences, Fudan University, Shanghai, China, [4] Department of Otorhinolaryngology, Affiliated Eye and ENT Hospital of Fudan University, Shanghai, China, [5] The State Key Laboratory of Medical Neurobiology, The Institutes of Brain Science and the Collaborative Innovation Center for Brain Science, Fudan University, Shanghai, China

Edited by:
Michael E. Smith,
Western Kentucky University, USA

Reviewed by:
Paola Bovolenta,
Consejo Superior de Investigaciones Científicas, Spain
Andy Groves,
Baylor College of Medicine, USA

***Correspondence:**
Huawei Li,
Department of Otorhinolaryngology, Affiliated Eye and ENT Hospital of Fudan University, Room 611, Building 9, No. 83, Fenyang Road, Xuhui District, Shanghai 200031, China
hwli@shmu.edu.cn

† These authors have contributed equally to this work.

The Wnt/β-catenin signaling pathway plays important roles in mammalian inner ear development. *Lgr5*, one of the downstream target genes of the Wnt/β-catenin signaling pathway, has been reported to be a marker for inner ear hair cell progenitors. *Lgr6* shares approximately 50% sequence homology with *Lgr5* and has been identified as a stem cell marker in several organs. However, the detailed expression profiles of *Lgr6* have not yet been investigated in the mouse inner ear. Here, we first used Lgr6-EGFP-Ires-CreERT2 mice to examine the spatiotemporal expression of Lgr6 protein in the cochlear duct during embryonic and postnatal development. Lgr6-EGFP was first observed in one row of prosensory cells in the middle and basal turn at embryonic day 15.5 (E15.5). From E18.5 to postnatal day 3 (P3), the expression of Lgr6-EGFP was restricted to the inner pillar cells (IPCs). From P7 to P15, the Lgr6-EGFP expression level gradually decreased in the IPCs and gradually increased in the inner border cells (IBCs). At P20, Lgr6-EGFP was only expressed in the IBCs, and by P30 Lgr6-EGFP expression had completely disappeared. Next, we demonstrated that Wnt/β-catenin signaling is required to maintain the Lgr6-EGFP expression *in vitro*. Finally, we demonstrated that the Lgr6-EGFP-positive cells isolated by flow cytometry could differentiate into myosin 7a-positive hair cells after 10 days in-culture, and this suggests that the Lgr6-positive cells might serve as the hair cell progenitor cells in the cochlea.

Keywords: Wnt, regeneration, hair cells, Lgr6, inner pillar cell, inner border cell, hair cell progenitor

Introduction

The mammalian inner ear cochlea is a very sophisticated organ. The organ of Corti in the inner ear is responsible for hearing in mammals and contains two types of mechanosensory hair cells (inner hair cells and outer hair cells) and six types of supporting cells [Deiters' cells, Hensen's cells, Claudius' cells, pillar cells, inner phalangeal cells, and inner border cells (IBCs)] (Chai et al., 2012). Cell proliferation and differentiation are coordinated in the development of the organ of Corti, but many molecular mechanisms involved in regulating this proliferation and differentiation remain undiscovered (Cremisi et al., 2003; Pagano and Jackson, 2004). During the development of the mouse cochlea, the otic placode—which will give rise to the auditory and vestibular sensory organs of the inner ear (Fritzsch et al., 1998)—forms on embryonic day 8.5 (E8.5). The placode invaginates to form the otocyst on E11. By this time, the regions that will give rise to sensory neuroepithelia have already been specified (Morsli et al., 1998). At E12, the progenitors of hair cells and supporting cells are still dividing (Ruben, 1967). At E12.5, apical progenitors begin to exit the cell cycle, and this is followed by the progenitor cells in the base of the cochlea. By E14, all progenitor cells of the inner ear have exited the cell cycle (Ruben, 1967; Lee et al., 2006). Hair cell differentiation first appears in the mid-basal region of the cochlea at E13.5 and spreads bidirectionally during the development of the organ of Corti (Chen et al., 2002). Hair cell differentiation finishes between E17 and E18 (Sher, 1971; Li and Ruben, 1979; Lim and Anniko, 1985; Chen et al., 2002).

The Wnt/β-catenin signaling pathway is reported to play important roles in mammalian cochlear development and hair cell regeneration by regulating both proliferation and differentiation of prosensory cells. The Wnt/β-catenin signaling pathway is also critical for otocyst induction, dorsal patterning of the otocyst, and the eventual formation of the vestibular organs (Hollyday et al., 1995; Jasoni et al., 1999; Riccomagno et al., 2005; Lillevali et al., 2006; Ohyama et al., 2006; Rakowiecki and Epstein, 2013). Wnt/β-catenin signaling also plays a key role in hair cell formation in the cochlea, and this is clearly demonstrated by the inability of hair cells to differentiate from sensory progenitors when Wnt/β-catenin is knocked out (Jacques et al., 2012; Shi et al., 2014).

Recently, the Wnt/β-catenin downstream target genes *Lgr5* and *Axin2* have been reported to be markers for inner ear hair cell progenitors. The Lgr5-positive hair cell progenitors can self-renew to regenerate hair cells after isolation by flow cytometry *in vitro*, and they can also spontaneously regenerate hair cells after hair cell loss in neonatal mouse cochleae *in vivo* (Chai et al., 2011, 2012; Shi et al., 2012, 2013; Jan et al., 2013; Cox et al., 2014). Recent studies also showed that Wnt/β-catenin signaling plays dual roles in controlling the proliferation and differentiation of hair cell progenitor cells (Jacques et al., 2012; Shi et al., 2014). Lgr6 is a member of the leucine-rich repeat-containing G-protein-coupled receptors (LGRs) (Barker and Clevers, 2010). In other organs, including the skin, taste buds, and lungs, Lgr6 has been identified as a stem cell marker (Snippert et al., 2010; Oeztuerk-Winder et al., 2012; Ren et al., 2014), and these Lgr6-positive stem cells have been reported to be involved in wound repair and hair follicle development (Barker and Clevers, 2010; Snippert et al., 2010; Leushacke and Barker, 2012). Lgr6 expression is sometimes up-regulated in gastric cancer, and Lgr6 expression is significantly correlated with patient survival; patients with Lgr6-positive tumors tend to live longer than patients with Lgr6-negative tumors (Krejs, 2010; Garlipp et al., 2011).

Lgr6 shares approximately 50% sequence homology with Lgr5, which is a marker of Wnt-regulated hair cell progenitor cells in the postnatal mouse cochleae. The expression pattern and characterization of Lgr5 have been well studied in the mouse inner ear (Chai et al., 2011, 2012; Shi et al., 2012, 2013; Jan et al., 2013; Cox et al., 2014). At E15.5, Lgr5 is expressed in the whole prosensory region of the cochlear duct, and the expression continues to decrease during development. From E18.5 to neonatal ages, Lgr5 expression is restricted to the third row of Deiters' cells, inner pillar cells (IPCs), medial inner phalangeal cells, and the lateral GER (greater epithelium region). By P30, Lgr5 expression is only detectable in the third row of Deiters' cells (Chai et al., 2011). However, the detailed expression profiles of the homologous Lgr6 protein during development have not yet been investigated in the mouse inner ear. In the gastrointestinal and integumentary systems, Lgr5 expression is regulated by Wnt signaling (Jaks et al., 2008; Ootani et al., 2009). In the inner ear, Wnt activation increases Lgr5 expression, and Wnt inhibition decreases Lgr5 expression (Chai et al., 2011, 2012; Shi et al., 2012, 2013). However, whether Wnt signaling can regulate the expression of Lgr6 has remained unknown. In mouse cochleae, the Lgr5-positive cells can regenerate hair cells both *in vivo* and *in vitro* and thus, serve as the inner ear hair cell progenitor cells (Chai et al., 2012; Shi et al., 2012, 2013; Cox et al., 2014; Li et al., 2015). However, the characterization of the Lgr6-positive cells has not been investigated in the mouse inner ear.

In this study, we first utilized transgenic Lgr6-EGFP-Ires-CreERT2 reporter mice to characterize the spatiotemporal expression of Lgr6 in the embryonic and postnatal mammalian cochlear duct. Next, we showed that Wnt signaling is required to maintain the expression of Lgr6. Last, we isolated the Lgr6-positive cells by flow cytometry and demonstrated that Lgr6-positive cells could differentiate into hair cells *in vitro.*

Methods

Animals

Lgr6-EGFP-Ires-CreERT2 mice in a C57BL/6J background were purchased from the Jackson Laboratory (stock no. 016934). These mice were generated by homologous recombination in embryonic supporting cells that placed an EGFP-Ires-CreERT2 cassette at the transcriptional start site of the *Lgr6* gene. Insertion of the EGFP-Ires-CreERT2 into the transcriptional start site of the gene enabled green fluorescent labeling of cells that normally express Lgr6. All of the transgenic mice used for our research were heterozygotes. All animal procedures were performed according to protocols approved by the Animal Care and Use Committee of Fudan University and were consistent with the National Institutes of Health Guide for the Care and Use of Laboratory Animals. All efforts were made to minimize the number of animals used and to prevent their suffering.

Genotyping, RT-PCR, and qPCR

Genomic DNA was isolated from transgenic mouse tails using a DNA extraction kit (pc 3202, Biomed) according to the manufacturer's instructions. We used the following genotyping primers: wild-type Lgr6 (forward) CTG TGG CTT TGC GCT GTG; (reverse) AAG GGC ACC AAA CGA GTG T; mutant Lgr6 (forward) GCC CAC CGA CGG CGC AGC CC; (reverse) GCT GAA CTT GTG CCG TTT A.

The total RNA from the cochlear sensory epithelium was processed with an RNeasy micro kit (Cat. #74004, Qiagen). cDNA was synthesized from 1 μg total RNA by reverse transcription using random primers (Promega) and Superscript III reverse transcriptase (Life Technologies). Quantitative real-time PCR (qPCR) was performed using SYBR Green PCR Master Mix (Life Technologies) on an AB 7500 Real-Time PCR System (Life Technologies). Each PCR reaction was carried out in triplicate, and the relative quantification of gene expression was analyzed using the ΔΔCT method with GAPDH as the endogenous reference. Primer pairs for the qPCR were designed using the online Primer3 software. *Lgr6*: (forward) GTA TGA ACA ACC TCA CGG AGC; (reverse) TTG GAG GCC AGA GAA TGC C; *Sox2*: (forward) ATG AAC GGC TGG AGC AAC GGC A; (reverse) TCA CAT GTG CGA CAG GGG CAG T; *GAPDH*: (forward) AAC GGG AAG CCC ATC ACC ATC TT; (reverse) CAG CCT TGG CAG CAC CAG TGG; *Lgr5*: (forward) TCT TCA CCT CCT ACC TGG ACC T; (reverse) GGC GTA GTC TGC TAT GTG GTG T; *Brn3.1*: (forward) CCC AAA TTC TCC AGC CTA CAC; (reverse) GGC GAG ATG TGC TCA AGT AAG T.

Cryosectioning

Heads from E15.5 mice and the otic bullae from E18.5–postnatal day 3 (P3) mice were isolated and fixed with 4% paraformaldehyde (Sigma-Aldrich) in 0.01 M phosphate-buffered saline (PBS, pH 7.4) at 4°C overnight. For P7 and older animals, decalcification was performed with 10% EDTA in PBS for 1–3 days at 4°C. Samples were immersed in 15% and then 30% sucrose in PBS at 4°C overnight, and then embedded in OCT compound (Sakura Finetek) at 4°C overnight. Serial frozen sections of 10–12 μm thickness were made with a Leica CM3050 cryostat (Leica).

Cell Sorting by Flow Cytometry

Cochleae from P3 Lgr6-EGFP-Ires-CreERT2 mice were dissected out and the stria vascularis and spiral ganglia were removed. The cochleae were incubated in 0.125% trypsin (Invitrogen) at 37°C for 8 min, and the same volume of 10 mg/mL trypsin inhibitor (Worthington Biochem) was added. Following trituration, cells were passed through a 40 μm filter (BD Biosciences) and labeled with 1 μg/mL propidium iodide (Sigma) to remove the dead cells. Wild-type cochleae were used to determine the background labeling levels in each sorting. The dissociated cells were sorted on a MoFlo® SX FACS cytometer (Beckman Coulter) using the channels for GFP, and the positive fractions were collected. We consistently achieved over 90% cell viability and over 95% purity for sorted cells. The purity of the sorted cells was assessed by re-sort analysis, immunohistochemistry, and quantitative RT-PCR. For staining, sorted cells were plated on fibronectin-coated slides (Sigma) and incubated for 1 h at 37°C before fixation and immunohistochemistry.

Culture of Sorted Cells

Flow cytometry-isolated Lgr6-positive cells (2000 cells with a density of 20 cells/μL) were plated on a laminin-coated 4-well dish and cultured for 10 days in DMEM/F12 media with 2% B27, 1% N2, EGF (20 ng/mL, Chemicon), bFGF (10 ng/mL, NIH), IGF-1 (50 ng/mL, Chemicon), and heparin sulfate (50 ng/mL, Sigma). The cells were fixed and immunostained for hair cell markers after 10 days of culture.

Tissue Cultures

P1 mice were sacrificed and their cochleae were carefully dissected to separate the organs of Corti from the spiral ganglia, the stria vascularis, and Reissner membranes under sterile conditions with fine forceps. Whole-mount cochleae were then transferred onto 10-mm coverslips (Fisher Scientific) pre-coated with poly-L-lysine (Sigma-Aldrich). Whole organs were cultured in DMEM/F12 (Invitrogen) supplemented with N2 (Invitrogen), B27 (Invitrogen), and ampicillin (50 μg/mL; Sigma-Aldrich) in four-well Petri dishes (Greiner Bio-one). After 12 h, Bio (5 μM, Sigma) or IWP-2 (25 mM, Sigma) was added to the culture medium for 3 days. Culture media were replenished every day. After this final culture, the basal membranes were fixed with 4% paraformaldehyde for 30 min at room temperature.

Immunofluorescence, Image Acquisition, and Image Analysis

Immunofluorescence was performed as reported previously (Jiang et al., 2014). Fixed tissues were blocked with 10% donkey serum in 10 mM PBS (pH 7.4) with 1% Triton X-100 (Sangon Biotech) for 1 h at room temperature and then incubated with primary antibodies overnight at 4°C in a humidified chamber. The following day, tissues were rinsed with PBS and then incubated with secondary antibodies for 1 h at room temperature. After washing with PBS, tissues were mounted in antifade fluorescence mounting medium (DAKO) and coverslipped. The primary antibodies included anti-Lgr6 (1:500 dilution, Santa Cruz Biotechnology), anti-myosin 7a (1:1000 dilution, Proteus Bioscience), anti-GFP (1:1000 dilution, Abcam), and anti-Sox2 (1:500 dilution, Santa Cruz Biotechnology). The secondary antibodies were conjugated with FITC, Cy3, or Cy5 (1:500 dilution, Jackson ImmunoResearch). The nuclei were stained with 4,6-diamidino-2-phenylindole (DAPI, 1:800 dilution, Sigma-Aldrich) for 15 min at room temperature. Negative control experiments were performed as above by omitting the primary antibodies. Cochleae were dissected into the apical, middle, and basal turns, and photographs were taken using a Leica SP5 confocal fluorescence microscope (Leica) and analyzed with Photoshop CS4 (Adobe Systems).

Auditory Brainstem Responses

The auditory brainstem response (ABR) was measured to determine the hearing threshold of the mice. P30 mice were anaesthetized with ketamine (100 mg/kg) and xylazine (25 mg/kg; i.p.) and then placed on a thermostatic heating pad in a sound-attenuating chamber to maintain their body temperatures at 38°C. Electrodes were placed on the scalp of the mouse to record the electrical activity of the brain in response to sound. Four frequencies (8, 16, 24, and 32 kHz) were assessed with a TDT system 3 device (Tucker Davies Technologies).

Cell Counts

To quantify the Lgr6-positive cells in the three turns of the cochlea, we imaged the entire cochlea using a 40× objective and counted the EGFP-positive cells. For all experiments, only one cochlea from each mouse was used for immunofluorescence and quantification. Thus, *n* represents the number of mice examined.

Statistical Analysis

Statistical analyses were conducted using Microsoft Excel (Microsoft) and GraphPad Prism v5.0.3. The data were expressed as the mean ± SD. Immunofluorescence analysis was performed with a two-tailed, unpaired Student's t-test when comparing two groups or with a one-way ANOVA followed by a Dunnett's multiple comparisons test when comparing more than two groups. $P < 0.05$ was considered statistically significant.

Results

Lgr6 Expression in the Embryonic Cochlear Duct

We first investigated the expression pattern of the Wnt downstream target gene *Lgr6*. Here we took advantage of the Lgr6-EGFP-Ires-CreERT2 transgenic mice in which EGFP-Ires-CreERT2 is inserted into the transcriptional start site of the *Lgr6* gene. The cells in these mice that normally express Lgr6 are labeled with green fluorescent protein. At E13.5, we did not observe any Lgr6-EGFP-positive cells in the organ of Corti (data not shown). Two days later, at E15.5, we detected Lgr6-EGFP expression in one row of Sox2-positive progenitor cells, and the Lgr6 expression appeared as a gradient from the base to the apex in the cochlear duct floor epithelium (**Figures 1B**, **2A**). Lgr6-EGFP was mainly expressed in the middle and basal turns of the organ of Corti, and no Lgr6-EGFP was observed in the apical turn (n = 4) (**Table 1**). Starting at E15.5, myosin 7a, one of the hair cell-specific markers, was expressed in the base of the organ of Corti, and Sox2, the prosensory cell marker, was expressed in the prosensory region that gives rise to the organ of Corti (Kiernan et al., 2005; Dabdoub et al., 2008). In the basal turn, Lgr6-EGFP expression was only seen in one row of prosensory cells between the inner hair cells and outer hair cells (**Figure 1B**).

Hair cells complete their differentiation between E17 and E18. We examined the E18.5 cochlear duct and found a similar Lgr6-EGFP expression pattern with a gradient from base to apex as seen at E15.5. Lgr6-EGFP was expressed in the IPCs in the middle and basal turns (**Figure 1A**), and the Lgr6-EGFP expression was increased compared to E15.5 (n = 4) (**Figures 1**, **2**, and **Table 1**). The percentage of Lgr6-EGFP-positive cells out of the total IPCs was 24.42 ± 4.43% and 65.33 ± 5.13% in the middle and basal turns, respectively. We did not detect any Lgr6-EGFP-positive cells in the apical turn. At this development stage, we detected four rows of myosin 7a-positive hair cells in the organ of Corti (**Figure 2A**). In the apical and middle turn, Sox2 was expressed in hair cells, the adjacent supporting cells, and the GER medially (**Figure 1B**). This hair cell-bearing area at this stage is henceforth referred to as the prosensory region. Sox2 levels were down-regulated in more differentiated hair cells in the basal region (**Figure 1B**), and this down-regulation of Sox2 in hair cells was consistent with previous reports (Hume et al., 2007).

Lgr6-EGFP Expression is Restricted to the IPCs in the Cochlea at P1 and P3

Like the E18.5 cochlear duct, Lgr6-EGFP was also expressed in the IPCs in the middle and basal turns of P1 and P3 cochleae (**Figures 3A,C,D** and **Table 2**). There was no Lgr6-EGFP expression in the apical turn. At P1, Lgr6 expression increased in both the middle and basal turns compared to E18.5 (n = 4) (**Tables 1**, **2**). To confirm the expression of Lgr6, we stained the P1 cochleae with the Lgr6 antibody and found that the Lgr6 expression detected by immunohistochemical staining was identical to the Lgr6-EGFP reporter expression (**Figure 3B**). At P3, the Lgr6 expression decreased in both the basal and middle turns of the organ of Corti compared to the expression at P1 (n = 4) (**Figure 3C**, **Figure S1**, and **Table 2**).

Lgr6-EGFP Expression is Restricted to Both IPCs and IBCs from P7 to P15

Interestingly, at P7 we found that the Lgr6-EGFP expression was not only in the IPCs but also in the IBCs in both the middle and basal turns. There was no EGFP expression in the apical turn. The Lgr6 expression in the IPCs decreased at P7 compared to that of P3 (n = 4) (**Figure 6D**, **Table 2**). The Lgr6 expression in IBCs was similar to that in IPCs (n = 4) (**Figures 4**, **5A,B**, **6E** and **Table 3**). The percentage of Lgr6-EGFP-positive IPCs was 40 ± 3.6% and 85 ± 4.7% in the middle and basal turns, respectively. The percentage of Lgr6-EGFP-positive IBCs was 41.5 ± 4.1% and 87.3 ± 3.53% in the middle and basal turns, respectively.

At P10, Lgr6-EGFP expression in the middle and basal turns was similar to P7 (n = 4) (**Figures 4**, **5**, **6D,E**, **Tables 2**, **3**). The percentage of Lgr6-EGFP-positive IPCs was 15.19 ± 3.56% and 76.53 ± 4.12% in the middle and basal turns, respectively. The percentage of Lgr6-EGFP-positive IBCs was 92.1 ± 4.78% and 95.08 ± 4.61% in the middle and basal turns, respectively. However, Lgr6-EGFP expression also appeared in the IBCs of the apical turn (n = 4) (**Table 3**), and the percentage of Lgr6-EGFP-positive IBCs was 91.76 ± 3.53% in the apical turn.

At P15, the Lgr6-EGFP expression in the middle and basal turns was similar to the expression at P10 (n = 4) (**Figures 4**, **5**, **6D,E**, **Tables 2**, **3**). The percentage of Lgr6-EGFP-positive IPCs was 14.21 ± 3.43% and 70.32 ± 5.12% in the middle and basal turns, respectively. The percentage of Lgr6-EGFP-positive IBCs was 99.79 ± 3.56% and 98.34 ± 4.12% in the middle and basal turns, respectively. In the apical turn, Lgr6-EGFP was expressed only in the IBCs (n = 4) (**Table 3**), and the percentage of Lgr6-EGFP-positive IBCs was 98.12 ± 4.1%.

Lgr6-EGFP Expression is only seen in IBCs at P20 and Completely Disappears at P30

At P20, Lgr6-EGFP was expressed only in the IBCs, not in the IPCs, in all three turns. The Lgr6 expression level decreased gradually from the basal to apical turn (n = 4) (**Figure 6** and **Table 3**). The percentage of Lgr6-EGFP-positive IBCs was 19.23 ± 3.49%, 59.43 ± 4.23%, and 90.67 ± 5.01% in the apical, middle, and basal turns, respectively. At P30, we did not detect any Lgr6-EGFP expression in any cells in any of the turns (n = 4) (**Figure 6**).

Heterozygous Lgr6-EGFP-Ires-CreERT2 Mice have Normal Hearing

Heterozygous Lgr6-EGFP-Ires-CreERT2 mice have been reported to be healthy (Snippert et al., 2010), but data about their auditory function have not yet been provided. According to our ABR measurements, there was no

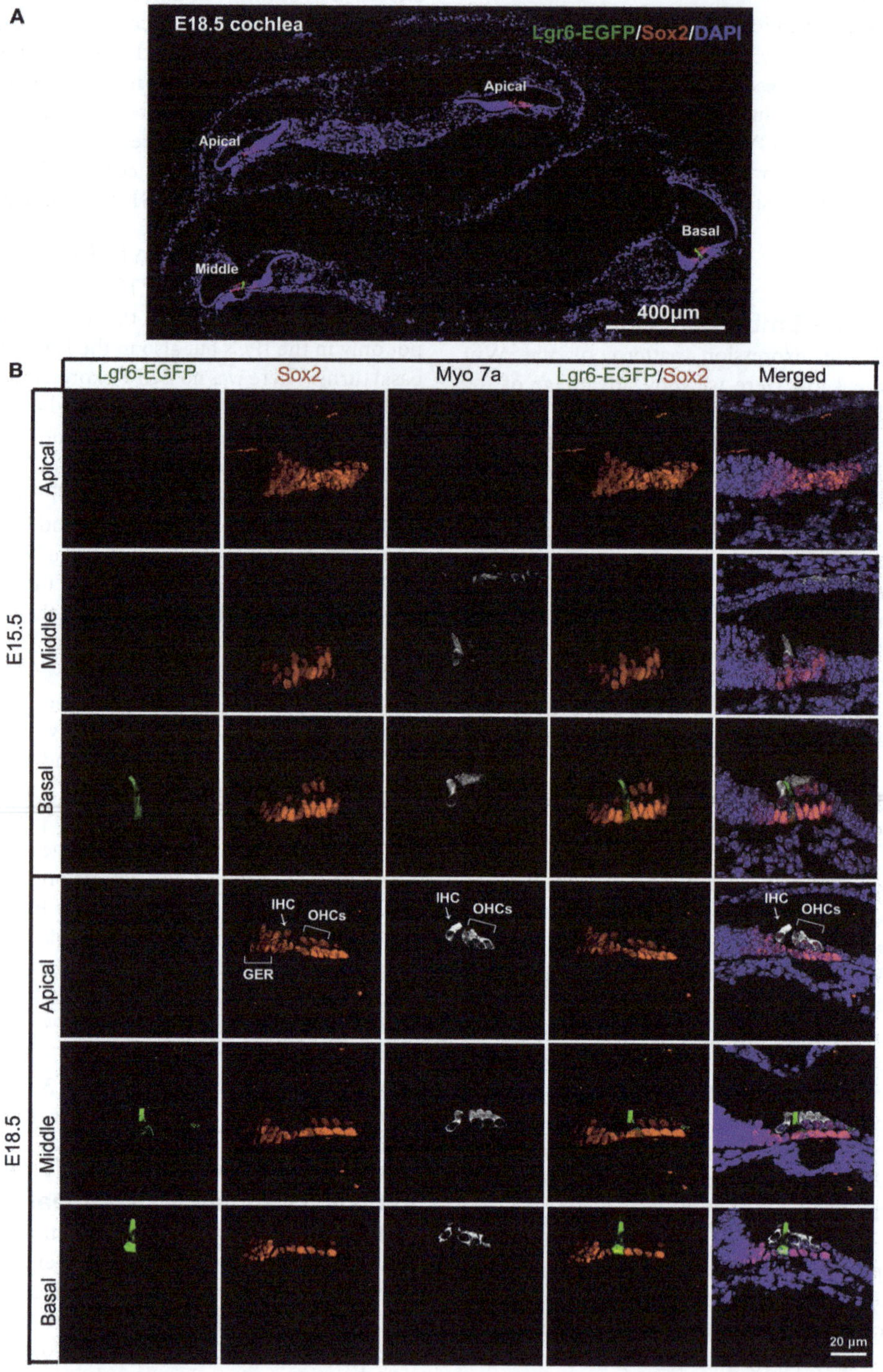

FIGURE 1 | Expression of Lgr6-EGFP in cochlear cryosections at E15.5 and E18.5. (A) At low magnification, expression of Lgr6-EGFP at E18.5 was restricted to one supporting cell in the middle and basal turns, and no expression was seen in the apical turn. **(B)** Lgr6-EGFP was expressed in one supporting cell in the middle and basal turns of the organ of Corti at E15.5. At E18.5, Lgr6-EGFP was expressed in the inner pillar cells in the middle and basal turns. IHC, inner hair cell; OHCs, outer hair cells; GER, greater epithelium region.

significant threshold difference between the heterozygous Lgr6-EGFP-Ires-CreERT2 mice and their age-matched wild-type littermates at P30 (One-Way ANOVA, $P = 0.79$) (**Figure 6C**).

Wnt Signaling is Required to Maintain the Expression of Lgr6

To investigate whether Wnt signaling can regulate Lgr6 expression, we dissected out the cochlea from P3

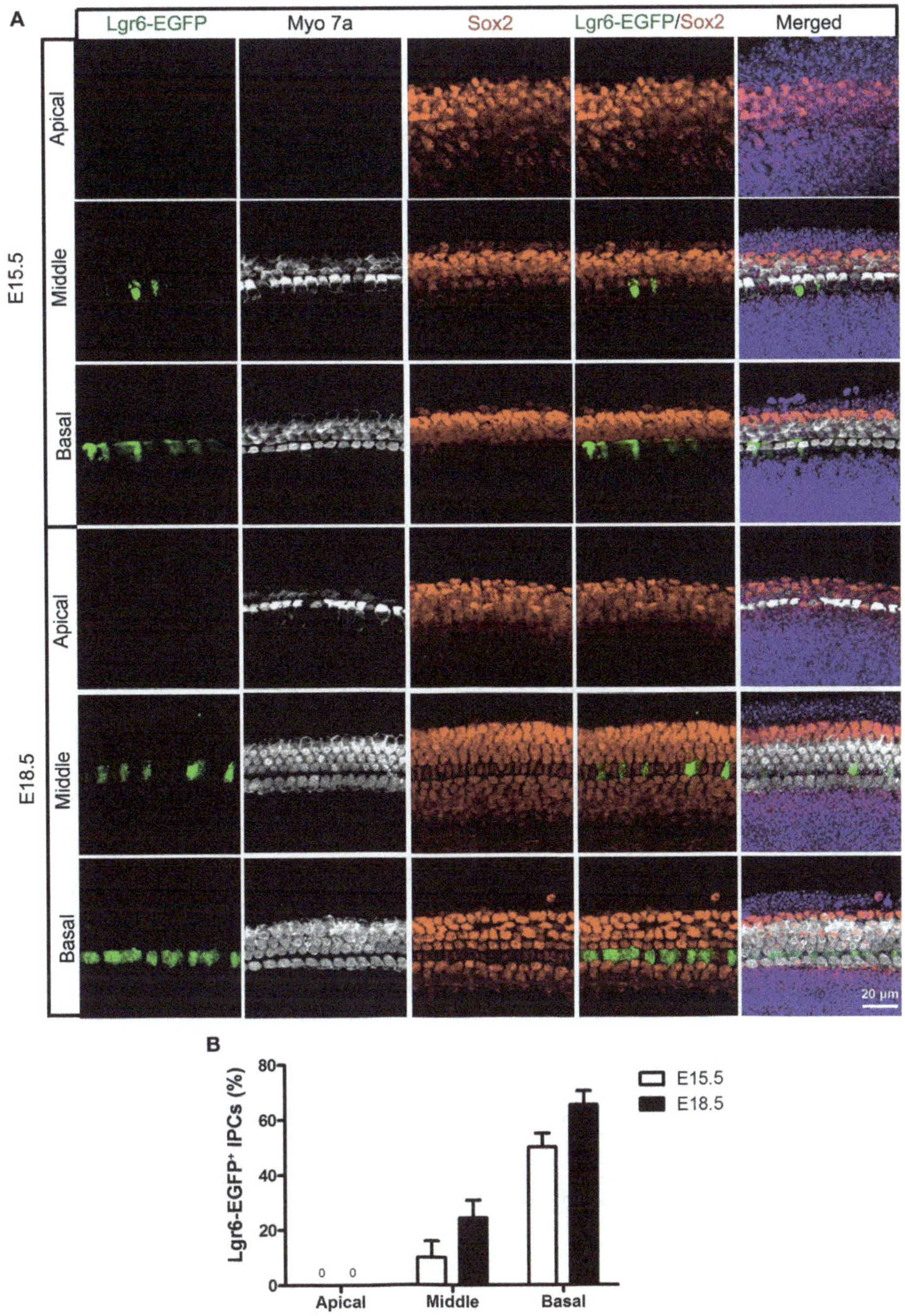

FIGURE 2 | Lgr6-EGFP expression in the whole mount cochleae of mouse embryos at E15.5 and E18.5. (A) Lgr6-EGFP was expressed in one row of supporting cells in the middle and basal turns of the organ of Corti at E15.5 and E18.5. There was no Lgr6-EGFP expression in the apical turn. **(B)** The percentage of Lgr6-EGFP-positive IPCs at E15.5 and E18.5. The Lgr6-EGFP expression increased in both the middle and basal turns of the organ of Corti from E15.5 to E18.5 ($n = 4$). IPCs, inner pillar cells.

Lgr6-EGFP-Ires-CreERT2 mice and treated the cochlear explants with the Wnt agonist Bio (5 μM) or the Wnt antagonist IWP-2 (25 μM) for 3 days. DMSO treatment was the vehicle control. In control cochleae, there were no Lgr6-EGFP-positive cells in the apical turn. When treated with the Wnt agonist Bio, the number of Lgr6-EGFP-positive cells increased significantly in the apical turn ($n = 4$, $P < 0.01$) (**Figures 7A,C** and **Table 4**); however, the Lgr6-EGFP-positive cell numbers in the middle and basal turns did not change significantly compared to controls ($n = 4$, $P = 0.25$, and $P = 0.95$, respectively) (**Figures 7A,C** and **Table 4**). When treated with the Wnt antagonist IWP-2, the Lgr6-EGFP-positive cell number decreased significantly both in the middle and basal turns compared to controls ($n = 4$, $P < 0.01$) (**Figures 7A,C** and **Table 4**). qPCR experiments showed similar results. We found that Bio treatment increased the Lgr6 expression level, but the increase was not statistically significant ($n = 4$, $P = 0.76$) (**Figure 7B**), while IWP-2 significantly decreased the Lgr6 expression level ($n = 4$, $P < 0.01$) (**Figure 7B**). These results suggested that Wnt signaling is required to maintain the expression of Lgr6 *in vitro*.

TABLE 1 | Quantification of Lgr6-EFGP/Sox2 double-positive inner pillar cells per 100 μm cochlear length at E15.5 and E18.5.

Embryonic	Apical	Middle	Basal
E15.5	0	2.53 ± 0.50	10.13 ± 0.71
E18.5	0	4.12 ± 0.83	12.08 ± 0.50

All the data are shown as the average ± S.D. n = 4 for all the samples.

Lgr6-Positive Cells Isolated by Flow Cytometry can Generate Hair Cells *In Vitro*

To further characterize the Lgr6-positive cells, we isolated these cells with FACS (florescence-activated cell sorting) and cultured

TABLE 2 | Quantification of Lgr6-EFGP/Sox2 double-positive inner pillar cells per 100 μm cochlear length from P1 to P30.

Age	Apical	Middle	Basal
P1	0	9.67 ± 0.35	15.03 ± 0.25
P3	0	7.03 ± 0.25	12.00 ± 0.30
P7	0	4.57 ± 0.26	10.40 ± 0.31
P10	0	2.20 ± 0.30	8.37 ± 0.25
P15	0	2.11 ± 0.28	7.87 ± 0.18
P20	0	0	0
P30	0	0	0

All the data are shown as the average ± S.D. n = 4 for all the samples.

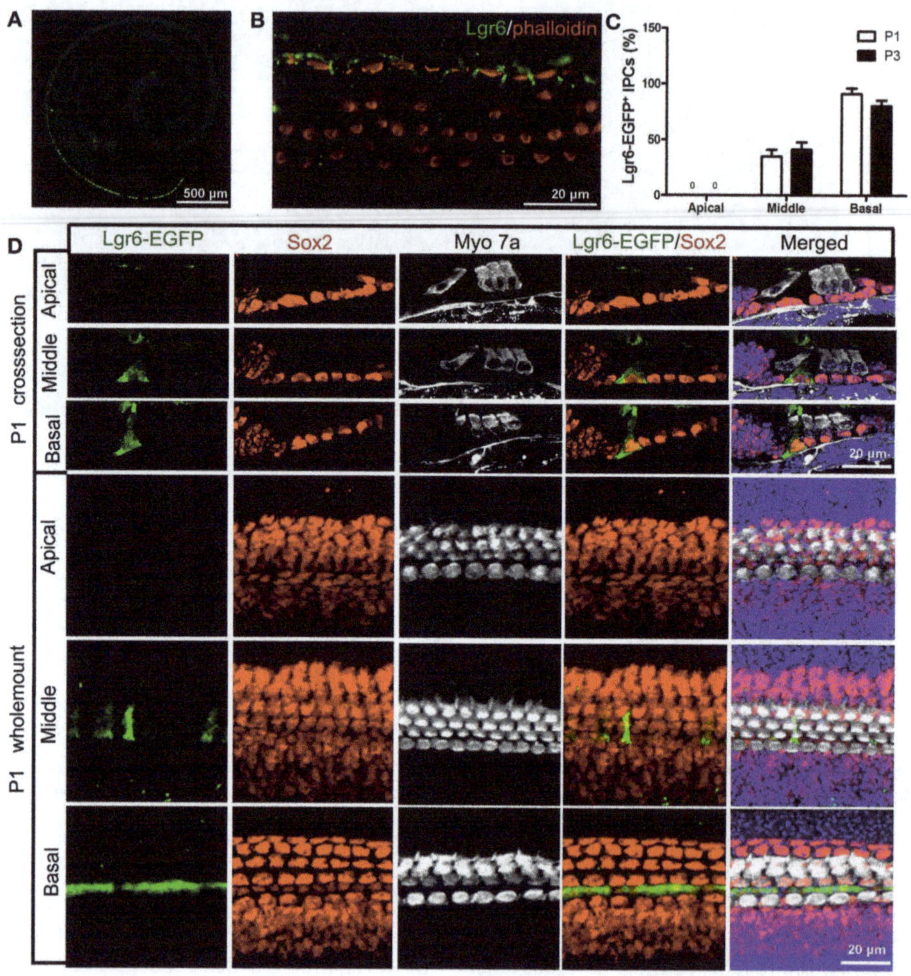

FIGURE 3 | Lgr6-EGFP expression is restricted to the IPCs in the cochlea at P1. (A) At low magnification, only one row of Lgr6-EGFP-positive cells was detected, and Lgr6-EGFP was only expressed in the middle and basal turns in the cochlear epithelium at P1. **(B)** Immunostaining with an anti-Lgr6 antibody in wild-type cochlea showed that Lgr6 expression was restricted to the IPCs at P1. **(C)** The percentage of Lgr6-EGFP-positive IPCs (IPCs) at P1 and P3 ($n = 4$). **(D)** At P1, Lgr6-EGFP was expressed only in the IPCs in the middle and basal turns. IPCs, inner pillar cells.

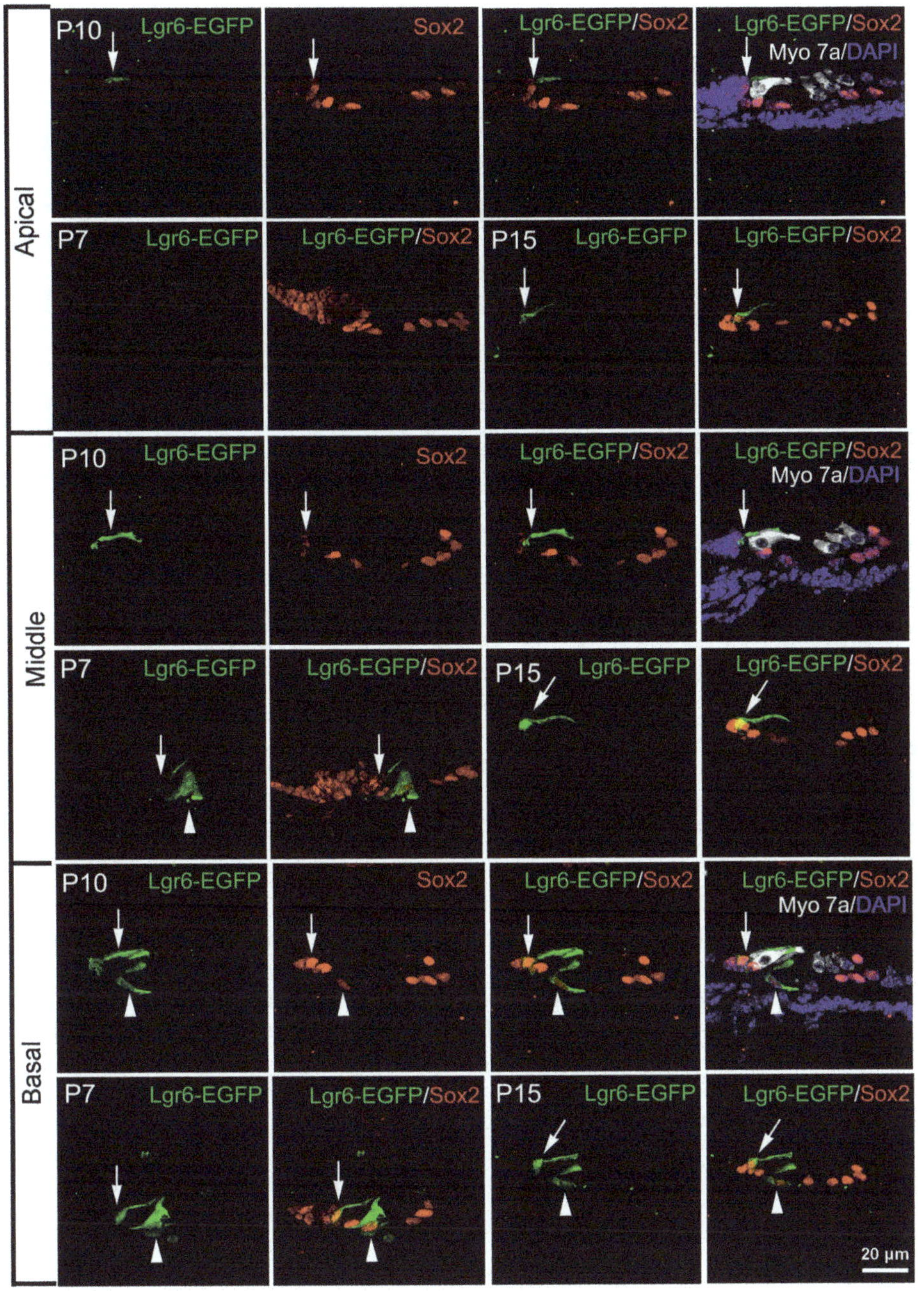

FIGURE 4 | Lgr6-EGFP expression is restricted to both inner pillar cells (IPCs) and inner border cells (IBCs) from P7 to P15. At P7, Lgr6-EGFP was expressed both in the IPCs (arrow head) and IBCs (arrow) in the middle and basal turns, and there was no Lgr6-EGFP expression in the apical turn. Between P10 and P15, Lgr6-EGFP was expressed only in the IPCs (arrow head), but in the basal turn Lgr6-EGFP was expressed in both the IPCs (arrow head) and IBCs (arrow).

them to test whether the Lgr6-positive cells could generate hair cells *in vitro*. In this experiment, we dissected out the cochlea from 40 to 50 Lgr6-EGFP-Ires-CreERT2 mice and purified the Lgr6-EGFP-positive cells by FACS. We found that around 0.8% of the cells were Lgr6-EGFP-positive ($n = 3$) (**Figure 8A**). Immunohistochemical staining showed that 94.43 ± 3.67% of the Lgr6-positive cells sorted by flow cytometry were also EGFP positive ($n = 3$). Isolated Lgr6-EGFP-positive cells showed no staining for the hair cell marker myosin 7a ($n = 3$) (**Figure 8D**), but almost all cells were positive for the supporting cell marker Sox2 (95.65 ± 44.35%, $n = 3$) (**Figure 8D**). qPCR data also showed that the Lgr6-EGFP-positive cells had significantly higher Lgr6 expression ($P < 0.001$), slightly higher Sox2 expression ($P < 0.05$), and significantly lower hair cell marker Brn3.1 expression ($P < 0.001$) compared to the EGFP-negative cells ($n = 3$) (**Figure 8B**). We then cultured the flow

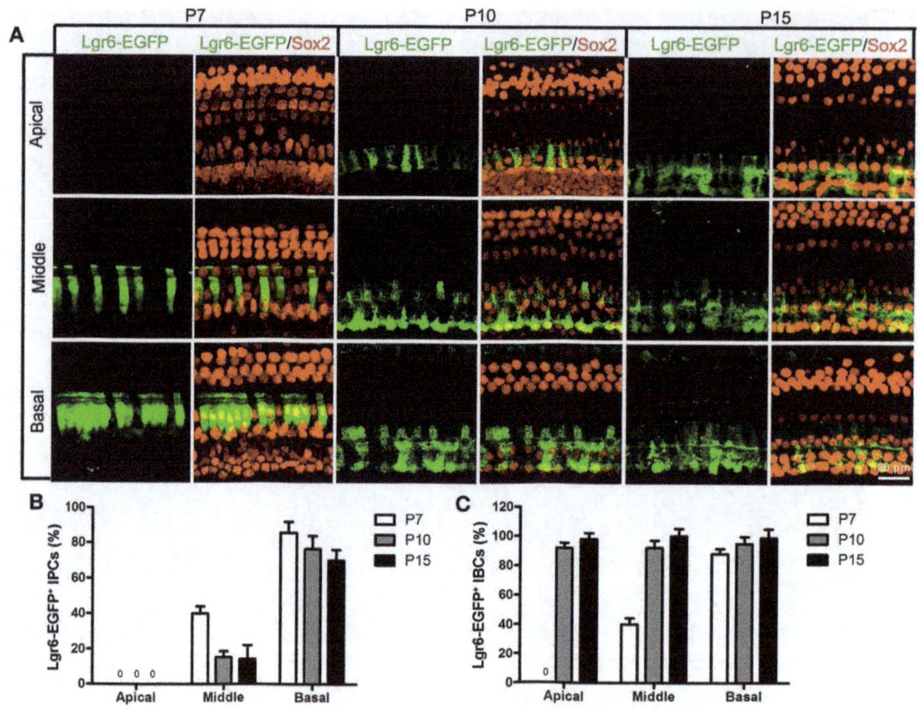

FIGURE 5 | Lgr6-EGFP expression decreased in the IPCs and increased in the IBCs from P7 to P15. (A) From P7 to P15, Lgr6-EGFP was expressed in both the IPCs and IBCs in the middle and basal turns. In the apical turn, there was no Lgr6-EGFP expression at P7, and Lgr6-EGFP was only expressed in the IBCs at P10 and P15. **(B)** From P7 to P15, the percentage of Lgr6-EGFP-positive IPCs gradually decreased ($n = 4$), **(C)** From P7 to P15, the percentage of Lgr6-EGFP-positive IBCs gradually increased ($n = 4$). IPCs, inner pillar cells; IBCs, inner border cells.

cytometry-isolated Lgr6-EGFP-positive cells at a density of 20 cells/μL for 10 days and found that these Lgr6-EGFP-positive cells could generate myosin 7a-positive hair cells. After 10 days of culture, 2000 Lgr6-EGFP-positive cells could generate 802 ± 27 myosin 7a-positive hair cells. In contrast, 2000 Lgr6-negative cells could only generate around 9 ± 2 myosin 7a-positive hair cells ($n = 3$) (**Figures 8C,E**). This result indicated that Lgr6-positive cells might also have the ability to serve as hair cell progenitors.

Discussion

In this study, we used Lgr6-EGFP-Ires-CreERT2 knock-in mice to determine the expression pattern of the *Lgr6* gene. During embryonic development, Lgr6 was first observed at E15.5 in one row of Sox2-positive progenitor cells. We observed the highest level of expression in the basal turn of the organ of Corti followed by reduced expression in the middle turn and no expression in the apical turn. Lgr6 expression in the IPCs increased from E15.5 to P1 at which time it began to decrease. From P7 to P15, we observed Lgr6-EGFP expression not only in the IPCs but also in the IBCs. From P7 to P15, the Lgr6 expression level gradually decreased in the IPCs and gradually increased in the IBCs. At P20, Lgr6 expression in the IPCs disappeared and Lgr6 expression was only observed in the IBCs with a gradient from the basal to apical turns. At P30, Lgr6 expression had completely disappeared in all three turns.

The *Lgr6* gene is homologous to *Lgr5*. Previous studies reported that *Lgr5* is expressed in the prosensory region during embryonic development and is expressed in the third row of Deiters' cells, the IPCs, the medial inner phalangeal cells, and the lateral GER at P3. From P3 to P7, the level of Lgr5-EGFP expression gradually decreased in the IPCs, the inner phalangeal cells, and the lateral GER. At P15, only the third row of Deiters' cells expressed Lgr5-EGFP (Chai et al., 2011; Shi et al., 2012). In this study, when we compared the gene expression of *Lgr6* and *Lgr5*, we found different expression patterns during the development and maturation of the organ of Corti. Generally speaking, during embryonic development Lgr6 is expressed in a sub-population of Lgr5-positive prosensory cells, and we observed Lgr6 expression in the Lgr5-positive IPCs from E18.5 to P3. From P7 to P15, Lgr5 expression in the IPCs, the medial inner phalangeal cells, and the lateral GER almost completely disappeared and Lgr5 expression was restricted to the third row of Deiters' cell. However, at the same developmental stage Lgr6 was expressed in both the IPCs and IBCs. At P20, Lgr5 was restricted to the third row of Deiters' cells and Lgr6 was restricted to the IBCs. At P30, Lgr5 was still expressed in the third row of Deiters' cells, but Lgr6 expression completely disappeared. The other difference between Lgr5 and Lgr6 expression is the expression pattern along the apical—basal axis. Lgr6 expression had a clear gradient from the basal to apical turns, and prior to P7 Lgr6 expression was restricted to the middle and basal turns

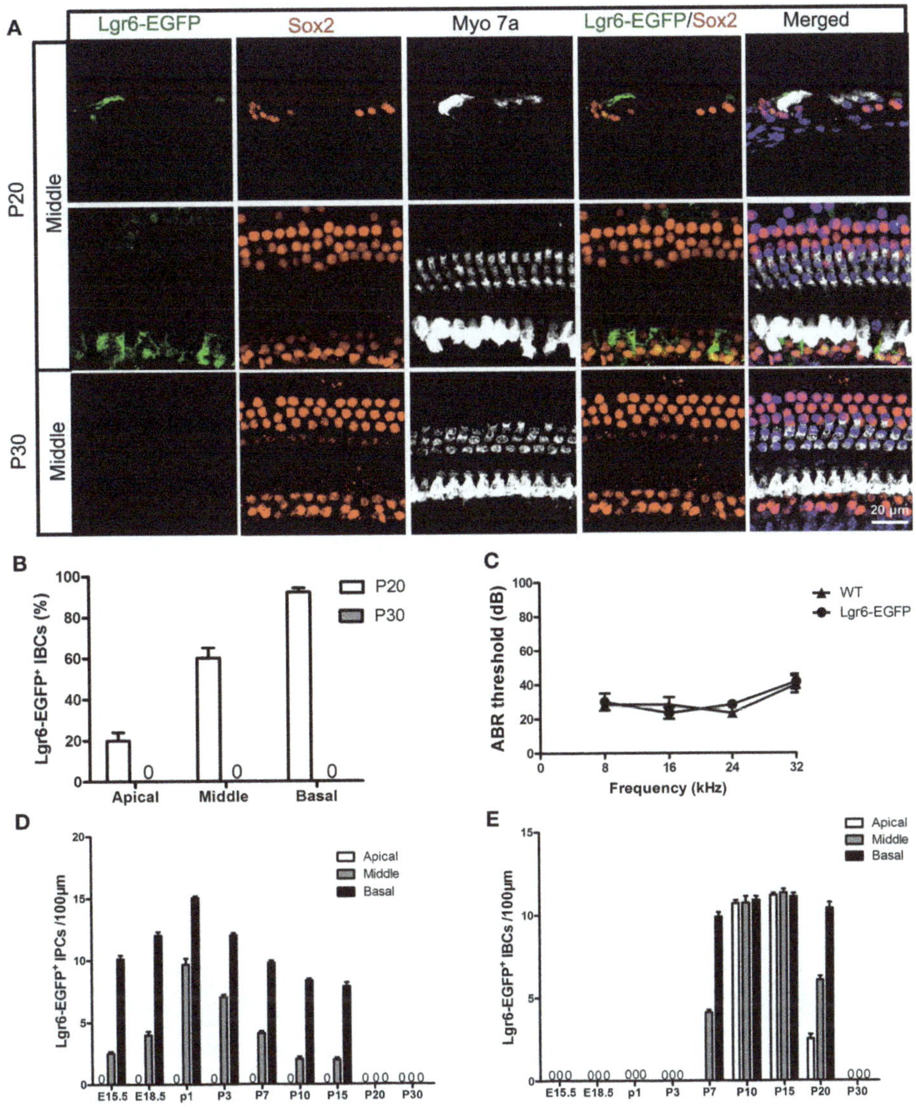

FIGURE 6 | Lgr6-EGFP expression was restricted to IBCs at P20 and completely disappeared at P30. (A) Lgr6-EGFP was expressed only in the IBCs at P20, and Lgr6-EGFP expression disappeared at P30. **(B)** Lgr6-EGFP expression decreased gradually from the basal to apical turn at P20 ($n = 4$). **(C)** The P30 heterozygous Lgr6-EGFP-Ires-CreERT2 mice had normal hearing. **(D)** The number of Lgr6-EGFP-positive IPCs per 100 μm cochlear epithelium from E15.5 to P30. The number of Lgr6-EGFP-positive IPCs started to increase at E15.5, peaked at P1, and then gradually decreased and disappeared by P20 ($n = 4$). **(E)** The number of Lgr6-EGFP-positive IBCs per 100 μm cochlear epithelium from E15.5 to P30. The Lgr6-EGFP-positive IBCs first appeared at P7. The number of cells increased and reached a peak at P15 and then decreased and disappeared by P30 ($n = 4$). IPCs, inner pillar cells; IBCs, inner border cells.

and no Lgr6 was expressed in the apical turn. However, Lgr5 was expressed in all three turns with no clear difference between the turns.

The canonical Wnt/β-catenin signaling pathway is known to play crucial roles in cochlear duct development by regulating proliferation and hair cell differentiation (Jacques et al., 2012; Shi et al., 2014). Wnt/β-catenin signaling regulates the expression of downstream target genes, including *Lgr5* and *Axin2*, and modulates the proliferation of Lgr5-positive and Axin2-positive progenitor cells (Chai et al., 2011, 2012; Shi et al., 2012, 2013). In cell cultures, the Wnt agonist Wnt3a increases the *Lgr5* mRNA expression *in vitro*, and exogenous Wnt3a prevents the decline of Lgr5-EGFP expression in cultured P6 Lgr5-EGFP cochleae. In addition, the Wnt antagonist Fz8CRD decreases *Lgr5* mRNA expression *in vitro*; in P3 Lgr5-EGFP cochleae, Lgr5-EGFP expression cannot be detected when treated with Fz8CRD, suggesting Lgr5-EGFP expression is dependent on active Wnt signaling (Chai et al., 2011). In this study, we investigated the effect of Wnt/β-catenin signaling on another Wnt downstream gene, *Lgr6*. We found that activating Wnt/β-catenin signaling with the exogenous Wnt agonist Bio significantly increased Lgr6 expression in the apical turn, but Lgr6 expression in the middle and basal turns was not significantly changed. On the other hand, inhibition of Wnt/β-catenin signaling with Iwp2 significantly reduced Lgr6 expression in the cochleae suggesting that Wnt signaling is required to maintain the expression of Lgr6.

Lgr6 has been reported to be a stem cell marker in numerous organs, including the skin, taste buds, and lungs (Snippert et al., 2010; Oeztuerk-Winder et al., 2012; Ren et al., 2014). In hair follicles, Lgr6 is expressed in a stem cell population above the follicle bulge, and these Lgr6-positive stem cells have the ability to generate all cell lineages found in the skin (Snippert et al., 2010). In taste buds, both Lgr5 and Lgr6 mark the stem cells, and the individually Lgr5-positive or Lgr6-positive cells can regenerate functional taste cells *ex vivo* (Ren et al., 2014). In the inner ear, previous studies have demonstrated that the Wnt downstream target gene *Lgr5* marks the inner ear progenitor cells and the Lgr5-positive cell can generate hair cells both *in vitro* and *in vivo*. After hair cell damage, these Lgr5-positive progenitors also have the ability to regenerate new hair cells via both mitotic regeneration and direct differentiation (Chai et al., 2012; Shi et al., 2012, 2013; Jan et al., 2013; Cox et al., 2014). In this study, we used Lgr6-EGFP-Ires-CreERT2 mice and flow cytometry to characterize the identity of Lgr6-positive cells. We found that Lgr6-positive cells isolated by FACS also have the ability to differentiate into hair cells *in vitro*, and this suggests that Lgr6 might also mark hair cell progenitors in the organ of Corti. The detailed identity of the Lgr6-positive cells and the mechanisms involved in regulating these cells are worthy of study in the future.

In summary, we have determined the detailed expression pattern of the Wnt downstream target gene *Lgr6* in the

TABLE 3 | Quantification of Lgr6-EFGP/Sox2 double-positive inner border cells per 100 μm cochlear length from P1 to P30.

Age	Apical	Middle	Basal
P1	0	0	0
P3	0	0	0
P7	0	4.30 ± 0.23	9.9 ± 0.31
P10	10.72 ± 0.39	10.78 ± 0.36	10.92 ± 0.19
P15	11.17 ± 0.35	11.25 ± 0.45	11.20 ± 0.15
P20	2.53 ± 0.45	6.07 ± 0.40	10.60 ± 0.25
P30	0	0	0

All the data are shown as the average ± S.D. n = 4 for all the samples.

TABLE 4 | Quantification of Lgr6-EFGP/Sox2 double-positive inner pillar cells per 100 μm cochlear length after Wnt agonist/antagonist treatment.

Treatment	Apical	Middle	Basal
Vehicle	0	1.05 ± 0.39	14.80 ± 0.88
Bio	0.88 ± 0.18	10.67 ± 0.25	14.03 ± 0.37
IWP-2	0	3.95 ± 0.36	9.65 ± 0.33

All the data are shown as the average ± S.D. n = 4 for all the samples.

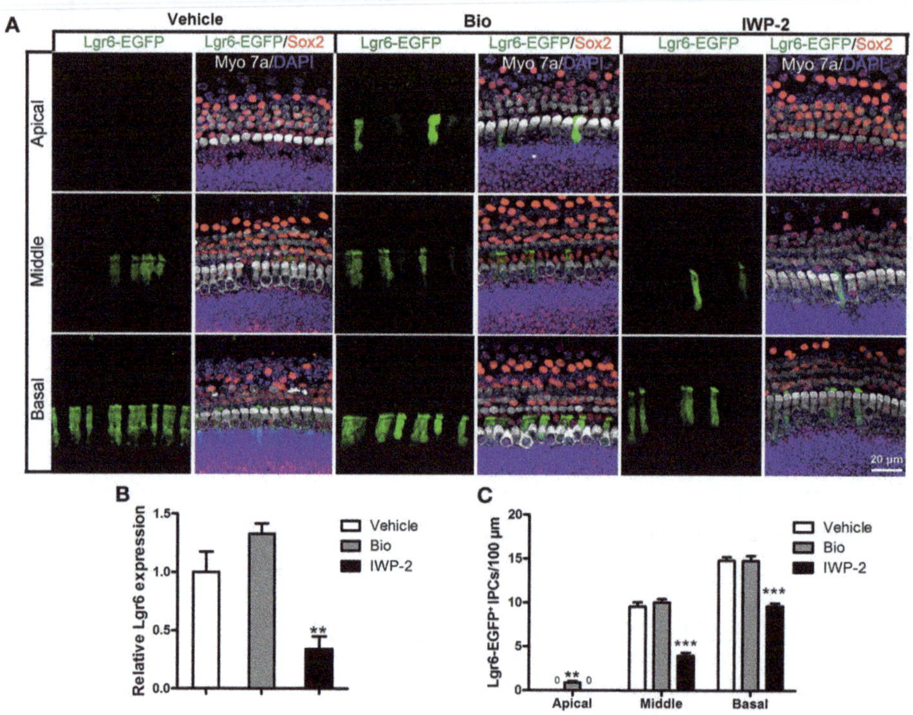

FIGURE 7 | Wnt signaling regulates the expression of Lgr6. (A) Bio treatment significantly increased Lgr6-EGFP expression in the apical turn, but the Lgr6-EGFP expression level did not change in the middle and basal turns compared with the PBS vehicle group. IWP-2 treatment significantly decreased Lgr6-EGFP expression in both the middle and basal turns. **(B)** Quantitative PCR results showed Bio treatment slightly increased *Lgr6* expression and IWP-2 treatment significantly decreased *Lgr6* expression. **(C)** The quantification of Lgr6-EGFP-positive inner pillar cells per 100 μm cochlear epithelium. $^{**}p < 0.01$, $^{***}p < 0.001$.

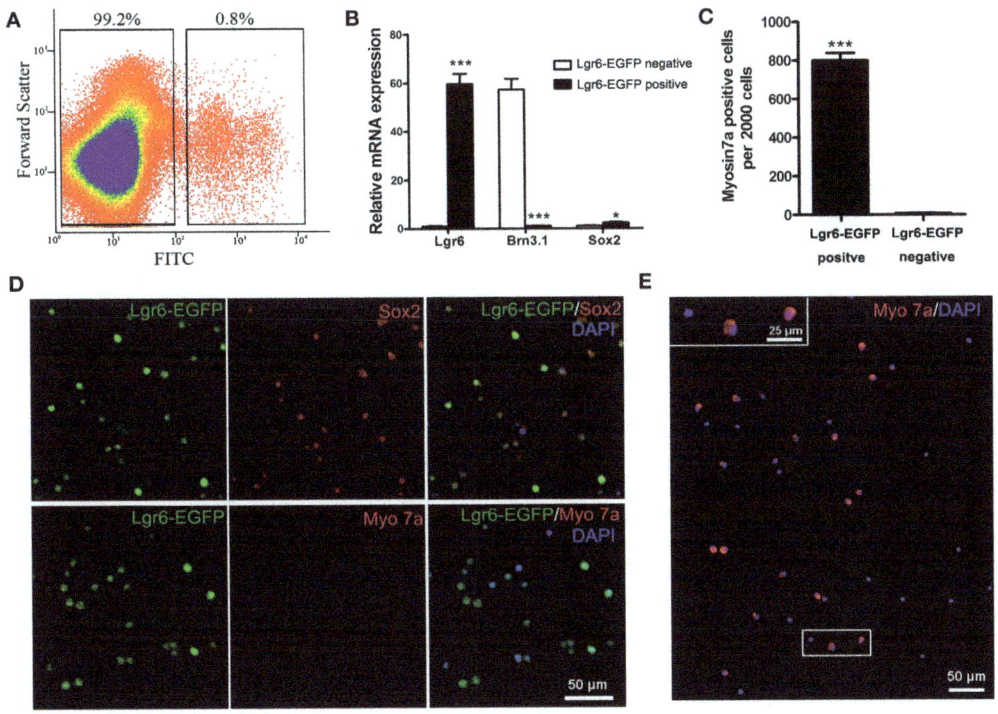

FIGURE 8 | Flow cytometry-isolated Lgr6-positive cells can generate hair cells *in vitro*. (A) Lgr6-GFP-positive and Lgr6-GFP-negative cells were isolated using flow cytometry. **(B)** Quantitative PCR showed that isolated Lgr6-EGFP-positive cells had significantly higher Lgr6 expression, slightly higher Sox2 expression, and significantly lower Brn3.1 expression compared to the Lgr6-EGFP-negative cells. **(C)** Isolated Lgr6-EGFP-positive cells generated significantly more myosin 7a-positive cells than Lgr6-EGFP-negative cells. **(D)** Immunostaining showed that among the hair cells that developed from isolated Lgr6-EGFP-positive cells, 95% were Lgr6-EGFP-positive, 96% were Sox2-positive, and none were myosin 7a-positive. **(E)** Isolated Lgr6-GFP-positive cells can generate myosin 7a+ hair cells after 10 days of *in vitro* culture. $^{*}p < 0.05$, $^{***}p < 0.001$.

mouse cochlear duct from embryonic to adult ages, and we demonstrated that Wnt signaling is required to maintain the expression of Lgr6 in whole organ cultures *in vitro*. In addition, we demonstrated that when isolated by FACS, Lgr6-positive cells can differentiate into hair cells *in vitro*, indicating that Lgr6-positive cells might have the potential to be inner ear hair cell progenitors. These findings suggest that the Lgr6-positive cells might also serve as candidate therapeutic targets for hair cell regeneration.

Author Contributions

Conceived and designed the experiments: HL. Performed the experiments: YZ, YC, LX, and LL. Analyzed the data: YZ, YC, and HL. Wrote the paper: YZ, YC, and HL.

Acknowledgments

This work was supported by grants from the Major State Basic Research Development Program of China (973 Program) (2011CB504506, 2015CB965000), the National Natural Science Foundation of China (81371094, 81230019, and 81470692), the Innovation Programme of Major Basic Research Projects, the Science and Technology Commission of Shanghai Municipality (14DJ1400203), the Shanghai Rising-Star Program (12QA1400500), the Jiangsu Province Natural Science Foundation (BK20140620), the Fundamental Research Funds for the Central Universities (2242014R30022, NO2013WSN085), the Construction Program of Shanghai Committee of Science and Technology (12DZ2251700), and the Major Program of Shanghai Committee of Science and Technology (11441901000). We thank Chuijin Lai and Tianfeng Wang for their excellent technique support and Jin Li and Yalin Huang (IBS, Fudan University) for help with the confocal microscope.

References

Barker, N., and Clevers, H. (2010). Leucine-rich repeat-containing G-protein-coupled receptors as markers of adult stem cells. *Gastroenterology* 1681–1696. doi: 10.1053/j.gastro.2010.03.002

Chai, R., Kuo, B., Wang, T., Liaw, E. J., Xia, A., Jan, T. A., et al. (2012). Wnt signaling induces proliferation of sensory precursors in the postnatal mouse cochlea. *Proc. Natl. Acad. Sci. U.S.A.* 109, 8167–8172. doi: 10.1073/pnas.1202774109

Chai, R., Xia, A., Wang, T., Jan, T. A., Hayashi, T., Bermingham-McDonogh, O., et al. (2011). Dynamic expression of Lgr5, a Wnt target gene, in the developing and mature mouse cochlea. *J. Assoc. Res. Otolaryngol.* 12, 455–469. doi: 10.1007/s10162-011-0267-2

Chen, P., Johnson, J. E., Zoghbi, H. Y., and Segil, N. (2002). The role of Math1 in inner ear development: uncoupling the establishment of the sensory primordium from hair cell fate determination. *Development* 129, 2495–2505.

Cox, B. C., Chai, R., Lenoir, A., Liu, Z., Zhang, L., Nguyen, D. H., et al. (2014). Spontaneous hair cell regeneration in the neonatal mouse cochlea *in vivo*. *Development* 141, 816–829. doi: 10.1242/dev.103036

Cremisi, F., Philpott, A., and Ohnuma, S. (2003). Cell cycle and cell fate interactions in neural development. *Curr. Opin. Neurobiol.* 13, 26–33. doi: 10.1016/S0959-4388(03)00005-9

Dabdoub, A., Puligilla, C., Jones, J. M., Fritzsch, B., Cheah, K. S., Pevny, L. H., et al. (2008). Sox2 signaling in prosensory domain specification and subsequent hair cell differentiation in the developing cochlea. *Proc. Natl. Acad. Sci. U.S.A.* 105, 18396–18401. doi: 10.1073/pnas.0808175105

Fritzsch, B., Barald, K. F., and Lomax, M. I. (1998). "Early development of the vertebrate ear," in *Development of the Auditory System*, eds E. W. Rubel and A. N. P. A. R. R. Fay (New York, NY: Springer-Verlag), 80–145.

Garlipp, B., Schwalenberg, J., Adolf, D., Lippert, H., and Meyer, F. (2011). Epidemiology, surgical management and early postoperative outcome in a cohort of gastric cancer patients of a tertiary referral center in relation to multi-center quality assurance studies. *Pol. Przegl. Chir.* 83, 123–134. doi: 10.2478/v10035-011-0020-x

Hollyday, M., McMahon, J. A., and McMahon, A. P. (1995). Wnt expression patterns in chick embryo nervous system. *Mech. Dev.* 52, 9–25. doi: 10.1016/0925-4773(95)00385-E

Hume, C. R., Bratt, D. L., and Oesterle, E. C. (2007). Expression of LHX3 and SOX2 during mouse inner ear development. *Gene Expr. Patterns* 7, 798–807. doi: 10.1016/j.modgep.2007.05.002

Jacques, B. E., Puligilla, C., Weichert, R. M., Ferrer-Vaquer, A., Hadjantonakis, A. K., Kelley, M. W., et al. (2012). A dual function for canonical Wnt/beta-catenin signaling in the developing mammalian cochlea. *Development* 139, 4395–4404. doi: 10.1242/dev.080358

Jaks, V., Barker, N., Kasper, M., van Es, J. H., Snippert, H. J., Clevers, H., et al. (2008). Lgr5 marks cycling, yet long-lived, hair follicle stem cells. *Nat. Genet.* 40, 1291–1299. doi: 10.1038/ng.239

Jan, T. A., Chai, R., Sayyid, Z. N., van Amerongen, R., Xia, A., Wang, T., et al. (2013). Tympanic border cells are Wnt-responsive and can act as progenitors for postnatal mouse cochlear cells. *Development* 140, 1196–1206. doi: 10.1242/dev.087528

Jasoni, C., Hendrickson, A., and Roelink, H. (1999). Analysis of chicken Wnt-13 expression demonstrates coincidence with cell division in the developing eye and is consistent with a role in induction. *Dev. Dyn.* 215, 215–224.

Jiang, M., Wang, Q., Karasawa, T., Koo, J. W., Li, H., Steyger, P. S., et al. (2014). Sodium-glucose transporter-2 (SGLT2; SLC5A2) enhances cellular uptake of aminoglycosides. *PLoS ONE* 9:e108941. doi: 10.1371/journal.pone.0108941

Kiernan, A. E., Cordes, R., Kopan, R., Gossler, A., and Gridley, T. (2005). The Notch ligands DLL1 and JAG2 act synergistically to regulate hair cell development in the mammalian inner ear. *Development* 132, 4353–4362. doi: 10.1242/dev.02002

Krejs, G. J. (2010). Gastric cancer: epidemiology and risk factors. *Dig. Dis.* 28, 600–603. doi: 10.1159/000320277

Lee, Y. S., Liu, F., and Segil, N. (2006). A morphogenetic wave of p27Kip1 transcription directs cell cycle exit during organ of Corti development. *Development* 133, 2817–2826. doi: 10.1242/dev.02453

Leushacke, M., and Barker, N. (2012). Lgr5 and Lgr6 as markers to study adult stem cell roles in self-renewal and cancer. *Oncogene* 31, 3009–3022. doi: 10.1038/onc.2011.479

Li, C. W., and Ruben, R. J. (1979). Further study of the surface morphology of the embryonic mouse cochlear sensory epithelia. *Otolaryngol. Head Neck Surg.* 87, 479–485.

Li, W., Wu, J., Yang, J., Sun, S., Chai, R., Chen, Z. Y., et al. (2015). Notch inhibition induces mitotically generated hair cells in mammalian cochleae via activating the Wnt pathway. *Proc. Natl. Acad. Sci. U.S.A.* 112, 166–171. doi: 10.1073/pnas.1415901112

Lillevali, K., Haugas, M., Matilainen, T., Pussinen, C., Karis, A., and Salminen, M. (2006). Gata3 is required for early morphogenesis and Fgf10 expression during otic development. *Mech. Dev.* 123, 415–429. doi: 10.1016/j.mod.2006.04.007

Lim, D. J., and Anniko, M. (1985). Developmental morphology of the mouse inner ear. A scanning electron microscopic observation. *Acta Otolaryngol. Suppl.* 422, 1–69. doi: 10.3109/00016488509121766

Morsli, H., Choo, D., Ryan, A., Johnson, R., and Wu, D. K. (1998). Development of the mouse inner ear and origin of its sensory organs. *J. Neurosci.* 18, 3327–3335.

Oeztuerk-Winder, F., Guinot, A., Ochalek, A., and Ventura, J. J. (2012). Regulation of human lung alveolar multipotent cells by a novel p38alpha MAPK/miR-17-92 axis. *EMBO J.* 31, 3431–3441. doi: 10.1038/emboj.2012.192

Ohyama, T., Mohamed, O. A., Taketo, M. M., Dufort, D., and Groves, A. K. (2006). Wnt signals mediate a fate decision between otic placode and epidermis. *Development* 133, 865–875. doi: 10.1242/dev.02271

Ootani, A., Li, X., Sangiorgi, E., Ho, Q. T., Ueno, H., Toda, S., et al. (2009). Sustained *in vitro* intestinal epithelial culture within a Wnt-dependent stem cell niche. *Nat. Med.* 15, 701–706. doi: 10.1038/nm.1951

Pagano, M., and Jackson, P. K. (2004). Wagging the dogma; tissue-specific cell cycle control in the mouse embryo. *Cell* 118, 535–538. doi: 10.1016/j.cell.2004.08.013

Rakowiecki, S., and Epstein, D. J. (2013). Divergent roles for Wnt/beta-catenin signaling in epithelial maintenance and breakdown during semicircular canal formation. *Development* 140, 1730–1739. doi: 10.1242/dev.092882

Ren, W., Lewandowski, B. C., Watson, J., Aihara, E., Iwatsuki, K., Bachmanov, A. A., et al. (2014). Single Lgr5- or Lgr6-expressing taste stem/progenitor cells generate taste bud cells *ex vivo*. *Proc. Natl. Acad. Sci. U.S.A.* 111, 16401–16406. doi: 10.1073/pnas.1409064111

Riccomagno, M. M., Takada, S., and Epstein, D. J. (2005). Wnt-dependent regulation of inner ear morphogenesis is balanced by the opposing and supporting roles of Shh. *Genes Dev.* 19, 1612–1623. doi: 10.1101/gad.1303905

Ruben, R. J. (1967). Development of the inner ear of the mouse: a radioautographic study of terminal mitoses. *Acta Otolaryngol. Suppl.* 220, 221–244.

Sher, A. E. (1971). The embryonic and postnatal development of the inner ear of the mouse. *Acta Otolaryngol. Suppl.* 285, 1–77.

Shi, F., Hu, L., and Edge, A. S. (2013). Generation of hair cells in neonatal mice by beta-catenin overexpression in Lgr5-positive cochlear progenitors. *Proc. Natl. Acad. Sci. U.S.A.* 110, 13851–13856. doi: 10.1073/pnas.1219952110

Shi, F., Hu, L., Jacques, B. E., Mulvaney, J. F., Dabdoub, A., and Edge, A. S. (2014). beta-Catenin is required for hair-cell differentiation in the cochlea. *J. Neurosci.* 34, 6470–6479. doi: 10.1523/JNEUROSCI.4305-13.2014

Shi, F., Kempfle, J. S., and Edge, A. S. (2012). Wnt-responsive lgr5-expressing stem cells are hair cell progenitors in the cochlea. *J. Neurosci.* 32, 9639–9648. doi: 10.1523/JNEUROSCI.1064-12.2012

Snippert, H. J., Haegebarth, A., Kasper, M., Jaks, V., van Es, J. H., Barker, N., et al. (2010). Lgr6 marks stem cells in the hair follicle that generate all cell lineages of the skin. *Science* 327, 1385–1389. doi: 10.1126/science.1184733

7

Age-related hearing impairment and the triad of acquired hearing loss

Chao-Hui Yang[1,2], *Thomas Schrepfer*[1] *and Jochen Schacht*[1]*

[1] *Department of Otolaryngology, Kresge Hearing Research Institute, University of Michigan, Ann Arbor, MI, USA,* [2] *Division of Otology, Department of Otolaryngology, Kaohsiung Chang Gung Memorial Hospital, Chang Gung University College of Medicine, Kaohsiung, Taiwan*

Edited by:
Andy Groves,
Baylor College of Medicine, USA

Reviewed by:
Allison B. Coffin,
Washington State University, USA
Peter S. Steyger,
Oregon Health & Science University, USA

***Correspondence:**
Jochen Schacht,
Department of Otolaryngology, Kresge Hearing Research Institute, University of Michigan, Medical Sciences I Building, Rm. 5315, 1150 West Medical Center Drive, Ann Arbor, MI 48109-5616, USA
schacht@umich.edu

Understanding underlying pathological mechanisms is prerequisite for a sensible design of protective therapies against hearing loss. The triad of age-related, noise-generated, and drug-induced hearing loss displays intriguing similarities in some cellular responses of cochlear sensory cells such as a potential involvement of reactive oxygen species (ROS) and apoptotic and necrotic cell death. On the other hand, detailed studies have revealed that molecular pathways are considerably complex and, importantly, it has become clear that pharmacological protection successful against one form of hearing loss will not necessarily protect against another. This review will summarize pathological and pathophysiological features of age-related hearing impairment (ARHI) in human and animal models and address selected aspects of the commonality (or lack thereof) of cellular responses in ARHI to drugs and noise.

Keywords: acquired hearing loss, ototoxicity, noise trauma, presbycusis, aminoglycoside antibiotics

Introduction

Acquired hearing loss is the most common hearing impairment in modern societies. Not all of its causes, however, are of modern origin. Of the major contributing entities, presbycusis or age-related hearing impairment (ARHI) has been recognized by physicians and societies since ancient times. The environmental overload with damaging noise levels, beginning with the industrial revolution, and the introduction of ototoxic antibiotics and anti-cancer agents in the last century added to the spectrum of hazards to the auditory system and established the current triad of drug-induced, noise-induced and age-related hearing losses.

Medical science and research over the last centuries have given us an excellent knowledge of inner ear pathologies and their functional consequences. Recent advances have added insights into molecular pathways, their physiological control mechanisms, and their modulation by environmental and genetic influences. Intriguing biochemical and molecular parallels began to surface, leading to speculation of a common underlying mechanism of acquired hearing loss and the prospect for a unified pharmacological protection. However, details about the individuality of cell death and homeostatic pathways and differentiated responses to attempted protection soon dispelled this notion. This review will focus on ARHI and compare its biochemical and molecular characteristics to ototoxic hair cell death and noise trauma. While the overall pattern of presbycusis is also shaped by changes in central auditory pathways, we will limit our considerations to the cochlea.

Age-Related Hearing Impairment (ARHI)

Prevalence

ARHI is the most prevalent form of hearing loss in humans. It is characterized by decreased hearing sensitivity, decreased ability to understand speech in a noisy environment, slowed central processing of acoustic stimuli, and impaired sound localization (Gates and Mills, 2005). Based on a survey from 2001 through 2008, Lin et al. (2011) estimated that 30 million, or 12.7% of U.S. Americans of 12 years and older had bilateral hearing loss with elevated thresholds of >25 dB in the better hearing ear for a speech-frequency pure-tone average at 0.5, 1, 2 and 4-kHz. The percentage of the afflicted population increased dramatically in the elderly. Sixty-three percent of male and 48% of female adults aged between 70 and 79 years were affected. Similar data for Europe indicated that 30% of men and 20% of women had a hearing loss of 30 dB or more at the age of 70 years, and 55% of men and 45% of women at the age of 80 years (Roth, 2015).

First signs of ARHI in males may already be evident at an age of 30–39 years, beginning at the highest frequency range of 10–16 kHz; by 40–49 years hearing impairment has progressed to frequencies of 6–8 kHz. Presbycusis in females generally begins a decade later, and the principal speech band (0.5–4 kHz) is affected in both genders by 60–69 years (Sharashenidze et al., 2007). Besides gender differences, epidemiological studies in the USA have established a higher prevalence in Caucasians than in African-Americans (Lin et al., 2011).

Genetics

ARHI is shaped by the interplay between genes that govern cochlear integrity and noxious environmental events on the inner ear. Intrinsic factors contributing to presbycusis include genetic disorders rooted in mutations of both nuclear and mitochondrial DNA, hypertension, diabetes mellitus, and other metabolic and systemic diseases (Lee, 2013; Perry et al., 2014). Noise exposure, ototoxic medications, and diet—while being able to cause hearing loss independently—are modulating extrinsic factors of ARHI. The overall impact of individual genetic factors in the development of ARHI in humans remains uncertain but there is evidence for their major contribution in familial aggregation of presbycusis (Raynor et al., 2009). Siblings of individuals with hearing loss had more than four times higher odds of also having hearing loss than siblings of individuals without hearing loss; the risk ratio was greater in women than men. Overall, about half of the variance in this cluster of ARHI could be ascribed to genetic factors the precise nature of which remains elusive. ARHI seems to be polygenic but no major common genetic variants have been identified (Fransen et al., 2015). In agreement with human findings, recent animal studies suggest multiple genetic influences on the progression of ARHI and on the interaction of age with noise in mice (Noben-Trauth and Johnson, 2009; Ohmen et al., 2014). Results from the offspring of 4-way-cross mice provided evidence for several specific alleles that affected hearing at select frequencies, ages, or following noise trauma (Schacht et al., 2012a).

An intriguing question is a potential relationship between presbycusis and late-onset hearing loss due to highly penetrant monogenic mutations. The age of onset of both is fluid but a late-onset hearing loss is generally evident by young adulthood. Any genetic similarities or differences are yet to be determined.

Impact of Lifestyle and Disease

Lifestyle may influence auditory performance at any age as well as the progression of presbycusis. In a cross-sectional analysis of 164,770 participants, smoking and passive smoking was associated with increased odds of hearing loss in a dose-dependent manner (Dawes et al., 2014). In contrast, moderate use of alcohol was associated with better hearing in the elderly in three independent studies (Popelka et al., 2000; Fransen et al., 2008; Gopinath et al., 2010a), an effect in line with observations that low alcohol intake can be beneficial for general health. Heavy drinkers, in contrast, as well as those with a high body mass index, had a tendency toward more pronounced high-frequency hearing loss. Such differential influences of lifestyle might be related to overall health, especially in association with cardiovascular disease. A cause of microvascular abnormalities that also might affect hearing is type 2 diabetes mellitus (Mitchell et al., 2009). Type 2 diabetes, often associated with overweight and obese body habitus in adults as well as in youth, is a common metabolic disease that causes impairment of various organ systems. Data from a large longitudinal cohort study indicate that type 2 diabetes is associated with prevalent hearing loss and a significant accelerated progression of hearing loss in patients with newly diagnosed diabetes (Mitchell et al., 2009).

Since diet is one of the few potentially modifiable risk factors for age-related hearing loss, the impact of nutritional behavior has frequently been investigated (Gopinath et al., 2010a, 2011b). Both a high-carbohydrate diet and a high dietary intake of cholesterol were associated with ARHI. In contrast, treatment with 3-hydroxy-3-methyl-glutaryl (HMG) CoA reductase drugs (statins) and consumption of monounsaturated fats and cereal fibers inclined toward a lower prevalence of hearing loss. We will discuss more aspects of dietary manipulations of ARHI in the "Antioxidants and Vitamins in Human Hearing and Prevention of Hearing Loss" Section.

Cochlear Pathology in Humans and Animal Models

A hallmark of human ARHI is the variability of its pathology. Although high-frequency hearing loss appears to be a prevalent form, some individuals may also show a gradually sloping or a flat audiometric curve (Suga and Lindsay, 1976). Moreover, different structural elements can be affected such as hair cells, neurons, lateral wall tissues, or a combination thereof (Nelson and Hinojosa, 2006). This variability has been ascribed to genetic susceptibility modified by environmental effects of noise exposure, disease, and lifestyle. In practice, ARHI is largely an umbrella term for multiple forms of auditory pathology manifest in aging individuals.

In contrast, drug- and noise-induced hearing loss tend to present a well-defined pattern of damage in both human and experimental animals. Both aminoglycoside antibiotics and cisplatin primarily damage outer hair cells in a predictable base-to-apex progression. Noise trauma may initially affect fibrocytes of the spiral ligament (Hirose and Liberman, 2003) and will—at higher intensities or longer duration—damage hair cells in relation to the frequency and intensity of the stimulus.

Sensorineural Elements

Sensory hair cell loss has been documented in temporal bones of patients with ARHI but does not appear to be its only determining cause. The area of destruction was usually located in the basal end of the cochlea causing a threshold elevation at 8 kHz but rarely extended towards the apex far enough to involve speech frequencies (Schuknecht and Gacek, 1993). More recent studies of temporal bones have expanded this view by showing significant degeneration of multiple cochlear elements including stria vascularis and spiral ganglion cells that better correlate with the severity of hearing loss (Nelson and Hinojosa, 2006). Specifically, the extent of ganglion cell degeneration was associated with the slope of the descending high-frequency component of the audiogram. In addition, several reports have indicated nerve damage in the presence of apparently intact hair cells in ARHI (Sone et al., 1998; van Ruijven et al., 2005; Linthicum and Fayad, 2009).

Animal models that reflect a sensorineural ARHI with loss of outer and, later, inner hair cells include aging rats and mice. CBA/J mice as well as the CBA/CaJ and CAST strains present little evidence of hearing loss until 18 months of age, i.e., long into their lifespan, when they begin to show hair cell loss and elevated auditory thresholds (Li and Borg, 1991; Sha et al., 2008). In contrast, the C57BL/6, BALB and DBA/J strains develop a severe high-frequency sensorineural hearing loss as early as 5 weeks in DBA or 3 months of age in C57BL/6 (Zheng et al., 1999). Those strains carry a mutation of the cadherin 23 (*Cdh23*) gene at the *ahl* locus predisposing them to accelerated hearing loss, distinct from the late-life age-related changes in other mouse strains and in human. Indeed, no convincing evidence yet exists associating variants in human *CDH23* with ARHI. For example, a recent study of 310 aging participants with poor hearing vs. 308 participants with good hearing found no association of a common *CDH23* variant with presbycusis (Hwang et al., 2012b). These facts should therefore disqualify strains carrying the $Cdh23^{ahl}$ allele as models of typical ARHI in human. Likewise, mouse models with defective mitochondrial DNA repair mechanisms may show an accelerated hearing loss that does not reflect human presbycusis (see "Involvement of Mitochondria" Section).

Degeneration of spiral ganglion cells can also be observed in animal models of aging. The degeneration may follow the loss of hair cells but may also occur independently (Keithley et al., 1989; Sha et al., 2008). Conversely, spiral ganglion cells may be preserved in the presence of a degenerated cochlea (White et al., 2000). More recently there has been evidence for synaptopathy as a pathophysiological process underlying supra-threshold deficits. In mice, degeneration of cochlear synapses in age-related hearing loss preceded both cochlear nerve degeneration and hair cell loss and occurred long before a threshold elevation was measurable (Kujawa and Liberman, 2015). In fact, these observations may relate to a report by Crowe et al. (1993) on "dendritic presbycusis" in which human temporal bones presented a normal cochlea but a loss of dendritic processes of the spiral ganglion (Rizk and Linthicum, 2012).

Synaptopathy may also be a consequence of noise exposure or aminoglycoside treatment. Following a noise exposure regimen that initially only led to a temporary threshold shift as assessed by auditory brainstem response (ABR), compound action potential and distortion-product otoacoustic emission (DPOAE; Kujawa and Liberman, 2009), the synapses from the afferent nerve fibers to the inner hair cells were the most vulnerable elements at a later age, not the hair cells, resulting in an attenuation of supra-threshold neural responses. Threshold elevations without a reduction in hair cell counts have also been observed after kanamycin administration in guinea pigs (Nicol et al., 1992). In a mouse model of enhanced endoplasmic reticulum stress (Oishi et al., 2015) gentamicin caused synaptopathy; spiral ganglion cells and inner hair cell synapses were reduced while hair cells remained intact by morphology and DPOAE measurements.

The complexity of age-related changes clearly calls for carefully selected animal models and detailed assessments of auditory pathophysiology. Appropriate animal models would develop hearing loss with advanced age and not be confounded by mutations that disrupt the physiological aging process. In addition to loss of hair cells, neuronal elements including synaptic connections need to be evaluated. As a physiological measure, ABR thresholds are insufficient just as a pure-tone audiogram would be insensitive to diffuse neural degeneration and an impaired understanding of complex sounds in humans. Therefore animal experimentation needs to consider supra-threshold deficits and performance in simple behavioral tasks such as gap detection (Altschuler et al., 2015).

Stria Vascularis and Spiral Ligament

As briefly mentioned in the preceding section, age also changes the morphology of cochlear supporting tissues. For example, the volume of stria vascularis and spiral ligament was significantly lower in temporal bones of older (64–84 years old) than in younger (15–38 years old) subjects (Ishiyama et al., 2007). More to the point, strial atrophy was a frequent occurrence in temporal bones of individuals that had been diagnosed with ARHI (Schuknecht et al., 1974; Suga and Lindsay, 1976; Nelson and Hinojosa, 2006). However, there is no indication that strial pathology can be a sole cause of hearing loss. In fact, the best correlation between the severity of ARHI and morphological changes was established for the extent of degeneration of all four cochlear elements, namely stria vascularis, spiral ganglion cell, inner and outer hair cells (Nelson and Hinojosa, 2006). The observation that ABR thresholds were not associated with a single peripheral deficit was also made from a study of age-related hearing loss in rhesus monkeys (Engle et al., 2013). Spiral ganglion density and loss of outer hair cells contributed to the audiometric impairments but neither did decreases in inner hair cell numbers or thickness of stria vascularis. The strongest correlation was seen with the number of different pathologies present.

Human studies cannot evaluate the metabolic consequences of strial pathology on the endocochlear potential. Animal models indicate strial dysfunction is not a prerequisite for loss of hair cells. Although CBA/CaJ mice may display a gradual decline in endocochlear potential during aging, other strains such as CBA/J maintain a stable potential (Sha et al., 2008; Ohlemiller et al., 2010) while developing ARHI. Conversely, however, a significant decline in endocochlear potential should lead to impaired auditory processing. Among animals, the Mongolian gerbil is considered a model for a strial contribution to hearing loss with age. Strial atrophy was variable but Na, K-ATPase activity and the endocochlear potential tended to decrease (Schulte and Schmiedt, 1992).

Morphological changes in the stria may also be associated with treatment by drugs and noise but may not be causal to hearing loss. Strial pathology can be observed after aminoglycoside challenge (Forge et al., 1987), but the endocochlear potential remains stable until late in ototoxic treatment (Komune et al., 1987; Xiong et al., 2011), negating a functional consequence of such alterations. Cisplatin may affect both strial morphology and function (Laurell et al., 2007) but at least some of these changes are reversible (Klis et al., 2000) and therefore not a direct cause of hair cell loss. The effects of noise on lateral wall tissues are variable, probably determined by the intensity of the treatment or species differences, but noise trauma caused degeneration of fibrocytes and edema with temporary changes to the endocochlear potential (Hirose and Liberman, 2003). Considering the sum of the evidence it appears that strial pathology, although seen to some extent in the aging and drug- or noise-treated cochlea, is not a primary or decisive cause of acquired hearing loss.

Molecular Pathology

Oxidative Stress

Potentially detrimental reactive oxygen species (ROS) are produced in every cell by enzymatic reactions and mitochondrial respiratory mechanisms. However, only their excess—either via overproduction or insufficient detoxification—will create oxidative stress and potentially trigger cell death. A well-maintained redox balance is important for the cochlea as for any other tissue. Transgenic mice with deficiencies in antioxidant systems, lacking the enzyme copper/zinc superoxide dismutase, lost hair cells and auditory neurons to a greater extent than their normal littermates (McFadden et al., 1999; Keithley et al., 2005). Outer hair cells, especially those in the base of cochlea, appear to be highly sensitive to ROS damage as compared to supporting cells (Sha et al., 2001).

Human studies have only been able to approach a potential link between oxidative stress and hearing performance indirectly via the determination of stress markers in serum. A group of 63 subjects with diabetes mellitus and diabetic hearing impairment showed significant increases in serum levels of oxidation markers and enzymes such as glutathione peroxidase and superoxide dismutase (Aladag et al., 2009). Serum levels of several ROS species were also determined in a cross-sectional study on 302 subjects aged 40–77 years with or without clinically diagnosed age-related sensorineural hearing loss (Hwang et al., 2012a). Assays reflecting the combined concentrations of hydrogen peroxide, hypochloride and hydroxyl radicals showed a significant positive association between their elevated levels and pure-tone thresholds at low (250–1,000 Hz) and high frequencies (2,000–8,000 Hz). An indicator for superoxide, in contrast, only implied an association with low-frequency thresholds. While such associations are intriguing they cannot provide information on potential causal relationships or the redox status of the auditory system. Interestingly, the use of antioxidant supplementation (vitamins C and E, folate, coffee, and tea), which was reported by 66% of the participants in the latter study, had no influence on auditory performance.

Animal studies, unfortunately, do not resolve the question of how oxidative stress relates to the development of ARHI. In a CBA mouse model of age-related hearing loss (Jiang et al., 2007) markers of oxidation began to appear at 12–18 months of age in the organ of Corti and later (at 23 months) in spiral ganglion cells, stria vascularis and spiral ligament. Conversely, components of cellular antioxidant systems had decreased by 18 months in the organ of Corti. This evidence of an imbalanced redox system resembles the pattern of oxidative stress in animal models of drug-induced hearing loss and noise trauma. A striking contrast, however, is the fact that a case can be made for a causal relationship in the latter two pathologies but not in ARHI: dietary manipulations reducing oxidative stress effectively protect against aminoglycoside ototoxicity and the permanent effects of noise trauma but not against AHRI (Oishi and Schacht, 2011; Xie et al., 2011).

The complexity of mechanisms underlying age-related cochlear pathology and pathophysiology were further illustrated by studies employing caloric restriction in mice. Caloric restriction is a well-established regimen to increase stress-resistance by curbing ROS (Sohal and Weindruch, 1996). Such a diet can extend longevity, slow age-related physiological declines, and decrease tumor and disease burden in a variety of animal species. Willott et al. (1995) evaluated ARHI in 15 different mouse strains maintained on a well-controlled calorically restricted diet beginning at a young age. The results varied profoundly between strains. They ranged from an amelioration of age-related hearing loss (as measured by auditory brainstem response or cochlear pathology) to no apparent effect and to an acceleration and exacerbation of hearing loss. Hence, genetic heterogeneity had a greater influence on auditory performance than caloric restriction. By extension, genetics can be expected also to influence the outcome of dietary manipulations with antioxidants.

From the sum of these results, we can postulate that oxidative stress can accompany but is not an obligatory condition for ARHI. The "Antioxidant Protection in Animal Models" Section will further explore this notion.

Involvement of Mitochondria

A decisive role of mitochondria in the aging process in general seems firmly established. Mitochondria are particularly vulnerable to the cumulative effects of genetic or environmental damage because mitochondria, in contrast to nuclei, lack an efficient DNA-repair system and protective histones. Hence, mutations in the mitochondrial DNA (mtDNA) for the 13 proteins that it encodes are more likely to occur and persist in a lifetime than mutations in nuclear DNA. As a consequence, mitochondrial function may be compromised and pathology can become evident, varying with cell type and the type of mutation (Lee and Wei, 2012). While much emphasis has been placed on the formation of ROS by mitochondria, recent evidence expands the spectrum of mitochondrial dysfunction to their turnover (fusion and fission) and energetics, regulation of calcium dynamics and apoptosis (Gonzalez-Freire et al., 2015).

An involvement of mitochondria in ARHI is supported by several lines of evidence. Patterns of maternal inheritance of presbycusis are one indication (Hutchin and Cortopassi, 2000). Likewise, a considerable literature confirms mitochondrial mutations in the temporal bones of patients with presbycusis (Fischel-Ghodsian et al., 1997). Such mtDNA mutations are highly variable, targeting different segments of the DNA, and often involving large-scale deletions in genes necessary for energy metabolism (Chen and Tang, 2014). Specifically, a mtDNA4977 deletion was more prevalent in temporal bones from patients with presbycusis than in individuals with normal audiograms (Bai et al., 1997) or in age-matched controls and young and middle-aged groups (Dai et al., 2004). A comparison of individual audiometric thresholds with levels of the mtDNA4977 deletion in archival human cochlear tissue (quantified by polymerase chain reaction) was able to establish a significant correlation between the severity of presbycusis and the deletion (Markaryan et al., 2009). While this evidence is solid, another study indicated that mitochondrial mutations *per se* do not determine the rate of age-related deterioration of hearing. An analysis of the mitochondrial genome of 200 individuals with normal hearing and 200 with significantly elevated thresholds (Bonneux et al., 2011) found a lack of an association between the mutation load of inherited mitochondrial variants and ARHI. A combination of mitochondrial defects with other environmental or genetic influences on the inner ear has to be postulated in these cases.

As animal models reflecting mitochondrial pathology, mouse mutants deficient in mitochondrial proofreading have been suggested (Kujoth et al., 2005). However, these animals are afflicted with dramatic degenerative changes in phenotype with devastating effects on the animals' health that are not shared by late-life wild-type mice. Such "catastrophic mutations" do not represent a normal aging process (Gershon, 2005; Miller, 2005) and we have to treat results from these mouse strains with caution. Another example of a confounding mitochondrial mutation is the DBA/2 mouse which, in addition to harboring the *Cdh23*^{ahl} allel, presents defects in the respiratory chain (Someya et al., 2007; Johnson et al., 2008). It is yet to be established whether information derived from these models contributes to or distracts from our understanding of ARHI.

Among the other forms of acquired hearing loss, a direct effect on mitochondria can be deduced for aminoglycoside ototoxicity: the decoding site of mitochondrial RNA is structurally highly similar to the corresponding decoding site in bacteria, where aminoglycosides bind and inhibit protein synthesis. Drug affinity to mitochondrial RNA has indeed been correlated with ototoxicity (Shulman et al., 2014) and non-ototoxic aminoglycosides have been developed on the basis of differential binding to bacterial and mitochondrial RNA (Duscha et al., 2014). As a consequence (or independently) the drugs may disrupt the respiratory complexes (Jensen-Smith et al., 2012) compromising energy metabolism or initiating cell death pathways.

The mechanism by which mitochondria might participate in acute noise damage may have several components. A reduction in cochlear blood flow and oxygen availability would lead to inefficient oxidative phosphorylation and a rapid depletion of ATP levels (Chen et al., 2012). This impairment of mitochondrial function may be coupled with a "reperfusion effect" when blood flow resumes, causing excess ROS formation. An elevation of intracellular free calcium following noise exposure (Fridberger et al., 1998) is another potential trigger of mitochondrial dysfunction. Although calcium does not directly affect the respiratory chain, it may affect mitochondrial membrane permeability in addition to activating cell-damaging lipid peroxidation or protein kinase pathways.

In summary, there is clear evidence that mitochondria play a role in all three forms of acquired hearing loss (Böttger and Schacht, 2013). However, the detailed mechanisms diverge between these pathologies, perhaps even with only little overlap. Primary disruptions appear to be mtDNA deletions (in ARHI), dysfunction of mtRNA processes (aminoglycosides), and a compromised respiratory metabolism (noise trauma), providing examples of the multifaceted contributions of a single organelle.

Cell Death Pathways in Animal Models

Following a lethal insult, cells will undergo a controlled demise. The classical forms of cell death, apoptosis and necrosis, and related pathways have been documented for ARHI in animal models where they may operate in parallel or sequentially. Apoptosis was evident in aging rat cochleae and in outer hair cells of both middle-aged (12-month-old) and old (18–26-month-old) CBA/J mice with hearing deficits. The middle-aged mice also bore nuclei with necrotic features, which were absent from old mice (Hu et al., 2008; Sha et al., 2009).

Essential effectors of intrinsic apoptosis are the caspases, proteases that are sometimes termed "executioner" proteins. Their activities are modulated by the Bcl-2 family of apoptosis regulators. Bax and Bak, pro-apoptotic proteins in the Bcl-2 family, translocate to mitochondria and lead to an increase of mitochondrial membrane permeability resulting in the release of cytochrome c; activated caspase-9 and caspase-3 then initiate signaling pathways towards cell death. These caspase-dependent pathways and the participation of Bcl family of proteins have been established for age-related hearing loss *in vivo* in the gerbil, the rat, and the mouse (Alam et al., 2001; Hu et al., 2008; Sha et al., 2009). Commensurate with apoptotic events is the translocation of endonuclease G in animal models of ARHI (Sha et al., 2009). Apoptosis-inducing factor and endonuclease G translocate from mitochondria to the nucleus, promoting chromatin condensation and DNA fragmentation.

Another route to cell death associated with ARHI is the MAPK pathway. Mitogen-activated protein kinases

(MAPKs) are a family of kinases that include c-jun NH2-terminal kinases (JNK), p38 MAPKs, and other extracellular signal-regulated kinases. Immunohistochemical analyses in the cochlea of aging CBA/J mice demonstrated increased phosphorylation (i.e., activation) of JNK and p38 MAPK in outer hair cells (Sha et al., 2009). A screen for gene expression patterns in the aging CBA mouse cochlea (Tadros et al., 2008) likewise found significant changes with age that included the family of caspases, MAP kinases, and calpains.

Calpains and cathepsins are calcium-dependent proteases that activate downstream pathways by proteolysis of target proteins. They are components of caspase-independent signaling to cell death, released from lysosomes in response to increased intracellular calcium, and implicated in apoptotic and necrotic cell death. Both of these proteases are activated in the aging mouse cochlea (Sha et al., 2009). In addition, the same study also demonstrated cytochrome c release, activation of caspase-9, translocation of endonuclease G and the involvement of the MAPK pathway, indicating that multiple cell death pathways can be proceeding concurrently.

There is considerable overlap in cell death pathways between the three pathologies. Apoptotic markers have been demonstrated for aminoglycoside ototoxicity in guinea pig cochlear and vestibular sensory epithelia (Lang and Liu, 1997; Nakagawa et al., 1998), for cisplatin ototoxicity in the gerbil (Alam et al., 2000), and for noise-induced hearing loss in the guinea pig and chinchilla (Yang et al., 2004). Necrotic hair cells appeared in response to aminoglycosides in CBA/J mice (Jiang et al., 2006a) and following noise exposure in the chinchilla, but have rarely been observed as a result of cisplatin ototoxicity. Active caspase-3 and caspase-9 or cytochrome c release may accompany hair cell death in response to aminoglycosides in various model systems (Cunningham et al., 2002; Wei et al., 2005), to cisplatin *in vivo* (Devarajan et al., 2002), and following noise exposure (Nicotera et al., 2003). Upstream of caspases, Bcl-2 family proteins were induced by aminoglycosides in the zebra fish lateral line (Coffin et al., 2013), by cisplatin in the gerbil, and by noise in the CBA/J mouse and the guinea pig (Vicente-Torres and Schacht, 2006; Yamashita et al., 2008). Translocation of endonuclease G is also evident in animal models of aminoglycoside ototoxicity (Jiang et al., 2006a) and noise-induced hearing loss (Yamashita et al., 2004). Further extending the similarities, p38 MAPK and JNK are involved in aminoglycoside ototoxicity (Pirvola et al., 2000; Wei et al., 2005) and noise trauma (Wang et al., 2003; Jamesdaniel et al., 2011). Finally, both calpain and cathepsin were activated in response to aminoglycoside treatment *in vivo* (Jiang et al., 2006a) and calpain in response to noise exposure (Wang et al., 1999).

This commonality of cellular responses reflects the fact that even widely different initial insults to cell integrity will converge into a few final pathways of cell death. Intimately linked to the emergence of such pathways is the recruitment of survival mechanisms. The balance between these competing forces will ultimately decide cell fate.

Protection from Cochlear Pathology and Pathophysiology

Homeostatic (Cell Rescue) Pathways in Animal Models

A first response of cells under attack by potentially injurious stimuli will be to maintain their integrity by evoking homeostatic pathways. In the case of acquired hearing loss, upregulation of antioxidant defenses appears to be a ubiquitous response. In fact, in a direct comparison, Chen et al. (2013) demonstrated the upregulation of the antioxidant peroxiredoxin 3 in mice *in vivo* after acute noise exposure, after a 2 week treatment with kanamycin, and in the cochlea of 19-month-old animals. Likewise, heat shock proteins which stabilize protein structure against cell stress will attenuate loss of hair cells or auditory function by drugs (Taleb et al., 2009), noise (Yoshida et al., 1999), and age (Mikuriya et al., 2008). Another canonical protective pathway mediated by phosphatidylinositol 3,4,5-trisphosphate/Akt signaling has been documented for aminoglycoside ototoxicity (Chung et al., 2006; Jiang et al., 2006b) and ARHI (Sha et al., 2010). Both the knowledge of cell death and molecular rescue pathways can provide a rational basis for the choice of pharmacological agents to prevent or attenuate acquired hearing loss.

Antioxidant Protection in Animal Models

There was early tantalizing support for antioxidant protection against ARHI. A prospective randomized study had suggested that dietary supplementation might delay or mitigate auditory damage. Treated Fischer 344 rats had improved auditory sensitivities in old age but the improvements were small and differed with different antioxidants while the number of long-term surviving animals was low (Seidman, 2000). Later studies using a variety of different approaches yielded ambiguous results or were met with failure, shedding doubt on the general applicability of such an intervention.

The deterioration of auditory neurons and stria vascularis was reduced in beagle dogs that were fed an antioxidant-enriched diet (supplemented with vitamin E, l-carnitine, lipoic acid, and vitamin C) for the last 3 years of their lives (Le and Keithley, 2007). Unfortunately, the study was confounded by excessive noise in the dog kennel and it could not be ruled out that some of the pathology attenuated by the diet had been noise-induced. The same authors investigated transgenic mice overexpressing mitochondrial superoxide dismutase (SOD2) as a means to reduce oxidative stress. Contrary to expectation, hearing loss at 20 months of age was greater in transgenics than in the parent strain of B6 mice. This result complemented an earlier study (Keithley et al., 2005) in which the overexpression of cytosolic copper-zinc superoxide dismutase (SOD1) also did not prevent age-related hearing loss.

Outright failures of dietary intervention were observed in an attempt to lower oxidative stress by strengthening mitochondrial energy metabolism with acetyl L-carnitine in 15- to 24-months old rats (Bielefeld et al., 2008). Auditory performance was not affected although it could be argued that the duration of intervention of up to 90 days might have been insufficient. Sha et al. (2012) subjected CBA/J mice to a long-term dietary treatment from 10 to 22 months of age, spanning a period from normal auditory thresholds to significant hearing loss. Food enriched with a combination of vitamins A, C, E and α-lipoic acid did not delay or attenuate age-related hearing loss.

In striking contrast to ARHI, reliably positive results have been achieved with antioxidants in preventing hearing loss caused by drugs or noise. Recent review articles have extensively discussed mechanisms and therapeutic approaches to reduce the ototoxic impact of cisplatin and aminoglycosides (Huth et al., 2011; Xie et al., 2011; Schacht et al., 2012b) as well as noise trauma (Oishi and Schacht, 2011). This contrast in efficacious protection reinforces the conclusion put forth in the "Oxidative Stress" Section that oxidative stress can accompany ARHI but cannot its sole cause.

Antioxidants and Vitamins in Human Hearing and Prevention of Hearing Loss

Lifestyle and diet influence both our general health and our sense of hearing (see "Impact of Lifestyle and Disease" Section). To what extend these two effects can be distinguished is an interesting theoretical question but of no practical consequence. Diet is an easily modifiable factor and any delay in ARHI would have important implications for public health. Unfortunately, there is no simple remedy.

Influence of Vitamins on the Prevalence of Hearing Loss

An adequate intake of vitamins is essential for normal auditory function as a number of cross-sectional studies have demonstrated. Spankovich et al. (2011) compared pure-tone audiometry and otoacoustic emissions with dietary data for 2,111 adults, aged 49–99 years of age. Better hearing was associated with higher reported intake of vitamin C, vitamin E, riboflavin (vitamin B_2), magnesium, and lycopene (a carotenoid antioxidant). Similarly, an epidemiological study of 1,910 Korean subjects aged 50–80 years compared their hearing thresholds with self-reported intake of dietary supplements (Kang et al., 2014). The intake of vitamin C, and to a lesser extent retinol (a vitamin A analog), riboflavin (vitamin B_2), and niacin (vitamin B_3) positively correlated with better thresholds. A survey of a general population in the USA aged 20–69 years (2,592 subjects) likewise found that diets high in vitamin C, beta-carotene, and magnesium were correlated with better hearing (Choi et al., 2014).

However, results from surveys of different populations do not always agree. For example, auditory thresholds were impaired in subjects (55 women aged 60–71 years) with low serum levels of folic acid (vitamin B_9) and vitamin B_{12} (Houston et al., 1999). Another cross-sectional study of presbycusic subjects confirmed that low serum folate levels (<11 nmol/L) increased the odds of prevalent mild hearing loss (Gopinath et al., 2010b). In contrast, Berner et al. (2000) failed to demonstrate any association between hearing level and vitamin B_{12} or folic acid in 91 elderly subjects. A poor vitamin B_{12} status was also evident in 93 older adults with hearing loss (Park et al., 2006) but short-term dietary supplementation with vitamin B_{12} did not affect their hearing.

Another caveat is that an overuse of vitamins may be detrimental to the auditory system. Higher vitamin A intake (Spankovich et al., 2011) and higher serum levels of vitamin D (Kang et al., 2014) have been associated with worse hearing.

Influence of Vitamins on the Incidence of Hearing Loss

Even if a balanced or fortified diet generally promotes good health and hearing, a direct impact of nutritional supplements on the progression of ARHI remains debatable. A good example of a discord between the influence of nutrition on prevalence and on incidence of hearing loss comes from cross-sectional and longitudinal analyses of 2,956 participants of age 50 and older (Gopinath et al., 2011a). A segment of the study group that took dietary vitamin E or vitamin A had a 14% and a 47% reduced risk, respectively, of prevalence of a moderate (or greater) hearing loss. Over a 5-year follow-up period, however, an increased dietary intake had no influence on the incidence of ARHI during that time.

A prospective cohort study of 26,273 men aged 40–74 years reported a similar lack of benefits (Shargorodsky et al., 2010). The group was followed for 18 years and 3,559 cases of hearing loss were documented. There was no significant association between the risk of hearing loss and the self-reported intake of Vitamin B12, vitamin C, vitamin E, or beta carotene.

The utility of antioxidant treatments was further cast in doubt in a recent prospective, placebo-controlled, double-blind and randomized trial with 120 participants of 60 years of age or older (Polanski and Cruz, 2013). The subjects were treated for 6 months with one of four regimens: α-lipoic acid plus vitamin C, papaverine chlorhydrate plus vitamin E, gingko extract, or placebo. The various supplements had no effect on pure tone audiometry, speech recognition threshold, or percentage index of speech recognition, regardless whether measured between groups or longitudinally over time.

A possible exception to this scenario of failures is folic acid. A double-blind randomized and placebo-controlled study in 728 older men and women (Durga et al., 2007) provided evidence for the efficacy of folic acid supplementation. Over a 3-year period, the decline in low-frequency hearing was significantly attenuated in elderly participants compared with a placebo group. However, the effect was modest (0.7 dB) and high-frequency hearing was not rescued. A caveat applies: the study was conducted in the Netherlands where food products are not fortified with folic acid. In many industrialized countries, folic acid is added to flour in order to prevented neural tube defects in infants. However, confirmative data were obtained in the prospective cohort study cited above (Shargorodsky et al., 2010). Folate reduced the risk of hearing loss in men older than 60 years when comparing the highest quintile vs. lowest quintile of intake. The authors offer the explanation that high folic acid intake is necessary to overcome an age-related increased prevalence of folate malabsorption and folate depletion.

Antioxidants as Protection Against Drugs and Noise

The reliable protection achieved with antioxidants against drugs and noise trauma in animal models has prompted several trials in humans. Based on the efficacy of salicylate in a guinea pig model of ototoxicity (Sha and Schacht, 1999), aspirin (acetyl salicylate) was co-administered with gentamicin in a randomized double-blind clinical trial involving 195 patients (Sha et al., 2006). Fourteen of 106 subjects in the control group but only 3 of 89 in the aspirin group met the criteria of hearing loss ($\geq$15 dB threshold shift at both 6 and 8 kHz unilaterally or bilaterally), representing a 75% reduction of the incidence of hearing loss. This study provided the first proof-of-principle that it is possible to translate animal experiments in the field of acquired hearing loss to the clinic. An independent follow-up trial with 30 patients per group confirmed the efficacy of aspirin (Behnoud et al., 2009). Another antioxidant, N-acetylcysteine (NAC) also attenuated ototoxicity caused by aminoglycosides in patients with bacteremia receiving hemodialysis (Feldman et al., 2007). Of 20 patients in the control group, 11 showed elevated pure-tone hearing thresholds at the follow-up examination as opposed to only 2 of 20 patients in the NAC group. In contrast, a small-scale study of vitamin E in the prevention of aminoglycoside ototoxicity was not successful (Kharkheli et al., 2007).

Therapeutic agents to mitigate noise-induced hearing loss in human subjects have included magnesium which is primarily a vasodilator, not an antioxidant (Attias et al., 1994), and NAC. In an attempt to reduce temporary threshold shifts after exposure to loud music in 31 normal subjects, NAC was not effective in protecting pure-tone thresholds and distortion product otoacoustic emissions (Kramer et al., 2006). Likewise, Lindblad et al. (2011) found no significant differences in temporary noise-induced threshold shifts and DPOAE amplitude in military personnel after a shooting exercise. However, more sensitive supra-threshold measurements (psycho-acoustical modulation

TABLE 1 | Selected features of acquired hearing loss.

	Age	Drugs	Noise
Pathology			
Organ of Corti	Loss of hair cells in sensorineural hearing loss	Loss of (primarily outer) hair cells	Dislocation of tectorial membrane from stereocilia; breaking of tip links; loss of hair cells
Stria vascularis (and spiral ligament)	Compromised structure and possibly function in some forms of hearing loss	Aminoglycosides: endolymphatic potential (EP) unaffected Cisplatin: EP may be decreased	May reduce EP; loss of fibrocytes
Spiral ganglion and auditory nerve	Reduced in sensorineural hearing loss; loss of synaptic connections	Loss considered mostly secondary; loss of synaptic connections possible	Loss of synaptic connections
Reactive oxidant species			
Evidence	Causal relation largely not supported	+	+
Likely sources	Mitochondria	Aminoglycosides: non-enzymatic; mitochondria; NADPH oxidase Cisplatin: mitochondria, NADPH oxidase	mitochondria; NADPH oxidase; calcium influx may cause oxidative stress
Effects on mitochondria			
	mtDNA mutations might impair auditory function; specific mutations correlate with presbycusis in human	Aminoglycosides: Bind to mtRNA and impair mitochondrial protein synthesis and function; inhibition of the electron transport chain	Reduced blood flow may impair oxidative phosphorylation
Potential cell death pathways			
Apoptosis	+	+	+
Necrosis	+	Aminoglycosides: + Cisplatin: ?	+
MAPK pathway	+	Aminoglycosides: + Cisplatin: JNK ?	+
Caspase-dependent	?	Evidence mostly from *in vitro* studies	+
Caspase-independent	?	*In vivo* +	+
Potential cell rescue pathways			
Homeostasis (e.g., Prx3)	+	+	+
NF-κB	Not determined	Aminoglycosides: +	+
PI3-kinase	+	Aminoglycosides: +	?
Heat shock proteins	+	+	+
Prevention			
Nutritional supplements	Inconsistent in animals Inconclusive evidence in clinical trials and epidemiological studies	Aminoglycosides: Consistent protection in animals; successful clinical trials. Cisplatin: success in animal studies	Mostly protective in animal studies Inconclusive in clinical or field trials, which are largely of temporary hearing loss

+, supporting evidence exists; ?, not known or inconclusive. For drug-induced hearing loss, preference was given to results from studies in vivo or with cochlear tissues in vitro; for age-related hearing loss, results from confounded models (See text: mice with Cdh23 mutations or catastrophic mitochondrial mutations) were de-emphasized.

transfer functions) were compromised in 23 noise-exposed controls but not in 11 subjects receiving NAC. Another double-blind cross-over study assessed the efficacy of NAC in 53 male Taiwanese steel workers that were also genotyped for deficiencies in glutathione S-transferases, enzymes that protect against oxidative stress (Lin et al., 2010). Noise-induced temporary threshold shifts were small, averaging ~3 dB at high frequencies (3,000–6,000 Hz). NAC reduced the threshold shifts only in a subset of workers with specific null genotypes (GSTT1 and GSTM1) of glutathione S-transferases.

The Conundrum of Therapeutic Protection

A conclusion that can be drawn from human studies is that antioxidants are viable therapeutic agents against drug- and noise-induced hearing loss. To what extent dietary manipulation can attenuate presbycusis, however, remains to be established. But even for ototoxicity and noise trauma the situation may not be predictable. Individual genetic predisposition and the physiological (nutritional) state are confounding factors that are capable of influencing the success of therapeutic interventions. Furthermore, subtle forms of auditory damage may escape simple audiometric tests and a final verdict on success or failure of protective strategies may have to await more sophisticated audiological assessments.

There is another unresolved question. While a short-term administration of antioxidants or vitamins might be safe for drug and noise exposure, the hazards of a life-long regimen of nutritional supplements are unknown. Studies in animals as well as clinical trials have warned of a potentially increased risk of cancer and mortality associated with prolonged consumption of antioxidants or vitamins. Specifically, meta-analyses of clinical trials singled out beta-carotene, vitamin A, and vitamin E as associated with increased overall mortality (Miller et al., 2005; Bjelakovic et al., 2014). A well-balanced diet might be all that is needed to maintain health and hearing into old age (Halliwell, 2011).

Outlook

When we compare the mechanisms of drug, noise, and age-related hearing loss, there appear to be more similarities between drug- and noise-induced hearing loss than between those two and age (**Table 1**). One of the reasons might be that age-related hearing loss is complexly influenced by genetics and a lifetime of environmental factors that render its mechanisms and manifestations highly variable. For preventive treatments, it appears that supra-normal doses of protective agents are successful to combat the acute damage of noise or drug trauma but generally fail when given over the long term in an attempt to curb the auditory deficiencies in aging.

Looking ahead, regeneration of human hair cells seems decades away but other approaches may provide new directions. Some aspects of ARHI may relate to the phenomenon of cochlear synaptopathy, causing "hidden hearing loss" by the loss of auditory nerve fiber/hair cell connections (Kujawa and Liberman, 2015). In a noise-induced synaptopathy model, the administration and the overexpression of the neurotrophins NT-3 partially rescued the synaptopathy phenotype in mice (Wan et al., 2014). If an appropriate diagnostic method and drug application can be identified for ARHI, the regeneration of the terminal nerve fibers might be a suitable therapeutic option for at least a selected group of patients.

Acknowledgments

The authors wish to thank the reviewers of this manuscript for thoughtful and constructive comments and Andra E. Talaska for expert editorial help. Dr. Schacht's work on age-related hearing impairment was funded by grant P01 AG-025164 and work on drug-induced hearing loss is supported by grant R01 DC003685 from the National Institute on Aging and National Institute on Deafness and Other Communication Disorders, respectively, National Institutes of Health.

References

Aladag, I., Eyibilen, A., Güven, M., Atis, O., and Erkorkmaz, U. (2009). Role of oxidative stress in hearing impairment in patients with type two diabetes mellitus. *J. Laryngol. Otol.* 123, 957–963. doi: 10.1017/S0022215109004502

Alam, S. A., Ikeda, K., Oshima, T., Suzuki, M., Kawase, T., Kikuchi, T., et al. (2000). Cisplatin-induced apoptotic cell death in Mongolian gerbil cochlea. *Hear Res.* 141, 28–38. doi: 10.1016/s0378-5955(99)00211-7

Alam, S. A., Oshima, T., Suzuki, M., Kawase, T., Takasaka, T., and Ikeda, K. (2001). The expression of apoptosis-related proteins in the aged cochlea of Mongolian gerbils. *Laryngoscope* 111, 528–534. doi: 10.1097/00005537-200103000-00026

Altschuler, R. A., Dolan, D. F., Halsey, K., Kanicki, A., Deng, N., Martin, C., et al. (2015). Age-related changes in auditory nerve-inner hair cell connections, hair cell numbers, auditory brain stem response and gap detection in UM-HET4 mice. *Neuroscience* 292, 22–33. doi: 10.1016/j.neuroscience.2015.01.068

Attias, J., Weisz, G., Almog, S., Shahar, A., Wiener, M., Joachims, Z., et al. (1994). Oral magnesium intake reduces permanent hearing loss induced by noise exposure. *Am. J. Otolaryngol.* 15, 26–32. doi: 10.1016/0196-0709(94)90036-1

Bai, U., Seidman, M. D., Hinojosa, R., and Quirk, W. S. (1997). Mitochondrial DNA deletions associated with aging and possibly presbycusis: a human archival temporal bone study. *Am. J. Otol.* 18, 449–453.

Behnoud, F., Davoudpur, K., and Goodarzi, M. T. (2009). Can aspirin protect or at least attenuate gentamicin ototoxicity in humans? *Saudi Med. J.* 30, 1165–1169.

Berner, B., Odum, L., and Parving, A. (2000). Age-related hearing impairment and B vitamin status. *Acta Otolaryngol.* 120, 633–637. doi: 10.1080/000164800750000469

Bielefeld, E. C., Coling, D., Chen, G. D., and Henderson, D. (2008). Multiple dosing strategies with acetyl L-carnitine (ALCAR) fail to alter age-related hearing loss in the Fischer 344/NHsd rat. *J. Negat. Results Biomed.* 7:4. doi: 10.1186/1477-5751-7-4

Bjelakovic, G., Nikolova, D., and Gluud, C. (2014). Antioxidant supplements and mortality. *Curr. Opin. Clin. Nutr. Metab. Care* 17, 40–44. doi: 10.1097/MCO.0000000000000009

Bonneux, S., Fransen, E., Van Eyken, E., Van Laer, L., Huyghe, J., Van de Heyning, P., et al. (2011). Inherited mitochondrial variants are not a major cause of age-related hearing impairment in the European population. *Mitochondrion* 11, 729–734. doi: 10.1016/j.mito.2011.05.008

Böttger, E. C., and Schacht, J. (2013). The mitochondrion: a perpetrator of acquired hearing loss. *Hear Res.* 303, 12–19. doi: 10.1016/j.heares.2013.01.006

Chen, H., and Tang, J. (2014). The role of mitochondria in age-related hearing loss. *Biogerontology* 15, 13–19. doi: 10.1007/s10522-013-9475-y

Chen, F. Q., Zheng, H. W., Hill, K., and Sha, S. H. (2012). Traumatic noise activates Rho-family GTPases through transient cellular energy depletion. *J. Neurosci.* 32, 12421–12430. doi: 10.1523/jneurosci.6381-11.2012

Chen, F. Q., Zheng, H. W., Schacht, J., and Sha, S. H. (2013). Mitochondrial peroxiredoxin 3 regulates sensory cell survival in the cochlea. *PLoS One* 8:e61999. doi: 10.1371/journal.pone.0061999

Choi, Y. H., Miller, J. M., Tucker, K. L., Hu, H., and Park, S. K. (2014). Antioxidant vitamins and magnesium and the risk of hearing loss in the US general population. *Am. J. Clin. Nutr.* 99, 148–155. doi: 10.3945/ajcn.113.068437

Chung, W. H., Pak, K., Lin, B., Webster, N., and Ryan, A. F. (2006). A PI3K pathway mediates hair cell survival and opposes gentamicin toxicity in neonatal rat organ of Corti. *J. Assoc. Res. Otolaryngol.* 7, 373–382. doi: 10.1007/s10162-006-0050-y

Coffin, A. B., Rubel, E. W., and Raible, D. W. (2013). Bax, Bcl2 and p53 differentially regulate neomycin- and gentamicin-induced hair cell death in the zebrafish lateral line. *J. Assoc. Res. Otolaryngol.* 14, 645–659. doi: 10.1007/s10162-013-0404-1

Crowe, S. J., Guild, S. R., and Polvogt, L. M. (1993). Observations on the pathology of high-tone deafness. *Bull. Johns Hopkins Hosp.* 54, 315–379.

Cunningham, L. L., Cheng, A. G., and Rubel, E. W. (2002). Caspase activation in hair cells of the mouse utricle exposed to neomycin. *J. Neurosci.* 22, 8532–8540.

Dai, P., Yang, W., Jiang, S., Gu, R., Yuan, H., Han, D., et al. (2004). Correlation of cochlear blood supply with mitochondrial DNA common deletion in presbyacusis. *Acta Otolaryngol.* 124, 130–136. doi: 10.1080/00016480410016586

Dawes, P., Cruickshanks, K. J., Moore, D. R., Edmondson-Jones, M., Mccormack, A., Fortnum, H., et al. (2014). Cigarette smoking, passive smoking, alcohol consumption and hearing loss. *J. Assoc. Res. Otolaryngol.* 15, 663–674. doi: 10.1007/s10162-014-0461-0

Devarajan, P., Savoca, M., Castaneda, M. P., Park, M. S., Esteban-Cruciani, N., Kalinec, G., et al. (2002). Cisplatin-induced apoptosis in auditory cells: role of death receptor and mitochondrial pathways. *Hear Res.* 174, 45–54. doi: 10.1016/s0378-5955(02)00634-2

Durga, J., Verhoef, P., Anteunis, L. J., Schouten, E., and Kok, F. J. (2007). Effects of folic acid supplementation on hearing in older adults: a randomized, controlled trial. *Ann. Intern. Med.* 146, 1–9. doi: 10.7326/0003-4819-146-1-200701020-00003

Duscha, S., Boukari, H., Shcherbakov, D., Salian, S., Silva, S., Kendall, A., et al. (2014). Identification and evaluation of improved 4′-O-(alkyl) 4,5-disubstituted 2-deoxystreptamines as next-generation aminoglycoside antibiotics. *MBio* 5:e01827-14. doi: 10.1128/mbio.01827-14

Engle, J. R., Tinling, S., and Recanzone, G. H. (2013). Age-related hearing loss in rhesus monkeys is correlated with cochlear histopathologies. *PLoS One* 8:e55092. doi: 10.1371/journal.pone.0055092

Feldman, L., Efrati, S., Eviatar, E., Abramsohn, R., Yarovoy, I., Gersch, E., et al. (2007). Gentamicin-induced ototoxicity in hemodialysis patients is ameliorated by N-acetylcysteine. *Kidney Int.* 72, 359–363. doi: 10.1038/sj.ki.5002295

Fischel-Ghodsian, N., Bykhovskaya, Y., Taylor, K., Kahen, T., Cantor, R., Ehrenman, K., et al. (1997). Temporal bone analysis of patients with presbycusis reveals high frequency of mitochondrial mutations. *Hear Res.* 110, 147–154. doi: 10.1016/s0378-5955(97)00077-4

Forge, A., Wright, A., and Davies, S. J. (1987). Analysis of structural changes in the stria vascularis following chronic gentamicin treatment. *Hear Res.* 31, 253–265. doi: 10.1016/0378-5955(87)90195-x

Fransen, E., Bonneux, S., Corneveaux, J. J., Schrauwen, I., Di Berardino, F., White, C. H., et al. (2015). Genome-wide association analysis demonstrates the highly polygenic character of age-related hearing impairment. *Eur. J. Hum. Genet.* 23, 110–115. doi: 10.1038/ejhg.2014.56

Fransen, E., Topsakal, V., Hendrickx, J. J., Van Laer, L., Huyghe, J. R., Van Eyken, E., et al. (2008). Occupational noise, smoking and a high body mass index are risk factors for age-related hearing impairment and moderate alcohol consumption is protective: a European population-based multicenter study. *J. Assoc. Res. Otolaryngol.* 9, 264–276; discussion 261–263. doi: 10.1007/s10162-008-0123-1

Fridberger, A., Flock, A., Ulfendahl, M., and Flock, B. (1998). Acoustic overstimulation increases outer hair cell Ca2+ concentrations and causes dynamic contractions of the hearing organ. *Proc. Natl. Acad. Sci. U S A* 95, 7127–7132. doi: 10.1073/pnas.95.12.7127

Gates, G. A., and Mills, J. H. (2005). Presbycusis. *Lancet* 366, 1111–1120. doi: 10.1016/S0140-6736(05)67423-5

Gershon, D. (2005). Evaluating evidence for aging. *Science* 310, 441–443. doi: 10.1126/science.310.5747.441

Gonzalez-Freire, M., de Cabo, R., Bernier, M., Sollott, S. J., Fabbri, E., Navas, P., et al. (2015). Reconsidering the role of mitochondria in aging. *J Gerontol. A Biol. Sci. Med. Sci.* doi: 10.1093/gerona/glv070 [Epub ahead of print].

Gopinath, B., Flood, V. M., McMahon, C. M., Burlutsky, G., Brand-Miller, J., and Mitchell, P. (2010a). Dietary glycemic load is a predictor of age-related hearing loss in older adults. *J. Nutr.* 140, 2207–2212. doi: 10.3945/jn.110.128462

Gopinath, B., Flood, V. M., McMahon, C. M., Burlutsky, G., Spankovich, C., Hood, L. J., et al. (2011a). Dietary antioxidant intake is associated with the prevalence but not incidence of age-related hearing loss. *J. Nutr. Health Aging* 15, 896–900. doi: 10.1007/s12603-011-0119-0

Gopinath, B., Flood, V. M., Rochtchina, E., McMahon, C. M., and Mitchell, P. (2010b). Serum homocysteine and folate concentrations are associated with prevalent age-related hearing loss. *J. Nutr.* 140, 1469–1474. doi: 10.3945/jn.110.122010

Gopinath, B., Flood, V. M., Teber, E., Mcmahon, C. M., and Mitchell, P. (2011b). Dietary intake of cholesterol is positively associated and use of cholesterol-lowering medication is negatively associated with prevalent age-related hearing loss. *J. Nutr.* 141, 1355–1361. doi: 10.3945/jn.111.138610

Halliwell, B. (2011). Free radicals and antioxidants - quo vadis? *Trends Pharmacol. Sci.* 32, 125–130. doi: 10.1016/j.tips.2010.12.002

Hirose, K., and Liberman, M. C. (2003). Lateral wall histopathology and endocochlear potential in the noise-damaged mouse cochlea. *J. Assoc. Res. Otolaryngol.* 4, 339–352. doi: 10.1007/s10162-002-3036-4

Houston, D. K., Johnson, M. A., Nozza, R. J., Gunter, E. W., Shea, K. J., Cutler, G. M., et al. (1999). Age-related hearing loss, vitamin B-12 and folate in elderly women. *Am. J. Clin. Nutr.* 69, 564–571.

Hu, B. H., Yang, W. P., Bielefeld, E. C., Li, M., Chen, G. D., and Henderson, D. (2008). Apoptotic outer hair cell death in the cochleae of aging Fischer 344/NHsd rats. *Hear Res.* 245, 48–57. doi: 10.1016/j.heares.2008.08.006

Hutchin, T. P., and Cortopassi, G. A. (2000). Mitochondrial defects and hearing loss. *Cell. Mol. Life Sci.* 57, 1927–1937. doi: 10.1007/pl00000673

Huth, M. E., Ricci, A. J., and Cheng, A. G. (2011). Mechanisms of aminoglycoside ototoxicity and targets of hair cell protection. *Int. J. Otolaryngol.* 2011:937861. doi: 10.1155/2011/937861

Hwang, J. H., Chen, J. C., Hsu, C. J., Yang, W. S., and Liu, T. C. (2012a). Plasma reactive oxygen species levels are correlated with severity of age-related hearing impairment in humans. *Neurobiol. Aging* 33, 1920–1926. doi: 10.1016/j.neurobiolaging.2011.10.012

Hwang, J. H., Liu, K. S., Wu, C. C., and Liu, T. C. (2012b). Association of cadherin23 single nucleotide polymorphism with age-related hearing impairment in Han Chinese. *Otolaryngol. Head Neck Surg.* 147, 531–534. doi: 10.1177/0194599812446904

Ishiyama, G., Tokita, J., Lopez, I., Tang, Y., and Ishiyama, A. (2007). Unbiased stereological estimation of the spiral ligament and stria vascularis volumes in aging and Ménière's disease using archival human temporal bones. *J. Assoc. Res. Otolaryngol.* 8, 8–17. doi: 10.1007/s10162-006-0057-4

Jamesdaniel, S., Hu, B., Kermany, M. H., Jiang, H., Ding, D., Coling, D., et al. (2011). Noise induced changes in the expression of p38/MAPK signaling proteins in the sensory epithelium of the inner ear. *J. Proteomics* 75, 410–424. doi: 10.1016/j.jprot.2011.08.007

Jensen-Smith, H. C., Hallworth, R., and Nichols, M. G. (2012). Gentamicin rapidly inhibits mitochondrial metabolism in high-frequency cochlear outer hair cells. *PLoS One* 7:e38471. doi: 10.1371/journal.pone.0038471

Jiang, H., Sha, S. H., Forge, A., and Schacht, J. (2006a). Caspase-independent pathways of hair cell death induced by kanamycin *in vivo*. *Cell Death Differ.* 13, 20–30. doi: 10.1038/sj.cdd.4401706

Jiang, H., Sha, S. H., and Schacht, J. (2006b). Kanamycin alters cytoplasmic and nuclear phosphoinositide signaling in the organ of Corti *in vivo*. *J. Neurochem.* 99, 269–276. doi: 10.1111/j.1471-4159.2006.04117.x

Jiang, H., Talaska, A. E., Schacht, J., and Sha, S. H. (2007). Oxidative imbalance in the aging inner ear. *Neurobiol. Aging* 28, 1605–1612. doi: 10.1016/j.neurobiolaging.2006.06.025

Johnson, K. R., Longo-Guess, C., Gagnon, L. H., Yu, H., and Zheng, Q. Y. (2008). A locus on distal chromosome 11 (ahl8) and its interaction with Cdh23 ahl underlie the early onset, age-related hearing loss of DBA/2J mice. *Genomics* 92, 219–225. doi: 10.1016/j.ygeno.2008.06.007

Kang, J. W., Choi, H. S., Kim, K., and Choi, J. Y. (2014). Dietary vitamin intake correlates with hearing thresholds in the older population: the Korean National Health and Nutrition Examination Survey. *Am. J. Clin. Nutr.* 99, 1407–1413. doi: 10.3945/ajcn.113.072793

Keithley, E. M., Canto, C., Zheng, Q.-Y., Wang, X., Fischel-Ghodsian, N., and Johnson, K. (2005). Cu/Zn superoxide dismutase and age-related hearing loss. *Hear Res.* 209, 76–85. doi: 10.1016/j.heares.2005.06.009

Keithley, E. M., Ryan, A. F., and Woolf, N. K. (1989). Spiral ganglion cell density in young and old gerbils. *Hear Res.* 38, 125–133. doi: 10.1016/0378-5955(89)90134-2

Kharkheli, E., Kevanishvili, Z., Maglakelidze, T., Davitashvili, O., and Schacht, J. (2007). Does vitamin E prevent gentamicin-induced ototoxicity? *Georgian Med. News* 146, 14–17.

Klis, S. F., O'Leary, S. J., Hamers, F. P., De Groot, J. C., and Smoorenburg, G. F. (2000). Reversible cisplatin ototoxicity in the albino guinea pig. *Neuroreport* 11, 623–626. doi: 10.1097/00001756-200002280-00037

Komune, S., Ide, M., Nakano, T., and Morimitsu, T. (1987). Effects of kanamycin sulfate on cochlear potentials and potassium ion permeability through the cochlear partitions. *ORL J. Otorhinolaryngol. Relat. Spec.* 49, 9–16. doi: 10.1159/000275900

Kramer, S., Dreisbach, L., Lockwood, J., Baldwin, K., Kopke, R., Scranton, S., et al. (2006). Efficacy of the antioxidant N-acetylcysteine (NAC) in protecting ears exposed to loud music. *J. Am. Acad. Audiol.* 17, 265–278. doi: 10.3766/jaaa.17.4.5

Kujawa, S. G., and Liberman, M. C. (2009). Adding insult to injury: cochlear nerve degeneration after "temporary" noise-induced hearing loss. *J. Neurosci.* 29, 14077–14085. doi: 10.1523/jneurosci.2845-09.2009

Kujawa, S. G., and Liberman, M. C. (2015). Synaptopathy in the noise-exposed and aging cochlea: primary neural degeneration in acquired sensorineural hearing loss. *Hear Res.* doi: 10.1016/j.heares.2015.02.009 [Epub ahead of print].

Kujoth, G. C., Hiona, A., Pugh, T. D., Someya, S., Panzer, K., Wohlgemuth, S. E., et al. (2005). Mitochondrial DNA mutations, oxidative stress and apoptosis in mammalian aging. *Science* 309, 481–484. doi: 10.1126/science.1112125

Lang, H., and Liu, C. (1997). Apoptosis and hair cell degeneration in the vestibular sensory epithelia of the guinea pig following a gentamicin insult. *Hear Res.* 111, 177–184. doi: 10.1016/s0378-5955(97)00098-1

Laurell, G., Ekborn, A., Viberg, A., and Canlon, B. (2007). Effects of a single high dose of cisplatin on the melanocytes of the stria vascularis in the guinea pig. *Audiol. Neurotol.* 12, 170–178. doi: 10.1159/000099020

Le, T., and Keithley, E. M. (2007). Effects of antioxidants on the aging inner ear. *Hear Res.* 226, 194–202. doi: 10.1016/j.heares.2006.04.003

Lee, K. Y. (2013). Pathophysiology of age-related hearing loss (peripheral and central). *Korean J. Audiol.* 17, 45–49. doi: 10.7874/kja.2013.17.2.45

Lee, H. C., and Wei, Y. H. (2012). Mitochondria and aging. *Adv. Exp. Med. Biol.* 942, 311–327. doi: 10.1007/978-94-007-2869-1_14

Li, H. S., and Borg, E. (1991). Age-related loss of auditory sensitivity in two mouse genotypes. *Acta Otolaryngol.* 111, 827–834. doi: 10.3109/00016489109138418

Lin, F. R., Niparko, J. K., and Ferrucci, L. (2011). Hearing loss prevalence in the United States. *Arch. Intern. Med.* 171, 1851–1852. doi: 10.1001/archinternmed.2011.506

Lin, C. Y., Wu, J. L., Shih, T. S., Tsai, P. J., Sun, Y. M., Ma, M. C., et al. (2010). N-Acetyl-cysteine against noise-induced temporary threshold shift in male workers. *Hear Res.* 269, 42–47. doi: 10.1016/j.heares.2010.07.005

Lindblad, A. C., Rosenhall, U., Olofsson, A., and Hagerman, B. (2011). The efficacy of N-acetylcysteine to protect the human cochlea from subclinical hearing loss caused by impulse noise: a controlled trial. *Noise Health* 13, 392–401. doi: 10.4103/1463-1741.90293

Linthicum, F. H. Jr., and Fayad, J. N. (2009). Spiral ganglion cell loss is unrelated to segmental cochlear sensory system degeneration in humans. *Otol. Neurotol.* 30, 418–422. doi: 10.1097/mao.0b013e31819a8827

Markaryan, A., Nelson, E. G., and Hinojosa, R. (2009). Quantification of the mitochondrial DNA common deletion in presbycusis. *Laryngoscope* 119, 1184–1189. doi: 10.1002/lary.20218

McFadden, S. L., Ding, D., Reaume, A. G., Flood, D. G., and Salvi, R. J. (1999). Age-related cochlear hair cell loss is enhanced in mice lacking copper/zinc superoxide dismutase. *Neurobiol. Aging* 20, 1–8. doi: 10.1016/s0197-4580(99)00018-4

Mikuriya, T., Sugahara, K., Sugimoto, K., Fujimoto, M., Takemoto, T., Hashimoto, M., et al. (2008). Attenuation of progressive hearing loss in a model of age-related hearing loss by a heat shock protein inducer, geranylgeranylacetone. *Brain Res.* 1212, 9–17. doi: 10.1016/j.brainres.2008.03.031

Miller, R. A. (2005). Evaluating evidence for aging. *Science* 310, 441–443. doi: 10.1126/science.310.5747.441

Miller, E. R. 3rd, Pastor-Barriuso, R., Dalal, D., Riemersma, R. A., Appel, L. J., and Guallar, E. (2005). Meta-analysis: high-dosage vitamin E supplementation may increase all-cause mortality. *Ann. Intern. Med.* 142, 37–46. doi: 10.7326/0003-4819-142-1-200501040-00110

Mitchell, P., Gopinath, B., Mcmahon, C. M., Rochtchina, E., Wang, J. J., Boyages, S. C., et al. (2009). Relationship of Type 2 diabetes to the prevalence, incidence and progression of age-related hearing loss. *Diabet. Med.* 26, 483–488. doi: 10.1111/j.1464-5491.2009.02710.x

Nakagawa, T., Yamane, H., Takayama, M., Sunami, K., and Nakai, Y. (1998). Apoptosis of guinea pig cochlear hair cells following chronic aminoglycoside treatment. *Eur. Arch. Otorhinolaryngol.* 255, 127–131. doi: 10.1007/s004050050027

Nelson, E. G., and Hinojosa, R. (2006). Presbycusis: a human temporal bone study of individuals with downward sloping audiometric patterns of hearing loss and review of the literature. *Laryngoscope* 116, 1–12. doi: 10.1097/01.mlg.0000236089.44566.62

Nicol, K. M. M., Hackney, C. M., Evans, E. F., and Pratt, S. R. (1992). Behavioural evidence for recovery of auditory function in guinea pigs following kanamycin administration. *Hear Res.* 61, 117–131. doi: 10.1016/0378-5955(92)90042-l

Nicotera, T. M., Hu, B. H., and Henderson, D. (2003). The caspase pathway in noise-induced apoptosis of the chinchilla cochlea. *J. Assoc. Res. Otolaryngol.* 4, 466–477. doi: 10.1007/s10162-002-3038-2

Noben-Trauth, K., and Johnson, K. R. (2009). Inheritance patterns of progressive hearing loss in laboratory strains of mice. *Brain Res.* 1277, 42–51. doi: 10.1016/j.brainres.2009.02.012

Ohlemiller, K. K., Dahl, A. R., and Gagnon, P. M. (2010). Divergent aging characteristics in CBA/J and CBA/CaJ mouse cochleae. *J. Assoc. Res. Otolaryngol.* 11, 605–623. doi: 10.1007/s10162-010-0228-1

Ohmen, J., Kang, E. Y., Li, X., Joo, J. W., Hormozdiari, F., Zheng, Q. Y., et al. (2014). Genome-wide association study for age-related hearing loss (AHL) in the mouse: a meta-analysis. *J. Assoc. Res. Otolaryngol.* 15, 335–352. doi: 10.1007/s10162-014-0443-2

Oishi, N., Duscha, S., Boukari, H., Meyer, M., Xie, J., Wei, G., et al. (2015). XBP1 mitigates aminoglycoside-induced endoplasmic reticulum stress and neuronal cell death. *Cell Death Dis.* 6:e1763. doi: 10.1038/cddis.2015.108

Oishi, N., and Schacht, J. (2011). Emerging treatments for noise-induced hearing loss. *Expert. Opin. Emerg. Drugs* 16, 235–245. doi: 10.1517/14728214.2011.552427

Park, S., Johnson, M. A., Shea-Miller, K., De Chicchis, A. R., Allen, R. H., and Stabler, S. P. (2006). Age-related hearing loss, methylmalonic acid and vitamin B12 status in older adults. *J. Nutr. Elder* 25, 105–120. doi: 10.1300/j052v25n03_08

Perry, B. P., Sebold, C., Hasi, M., Heard, P., Carter, E., Hill, A., et al. (2014). Sensorineural hearing loss in people with deletions of 18q: hearing in 18q. *Otol. Neurotol.* 35, 782–786. doi: 10.1097/mao.0000000000000363

Pirvola, U., Xing-Qun, L., Virkkala, J., Saarma, M., Murakata, C., Camoratto, A. M., et al. (2000). Rescue of hearing, auditory hair cells and neurons by CEP-1347/KT7515, an inhibitor of c-Jun N-terminal kinase activation. *J. Neurosci.* 20, 43–50.

Polanski, J. F., and Cruz, O. L. (2013). Evaluation of antioxidant treatment in presbyacusis: prospective, placebo-controlled, double-blind, randomised trial. *J. Laryngol. Otol.* 127, 134–141. doi: 10.1017/s0022215112003118

Popelka, M. M., Cruickshanks, K. J., Wiley, T. L., Tweed, T. S., Klein, B. E., Klein, R., et al. (2000). Moderate alcohol consumption and hearing loss: a protective effect. *J. Am. Geriatr. Soc.* 48, 1273–1278. doi: 10.1111/j.1532-5415.2000.tb02601.x

Raynor, L. A., Pankow, J. S., Miller, M. B., Huang, G. H., Dalton, D., Klein, R., et al. (2009). Familial aggregation of age-related hearing loss in an epidemiological study of older adults. *Am. J. Audiol.* 18, 114–118. doi: 10.1044/1059-0889(2009/08-0035)

Rizk, H. G., and Linthicum, F. H. Jr. (2012). Histopathologic categorization of presbycusis. *Otol. Neurotol.* 33, e23–e24. doi: 10.1097/mao.0b013e31821f84ee

Roth, T. N. (2015). Aging of the auditory system. *Handb. Clin. Neurol.* 129, 357–373. doi: 10.1016/B978-0-444-62630-1.00020-2

Schacht, J., Altschuler, R., Burke, D. T., Chen, S., Dolan, D., Galecki, A. T., et al. (2012a). Alleles that modulate late life hearing in genetically heterogeneous mice. *Neurobiol. Aging* 33, 1842.e15–1842.e29. doi: 10.1016/j.neurobiolaging.2011.12.034

Schacht, J., Talaska, A. E., and Rybak, L. (2012b). Cisplatin and aminoglycoside antibiotics: hearing loss and its prevention. *Anat. Rec. (Hoboken)* 295, 1837–1850. doi: 10.1002/ar.22578

Schuknecht, H. F., and Gacek, M. R. (1993). Cochlear pathology in presbycusis. *Ann. Otol. Rhinol Laryngol.* 102, 1–16.

Schuknecht, H. F., Watanuki, K., Takahashi, T., Belal, A. A. Jr., Kimura, R. S., Jones, D. D., et al. (1974). Atrophy of the stria vascularis, a common cause for hearing loss. *Laryngoscope* 84, 1777–1821. doi: 10.1288/00005537-197410000-00012

Schulte, B. A., and Schmiedt, R. A. (1992). Lateral wall Na,K-ATPase and endocochlear potentials decline with age in quiet-reared gerbils. *Hear. Res.* 61, 35–46. doi: 10.1016/0378-5955(92)90034-k

Seidman, M. D. (2000). Effects of dietary restriction and antioxidants on presbyacusis. *Laryngoscope* 110, 727–738. doi: 10.1097/00005537-200005000-00003

Sha, S. H., Chen, F. Q., and Schacht, J. (2009). Activation of cell death pathways in the inner ear of the aging CBA/J mouse. *Hear. Res.* 254, 92–99. doi: 10.1016/j.heares.2009.04.019

Sha, S. H., Chen, F. Q., and Schacht, J. (2010). PTEN attenuates PIP3/Akt signaling in the cochlea of the aging CBA/J mouse. *Hear. Res.* 264, 86–92. doi: 10.1016/j.heares.2009.09.002

Sha, S. H., and Schacht, J. (1999). Salicylate attenuates gentamicin-induced ototoxicity. *Lab. Invest.* 79, 807–813.

Sha, S. H., Kanicki, A., Dootz, G., Talaska, A. E., Halsey, K., Dolan, D., et al. (2008). Age-related auditory pathology in the CBA/J mouse. *Hear. Res.* 243, 87–94. doi: 10.1016/j.heares.2008.06.001

Sha, S. H., Kanicki, A., Halsey, K., Wearne, K. A., and Schacht, J. (2012). Antioxidant-enriched diet does not delay the progression of age-related hearing loss. *Neurobiol. Aging* 33, 1010.e15–1010.e16. doi: 10.1016/j.neurobiolaging.2011.10.023

Sha, S. H., Qiu, J. H., and Schacht, J. (2006). Aspirin to prevent gentamicin-induced hearing loss. *N. Engl. J. Med.* 354, 1856–1857. doi: 10.1056/nejmc053428

Sha, S. H., Taylor, R., Forge, A., and Schacht, J. (2001). Differential vulnerability of basal and apical hair cells is based on intrinsic susceptibility to free radicals. *Hear. Res.* 155, 1–8. doi: 10.1016/s0378-5955(01)00224-6

Sharashenidze, N., Schacht, J., and Kevanishvili, Z. (2007). Age-related hearing loss: gender differences. *Georgian Med. News* 144, 14–18.

Shargorodsky, J., Curhan, S. G., Eavey, R., and Curhan, G. C. (2010). A prospective study of vitamin intake and the risk of hearing loss in men. *Otolaryngol. Head Neck Surg.* 142, 231–236. doi: 10.1016/j.otohns.2009.10.049

Shulman, E., Belakhov, V., Wei, G., Kendall, A., Meyron-Holtz, E. G., Ben-Shachar, D., et al. (2014). Designer aminoglycosides that selectively inhibit cytoplasmic rather than mitochondrial ribosomes show decreased ototoxicity: a strategy for the treatment of genetic diseases. *J. Biol. Chem.* 289, 2318–2330. doi: 10.1074/jbc.m113.533588

Sohal, R. S., and Weindruch, R. (1996). Oxidative stress, caloric restriction and aging. *Science* 273, 59–63. doi: 10.1126/science.273.5271.59

Someya, S., Yamasoba, T., Prolla, T. A., and Tanokura, M. (2007). Genes encoding mitochondrial respiratory chain components are profoundly down-regulated with aging in the cochlea of DBA/2J mice. *Brain Res.* 1182, 26–33. doi: 10.1016/j.brainres.2007.08.090

Sone, M., Schachern, P. A., and Paparella, M. M. (1998). Loss of spiral ganglion cells as primary manifestation of aminoglycoside ototoxicity. *Hear. Res.* 115, 217–223. doi: 10.1016/s0378-5955(97)00191-3

Spankovich, C., Hood, L. J., Silver, H. J., Lambert, W., Flood, V. M., and Mitchell, P. (2011). Associations between diet and both high and low pure tone averages and transient evoked otoacoustic emissions in an older adult population-based study. *J. Am. Acad. Audiol.* 22, 49–58. doi: 10.3766/jaaa.22.1.6

Tadros, S. F., D'souza, M., Zhu, X., and Frisina, R. D. (2008). Apoptosis-related genes change their expression with age and hearing loss in the mouse cochlea. *Apoptosis* 13, 1303–1321. doi: 10.1007/s10495-008-0266-x

Suga, F., and Lindsay, J. R. (1976). Histopathological observations of presbycusis. *Ann. Otol. Rhinol Laryngol.* 85, 169–184. doi: 10.1177/000348947608500201

Taleb, M., Brandon, C. S., Lee, F. S., Harris, K. C., Dillmann, W. H., and Cunningham, L. L. (2009). Hsp70 inhibits aminoglycoside-induced hearing loss and cochlear hair cell death. *Cell Stress Chaperones* 14, 427–437. doi: 10.1007/s12192-008-0097-2

van Ruijven, M. W., De Groot, J. C., Klis, S. F., and Smoorenburg, G. F. (2005). The cochlear targets of cisplatin: an electrophysiological and morphological time-sequence study. *Hear. Res.* 205, 241–248. doi: 10.1017/s0022215106002945

Vicente-Torres, M. A., and Schacht, J. (2006). A BAD link to mitochondrial cell death in the cochlea of mice with noise-induced hearing loss. *J. Neurosci. Res.* 83, 1564–1572. doi: 10.1002/jnr.20832

Wan, G., Gomez-Casati, M. E., Gigliello, A. R., Liberman, M. C., and Corfas, G. (2014). Neurotrophin-3 regulates ribbon synapse density in the cochlea and induces synapse regeneration after acoustic trauma. *eLife* 3:e03564. doi: 10.7554/elife.03564

Wang, J., Ding, D., Shulman, A., Stracher, A., and Salvi, R. J. (1999). Leupeptin protects sensory hair cells from acoustic trauma. *Neuroreport* 10, 811–816. doi: 10.1097/00001756-199903170-00027

Wang, J., Van De Water, T. R., Bonny, C., De Ribaupierre, F., Puel, J. L., and Zine, A. (2003). A peptide inhibitor of c-Jun N-terminal kinase protects against both aminoglycoside and acoustic trauma-induced auditory hair cell death and hearing loss. *J. Neurosci.* 23, 8596–8607.

Wei, X., Zhao, L., Liu, J., Dodel, R. C., Farlow, M. R., and Du, Y. (2005). Minocycline prevents gentamicin-induced ototoxicity by inhibiting p38 MAP kinase phosphorylation and caspase 3 activation. *Neuroscience* 131, 513–521. doi: 10.1016/j.neuroscience.2004.11.014

White, J. A., Burgess, B. J., Hall, R. D., and Nadol, J. B. (2000). Pattern of degeneration of the spiral ganglion cell and its processes in the C57BL/6J mouse. *Hear. Res.* 141, 12–18. doi: 10.1016/s0378-5955(99)00204-x

Willott, J. F., Erway, L. C., Archer, J. R., and Harrison, D. E. (1995). Genetics of age-related hearing loss in mice. II. Strain differences and effects of caloric restriction on cochlear pathology and evoked response thresholds. *Hear. Res.* 88, 143–155. doi: 10.1016/0378-5955(95)00107-f

Xie, J., Talaska, A. E., and Schacht, J. (2011). New developments in aminoglycoside therapy and ototoxicity. *Hear. Res.* 281, 28–37. doi: 10.1016/j.heares.2011.05.008

Xiong, H., Chu, H., Zhou, X., Huang, X., Cui, Y., Zhou, L., et al. (2011). Simultaneously reduced NKCC1 and Na,K-ATPase expression in murine cochlear lateral wall contribute to conservation of endocochlear potential following a sensorineural hearing loss. *Neurosci. Lett.* 488, 204–209. doi: 10.1016/j.neulet.2010.11.030

Yamashita, D., Miller, J. M., Jiang, H. Y., Minami, S. B., and Schacht, J. (2004). AIF and EndoG in noise-induced hearing loss. *Neuroreport* 15, 2719–2722.

Yamashita, D., Minami, S. B., Kanzaki, S., Ogawa, K., and Miller, J. M. (2008). Bcl-2 genes regulate noise-induced hearing loss. *J. Neurosci. Res.* 86, 920–928. doi: 10.1002/jnr.21533

Yang, W. P., Henderson, D., Hu, B. H., and Nicotera, T. M. (2004). Quantitative analysis of apoptotic and necrotic outer hair cells after exposure to different levels of continuous noise. *Hear. Res.* 196, 69–76. doi: 10.1016/j.heares.2004.04.015

Yoshida, N., Kristiansen, A., and Liberman, M. C. (1999). Heat stress and protection from permanent acoustic injury in mice. *J. Neurosci.* 19, 10116–10124.

Zheng, Q. Y., Johnson, K. R., and Erway, L. C. (1999). Assessment of hearing in 80 inbred strains of mice by ABR threshold analyses. *Hear. Res.* 130, 94–107. doi: 10.1016/s0378-5955(99)00003-9

8

Protecting mammalian hair cells from aminoglycoside-toxicity: assessing phenoxybenzamine's potential

Paromita Majumder[1], Paulette A. Moore[1], Guy P. Richardson[2] and Jonathan E. Gale[1,3]**

[1] UCL Ear Institute, University College London, London, UK, [2] Sussex Neuroscience, School of Life Sciences, University of Sussex, Falmer, UK, [3] Department of Cell and Developmental Biology, University College London, London, UK

Edited by:
Peter S. Steyger,
Oregon Health & Science University,
USA

Reviewed by:
Allison B. Coffin,
Washington State University, USA
Federico Kalinec,
University of California, Los Angeles,
USA

***Correspondence:**
Paromita Majumder
paromita.majumder@gmail.com
Jonathan E. Gale
j.e.gale@ucl.ac.uk

Aminoglycosides (AGs) are widely used antibiotics because of their low cost and high efficacy against gram-negative bacterial infection. However, AGs are ototoxic, causing the death of sensory hair cells in the inner ear. Strategies aimed at developing or discovering agents that protect against aminoglycoside ototoxicity have focused on inhibiting apoptosis or more recently, on preventing antibiotic uptake by the hair cells. Recent screens for ototoprotective compounds using the larval zebrafish lateral line identified phenoxybenzamine as a potential protectant for aminoglycoside-induced hair cell death. Here we used live imaging of FM1-43 uptake as a proxy for aminoglycoside entry, combined with hair-cell death assays to evaluate whether phenoxybenzamine can protect mammalian cochlear hair cells from the deleterious effects of the aminoglycoside antibiotic neomycin. We show that phenoxybenzamine can block FM1-43 entry into mammalian hair cells in a reversible and dose-dependent manner, but pre-incubation is required for maximal inhibition of entry. We observed differential effects of phenoxybenzamine on FM1-43 uptake in the two different types of cochlear hair cell in mammals, the outer hair cells (OHCs) and inner hair cells (IHCs). The requirement for pre-incubation and reversibility suggests an intracellular rather than an extracellular site of action for phenoxybenzamine. We also tested the efficacy of phenoxybenzamine as an otoprotective agent. In mouse cochlear explants the hair cell death resulting from 24 h exposure to neomycin was steeply dose-dependent, with 50% cell death occurring at ~230 μM for both IHC and OHC. We used 250 μM neomycin in subsequent hair-cell death assays. At 100 μM with 1 h pre-incubation, phenoxybenzamine conferred significant protection to both IHCs and OHCs, however at higher concentrations phenoxybenzamine itself showed clear signs of ototoxicity and an additive toxic effect when combined with neomycin. These data do not support the use of phenoxybenzamine as a therapeutic agent in mammalian inner ear. Our findings do share parallels with the observations from the zebrafish lateral line model but they also highlight the necessity for validation in the mammalian system and the potential for differential effects on sensory hair cells from different species, in different systems and even between cells in the same organ.

Keywords: hair cells, cochlea, aminoglycosides, ototoxicity, FM 1-43, organotypic culture, mechanoelectrical transduction channels, inner ear

INTRODUCTION

Aminoglycosides (AGs) are widely used antibiotics because of their low cost and high efficacy against gram-negative bacterial infection. AGs are both nephrotoxic (Toubeau et al., 1986; Hock and Anderson, 1995) and ototoxic (Greenwood, 1959) affecting the vestibular and auditory organs (Matz et al., 2004). Among the AGs neomycin is highly toxic, particularly in the hearing organ, the cochlea (Forge and Schacht, 2000). In the cochlea, AGs first affect the high-frequency hair cells found at the basal end of the cochlea, subsequently extending to the lower-frequency regions at the apical end of cochlear spiral (Aran and Darrouzet, 1975; Stebbins et al., 1979; for review see Forge and Schacht, 2000).

In order to access the apical surface of hair cells AGs must first pass through the blood labyrinth barrier which is composed of a highly specialized capillary network in the stria vascularis (Shi, 2016). Studies with fluorescently-tagged gentamicin showed that it travels from the stria vascularis capillaries into marginal cells and then into the endolymph (Wang and Steyger, 2009; Wang et al., 2010) at which point it comes into contact with the apical surface of the hair cells. AGs can enter into hair cells via an endocytic route (Hashino and Shero, 1995) or via the mechanotransduction (MET) channels, located in the hair cell's stereociliary bundle (Gale et al., 2001; Marcotti et al., 2005; Dai et al., 2006; Wang and Steyger, 2009; Alharazneh et al., 2011) a route that is facilitated by the low calcium concentration of the endolymph (Marcotti et al., 2005).

When mammalian cochlear hair cells die there is no endogenous regenerative process that can replace them and thus hearing loss is permanent. Stem cell based therapies are being pursued and may well be available in the longer term. In the shorter term, however, it is important that we discover therapies that might protect hair cells from damage and death as a result of ototoxic medication, noise-induced hearing loss and aging.

New aminoglycoside antibiotics derived from the structural backbones of existing AGs are being produced to generate less ototoxicity whilst still being effective antibiotics (Matt et al., 2012; Duscha et al., 2014; Shulman et al., 2014; Huth et al., 2015). Until such antibiotics are available, a protective agent that could be applied along with any known ototoxin would be very advantageous. There have been a number of screens to identify compounds that might confer hair-cell protection during ototoxicity, including screens of FDA-approved drugs that could bypass some of the approval requirements (Ou et al., 2009). Many of these have used the zebrafish lateral line system as a screening model. One of the compounds that came through two separate screens using two different sets of FDA-approved compounds was phenoxybenzamine (also known as N-(2-chloroethyl)-N-(1-methyl-2-phenoxyethyl) benzylamine hydrochloride or dibenzyline) which was one of seven drugs which showed protection against aminoglycoside-induced hair-cell death potentially by blocking aminoglycoside uptake by hair cells (Ou et al., 2009; Vlasits et al., 2012). In zebrafish it was noted that pre-incubation of phenoxybenzamine was required to see efficacy in increasing hair-cell survival (Vlasits et al., 2012). Although phenoxybenzamine is a well characterized drug that is known to cross the blood brain barrier (Diop and Dausse, 1986) and so perhaps the blood labyrinth barrier, it has not been tested on mammalian cochlear hair cells.

Phenoxybenzamine is a well-known alpha-1-A and alpha-2-A adrenergic receptor antagonist (Thoenen et al., 1964). Among alpha 1-A and 2-A receptors, phenoxybenzamine has a slow onset and long lasting effect compared with other alpha adrenergic blockers and it is used to reduce the vasoconstriction caused by epinephrine (adrenaline) and norepinephrine. Phenoxybenzamine acts by covalently binding to the receptor resulting in the inhibition of ligand binding. It is used to reduce the hypertension caused by pheochromocytoma, for lower urinary tract problems (e.g., neurogenic bladder; Te, 2002), benign prostatic hyperplasia (Kumar and Dewan, 2000) and in complex regional pain syndrome (Inchiosa, 2013). Phenoxybenzamine is also known to block 5-HT2 serotonin receptors (Frazer and Hensley, 1999), in some cases acting as an irreversible blocker (Doggrell, 1995).

In this study we evaluated whether the protective effects of phenoxybenzamine that are observed in zebrafish hair cells (Ou et al., 2009; Vlasits et al., 2012) are also observed in mammalian inner hair cells (IHCs) and outer hair cells (OHCs). We first investigated the effects of phenoxybenzamine on the rapid FM1-43 entry into hair cells that occurs via the mechanoelectrical-transduction channels and mimics aminoglycoside entry (Gale et al., 2001). Second, we tested whether phenoxybenzamine could protect hair cells during neomycin ototoxicity.

MATERIALS AND METHODS

Materials

Phenoxybenzamine hydrochloride was obtained from Santa Cruz Biotechnology, Dallas, TX, USA and neomycin and ciprofloxacin from Sigma-Aldrich, UK. Leibovitz's L15 (L15), DMEM/F12, FM1-43FX and fetal bovine serum (FBS) were acquired from ThermoFisher scientific, UK and the cell and tissue adhesive Cell-Tak was supplied by BD Biosciences, UK. All other chemicals were obtained from Sigma-Aldrich, UK.

Postnatal Cochlea Isolation and Culture

In accordance with the United Kingdom Animals (Scientific Procedures) Act of 1986 (Schedule 1 procedures), cochleae were extracted from C57BL/6 wild-type mice at postnatal day 3–6 (P3-P6). The isolated cochleae were micro-dissected in Leibovitz L15 medium. The apical cochlear turn was discarded and the remaining 1.5 turns separated into "middle" and "basal" coils. The stria-vascularis was kept in place and Reissner's membrane was cut allowing the cochlear coils to be "fileted" open and then placed onto Cell-Tak® coated Matek (Ashland, MA, USA) dishes (Majumder et al., 2015). Explant cultures were incubated in DMEM/F12 supplemented with 1% FBS and ciprofloxacin (10 μg/ml) at 37°C in a 5% CO_2/95% air atmosphere overnight prior to experimentation.

Live FM1-43 Imaging and Analysis

All experiments were conducted at room temperature (20–22°C). FM1-43 (6 μM) was prepared from a 10 mM stock solution.

The control culture was loaded with 6 μM FM1-43 for 30 s and then immediately washed (five 10 s washes, followed by three slower, 2 min washes) in L15 or HBHBSS prior to imaging with a Zeiss 510NLO upright confocal microscope (excitation 488 nm, emission 500–550 nm) using a 40× (NA 0.8) water immersion objective. Confocal image stacks (~20 planes, 2 μm intervals) were acquired exactly 20 min after exposure to FM1-43. The confocal laser power and gain settings were identical for all live imaging experiments to enable data comparison. To evaluate whether phenoxybenzamine was more effective when pre-incubated, in a subset of experiments it was applied for 30 or 60 min prior to FM1-43 loading and the loading was performed in the continued presence of phenoxybenzamine (including the washout solution). To test for reversibility of the block, after 30 min of phenoxybenzamine incubation explants were washed for varying amounts of time before testing with FM1-43. Images were analyzed using ImageJ (NIH, USA). A running two frame average was applied to the *Z* planes and to maintain consistency ROIs were drawn two planes (i.e., ~4 μm) below the FM1-43 fluorescence signal from the hair-cell stereocilia. ROIs covered the extent of the cell body in that plane. Average intensities from the ROIs were recorded and the background fluorescence (measured in a non-cellular region) was subtracted. Measurements were taken from 30 OHCs and 10 IHCs per explant.

Ototoxic Hair Cell Death and Protection Assay

To determine a dose-response curve, middle and basal coil cochlear explants were exposed to 0, 10, 100, 200, 250, 400 or 1000 μM neomycin for 24 h. To determine whether phenoxybenzamine confers protection against neomycin ototoxicity, cochlear explants were pre-treated for 1 h in 0, 50, 100 or 200 μM phenoxybenzamine followed by 24 h co-treatment in phenoxybenzamine and 250 μM neomycin in DMEM/F12 media at 37°C in a 5% CO_2/95% air atmosphere. After all experiments, explants were fixed with 4% paraformaldehyde in 0.1 M phosphate buffered saline (PBS, pH 7.2) at room temperature for 30–45 min for immunostaining and later evaluation for pyknotic and surviving hair cells.

Immunohistochemistry, Image Acquisition and Analysis

After fixation the explants were rinsed three times with PBS and incubated in blocking solution (PBS, 10% secondary host antibody serum and 0.5% Triton X-100) for 2 h. Subsequently, the explants were incubated with a mouse monoclonal anti-myosin 7A antibody, deposited to the DSHB by Orten, D.J. (DSHB Hybridoma Product MYO7A 138-1, used at 1:250) or a rabbit polyclonal anti-myosin 7A (25–6790, Proteus BioScience, used at 1:1000) primary antibody in blocking solution overnight at 4°C. Samples were then washed in PBS and incubated for 2 h at room temperature with 4′,6′-diamidino-2-phenylindole (DAPI 1 μM), AlexaFluor647 phalloidin (33 nM) and goat anti-rabbit-Atto488 or goat anti-mouse-Atto488 secondary antibodies in blocking solution. The explants were rinsed three times with PBS and imaged using the multiphoton Zeiss 510 NLO upright confocal microscope. DAPI was imaged using the a two-photon Chameleon-XR Ti:Sapphire laser tuned to 720 nm (435–485 nm bandpass filter), Atto488 was imaged using the 488 nm (500–550 nm bandpass filter) and AlexaFluor647 phalloidin using the 633 nm (long pass filter 650 nm) laser lines. Images were acquired at 1.5 μm *Z* intervals using either Achroplan 40× (NA 0.8) or Achroplan 63× Vis-IR (NA 1.0) water immersion objectives.

Z stacks (25–30 planes, 1.5 μm intervals) were acquired from two different regions in each explant. Image stacks were visualized using ZEN Lite software (Carl Zeiss Ltd, Germany) to identify pyknotic and surviving hair cells. The hair cells were considered pyknotic when they presented with condensed and marginated chromatin in the nuclei (Li et al., 1995; Lahne and Gale, 2008). Here we have used the characteristic pattern of pyknosis that we observe with the DAPI and myosin 7A staining during the death of IHCs and OHCs (**Figure 1**).

Hair cells with normal nuclei were considered to be viable surviving hair cells. Counts from the two regions sampled were averaged so that each explant counted as one N sample. Images were independently evaluated by two individuals.

Statistics

For live imaging experiments, all the data are presented as the mean ± SEM and ANOVA was applied with *post hoc* Tukey-Kramer's with significance set at $p < 0.05$. For hair-cell survival and pyknosis, all the data are presented as the mean ± SEM and the statistical test used was Students's t-test with significance set as $p < 0.05$.

RESULTS

Phenoxybenzamine Blocks Rapid FM 1-43 Entry in Mammalian Hair Cells if Preincubated

To evaluate the nature of phenoxybenzamine's interaction with mammalian MET channels, we measured FM1-43 uptake by hair cells in cochlear explant cultures from postnatal day 3–6 mice. A brief (30 s) exposure to FM1-43 ensured that rapid entry through the MET channels was the primary uptake pathway as opposed to a slower endocytic mechanism. FM1-43 uptake was hair cell specific and irreversible with OHCs taking up approximately twice as much FM1-43 as IHCs as described previously (Gale et al., 2001). When 100 μM phenoxybenzamine was simply co-applied during FM-143 exposure there was no significant effect on FM1-43 uptake in either IHCs or OHCs. In contrast, when phenoxybenzamine was also pre-incubated for either 30 or 60 min, we found a significant reduction in FM1-43 uptake in OHCs, and a small reduction in uptake in IHCs that failed to reach significance (**Figures 2A,B**). Pre-incubation substantially reduced FM1-43 uptake to 28% of control levels in OHCs and 60% in IHCs respectively, significantly different to uptake both in the controls and in samples in which compounds were co-applied together (**Figure 2C**). The block of FM1-43 uptake was reversible upon washout although the recovery from block was not immediate. Comparing a 1 min washout with a 60 min

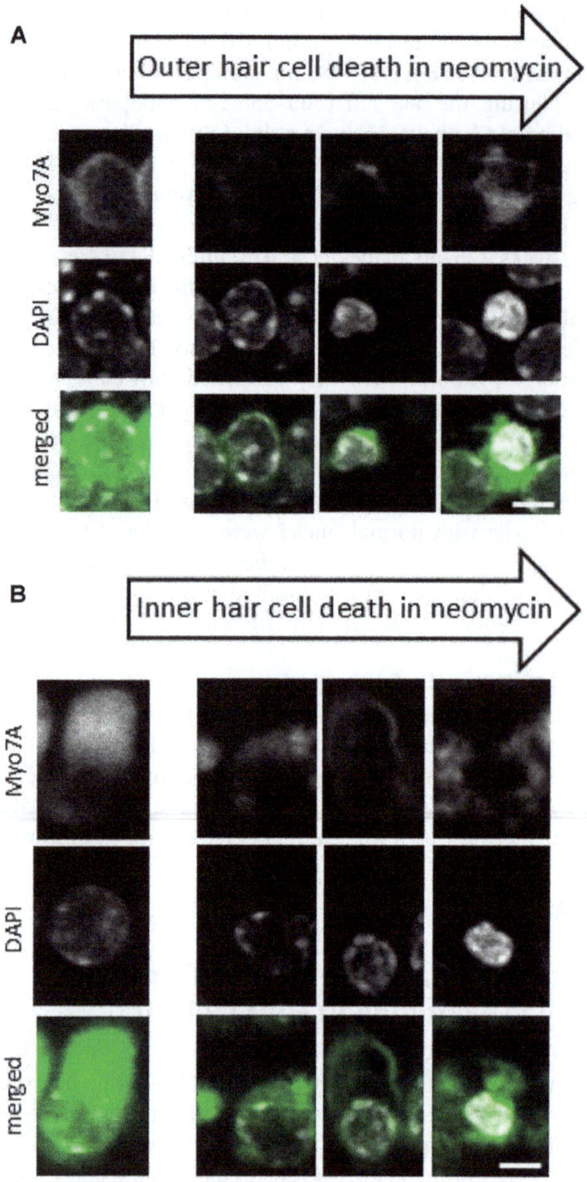

FIGURE 1 | Progression of neomycin-induced hair cell death. A sequence of images representing different stages of cell death that are observed after 24 h of neomycin exposure for both outer hair cells (OHCs) **(A)** and inner hair cells (IHCs) **(B)**. Anti-myosin 7A labeling (upper panel), 4′,6′-diamidino-2-phenylindole (DAPI) staining of nuclear chromatin (middle panel), Myo7A/DAPI merged image (lower panel). Since individual cells undergo cell death at different times each cell is at a different stage in the cell death process and the images have been compiled into a pseudo-time series as indicated by the arrows. Scale bar 5 μm.

washout we can see that the recovery was ~15% in OHCs after 1 min but was complete after 60 min (**Figure 3**). Recovery appeared to be faster but more variable in IHCs and on average we observed an overshoot in the recovery, but we note that the blocking effect of phenoxybenzamine was less robust in IHCs than in OHCs.

In order to determine whether the blockade of FM1-43 entry was dose-dependent, we varied the concentrations of phenoxybenzamine from 0 μM to 200 μM, pre-incubating for 30 min prior to FM1-43 application. The IC50 for the block of FM1-43 uptake by phenoxybenzamine differed slightly between OHC (logIC50 −4.185, 65 μM) and IHC (logIC50 −4.424, 38 μM) however, the Hill coefficient was strikingly different being 4 for OHC and 0.9 for IHC (**Figure 4**). One simple interpretation of these data is that there is a difference in the molecular nature of the MET channel in the two cochlear hair cell types. An alternative explanation is that the MET channel activity is reduced indirectly via a process that is affected by phenoxybenzamine and that is more prevalent in OHCs. We note that higher concentrations of phenoxybenzamine could not be tested due to problems with solubility that have been reported by others (Nisa et al., 2010).

Phenoxybenzamine Can Protect Hair Cells from Neomycin-Induced Ototoxicity

For the next experiments we set out to determine a concentration of neomycin that gave us ≥50% toxicity in our mouse cochlear explant culture model after 24 h of exposure. Cochlear explants were treated with neomycin at a range of concentrations from 0 μM to 1000 μM. At the end of the 24-h exposure explants were fixed and triple-labeled with DAPI, fluorescent phalloidin and antibodies to myosin 7A. *Z*-stack images were then collected using a confocal microscope (**Figure 5A**). Since hair cells are known to be able to survive without a hair bundle (Gale et al., 2002), we focused our analysis on the hair-cell soma and nuclear chromatin markers, as shown in **Figure 1**, to quantify the number of surviving hair cells, using the image stacks. A steep dose-dependence was observed for neomycin-induced hair cell death for both OHC and IHC (**Figure 5B**), with 50% cell death constants of 228 μM (log −3.642) and 232 μM (log −3.635) and different Hill coefficients of 4.7 and 1.9, respectively. Based on these experiments we decided to use 250 μM neomycin in subsequent experiments to test whether phenoxybenzamine could provide any protection in this 24 h ototoxicity model.

Given the requirement for drug pre-incubation, in test explants phenoxybenzamine (50, 100 or 200 μM) was applied for 1 h prior to the addition of neomycin in the presence of phenoxybenzamine. After 24 h explants were fixed, the same triple-labeling protocol was applied to all explants and image stacks collected and analyzed to quantify the number of surviving and pyknotic hair cells. At a concentration of 50 μM phenoxybenzamine did not offer significant protection against neomycin-induced ototoxicity (data not shown). In the presence of 100 μM phenoxybenzamine, however, the number of surviving OHC and IHC per 100 μm length of the cochlea was significantly higher, 27.9 ± 3.5 and 9.0 ± 1.0 respectively, compared to 17.6 ± 3.1 and 5.0 ± 1.4 with neomycin alone ($p < 0.05$). Using either the untreated control or phenoxybenzamine-treated alone explants to calculate the percent survival reveals that phenoxybenzamine increased OHC survival from 47% to 86% and IHC survival from 46% to 98% (**Figure 6**). Although phenoxybenzamine significantly reduced

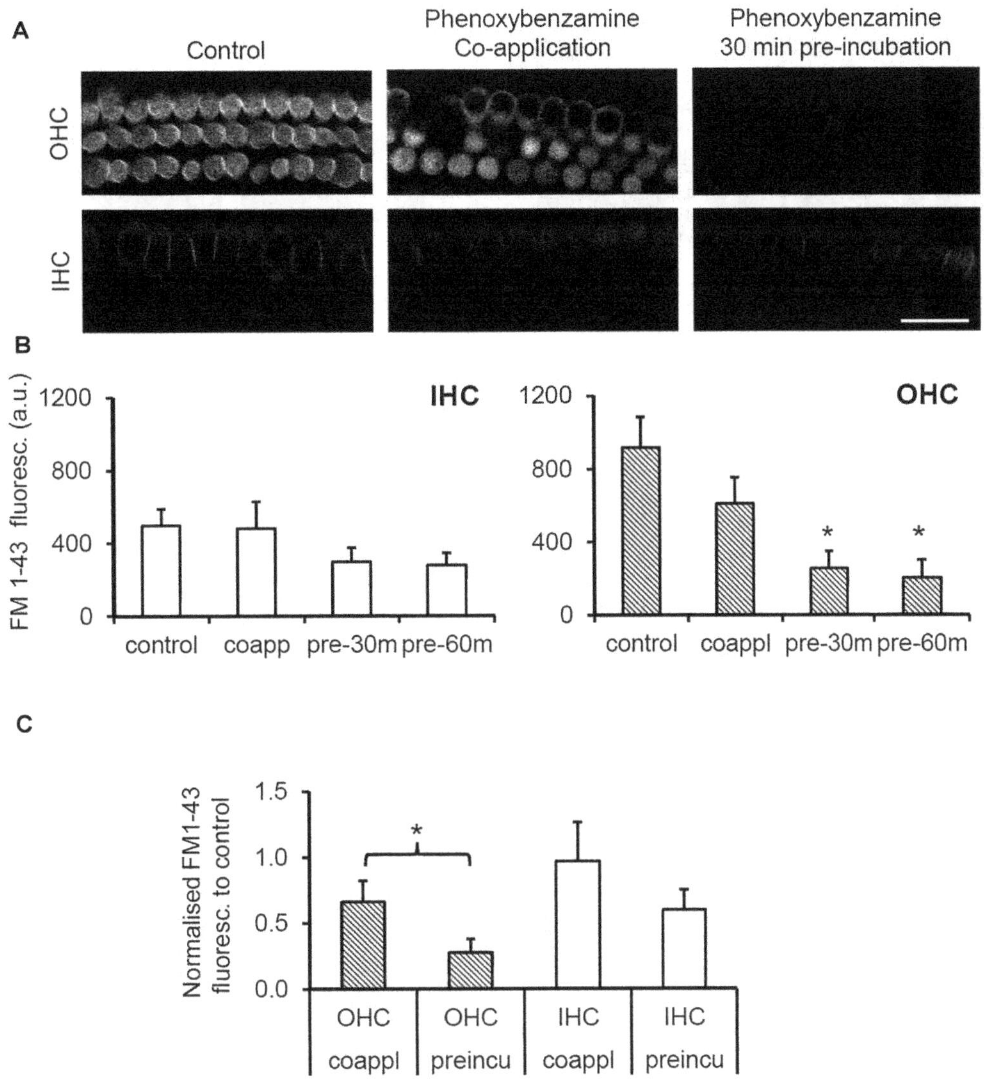

FIGURE 2 | Phenoxybenzamine (PB) significantly reduces rapid FM1-43 uptake in OHCs but not in inner cells. (A) Confocal images of FM1-43 uptake after brief exposure (30 s) in OHCs (upper panels) and IHCs (lower panel) under control conditions (left panel), either when co-applied with 100 μM PB (middle panel) or when explants were pre-incubated in PB for 30 min prior to FM1-43 application (right panel). **(B)** Quantification of FM1-43 fluorescence reveals that pre-incubation with phenoxybenzamine for 30 min or 60 min significantly reduces uptake in OHCs but not IHCs. Maximal inhibition of FM1-43 uptake is achieved in 30 min. **(C)** Pre-incubating with phenoxybenzamine is significantly more effective at blocking the rapid uptake of FM1-43. Expressed as a % of control, the uptake was reduced from 66% to 28% in OHCs and from 97% to 60% in IHCs. N numbers: control = 12; 100 μM PB-co-app = 6; 30 min pre-incubation = 9; 60 min pre-incubation = 6. Statistical test: ANOVA Tukey-Kramer's test, $^{*}p < 0.05$ in **(B)**; Student's t-test, $^{*}p < 0.05$ in **(C)**.

the number of neomycin-induced pyknotic OHC nuclei, we also observed a small but significant increase in pyknotic OHC and IHC nuclei when phenoxybenzamine was applied alone indicating the potential toxicity of the drug in the cochlea. The phenoxybenzamine-induced toxicity was more evident, particularly in OHCs at the highest concentration used (200 μM). In addition we observed that at 200 μM, rather than protecting hair cells against neomycin, phenoxybenzamine significantly enhanced the neomycin-induced toxicity in OHCs, whereas enhancement of toxicity was not observed in IHC (**Supplementary Figure S1**).

DISCUSSION

Phenoxybenzamine was one of a small number of compounds identified from two high-throughput drug screens for neomycin ototoxicity using zebrafish larvae (Ou et al., 2009; Vlasits et al., 2012). In zebrafish lateral line hair cells, the blockade of neomycin uptake into hair cells is thought to be the primary mode of action for the otoprotective effect of phenoxybenzamine (Ou et al., 2009). Here we used mammalian cochlear explant cultures from postnatal mice to evaluate the possible otoprotective effect of phenoxybenzamine. Testing

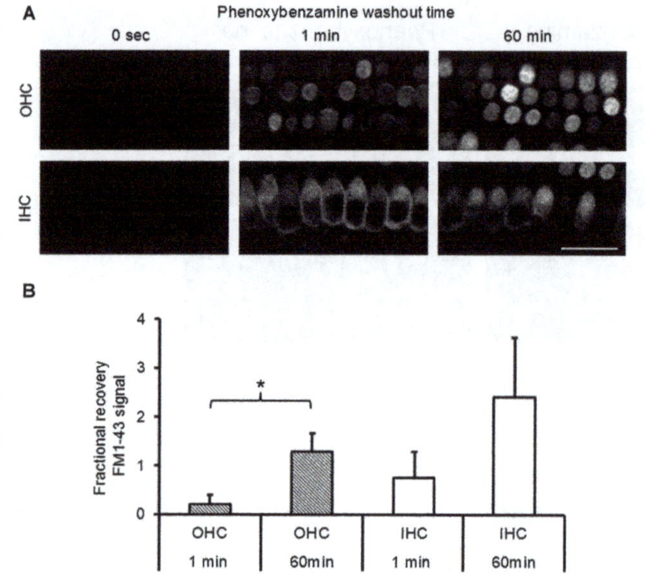

FIGURE 3 | Phenoxybenzamine block of FM1-43 entry is reversible. **(A)** After a 30 min pre-incubation in 100 μM phenoxybenzamine explants were washed for 1 min or 60 min in HBSS before being exposed to 6 μM FM1-43 for 30 s. Confocal images of the FM1-43 fluorescence signal in OHCs (upper panels) and IHCs (lower panel) when applied at 0 s, 1 min or 60 min after phenoxybenzamine washout. **(B)** The block by phenoxybenzamine is completely reversed 60 min after wash out. The fractional recovery of the FM1-43 signals was calculated from $F_{recov} = (F - F_{min})/(F_{max} - F_{min})$, where F_{min} is the signal from 30 min pre-incubation (n = 9) and F_{max} = control (no phenoxybenzamine) signal (n = 12) and F = 1 min (4) or 60 min (6). A F_{recov} value of 1 is equal to control (F_{max}). Student's t-test; *$p < 0.05$.

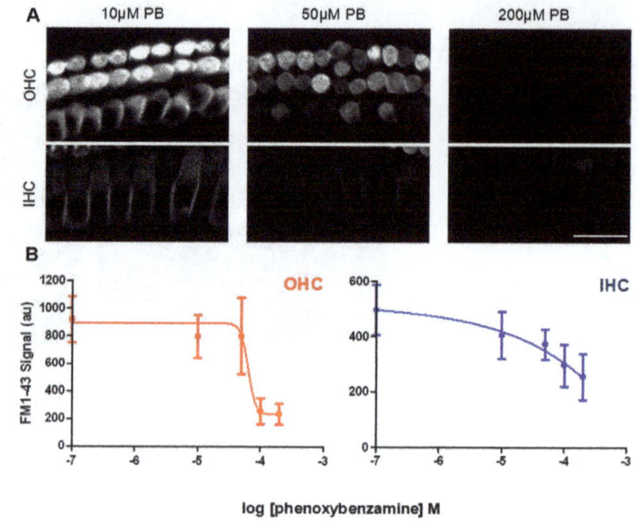

FIGURE 4 | Phenoxybenzamine block of FM1-43 entry is dose-dependent. **(A)** Confocal images of rapid FM-143 uptake assessed after 30 min of pre-incubation in 10, 50 or 200 μM phenoxybenzamine. Images at the focal planes of the OHC and IHC are shown. **(B)** Quantification of the rapid FM1-43 uptake in the presence of different concentrations of phenoxybenzamine reveal the reduction in FM1-43 uptake as a function of increasing phenoxybenzamine concentration in both OHC (red) and IHC (blue). The IC50 and Hill coefficient values from the curve fits are provided in the main text. N numbers: control (12); 10 μM PB (3); 50 μM PB (4); 100 μM (9); 200 μM (4). Scale bar: 20 μm.

compounds in the mammalian system is critical given the clear differences between the mammalian cochlea and the lateral line, not least because there are two distinctly different types of hair cell in the cochlea. We first characterized the effect of phenoxybenzamine on rapid FM1-43 uptake, which we use as mimic of neomycin entry since it permeates the mechanoelectrical transducer channels and has been shown to reduce the toxic effects of neomycin (Gale et al., 2001).

In zebrafish hair cells phenoxybenzamine blocks the uptake of both FM1-43 and gentamicin-Texas Red (Ou et al., 2009; Vlasits et al., 2012). We now show that phenoxybenzamine can block FM1-43 entry in both IHCs and OHCs in the mammalian cochlea. The IC50 for the blocking effect was quite similar between the two hair cell types (40–60 μM), however there was a ~4 fold difference in the Hill coefficient with the block in OHCs showing a steep dependence indicating cooperative binding, whereas in IHCs the coefficient was close to 1 suggesting non-cooperative binding of phenoxybenzamine. To better understand the mode of action, we compared pre-incubation of phenoxybenzamine with simple co-application and found that maximal inhibition was achieved by pre-incubation (**Figure 2**) as previously described in zebrafish (Vlasits et al., 2012). A 30 min pre-incubation was already maximal and no further block was observed when we extended the time of incubation to 60 min. Phenoxybenzamine is known to bind covalently to adrenergic receptors and serotonin receptors and in zebrafish the hair-cell survival effected by phenoxybenzamine persisted after phenoxybenzamine washout (Ou et al., 2009). In our live FM1-43 uptake assay, although the phenoxybenzamine effect remained for the first minute (at least in OHCs), the block was fully reversible after 60 min of washout. We observed differences in the effect of phenoxybenzamine on FM1-43 uptake in OHCs and IHCs. If the site of action of phenoxybenzamine in mammalian hair cells is within the mechanoelectrical transduction channel itself, this would suggest that there are significant differences in the structure of the channel between IHC and OHCs. Given the pre-incubation requirement, a simple explanation for this could that there is an intracellular binding site for phenoxybenzamine that is not present in IHCs. An alternative and perhaps more likely explanation is that there may be indirect effects of phenoxybenzamine on the mechanoelectrical transduction channels via regulatory molecules that are more prevalent in OHCs compared to IHCs.

We next examined whether the otoprotection seen in the lateral line with phenoxybenzamine is also observed in mammalian cochlear hair cells. The effects of AGs are both time and dose-dependent and we first set out to determine a neomycin-dose response curve for 24 h of exposure in our mouse cochlear explant model. We found a steep dose-dependence for neomycin-induced hair cell-death, particularly for OHCs (Hill coefficient of 4.7 compared to 1.9 in IHCs, **Figure 5**). The IC50 or

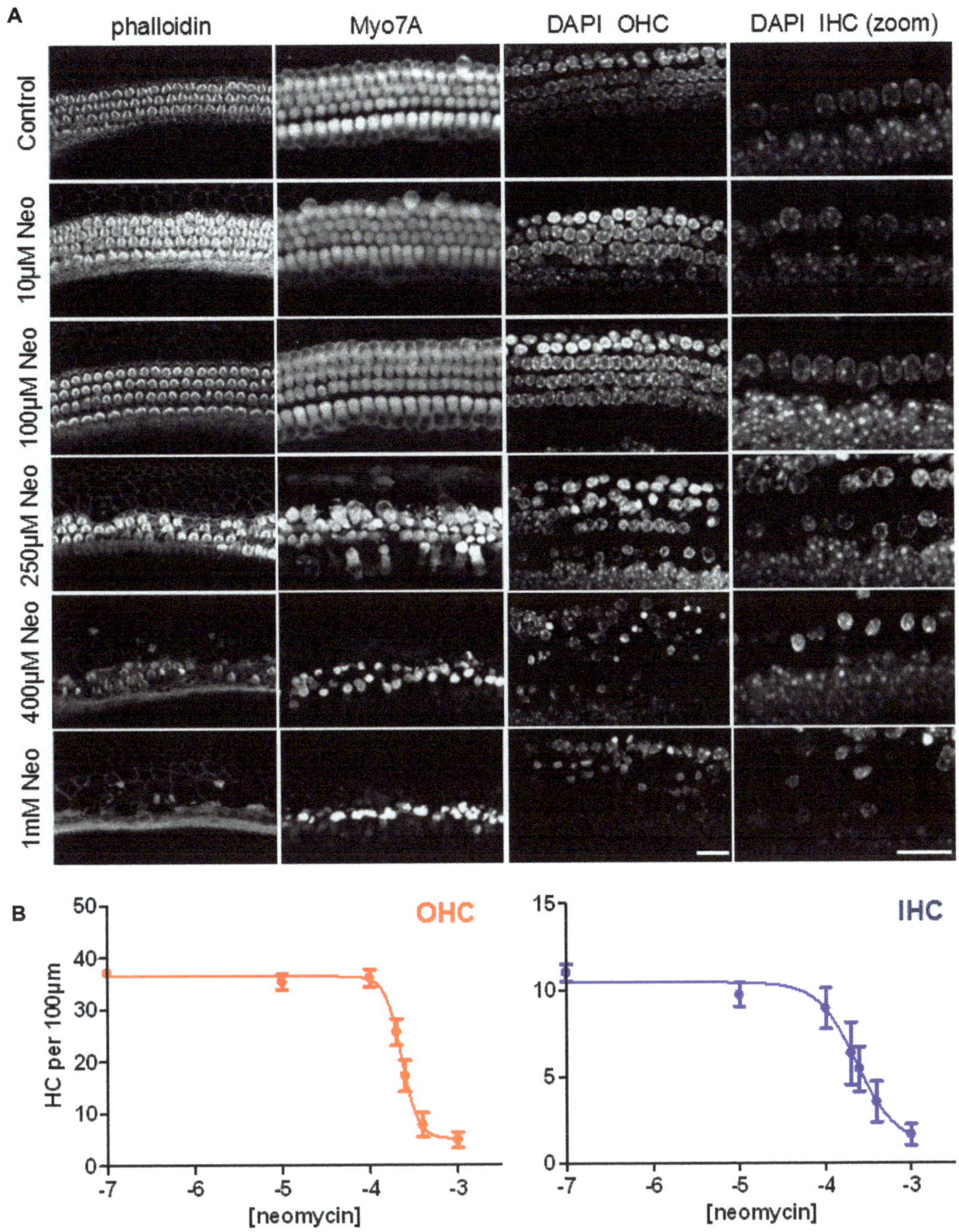

FIGURE 5 | Steep dose-dependent increase in hair-cell death after 24 h exposure to neomycin. (A) Confocal images of three different cellular markers: phalloidin, labeling F-actin; myosin7A (Myo7A), for the hair cell soma and DAPI which showing nuclear condensation and pyknosis in neomycin-treated examples. The right hand panels show a higher magnification (zoom) of the DAPI label in the IHC region. **(B)** Quantification of the numbers of surviving hair cells (expressed per 100 μm) reveals the steep dose-dependency of neomycin toxicity after 24 h of drug exposure. The 50% cell-death constants are similar between OHC (228 μM) and IHC (232 μM) but the Hill coefficients were quite different (4.7 and 1.9 respectively). N numbers: 0.1 μM (10); 10 μM (9); 100 μM (9); 200 μM (5); 250 μM (9); 400 μM (8); 1000 μM (10). Scale bar: 20 μm.

50% cell-death constant for neomycin was ~250 μM for both OHCs and IHCs and we used this concentration in subsequent assays in order to promote ~50% hair cell loss/survival, allowing either a protective effect or an enhancement of hair-cell death to be identified.

When used at a concentration of 100 μM phenoxybenzamine produced a significant protection of both OHC and IHCs, resulting in survival of both OHCs (86% survival) and IHCs (98% survival) relative to controls, i.e., phenoxybenzamine treatment alone. A small amount of toxicity was noted

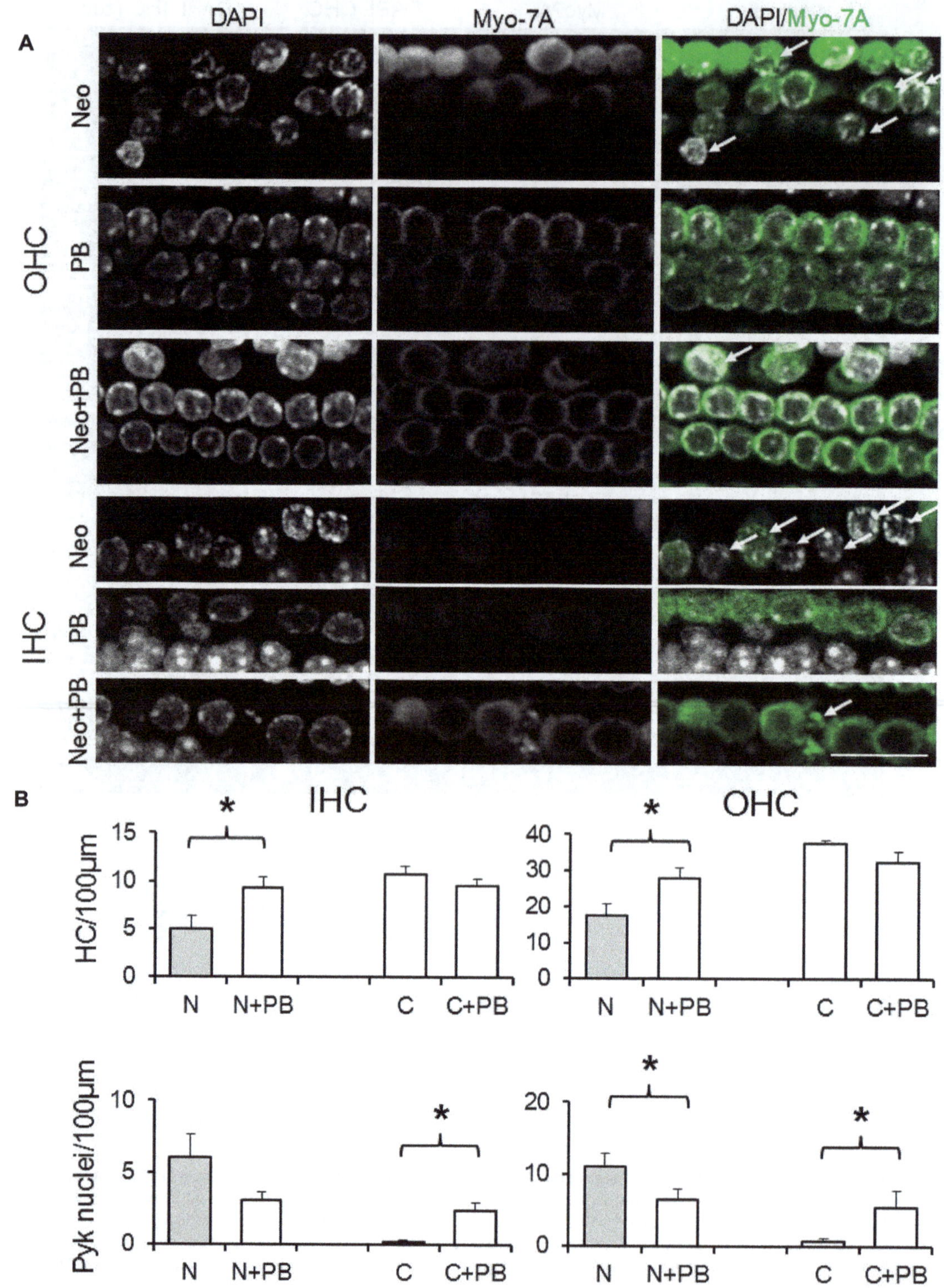

FIGURE 6 | Phenoxybenzamine confers protection against neomycin ototoxicity. (A) Representative confocal images showing the protective effect of the 100 μM phenoxybenzamine on the neomycin-induced hair cell death in both OHC and IHC. Images for phenoxybenzamine alone (PB), neomycin-alone for 250 μM for 24 h (Neo) or pre-incubation and continued presence of phenoxybenzamine during the neomycin exposure (Neo+PB). Images showing condensed chromation and pyknotic nuclei (DAPI staining, arrows) and the absence of the myosin7A labeling in missing/damaged hair cells. **(B)** Quantification of IHC and OHC survival (from myosin7A, upper graphs) and pyknotic hair cell nuclei (from DAPI images, lower graphs) in control C, 250 μM neomycin-treated (N), phenoxybenzamine alone (C+PB) or neomycin and phenoxybenzamine treated (N+PB) explants. N numbers: Neo (11); Neo+PB (8); PB alone (9); control (10). *$p < 0.05$ (compared to control). Scale bar, 20 μm.

in the phenoxybenzamine-alone controls, based on the assessment of nuclear chromatin and pyknosis (**Figures 1, 6**). At a higher concentration, 200 μM phenoxybenzamine in combination with neomycin produced different effects on the two types of hair cell. The IHCs were still protected but there was an enhancement of toxicity in OHCs indicating an additive effect of phenoxybenzamine and neomycin. When phenoxybenzamine was applied alone at 200 μM for 24 h it resulted in a small amount of OHC death but did not affect IHCs. The stronger block of FM1-43 uptake in OHCs compared to IHCs that we have shown could explain the differential toxicity if we assume that activity of the MET channels is essential for cell survival. Another possible explanation for the phenoxybenzamine-induced toxicity observed in OHCs is that it results from the differential expression of known phenoxybenzamine targets. We checked cochlear gene expression on gEAR portal[1] and found that both serotonin receptors and adrenergic receptors are differentially expressed by OHCs and IHCs (Liu et al., 2014) providing some support for this as an alternative hypothesis for the observed toxicity. Importantly, however, phenoxybenzamine protects both IHCs and OHCs from neomycin-induced toxicity and the simplest explanation is that this is due to a reduction in neomycin uptake via the MET channels, consistent with our FM1-43 uptake assay (a mimic for the neomycin uptake).

The lack of a significant effect of phenoxybenzamine on FM1-43 uptake in IHCs compared to OHCs, but the presence of a protective effect from neomycin suggests a greater complexity here. The primary pathway for the aminoglycoside entry into hair cells is now considered to be via the MET channels located at the top of the stereocilia, consistent with AGs acting as open-channel blockers (Kroese et al., 1989; Ricci, 2002; Marcotti et al., 2005) as described for FM1-43 (Gale et al., 2001). However, the contribution of other ion channels to the uptake of AGs into hair cells has been less well characterized. Channels such as the transient receptor potential (TRP) class members such as TRPC3, TRPV4, TRPA1 and PRPML3 which are expressed in the cochlea have not been ruled out as possible entry pathways (Castiglioni and García-Añoveros, 2007; Cuajungco et al., 2007; Asai et al., 2010; Stepanyan et al., 2011; Quick et al., 2012). AGs block a variety of ion channels such as large-conductance Ca^{2+}-activated K^+ channels (Nomura et al., 1990), N-type and P/Q type Ca^{2+} channels (Pichler et al., 1996), ryanodine receptors (Mead and Williams, 2002a,b), P2X receptors (Lin et al., 1993) and nicotinic acetylcholine receptors (Blanchet et al., 2000). Similar to its effects on the MET channels, FM1-43 is also known to block TRPC3/TRPC6 channels (Quick et al., 2012). Phenoxybenzamine could be affecting any of the above channels, however, investigating these different ion channels is outside of the remit of this current work. In these present experiments a somewhat unexpected result was the consistent difference we observed between IHC and OHCs. Differences in the nature of the MET channels between these two cell types have been described (Beurg et al., 2006, 2009) and although the our results were generated from a different type of assay, they support the possibility of there being alternative channel isoforms expressed in the two cell types.

In recent years high-throughput screening in non-mammalian models has proven to be very useful in identify new compounds for preventing hair-cell death. The data presented here indicate the importance of follow up studies in mammalian hair-cell models. Our study did identify consistency between results from zebrafish lateral line screens and the mammalian cochlea: from the mode of action of phenoxybenzamine on FM1-43 uptake to the requirement for pre-incubation to achieve maximal inhibition. The particular sensitivity of OHCs to phenoxybenzamine is, however, something that would tend to preclude its clinical use. Nonetheless, the differential effects of phenoxybenzamine on IHC and OHCs could turn out to be of significance in our understanding of the molecular mechanisms regulating MET channels.

[1]http://umgear.org/index.html

AUTHOR CONTRIBUTIONS

All authors contributed to the initial conception and design of the work. PM undertook the majority of data analysis and drafted the manuscript. JEG contributed to data analysis and to the writing and revision of the manuscript. PAM collected data and undertook data analysis as part of an undergraduate project in Sussex and a Masters project at UCL. GR contributed to initial experimental design and manuscript revision.

ACKNOWLEDGMENTS

PM was supported by an Action On Hearing Loss Pauline Ashley award (PA12 to PM), by a Conselho Nacional de Desenvolvimento Cientifico e Tecnológico (CNPq) fellowship (249335/2013-1 to PM) and by an Action On Hearing Loss International Grant (G52 to JG). PAM was a BSc Neuroscience student at the University of Sussex and an MSc Neuroscience student at UCL. The authors would like to thank Professor Jonathan Ashmore for helpful discussions.

SUPPLEMENTARY MATERIAL

FIGURE S1 | Higher concentrations of phenoxybenzamine confer some protection against neomycin ototoxicity for IHCs but are toxic to OHCs. (A) Quantification of hair cell survival in the presence of 200 μM phenoxybenzamine (PB) alone or in the presence of neomycin for both IHCs and OHCs. N numbers: Neo (11); control (4); Neo+PB 50 μM (4); 50 μM PB alone (4); Neo+PB 200 μM (5); 200 μM PB alone (4). $^*P < 0.05$ and $^{**}P < 0.005$. **(B)** Representative confocal images showing F-actin (phalloidin), myosin 7a (Myo7a), for the hair cell soma and DAPI showing nuclear condensation and pyknosis in neomycin-treated examples.

REFERENCES

Alharazneh, A., Luk, L., Huth, M., Monfared, A., Steyger, P. S., Cheng, A. G., et al. (2011). Functional hair cell mechanotransducer channels are required for aminoglycoside ototoxicity. *PLoS One* 6:e22347. doi: 10.1371/journal.pone.0022347

Aran, J. M., and Darrouzet, J. (1975). Observation of click-evoked compound VIII nerve responses before, during and over seven months after kanamycin treatment in the guinea pig. *Acta Otolaryngol.* 79, 24–32. doi: 10.3109/00016487509124650

Asai, Y., Holt, J. R., and Géléoc, G. S. (2010). A quantitative analysis of the spatiotemporal pattern of transient receptor potential gene expression in the developing mouse cochlea. *J. Assoc. Res. Otolaryngol.* 11, 27–37. doi: 10.1007/s10162-009-0193-8

Beurg, M., Evans, M. G., Hackney, C. M., and Fettiplace, R. (2006). A large-conductance calcium-selective mechanotransducer channel in mammalian cochlear hair cells. *J. Neurosci.* 26, 10992–11000. doi: 10.1523/JNEUROSCI.2188-06.2006

Beurg, M., Fettiplace, R., Nam, J.-H., and Ricci, A. J. (2009). Localization of inner hair cell mechanotransducer channels using high-speed calcium imaging. *Nat. Neurosci.* 12, 553–558. doi: 10.1038/nn.2295

Blanchet, C., Eróstegui, C., Sugasawa, M., and Dulon, D. (2000). Gentamicin blocks ACh-evoked K^+ current in guinea-pig outer hair cells by impairing Ca^{2+} entry at the cholinergic receptor. *J. Physiol.* 525, 641–654. doi: 10.1111/j.1469-7793.2000.t01-1-00641.x

Castiglioni, A. J., and García-Añoveros, J. (2007). MechanoTRPs and TRPA1. *Curr. Top. Membr.* 59, 171–189. doi: 10.1016/S1063-5823(06)59008-8

Cuajungco, M. P., Grimm, C., and Heller, S. (2007). TRP channels as candidates for hearing and balance abnormalities in vertebrates. *Biochim. Biophys. Acta* 1772, 1022–1027. doi: 10.1016/j.bbadis.2007.01.002

Dai, C. F., Mangiardi, D., Cotanche, D. A., and Steyger, P. S. (2006). Uptake of fluorescent gentamicin by vertebrate sensory cells *in vivo*. *Hear. Res.* 213, 64–78. doi: 10.1016/j.heares.2005.11.011

Diop, L., and Dausse, J. P. (1986). Specific binding of 3H-nicergoline in rat brain: comparison with the selective alpha 1-antagonist 3H-prazosin. *J. Pharmacol.* 17, 65–74.

Doggrell, S. A. (1995). Increase in affinity and loss of 5-hydroxytryptamine 2a-receptor reserve for 5- hydroxytryptamine on the aorta of spontaneously hypertensive rats. *J. Auton. Pharmacol.* 15, 371–377. doi: 10.1111/j.1474-8673.1995.tb00403.x

Duscha, S., Boukari, H., Shcherbakov, D., Salian, S., Silva, S., Kendall, A., et al. (2014). Identification and evaluation of improved 4'-*O*-(alkyl) 4,5-disubstituted 2-deoxystreptamines as next-generation aminoglycoside antibiotics. *MBio* 5:e01827. doi: 10.1128/mBio.01827-14

Forge, A., and Schacht, J. (2000). Aminoglycoside antibiotics. *Audiol. Neurootol.* 5, 3–22. doi: 10.1159/000013861

Frazer, A., and Hensley, J. (1999). "Serotonin receptors," in *Basic Neurochemistry: Molecular, Cellular and Medical Aspects*, 6th Edn. eds G. J. Siegel, B. W. Agranoff and R. W. Albers (Philadelphia: Lippincott-Raven), 263–292.

Gale, J. E., Marcotti, W., Kennedy, H. J., Kros, C. J., and Richardson, G. P. (2001). FM1-43 dye behaves as a permeant blocker of the hair-cell mechanotransducer channel. *J. Neurosci.* 21, 7013–7025.

Gale, J. E., Meyers, J. R., Periasamy, A., and Corwin, J. T. (2002). Survival of bundleless hair cells and subsequent bundle replacement in the bullfrog's saccule. *J Neurobiol.* 50, 81–92. doi: 10.1002/neu.10002

Greenwood, G. J. (1959). Neomycin ototoxicity; report of a case. *AMA Arch. Otolaryngol.* 69, 390–397. doi: 10.1001/archotol.1959.00730030400002

Hashino, E., and Shero, M. (1995). Endocytosis of aminoglycoside antibiotics in sensory hair cells. *Brain Res.* 704, 135–140. doi: 10.1016/0006-8993(95)01198-6

Hock, R., and Anderson, R. J. (1995). Prevention of drug-induced nephrotoxicity in the intensive care unit. *J. Crit. Care* 10, 33–43. doi: 10.1016/0883-9441(95)90029-2

Huth, M. E., Han, K.-H., Sotoudeh, K., Hsieh, Y.-J., Effertz, T., Vu, A. A., et al. (2015). Designer aminoglycosides prevent cochlear hair cell loss and hearing loss. *J. Clin. Invest.* 125, 583–592. doi: 10.1172/JCI77424

Inchiosa, M. A. Jr. (2013). Phenoxybenzamine in complex regional pain syndrome: potential role and novel mechanisms. *Anesthesiol. Res. Pract.* 2013:978615. doi: 10.1155/2013/978615

Kroese, A. B., Das, A., and Hudspeth, A. J. (1989). Blockage of the transduction channels of hair cells in the bullfrog's sacculus by aminoglycoside antibiotics. *Hear. Res.* 37, 203–217. doi: 10.1016/0378-5955(89)90023-3

Kumar, V. L., and Dewan, S. (2000). Alpha adrenergic blockers in the treatment of benign hyperplasia of the prostate. *Int. Urol. Nephrol.* 32, 67–71. doi: 10.1023/A:1007108201320

Lahne, M., and Gale, J. E. (2008). Damage-induced activation of ERK1/2 in cochlear supporting cells is a hair cell death-promoting signal that depends on extracellular ATP and calcium. *J. Neurosci.* 28, 4918–4928. doi: 10.1523/JNEUROSCI.4914-07.2008

Li, L., Nevill, G., and Forge, A. (1995). Two modes of hair cell loss from the vestibular sensory epithelia of the guinea pig inner ear. *J. Comp. Neurol.* 355, 405–417. doi: 10.1002/cne.903550307

Lin, X., Hume, R. I., and Nuttall, A. L. (1993). Voltage-dependent block by neomycin of the ATP-induced whole cell current of guinea-pig outer hair cells. *J. Neurophysiol.* 70, 1593–1605.

Liu, H., Pecka, J. L., Zhang, Q., Soukup, G. A., Beisel, K. W., and He, D. Z. Z. (2014). Characterization of transcriptomes of cochlear inner and outer hair cells. *J. Neurosci.* 34, 11085–11095. doi: 10.1523/JNEUROSCI.1690-14.2014

Majumder, P., Duchen, M. R., and Gale, J. E. (2015). Cellular glutathione content in the organ of Corti and its role during ototoxicity. *Front. Cell. Neurosci.* 9:143. doi: 10.3389/fncel.2015.00143

Marcotti, W., van Netten, S. M., and Kros, C. J. (2005). The aminoglycoside antibiotic dihydrostreptomycin rapidly enters mouse outer hair cells through the mechano -electrical transducer channels. *J. Physiol.* 567, 505–521. doi: 10.1113/jphysiol.2005.085951

Matt, T., Ng, C. L., Lang, K., Sha, S.-H., Akbergenov, R., Shcherbakov, D., et al. (2012). Dissociation of antibacterial activity and aminoglycoside ototoxicity in the 4-monosubstituted 2-deoxystreptamine apramycin. *Proc. Natl. Acad. Sci. U S A* 109, 10984–10989. doi: 10.1073/pnas.1204073109

Matz, G., Rybak, L., Roland, P. S., Hannley, M., Friedman, R., Manolidis, S., et al. (2004). Ototoxicity of ototopical antibiotic drops in humans. *Otolaryngol. Head Neck Surg.* 130, S79–S82. doi: 10.1016/j.otohns.2003.12.007

Mead, F., and Williams, A. J. (2002a). Block of the ryanodine receptor channel by neomycin is relieved at high holding potentials. *Biophys. J.* 82, 1953–1963. doi: 10.1016/s0006-3495(02)75544-6

Mead, F., and Williams, A. J. (2002b). Ryanodine-induced structural alterations in the RyR channel suggested by neomycin block. *Biophys. J.* 82, 1964–1974. doi: 10.1016/s0006-3495(02)75545-8

Nisa, N., Blokpoel, M. C., Robertson, B. D., Tyndall, J. D. A., Lun, S., Bishai, W. R., et al. (2010). Targeting the chromosome partitioning protein ParA in tuberculosis drug discovery. *J. Antimicrob. Chemother.* 65, 2347–2358. doi: 10.1093/jac/dkq311

Nomura, K., Maruse, K., Watanabe, K., and Sokabe, M. (1990). Aminoglycoside blockade of Ca^{2+}-activated K^+ channel from rat brain synaptosomal membranes incorporated into planar bilayers. *J. Membr. Biol.* 115, 241–251. doi: 10.1007/bf01868639

Ou, H. C., Cunningham, L. L., Francis, S. P., Brandon, C. S., Simon, J. A., Raible, D. W., et al. (2009). Identification of FDA-approved drugs and bioactives that protect hair cells in the zebrafish (*Danio rerio*) lateral line and mouse (*Mus musculus*) utricle. *J. Assoc. Res. Otolaryngol.* 10, 191–203. doi: 10.1007/s10162-009-0158-y

Pichler, M., Wang, Z., Grabner-Weiss, C., Reimer, D., Hering, S., Grabner, M., et al. (1996). Block of P/Q-type calcium channels by therapeutic concentrations of aminoglycoside antibiotics. *Biochemistry* 35, 14659–14664. doi: 10.1021/bi961657t

Quick, K., Zhao, J., Eijkelkamp, N., Linley, J. E., Rugiero, F., Cox, J. J., et al. (2012). TRPC3 and TRPC6 are essential for normal mechanotransduction in subsets of sensory neurons and cochlear hair cells. *Open Biol.* 2:120068. doi: 10.1098/rsob.120068

Ricci, A. (2002). Differences in mechano-transducer channel kinetics underlie tonotopic distribution of fast adaptation in auditory hair cells. *J. Neurophysiol.* 87, 1738–1748. doi: 10.1152/jn.00574.2001

Shi, X. (2016). Pathophysiology of the cochlear intrastrial fluid-blood barrier (review). *Hear. Res.* 338, 52–63. doi: 10.1016/j.heares.2016.01.010

Shulman, E., Belakhov, V., Wei, G., Kendall, A., Meyron-Holtz, E. G., Ben-Shachar, D., et al. (2014). Designer aminoglycosides that selectively inhibit cytoplasmic rather than mitochondrial ribosomes show decreased ototoxicity: a strategy for the treatment of genetic diseases. *J. Biol. Chem.* 289, 2318–2330. doi: 10.1074/jbc.M113.533588

Stebbins, W. C., Hawkins, J. E. Jr., Johnson, L. G., and Moody, D. B. (1979). Hearing thresholds with outer and inner hair cell loss. *Am. J. Otolaryngol.* 1, 15–27. doi: 10.1016/s0196-0709(79)80004-6

Stepanyan, R. S., Indzhykulian, A. A., Vélez-Ortega, A. C., Boger, E. T., Steyger, P. S., Friedman, T. B., et al. (2011). TRPA1-mediated accumulation of aminoglycosides in mouse cochlear outer hair cells. *J. Assoc. Res. Otolaryngol.* 12, 729–740. doi: 10.1007/s10162-011-0288-x

Te, A. E. (2002). A modern rationale for the use of phenoxybenzamine in urinary tract disorders and other conditions. *Clin. Ther.* 24, 851–861; discussion 837. doi: 10.1016/s0149-2918(02)80003-0

Thoenen, H., Hürlimann, A., and Haefely, W. (1964). Dual site of action of phenoxybenzamine in the cat's spleen: blockade of α-adrenergic receptors and inhibition of re-uptake of neurally released norepinephrine. *Experientia* 20, 272–273. doi: 10.1007/bf02151802

Toubeau, G., Laurent, G., Carlier, M. B., Abid, S., Maldague, P., Heuson-Stiennon, J. A., et al. (1986). Tissue repair in rat kidney cortex after short treatment with aminoglycosides at low doses. A comparative biochemical and morphometric study. *Lab. Invest.* 54, 385–393.

Vlasits, A. L., Simon, J. A., Raible, D. W., Rubel, E. W., and Owens, K. N. (2012). Screen of FDA-approved drug library reveals compounds that protect hair cells from aminoglycosides and cisplatin. *Hear. Res.* 294, 153–165. doi: 10.1016/j.heares.2012.08.002

Wang, Q., Kachelmeier, A., and Steyger, P. S. (2010). Competitive antagonism of fluorescent gentamicin uptake in the cochlea. *Hear. Res.* 268, 250–259. doi: 10.1016/j.heares.2010.06.008

Wang, Q., and Steyger, P. S. (2009). Trafficking of systemic fluorescent gentamicin into the cochlea and hair cells. *J. Assoc. Res. Otolaryngol.* 10, 205–219. doi: 10.1007/s10162-009-0160-4

9

Macrophage recruitment and epithelial repair following hair cell injury in the mouse utricle

Tejbeer Kaur[1], Keiko Hirose[1], Edwin W. Rubel[2] and Mark E. Warchol[1]*

[1] Department of Otolaryngology, Washington University School of Medicine, St. Louis, MO, USA, [2] The Virginia Merrill Bloedel Hearing Research Center and Department of Otolaryngology – Head and Neck Surgery, University of Washington School of Medicine, Seattle, WA, USA

Edited by:
Michael E. Smith,
Western Kentucky University, USA

Reviewed by:
Ruth Taylor,
University College London, UK
John Ramcharitar,
International American University,
Saint Lucia

***Correspondence:**
Mark E. Warchol,
Department of Otolaryngology,
Washington University School
of Medicine, 660 South Euclid
Avenue, Box 8115, St Louis,
MO 63110, USA
warcholm@ent.wustl.edu

The sensory organs of the inner ear possess resident populations of macrophages, but the function of those cells is poorly understood. In many tissues, macrophages participate in the removal of cellular debris after injury and can also promote tissue repair. The present study examined injury-evoked macrophage activity in the mouse utricle. Experiments used transgenic mice in which the gene for the human diphtheria toxin receptor (huDTR) was inserted under regulation of the Pou4f3 promoter. Hair cells in such mice can be selectively lesioned by systemic treatment with diphtheria toxin (DT). In order to visualize macrophages, Pou4f3–huDTR mice were crossed with a second transgenic line, in which one or both copies of the gene for the fractalkine receptor CX3CR1 were replaced with a gene for GFP. Such mice expressed GFP in all macrophages, and mice that were CX3CR1$^{GFP/GFP}$ lacked the necessary receptor for fractalkine signaling. Treatment with DT resulted in the death of ~70% of utricular hair cells within 7 days, which was accompanied by increased numbers of macrophages within the utricular sensory epithelium. Many of these macrophages appeared to be actively engulfing hair cell debris, indicating that macrophages participate in the process of ‘corpse removal’ in the mammalian vestibular organs. However, we observed no apparent differences in injury-evoked macrophage numbers in the utricles of CX3CR1$^{+/GFP}$ mice vs. CX3CR1$^{GFP/GFP}$ mice, suggesting that fractalkine signaling is not necessary for macrophage recruitment in these sensory organs. Finally, we found that repair of sensory epithelia at short times after DT-induced hair cell lesions was mediated by relatively thin cables of F-actin. After 56 days recovery, however, all cell-cell junctions were characterized by very thick actin cables.

Keywords: vestbular, auditory, hair cell, neuroimmunology, ototoxicity

Introduction

Hair cells are the sensory receptors of the inner ear. They detect sound vibrations and head movements, yielding information that is transmitted to the brain by auditory and vestibular afferent neurons. Within the various sensory epithelia of the ear, hair cells are completely surrounded by so-called supporting cells, which provide structural and trophic support to both hair cells and afferent neurons. Hair cells can be injured or lost as a result of noise exposure, ototoxicity, or as consequence of normal aging. The loss of hair cells can create cellular breaches within the sensory epithelia of the ear, leading to mixing of the inner ear fluids, and disruption of ionic homeostasis. As such, it is critical that such lesions are quickly repaired, and prior studies have shown that the loss of hair cells triggers adjoining supporting cells to undergo a coordinated and active cellular program, leading to removal of hair cell debris, and reformation of cell-cell junctions at the lumenal surface (e.g., Raphael and Altschuler, 1991; Meiteles and Raphael, 1994; Hordichok and Steyger, 2007; Bird et al., 2010; Anttonen et al., 2014).

Although most tissues and organ systems possess intrinsic cellular repair mechanisms, response to injury can also involve resident and recruited macrophages. These cells respond to injury by removing the debris of dead cells and can also secrete growth factors that evoke cell division and/or migration (Stefater et al., 2011). Prior studies have shown that the inner ear contains resident populations of macrophages and that hair cell injury leads to macrophage activation and recruitment (Warchol, 1997; Hirose et al., 2005; Warchol et al., 2012). However, the precise role of macrophages in the injured ear remains unknown. In the present study, we used novel transgenic mouse models to study the behavior of inner ear macrophages after selective ablation of vestibular hair cells. Our data indicate that the mouse utricle contains a resident population of macrophages, which are mainly confined to the stromal tissue below the sensory epithelium. Hair cell injury causes macrophages to enter the sensory epithelium, and some of those recruited cells appear to phagocytose hair cell debris. The signal(s) that promote macrophage recruitment are not known, but our data further suggest that signaling via fractalkine (CX3CL1/CX3CR1) is not required for macrophage entry into the injured vestibular epithelium. Notably, we also observed filamentous actin 'basket' structures within the injured epithelia, similar to those that have been shown to engulf hair cell debris in the avian utricle (Bird et al., 2010). Together, these results suggest that macrophages play an active role in the removal of dying hair cells, but that supporting cells may also contribute to this process.

Materials and Methods

Animals

All experimental protocols involving animals were approved by the Animal Studies Committee of the Washington University School of Medicine. Both of the transgenic mouse lines used in these studies have been described in previous publications. The Pou4f3–huDTR mouse line was generated by insertion of the gene for the human form of the diphtheria toxin receptor (huDTR, also known as HB-EGF) under regulation of the promoter for the Pou4f3 transcription factor. This factor, which is also known as Brn3.1 and Brn3c, is expressed only in developing and mature hair cells (Erkman et al., 1996; Xiang et al., 1997). As such, these mice express huDTR in hair cells and systemic administration of diphtheria toxin (DT) results in the selective death of hair cells in both the cochlea and vestibular organs (Tong et al., 2011, 2015; Golub et al., 2012; Mahrt et al., 2013; Cox et al., 2014).

C57BL6/J mice that were heterozygous for the Pou4f3–huDTR transgene were crossed with a second transgenic line in which one or both alleles of the gene for the fractalkine receptor (CX3CR1) was replaced with cDNA for GFP (provided by Dan Littmann, New York University, NY, USA). These mice express GFP in macrophages, monocytes, microglia, NK cells, and some T cells (Jung et al., 2000). In addition, $CX3CR1^{GFP/+}$ mice retain one copy of the gene for the fractalkine receptor and respond normally to the fractalkine ligand, while mice that are $CX3CR1^{GFP/GFP}$ lack this receptor and are not responsive to fractalkine. Experimental mice were either $CX3CR1^{+/GFP}:Pou4f3^{DTR/+}$ or $CX3CR1^{GFP/GFP}:Pou4f3^{DTR/+}$, while control mice lacked the Pou4f3–huDTR transgene but were heterozygous or homozygous for CX3CR1-GFP ($CX3CR1^{+/GFP}:Pou4f3^{+/+}$ or $CX_3CR1^{GFP}:Pou4f3^{+/+}$). Mice were housed in the animal facilities of the Division for Comparative Medicine at Washington University. They were kept on a 12 hr/day night light cycle and had free access to food and water.

Creation of Hair Cell Lesions

Adult mice (6–8 weeks) of either sex received a single intramuscular (i.m.) injection of (DT, 25ng/gm, Sigma-Aldrich). Mice then received daily intraperitoneal injections of lactated Ringer's solution (0.5 ml, for 3–6 days), and mouse food was supplemented with high-calorie gel (Tomlyn from Nutri-Cal). Mice were allowed to recover for 7, 14, or 56 days, at which time they were deeply anesthetized with Somnasol (0.1 ml/20 gm), and perfused transcardially with 4% paraformaldehyde in 0.1 M phosphate buffer (Electron Microscopy Sciences). Temporal bones were isolated and decalcified by treatment for 48–72 h in 0.1 M EDTA (at 4°C).

Histological Methods

Utricles were dissected from the decalcified temporal bones and rinsed in PBS. Non-specific antibody binding was reduced by treatment for 2 hr in PBS with 5% normal horse serum (NHS) and 0.2% Triton X-100. Specimens were incubated overnight at room temperature in primary antibodies. Hair cells were labeled with antibody against Myosin VI (goat polyclonal, Santa Cruz Biotechnology, 1:100) or otoferlin (mouse monoclonal, Abcam, 1:200). Intensity of macrophage-expressed GFP was amplified via labeling with an antibody against GFP (rabbit, Invitrogen, 1:500). After labeling with primary antibodies, specimens were thoroughly rinsed in PBS and incubated for 2 hr in secondaries (Alexa 546-anti-mouse or Alexa 546 anti-goat, and Alexa 488 anti-rabbit – Invitrogen). All specimens were also stained with Alexa-647 conjugated phalloidin (Invitrogen) and cell nuclei were labeled with DAPI. After labeling, specimens were mounted on microscope slides in glycerol/PBS (9:1), and coverslipped.

Cellular Imaging and Analysis

All specimens were imaged using a Zeiss LSM 700 confocal microscope. Volocity 3D image analysis software (Version 6.1.1, PerkinElmer) was used to reconstruct and process the images. Quantitative data were collected directly from these images and are presented as mean ± SD. Statistical tests were carried-out using Microsoft Excel software.

Results

Hair Cell Loss Following Diphtheria Toxin Treatment

All mice received a single 25 ng/gm injection of DT and were allowed to survive for 7, 14, or 56 days. Utricles of mice that possessed the Pou4f3–huDTR transgene displayed a significant hair cell lesion at 7 days after the DT injection (**Figure 1**). Hair cell loss was assessed by quantification of cells that displayed myosin VI or otoferlin immunoreactivity and also possessed phalloidin-labeled stereocilia bundles (**Figure 1**). Such cells were counted from six 50 μm × 50 μm regions, located in the central portion of the sensory epithelium, and the resulting values were normalized to hair cells/10,000 μm^2. Utricles from Pou4f3–huDTR mice contained 46.0 ± 12.8 HC/10,000 μm^2 (n = 7 utricles). In contrast, utricles from non-transgenic control mice (C57/Bl6 strain) appeared unaffected by DT treatment and contained 224.8 ± 16.0 hair cells/10,000 μm^2 (n = 6 utricles). Finally, utricles from Pou4f3–huDTR mice fixed at 14 days after DT injection contained 29.6 ± 10.4 hair cells/10,000 μm^2 (n = 7 utricles). These data indicate that a single injection of DT causes the death of ~85% of the hair cell population of the utricle within 14 days.

Remodeling of Epithelial Junctions Following Hair Cell Injury

The sensory epithelia of the inner ear form barriers between two fluid spaces of highly differing ionic composition (endolymph and perilymph). Repair of this epithelial barrier after injury or hair cell loss is critical to the maintenance of these fluids. Injury

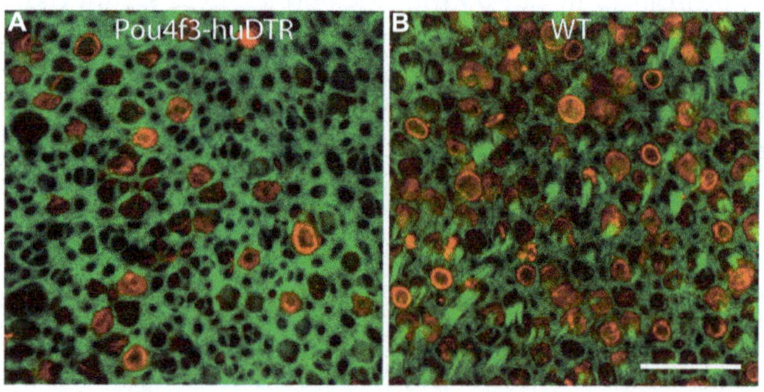

FIGURE 1 | Systemic treatment with diphtheria toxin (DT) lesions hair cells in the utricles of Pou4f3–huDTR (human form of the diphtheria toxin receptor) transgenic mice. Knock-in mice in which one copy of the gene for Pou4f3 was replaced with the gene for huDTR received a single 25 ng/gm injection of DT. After 7 days, mice were perfused and utricles were immunolabeled for myosin VI (red, hair cells) and also stained with phalloidin (green). A partial loss of hair cells was observed in the utricles of Pou4f3–huDTR mice **(A)**, when compared with littermates that did not possess the Pou4f3–huDTR transgene, but were also treated with DT **(B)**. Scale bar = 20 μm.

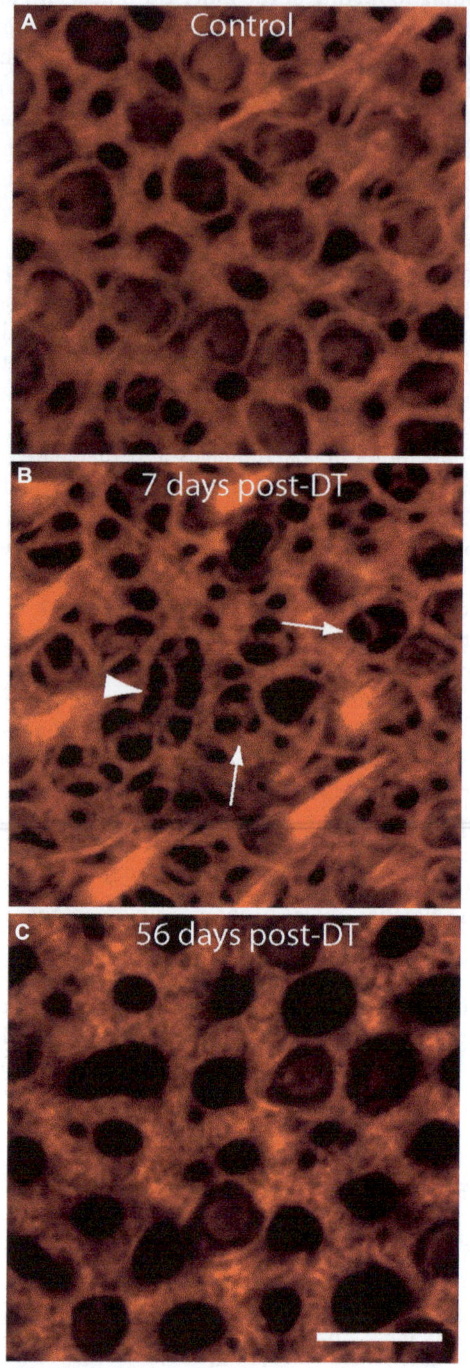

FIGURE 2 | Changes in the structure of actin bundles at cell–cell junctions following DT-mediated hair cell loss. All specimens were stained with phalloidin (red), which labels filamentous actin. **(A)** Junctions in undamaged utricles of control mice were comprised of thick actin bundles. Numerous stereocilia bundles were also apparent. **(B)** At 7 days after DT-induced hair cell injury, the epithelia contained many thin actin fibers, which are likely to be loci of epithelial repair after hair cell loss. Structures of thinner actin usually occupied a single cell-width (arrows), but some structures appeared to extend for several cell widths (arrow head). **(C)** Sensory epithelia of utricles examined at 56 days recovery from hair cell lesions contained very thick actin cables, suggesting nearly complete repair of the lumen. Scale bar = 10 μm.

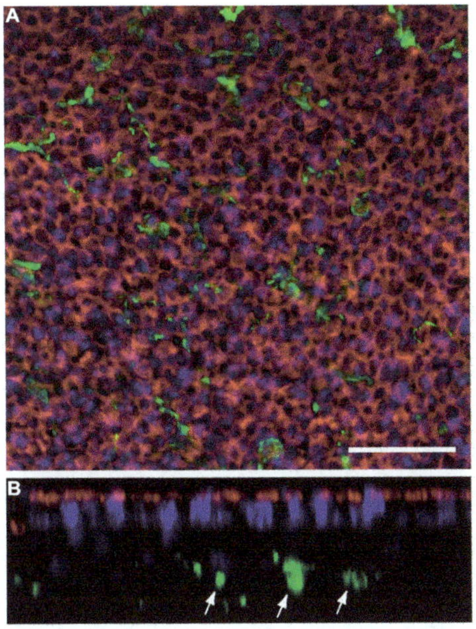

FIGURE 3 | Normal utricles contain resident populations of macrophages, which are primarily confined to the stromal tissue below the sensory epithelium. (A) Maximum intensity projection of a confocal stack collected from the central region of a histologically processed mouse utricle, to a depth of 20 µm. **(B)** Computationally reconstructed 'z-slice,' showing a slide view of the same image. Cell-cell junctions are labeled with phalloidin (red) and cell nuclei are stained with DAPI (blue). In addition, GFP-expressing macrophages (green) appear distributed throughout the specimen. However, examination of z-slice images reveals that nearly all macrophages reside in the stromal tissue, below the sensory epithelium (arrows). Scale bar = 30 µm.

to the vestibular epithelia of non-mammals leads to rapid reformation of cell-cell junctions by surviving supporting cells (e.g., Hordichok and Steyger, 2007; Bird et al., 2010). However, cellular junctions in the vestibular maculae of mammals are supported by thick bundles of filamentous actin (e.g., Burns et al., 2008), which may limit their ability to quickly reseal cellular lesions. In order to explore this issue, we examined the structure of actin cables at the lumenal surfaces of utricles after DT-induced hair cell loss. Specimens that were fixed at 7 days post-DT contained numerous thin actin bundles (**Figure 2**, arrows). Many of these were in the form of three radially directed thin actin bands (**Figure 2**, arrowhead). Such formations were previously described by Burns and Corwin (2014) and are likely to reflect epithelial repair after the loss of a single hair cell. However, we also noted more complex structures, which were comprised of thin actin bands that extended for several cell widths (arrow head, **Figure 2B**). These structures may have been created after the loss of 2–3 adjoining hair cells. Notably, at 56 days post-DT, the sensory epithelia appeared uniform and cell–cell junctions were characterized by very thick actin bundles (**Figure 2C**).

Hair Cell Loss Attracts Macrophages into the Sensory Epithelium

Prior studies have shown that the auditory organs of both birds and mammals contain resident populations of macrophages (e.g., Warchol, 1997; Hirose et al., 2005; Warchol et al., 2012), and macrophages are also present in the vestibular organs of mice (Zhang et al., 2013). Examination of undamaged utricles from CX3CR1$^{GFP/+}$ or CX3CR1$^{GFP/GFP}$ mice revealed numerous macrophages, which were mainly confined to the stromal tissue that underlies the sensory epithelium (**Figure 3**). In order to determine whether macrophages were recruited toward sites of hair cell injury, we quantified GFP-positive macrophages in the sensory epithelium of utricles from both normal and DT-lesioned animals. Confocal image stacks were obtained from whole-mount utricle specimens, and the numbers of macrophages within the sensory epithelium (i.e., within the same image planes as the DAPI-stained nuclei of hair

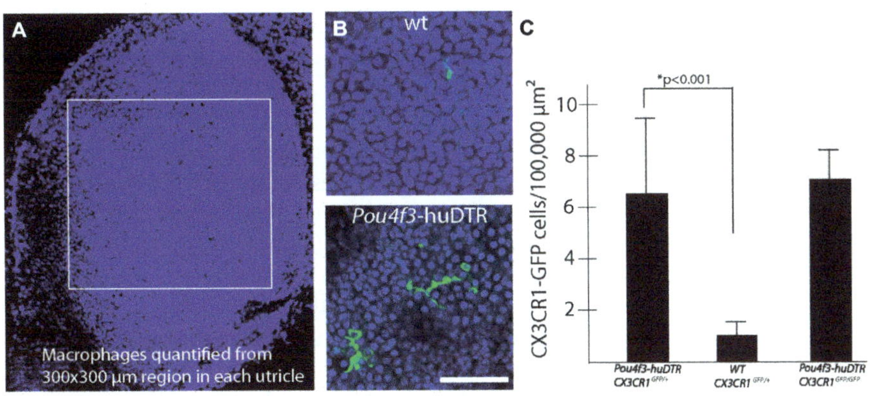

FIGURE 4 | Hair cell lesion increases the numbers of macrophages in the sensory epithelia of mouse utricles. (A) Confocal image stacks were obtained from 300 µm × 300 µm regions in the central portion of mouse utricles. **(B)** Examination of the DAPI-labeled nuclei of hair cells and supporting cells (blue) was used to determine the vertical extent of the sensory epithelium and the total number of GFP-labeled macrophages (green) within the sensory region was quantified. **(C)** Quantitative data revealed that injection of DT into Pou4f3–huDTR mice resulted in increased numbers of macrophages within the sensory epithelium, compared to normal C57/Bl6 mice that also received DT (*$p < 0.001$). However, the numbers of macrophages in the sensory epithelia of DT-treated Pou4f3–huDTR-CX3CR1$^{GFP/+}$ mice was nearly identical to that observed in the sensory epithelia of Pou4f3–huDTR-CX3CR1$^{GFP/GFP}$ mice.

cells and supporting cells) was quantified from a single field of 300 μm × 300 μm, located in the center of the utricle (**Figure 4A**). Resulting density data were then normalized to macrophages/100,000 μm^2. At 7 days after DT treatment, utricles from Pou4f3–huDTR-CX3CR1$^{GFP/+}$ mice contained 6.5 ± 3.2 GFP-labeled macrophages/100,000 μm^2 ($n = 8$), while utricles from DT-treated CX3CR1$^{GFP/+}$ mice that lacked the Pou4f3–huDTR transgene contained 1.0 ± 0.7 macrophages/100,000 μm^2 ($n = 8, p < 0.001$; **Figures 4B,C**). These findings indicate that the loss of hair cells leads to the recruitment of macrophages into the sensory epithelium. However, further quantification of epithelial macrophage numbers suggests that this increase is transitory. Specifically, at 14 days post-DT, utricles from Pou4f3–huDTR mice contained 1.9 ± 1.1 macrophages/100,000 μm^2 ($n = 7$ total: 2 CX3CR1$^{GFP/+}$ and 5 CX3CR1$^{GFP/GFP}$), while utricles from littermate mice that lacked the Pou4f3–huDTR transgene contained 1.4 ± 0.6 macrophages/100,000 μm^2 ($n = 4$ total: 1 CX3CR1$^{GFP/+}$ and 3 CX3CR1$^{GFP/GFP}$).

Genetic Deletion of CX3CR1 does Not Affect the Population of Utricular Macrophages

Macrophage recruitment to sites of tissue injury is mediated by a number of biological signals (Poon et al., 2014). One key modulator of macrophage recruitment and behavior is fractalkine (CX3CL1), a chemokine that is released by numerous cell phenotypes. Fractalkine interacts exclusively with the CX3CR1 receptor, which is expressed by macrophages, monocytes, and microglia (e.g., Ransohoff, 2009). Given the function of fractalkine signaling in other tissues, it was possible that disruption of fractalkine signaling (via deletion of the CX3CR1 receptor in CX3CR1$^{GFP/GFP}$ mice) might affect the recruitment of macrophages into the sensory epithelium after hair cell injury. To resolve this issue, we compared the numbers of macrophages in utricles from Pou4f3–huDTR-CX3CR1$^{GFP/+}$ (as reported above) with those observed at 7 days post-DT in utricles Pou4f3–huDTR-CX3CR1$^{GFP/GFP}$ mice ($n = 5$). Nearly identical macrophage numbers were observed in both genotypes (**Figure 4C**), suggesting that fractalkine signaling does not serve a critical role in the injury-evoked recruitment of macrophages into the utricular sensory epithelium.

Macrophages Within the Sensory Epithelium Phagocytose Hair Cell Debris

Removal of cellular debris after injury is essential for epithelial repair. In many epithelia, such debris clearance is mediated by a combination of nearby epithelial cells ('amateur phagocytes') and resident and/or recruited macrophages ('professional phagocytes'). Prior studies have shown that macrophages are mobilized after hair cell injury, but it was not clear whether those cells actually engulfed hair cell debris. In the present study, confocal imaging of utricles from Pou4f3–huDTR-CX3CR1$^{GFP/+}$ mice revealed numerous examples of GFP-labeled macrophages contacting labeled hair cells (**Figure 5**). Moreover, the incorporation of myosin VI and/or otoferlin-labeled material (i.e., hair cell constituents) into the GFP-labeled bodies of macrophages suggests that hair cell debris was being actively phagocytosed (**Figure 6**).

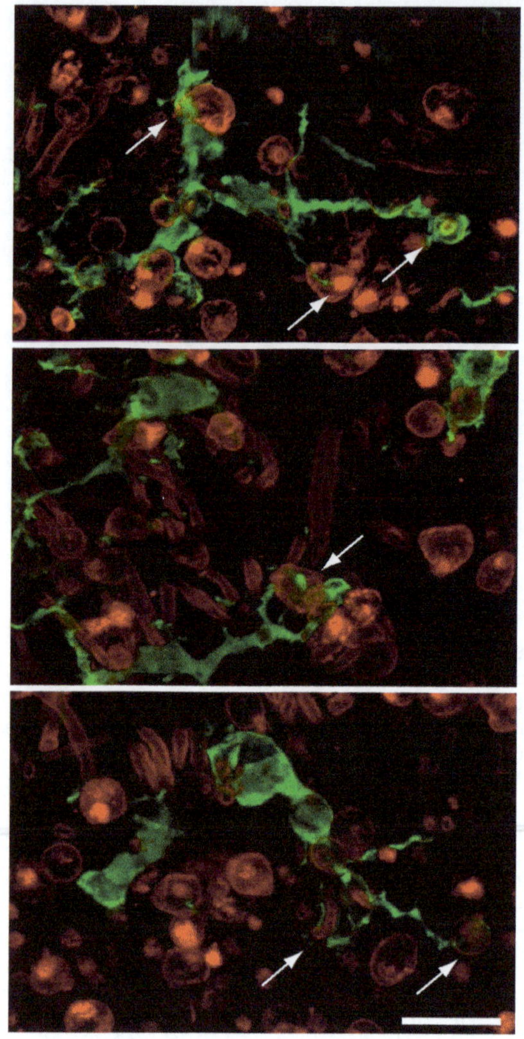

FIGURE 5 | Examples of GFP-expressing macrophages in the sensory epithelia of lesioned utricles. Processes of macrophages (green) frequently appeared to contact (arrows) immunolabeled hair cells (red, otoferlin), suggesting that apoptotic hair cells may attract macrophage pseudopodia. Scale bar = 20 μm.

This phenomenon was only observed in utricles from mice that possessed the huDTR transgene. In contrast, no phagocytic macrophages were observed in utricles taken from DT-treated wild-type (WT) mice.

Supporting Cells Form Actin Baskets Within the Sensory Epithelium

The sensory organs of the inner ear use a variety of strategies for the clearance of apoptotic hair cells. For example, dying hair cells in the chicken cochlea are extruded through the lumenal surface of the sensory epithelium (Cotanche and Dopyera, 1990; Duckert and Rubel, 1990; Janas et al., 1995; Hirose et al., 2004; Warchol et al., 2012), while outer hair cells in the mouse cochlea are engulfed by nearby Deiters cells (Anttonen et al., 2014), and apoptotic hair cells in the maculae

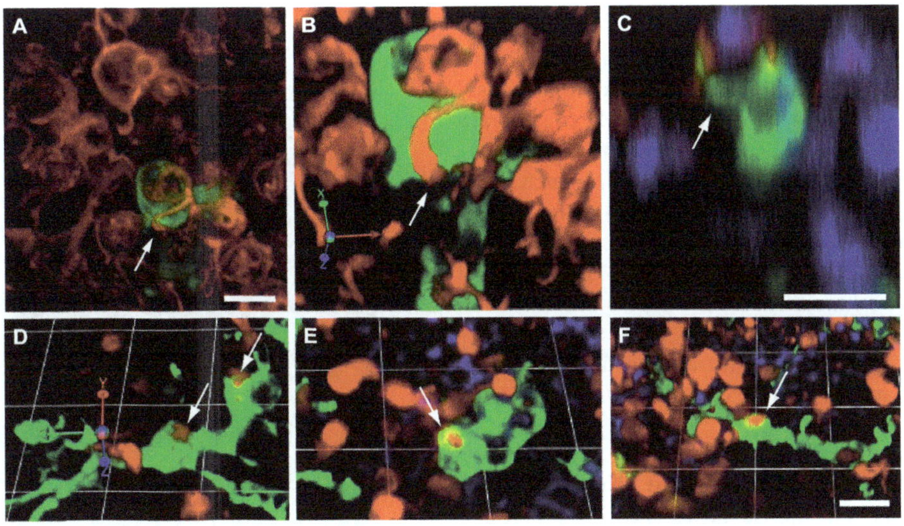

FIGURE 6 | Macrophage engulfment of hair cell debris. Confocal images of labeled hair cells and macrophages often revealed hair cells that were apparently enclosed within the processes of macrophages (arrows). **(A–C)** Three different renderings of the same confocal stack, showing an otoferlin-labeled hair cell (red) being engulfed by a calyx-like phagocytic process of a GFP-expressing macrophage (green). **(A)**: Maximum intensity projection. **(B)** 3-D rendering of same image stack, showing the macrophage surrounding the hair cell. **(C)** z-plane slice from the image stack, centered on the engulfed hair cell, which is enclosed by the macrophage process (green). Cell nuclei are also visible (DAPI, blue). **(D–F)** Three dimensional renderings of images showing the engulfment of hair cell debris (red) by GFP-expressing macrophages (green). In all cases, phagocytic events are indicated by arrows. All scale bars represent 10 μm.

of mammals are removed by a combination of these mechanisms (e.g., Li et al., 1995). Time-lapse imaging studies of the chick utricle have demonstrated that hair cell death triggers nearby supporting cells to form basket-shaped actin structures, which phagocytose the remnants of dying hair cells (Bird et al., 2010). Formation of similar structures has been observed in the vestibular organs of mice (e.g., Ball et al., 2013; Furrer et al., 2014; Monzack et al., 2015). In the present study, we frequently observed actin 'baskets,' which labeled strongly with phalloidin and were confined to the lower strata of the utricular sensory epithelia. These putative phagosomes were easily distinguished from phagocytic processes of macrophages, which expressed GFP but did not contain significant levels of F-actin (**Figure 7**).

Discussion

Hair cells can be lost from the inner ear after noise exposure, ototoxic injury, or as a consequence of normal aging. Because maintenance of the epithelial barrier is critical for separation of perilymph and endolymph, it is essential that the remaining cells quickly reseal the injured epithelium and remove cellular debris. These repair processes rely primarily on supporting cells, and appear to be mediated by different cellular mechanisms in the various hair cell epithelia of vertebrates. Specifically, supporting cells can undergo active and coordinated morphological changes, so as to extrude hair cell debris from the lumenal surface of the epithelium or to engulf such debris within the epithelium. Although macrophages are known to be present in the sensory organs of the inner ear, their role in epithelial repair and debris clearance is poorly understood. The present study characterized the behavior of macrophages in the mouse utricle in response to selective ablation of sensory hair cells. We found that the undamaged utricle possessed numerous resident macrophages, but that those cells resided in the stromal tissue below the sensory epithelium. However, hair cell death caused macrophages to enter the sensory epithelium, where they were observed to engulf hair cell debris.

Epithelial Repair and Actin Remodeling after Hair Cell Lesions

Supporting cells in the vestibular organs of mammals possess thick circumferential bundles of filamentous (F-) actin (e.g., Burns et al., 2008). In the utricles of mice, these structures develop during the first post-natal month and their formation correlates with diminished ability for cell spreading, proliferation, and plasticity (Collado et al., 2011). It is notable that these thick actin structures are unique to the vestibular organs of mammals; cell–cell junctions in the maculae of fish, amphibians, reptiles, and birds all possess much thinner actin belts (Burns et al., 2013). The vestibular organs of non-mammalian vertebrates are also capable of quickly regenerating lost hair cells, while the regenerative abilities of the mammalian vestibular organs are much more limited (e.g., Warchol, 2011). Based on these observations, it has been hypothesized that the thick actin bands of the mammalian ear may be an important inhibitor of its regenerative ability (e.g., Burns et al., 2008, 2013). In light of this suggestion, it is notable that we found that the initial phases of epithelial repair in the mouse utricle appear mediated by much thinner actin bands at cell–cell junctions. Similar structures were reported by Burns and Corwin (2014), who used time-lapse imaging of the mouse utricle to characterize the early cellular events that occur after hair cell loss. The Pou4f3–huDTR mouse strain permits characterization of this process *in vivo* and over longer time spans. Our data suggest that the thin actin bands are only present at early times after hair cell loss; cell–cell junctions at later recovery times display much thicker actin structures (e.g., **Figure 2C**). We speculate that the (transient) presence of thin actin cables in the injured epithelium may correspond to a period of partial plasticity of supporting cell phenotype, i.e., a time during which those supporting cells with thin actin cables may be able to change their identity into new hair cells. Partial regeneration via phenotypic change has been demonstrated in the vestibular organs of guinea pigs and mice (Forge et al., 1998; Lin et al., 2011).

Resident Macrophages in the Mouse Utricle

Our results confirm that the mouse utricle possesses a resident population of macrophages. In the uninjured utricle, resident macrophages appear to be confined to the stromal tissues below the sensory epithelium. Previous studies have suggested that many of these stromal macrophages are associated with small vessels or capillaries (Zhang et al., 2013). Although the functions of stromal macrophages are not known, the stromal is comprized of numerous cell phenotypes, many of which have been shown to interact with macrophages. For example, macrophages are known to release mitogens that stimulate proliferation of numerous cell types and they also participate in remodeling of the extracellular matrix (e.g., Chazaud, 2014). As such, it is likely that macrophages serve a number of distinct roles in the maintenance of inner ear stromal tissues. The notion is supported by the results of Warchol et al. (2012), who found that experimental depletion of macrophages from the avian cochlea resulted in reduced proliferation of the cells that reside immediately below the basilar membrane.

Macrophages Phagocytose Hair Cell Debris

Prior studies have shown that macrophages are present either within or near the auditory and vestibular organs of birds and mammals (Warchol, 1997; Bhave et al., 1998; Hirose et al., 2005), but the precise function of otic macrophages has been enigmatic. In many tissues, resident macrophages quickly remove the 'corpses' of apoptotic cells, in order to maintain tissue integrity, and prevent inflammation (Stefater et al., 2011). Although it is reasonable to assume that otic macrophages serve a similar role, previous studies have failed to provide direct evidence for macrophage-mediated phagocytosis of dying hair cells. Moreover, experimental depletion of macrophages from the avian basilar papilla (cochlea) did not affect the removal of hair cell debris from the sensory epithelium (Warchol et al., 2012). Previously, the only clear demonstration of phagocytosis of dead hair cells by recruited macrophages has come from time-lapse imaging studies of hair cell regeneration in lateral line neuromasts of axolotl salamanders (Jones and Corwin, 1996). The present study unequivocally shows that identified (i.e., CX3CR1-GFP) macrophages can engulf the remains of dead hair cells. It is notable, however, that we also observed the presence of F-actin phagosomes within the lesioned utricle. Similar basket-like structures have been shown to engulf hair cell debris following ototoxic injury in the avian utricle (Bird et al., 2010) and in the mouse utricle (Monzack et al., 2015). Although a complete study of theses structures is beyond the scope of the present study, our findings suggest that hair cell debris may be removed from the mammalian vestibular organs via (at least) two distinct cellular mechanisms.

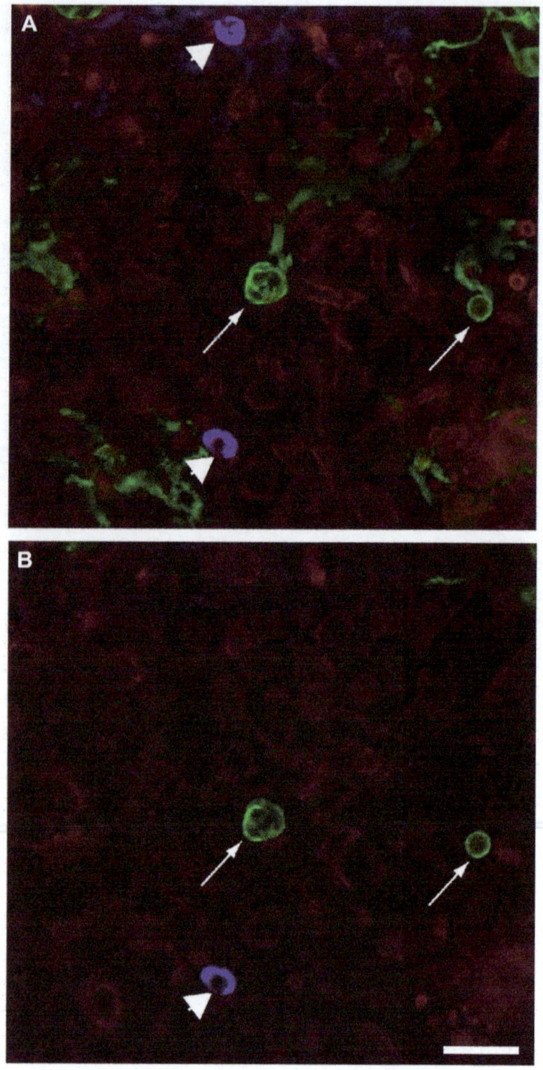

FIGURE 7 | Macrophages and actin basket phagosomes are simultaneously present in the injured mouse utricle. Calix-shaped phagocytic processes of GFP-expressing macrophages were observed in all lesioned sensory epithelia (arrows). Phalloidin staining (blue) also revealed F-actin phagosomes in these same epithelia (arrow heads). These basket-shaped structures could be distinguished from macrophages by their strong phalloidin labeling (blue). **(A)** Maximum intensity projection of full confocal stack. **(B)** Single z-section through this stack, showing a cross section through macrophage processes (green) and an F-actin phagosome (blue). Scale bar = 20 μm.

Role of Fractalkine in the Regulation of Vestibular Macrophages

Finally, our use of knock-in CX3CR1-GFP transgenic mice allowed us to evaluate the role of fractalkine signaling in regulating macrophage activity within the vestibular organs. Fractalkine (also known as CX3CL1) is a chemokine that plays a variety of roles in the regulation of immune cells and in the interaction between the innate immune system and the nervous system (e.g., Ransohoff, 2009). Fractalkine is expressed on cells as a membrane-bound protein. Under certain circumstances, fractalkine can be proteolytically cleaved near the extracellular membrane surface, releasing a diffusible fragment that can function as a macrophage chemoattractant (e.g., Ishida et al., 2008). Following DT-mediated hair cell lesions, we found that macrophage entry into the utricular sensory epithelium was nearly identical in mice with intact fractalkine signaling ($CX3CR1^{GFP/+}$) vs. those that lacked the fractalkine receptor ($CX3CR1^{GFP/GFP}$). Because of inter-specimen variability, it was not possible to quantify and compare the total numbers of macrophages within the stromal tissue of $CX3CR1^{GFP/+}$ and $CX3CR1^{GFP/GFP}$ mice. However, visual inspection of those specimens did not reveal any qualitative differences in macrophages between those two genotypes. Notably, a prior study has shown that genetic deletion of CX3CR1 leads to increased macrophage numbers in the ototoxically injured cochlea (Sato et al., 2010). Given these findings, we believe that the present data should be interpreted with caution. Specifically, our data suggest that lack of fractalkine signaling does not impede macrophages from entering the utricular sensory epithelium after selective hair cell injury. We speculate instead that other diffusible molecules that are released from dying hair cells and/or their adjoining supporting cells (e.g., ATP – Gale et al., 2004; Lahne and Gale, 2008) may attract macrophages to sites of hair cell injury. Future experiments will be necessary to resolve this issue.

References

Anttonen, T., Belevich, I., Kirjavainen, A., Laos, M., Brakebusch, C., Jokitalo, E., et al. (2014). How to bury the dead: elimination of apoptotic hair cells from the hearing organ of the mouse. *J. Assoc. Res. Otolaryngol.* 15, 975–992. doi: 10.1007/s10162-014-0480-x

Ball, G., May, L., Cunningham, L., and Gale, J. (2013). "Damage-induced responses in cochlear and vestibular supporting cells: a Jekyll and Hyde story in which ERK1/2 is necessary and sufficient?" *in Proceedings of the 36th Annual Midwinter Research Meeting of the Association for Research in Otolaryngology*, Baltimore, MD, Abstract 845.

Bhave, S. A., Oesterle, E. C., and Coltrera, M. D. (1998). Macrophage and microglia-like cells in the avian inner ear. *J. Comp. Neurol.* 475, 241–256. doi: 10.1002/(SICI)1096-9861(19980824)398:2<241::AID-CNE6>3.0.CO;2-0

Bird, J. E., Daudet, N., Warchol, M. E., and Gale, J. E. (2010). Rapid elimination of dying sensory hair cells maintains epithelial integrity in the avian inner ear. *J. Neurosci.* 30, 12545–12556. doi: 10.1523/JNEUROSCI.3042-10.2010

Burns, J. C., Christophel, J. J., Collado, M. S., Carfrae, M., and Corwin, J. T. (2008). Reinforcement of cell junctions correlates with the absence of hair cell regeneration in mammals and its occurrence in birds. *J. Comp. Neurol.* 511, 396–414. doi: 10.1002/cne.21849

Burns, J. C., Collado, M. S., Oliver, E. R., and Corwin, J. T. (2013). Specializations of intercellular junctions are associated with the presence and absence of hair cell regeneration in ears from six vertebrate classes. *J. Comp. Neurol.* 521, 1430–1448. doi: 10.1002/cne.23250

Burns, J. C., and Corwin, J. T. (2014). Responses to cell loss become restricted as the supporting cells in mammalian vestibular organs grow thick junctional actin bands that develop high stability. *J. Neurosci.* 34, 1998–2011. doi: 10.1523/JNEUROSCI.4355-13.2014

Chazaud, B. (2014). Macrophages: supportive cells for tissue repair and regeneration. *Immunobiology* 219, 172–178. doi: 10.1016/j.imbio.2013.09.001

Collado, M. S., Burns, J. C., Meyers, J. R., and Corwin, J. T. (2011). Variations in shape sensitive restriction points mirror differences in the regeneration capacities of avian and mammalian ears. *PLoS ONE* 6:e23861. doi: 10.1371/journal.pone.0023861

Cotanche, D. A., and Dopyera, C. E. J. (1990). Hair cell and supporting cell response to acoustic trauma in the chick cochlea. *Hear. Res.* 46, 29–40. doi: 10.1016/0378-5955(90)90137-E

Cox, B. C., Chai, R., Lenoir, A., Liu, Z., Zhang, L., Nguyen, D. H., et al. (2014). Spontaneous hair cell regeneration in the neonatal mouse cochlea *in vivo*. *Development* 141, 816–829. doi: 10.1242/dev.103036

Duckert, L. G., and Rubel, E. W. (1990). Ultrastructural observations on regenerating hair cells in the chick basilar papilla. *Hear. Res.* 48, 161–182. doi: 10.1016/0378-5955(90)90206-5

Erkman, L., McEvilly, R. J., Luo, L., Ryan, A. K., Hooshmand, F., O'Connell, S. M., et al. (1996). Role of transcription factors Brd-3.1 and Brn-3.2 in auditory and visual system development. *Nature* 381, 603–606. doi: 10.1038/381603a0

Forge, A., Li, L., and Nevill, G. (1998). Hair cell recovery in the vestibular sensory epithelia of mature guinea pigs. *J. Comp. Neurol.* 397, 69–88. doi: 10.1002/(SICI)1096-9861(19980720)397:1<69::AID-CNE6>3.0.CO;2-G

Furrer, S., Nguyen, T. B., Cox, B., Pujol, R., and Stone, J. (2014). "Hair cell death and clearance in undamaged adult mouse utricles," *in Proceedings of the 37th Annual Midwinter Research Meeting of the Association for Research in Otolaryngology*, San Diego, CA, Abstract PS-200.

Gale, J. E., Piazza, V., Ciubotaru, C. D., and Mammano, F. (2004). A mechanism for sensing noise damage in the inner ear. *Curr. Biol.* 14, 526–529. doi: 10.1016/j.cub.2004.03.002

Golub, T. S., Tong, L., Ngyuen, T. B., Hume, C. R., Palmiter, R. D., Rubel, E. W., et al. (2012). Hair cell replacement in adult mouse utricles after targeted ablation of hair cells with diphtheria toxin. *J. Neurosci.* 32, 15093–15105. doi: 10.1523/JNEUROSCI.1709-12.2012

Hirose, K., Discolo, C. M., Keasler, J. R., and Ransohoff, R. (2005). Mononuclear phagocytes migrate into the murine cochlea after acoustic trauma. *J. Comp. Neurol.* 489, 180–194. doi: 10.1002/cne.20619

Hirose, K., Westrum, L. E., Cunningham, D. E., and Rubel, E. W. (2004). Electron microscopy of degenerative changes in the chick basilar papilla after gentamicin exposure. *J. Comp. Neurol.* 470, 164–180. doi: 10.1002/cne.11046

Hordichok, A. J., and Steyger, P. S. (2007). Closure of supporting cell scar formations requires dynamic actin mechanisms. *Hear. Res.* 232, 1–19. doi: 10.1016/j.heares.2007.06.011

Ishida, Y., Gao, J. L., and Murphy, P. M. (2008). Chemokine receptor CX3CR1 mediates skin wound healing by promoting macrophage and fibroblast accumulation and function. *J. Immunol.* 180, 569–579. doi: 10.4049/jimmunol.180.1.569

Janas, J. D., Cotanche, D. A., and Rubel, E. W. (1995). Avian cochlear hair cell regeneration: stereological analyses of damage and recovery from a single high dose of gentamicin. *Hear. Res.* 92, 17–29. doi: 10.1016/0378-5955(95)00190-5

Jones, J. E., and Corwin, J. T. (1996). Regeneration of sensory cells after laser ablation in the lateral line system: hair cell lineage and macrophage behavior revealed by time-lapse video microscopy. *J. Neurosci.* 16, 649–662.

Jung, S., Aliberti, J., Graemmel, P., Sunshine, M. J., Kreutzberg, G. W., Sher, A., et al. (2000). Analysis of fractalkine receptor CX_3CR1 function by targeted deletion and green fluorescent protein reporter gene insertion. *Mol. Cell. Biol.* 20, 4106–4114. doi: 10.1128/MCB.20.11.4106-4114.2000

Lahne, M., and Gale, J. E. (2008). Damage-induced activation of ERK1/2 in cochlear supporting cells is a hair cell death promoting signal that depends on extracellular ATP and calcium. *J. Neurosci.* 28, 4918–4928. doi: 10.1523/JNEUROSCI.4914-07.2008

Li, L., Nevill, G., and Forge, A. (1995). Two modes of hair cell loss from the vestibular sensory epithelia of the guinea pig inner ear. *J. Comp. Neurol.* 355, 405–417. doi: 10.1002/cne.903550307

Lin, V., Golub, J. S., Nguyen, T. B., Hume, C. R., Oesterle, E. C., and Stone, J. S. (2011). Inhibition of Notch activity promotes nonmitotic regeneration of hair cells in the adult mouse utricle. *J. Neurosci.* 31, 15329–15339. doi: 10.1523/JNEUROSCI.2057-11.2011

Mahrt, E. J., Perkel, D. J., Tong, L., Rubel, E. W., and Portfors, C. V. (2013). Engineered deafness reveals that mouse courtship vocalizations do not require auditory experience. *J. Neurosci.* 33, 5573–5583. doi: 10.1523/JNEUROSCI.5054-12.2013

Meiteles, L. Z., and Raphael, Y. (1994). Scar formation in the vestibular sensory epithelium after aminoglycoside toxicity. *Hear. Res.* 79, 26–38. doi: 10.1016/0378-5955(94)90124-4

Monzack, E. L., May, L. A., Roy, S., Gale, J. E., and Cunningham, L. L. (2015). Live imaging the phagocytic activity of inner ear supporting cells in response to hair cell death. *Cell Death Differ.* (in press).

Poon, I. K., Lucas, C. D., Rossi, L. C., and Ravichandran, K. S. (2014). Apoptotic cells clearance: basic biology and therapeutic potential. *Nat. Rev. Immunol.* 14, 166–180. doi: 10.1038/nri3607

Ransohoff, R. M. (2009). Chemokines and chemokine receptors: standing at the crossroads of immunobiology and neurobiology. *Immunity* 31, 711–721. doi: 10.1016/j.immuni.2009.09.010

Raphael, Y., and Altschuler, R. A. (1991). Scar formation after drug-induced cochlear insult. *Hear. Res.* 51, 173–183. doi: 10.1016/0378-5955(91)90034-7

Sato, E., Shick, H. E., Ransohoff, R. M., and Hirose, K. (2010). Expression of fractalkine receptor CX3CR1 on cochlear macrophages influences survival of hair cells following ototoxic injury. *J. Assoc. Res. Otolaryngol.* 11, 223–234. doi: 10.1007/s10162-009-0198-3

Stefater, J. A., Ren, S., Lang, R. A., and Duffield, J. S. (2011). Metchnikoff's policemen: macrophages in development homeostasis and regeneration. *Trends Mol. Med.* 17, 743–752. doi: 10.1016/j.molmed.2011.07.009

Tong, L., Hume, C., Palmiter, R., and Rubel, E. W. (2011). "Ablation of mouse cochlear hair cells by activating the human diphtheria toxin receptor (DTR) gene targeted to the Pou4f3 locus," *in Proceedings of the 34th Annual Midwinter Research Meeting of the Association for Research in Otolaryngology*, Baltimore, MD, Abstract 836.

Tong, L., Strong, M. K., Kaur, T., Juiz, J. M., Oesterle, E. C., Hume, C., et al. (2015). Selective deletion of cochlear hair cells causes rapid age-dependent changes in spiral ganglion and cochlear nucleus neurons. *J. Neurosci.* (in press).

Warchol, M. E. (1997). Macrophage activity in the avian cochlea: demonstration of a resident population and recruitment to sites of hair cell lesions. *J. Neurobiol.* 33, 724–734. doi: 10.1002/(SICI)1097-4695(19971120)33:6<724::AID-NEU2>3.0.CO;2-B

Warchol, M. E. (2011). Sensory regeneration in the vertebrate inner ear: differences at the levels of cells and species. *Hear. Res.* 273, 72–29. doi: 10.1016/j.heares.2010.05.004

Warchol, M. E., Schwendener, R. A., and Hirose, K. (2012). Depletion of resident macrophages does not alter sensory regeneration in the avian cochlea. *PLoS ONE* 7:e51574. doi: 10.1371/journal.pone.0051574

Xiang, M., Gao, W. Q., Hasson, T., and Shin, J. J. (1997). Requirement for Brn-3c in maturation and survival, but not in fate determination of inner ear hair cells. *Development* 125, 3935–3946.

Zhang, F., Zhang, J., Neng, L., and Shi, X. (2013). Characterization and inflammatory response of perivascular-resident macrophage-like melanocytes in the vestibular system. *J. Assoc. Res. Otolaryngol.* 14, 635–643. doi: 10.1007/s10162-013-0403-2

10

Cellular glutathione content in the organ of Corti and its role during ototoxicity

Paromita Majumder[1], *Michael R. Duchen*[2] *and Jonathan E. Gale*[1,2*]

[1] *UCL Ear Institute, University College London, London, UK,* [2] *Department of Cell and Developmental Biology, University College London, London, UK*

Edited by:
Allison B. Coffin, Washington State University, USA

Reviewed by:
Peter S. Steyger, Oregon Health and Science University, USA
Robert Esterberg, University of Washington, USA

***Correspondence:**
Jonathan E. Gale, UCL Ear Institute, University College London, 332 Grays Inn Road, London, WXC1 8EE, UK
j.e.gale@ucl.ac.uk

Glutathione (GSH) is the major scavenger of reactive oxygen species (ROS) inside cells. We used live confocal imaging in order to clarify the role of GSH in the biology of the organ of Corti, the sensory epithelium of the cochlea, before, during and after the onset of hearing and in ~1 year old mice. GSH content was measured using monochlorobimane (MCB), a non-fluorescent cell permeant bimane that reacts with GSH, forming a fluorescent adduct through a reaction catalyzed by glutathione-S-transferase. GSH content increased significantly in inner hair cells during maturation in young adult animals, whereas there was no significant change in the outer hair cells. However, the GSH content in inner hair cells was significantly reduced in ~1 year old mice. The GSH content of supporting cells was comparatively stable over these ages. To test whether the GSH content played a significant protective role during ototoxicity, GSH synthesis was inhibited by buthionine sulfoximine (BSO) in organotypic cochlear explant cultures from immature mice. BSO treatment alone, which reduced GSH by 65 and 85% in inner hair cells and outer hair cells respectively, did not cause any significant cell death. Surprisingly, GSH depletion had no significant effect on hair cell survival even during exposure to the ototoxic aminoglycoside neomycin. These data suggest that the involvement of ROS during aminoglycoside-induced hair cell death is less clear than previously thought and requires further investigation.

Keywords: antioxidant, aging, ototoxicity, aminoglycosides, hair cells, organ of Corti, supporting cells, inner ear

Introduction

The tri-peptide gamma-glutamyl-cysteinyl-glycine (glutathione) is the major cellular antioxidant to combat reactive oxygen species (ROS). There are three major reservoirs of glutathione inside eukaryotic cells: ~90% in cytosol, ~10% in the mitochondria, and <1% in the endoplasmic reticulum. In cytoplasm, under normal physiological conditions, the ratio of reduced glutathione (GSH) to the oxidized disulphide form (GSSG) varies from 10:1 to 100:1 (Hwang et al., 1992; Lu, 1999). GSH is an antioxidant and a substrate for anti-oxidant enzymes such as selenium-dependent GSH peroxidase that neutralizes H_2O_2 and other free radicals. GSH is converted back to GSSG during this activity. A cellular

Abbreviations: GSH, reduced glutathione, glutathione, glutamylcysteinylglycine; GSSG, glutathione disulphide; MCB, monochlorobimane; ROS, reactive oxygen species; BSO, l-buthionime sulfoximine; CL, Claudius cells; HN, Hensen's cells; OHC, outer hair cells; DC, Deiters' cells; IHC, inner hair cells; HC, hair cells; OP, outer pillar cells; IP, inner pillars cell; IS, inner sulcus.

redox cycle is completed when GSSG is recycled back to its reduced form by GSSG-reductase at expense of NAPDH.

ROS are a natural side product of oxidative phosphorylation, being produced at many positions along the electron transport chain in the mitochondria (Gutteridge and Halliwell, 2000; Balaban et al., 2005). ROS molecules react with DNA, proteins and, lipids causing mutations and DNA–strand breaks, protein oxidation and, lipid peroxidation. A major contributor to the oxidative damage inside the cell is H_2O_2, which can be converted to superoxide ($\bullet O_2^-$) and the hydroxyl radical ($\bullet$OH).

In the inner ear, oxidative stress has long been associated with cellular damage that results from extracellular insults such as noise-induced hearing loss, aging and ototoxic drugs e.g. the aminoglycoside antibiotics and the cancer therapeutics, carboplatin and cisplatin (Yamane et al., 1995; Clerici et al., 1996). There is surprisingly little direct evidence that ROS formation is causal in cases of acquired hearing loss. Support for the ROS theory for hair cell loss comes from experiments in which antioxidants are found to ameliorate the effects of aminoglycoside ototoxicity and noise-induced hearing loss (Pierson and Gray, 1982; Hoffman et al., 1987; Quirk et al., 1994; Lautermann et al., 1995, 1997; Dehne et al., 2000). A number of mouse models also support the theory that ROS contribute significantly to acquired hearing loss including a targeted mutation of glutathione peroxidase-1 and a superoxide dismutase knockout (McFadden et al., 1999a,b; Ohlemiller et al., 2000). Nutrient deprivation, which is presumed to deplete the supply of GSH in hair cells, has been shown to enhance cell death during aminoglycoside ototoxicity, however as the authors indicated those results were correlative rather than direct (Lautermann et al., 1995). During aminoglycoside ototoxicity it has been proposed that aminoglycosides interact with transition metals inside the hair cell generating ROS and hydroxyl radicals due to the Fenton reaction (Priuska and Schacht, 1995) and the free radicals go on to trigger cell death pathways resulting in the apoptosis, see (Forge and Schacht, 2000).

An aim of this work was to evaluate the distribution of one of the primary sources of ROS buffering, GSH, in the organ of Corti, to assess the relative vulnerability of different cell types to oxidative damage. GSH content was measured in the organ of Corti at different ages through maturation of the organ into adulthood. In addition we assessed GSH content in aged (~1 year old) mice. We used live imaging in *ex vivo* auditory bullae preparations to quantify the fluorescent product of a reaction between monochlorobimane (MCB) and endogenous GSH. This allowed direct assessment of identifiable cells in a native, accessible environment in which the normal cell-cell interactions are maintained. In order to explore the role of GSH during aminoglycoside toxicity, we exposed organotypic cochlear explant cultures to the gamma-glutamylcysteine synthetase inhibitor buthionine sulfoximine (BSO) to deplete cellular GSH (Meister, 1983; Drew and Miners, 1984), then challenged with neomycin and evaluated hair cell survival.

Materials and Methods

Postnatal and Adult Cochlea Isolation and Culture

The animals were sacrificed in accordance with the United Kingdom Animals (Scientific Procedures) Act of 1986. Auditory bullae were isolated from C57BL/6 mice at postnatal days 4–6 (P4–P6), at hearing onset (P14–P16) and in both young (P33–P47) and aged (P357–P424, ~1 year old) adults. Auditory bullae were removed and transferred into Leibovitz's L15 (L15; LifeTech, UK) and then a window opened in the apical turn (Mammano and Ashmore, 1993); Reissner's membrane was peeled away and the stria vascularis removed in order to gain visual access to the organ of Corti. All acute experiments were performed in L15 solution.

For the aminoglycoside and BSO experiments that required longer incubations, cochleae from P4 to P6 mice were dissected out and placed in explant culture. Auditory bullae were removed and transferred into medium 199 (M199H, LifeTech, UK) supplemented with penicillin (10 U/ml) and fungizone (25 ng/ml). The cochleae were isolated from the surrounding cartilagenous capsule, Reissner's membrane was cut and removed but stria vascularis was maintained. The cochlea was cut into three and the apical, middle and basal turns then placed onto Cell-Tak® cell and tissue adhesive (BD Biosciences, UK)-coated Matek® (Ashland, MA, USA) culture dishes. Cell-Tak® was diluted in 0.1M $NaHCO_3$ to a final concentration of 70 μg/ml. Cochlear explants were subsequently incubated in DMEM/F-12 (LifeTech, UK) supplemented with 1% fetal bovine serum (FBS, LifeTech, UK) and maintained at 37°C in a 5% CO_2/95% air atmosphere.

During aminoglycoside exposure experiments, cochlear explant cultures were maintained in HEPES-buffered Hanks Balanced salt solution (10 mM HEPES) adjusted to pH 7.3 with NaOH.

Glutathione Staining and Imaging

Monochlorobimane (MCB) is a non-fluorescent bimane which is freely permeable across the cell membrane and forms a fluorescent adduct when combined with reduced glutathione (GSH) in a reaction catalyzed by glutathione s-transferase. MCB (Sigma-Aldrich, UK) was prepared as a 50 mM stock solution in DMSO and used at a final concentration of 50 μM. Our initial experiments confirmed that this reaction reached steady-state within 40 min (Supplementary Figure 1). Therefore, in all experiments MCB was applied for 40 min prior to imaging for cellular GSH measurement (Keelan et al., 2001). The conjugated GSH-MCB was imaged using multiphoton excitation from a Chameleon-XR Ti:Sapphire laser (Coherent, UK) tuned to 780 nm and fluorescence emission was captured using a 435–485 nm bandpass filter. The Zeiss 510NLO Axioskop and all other hardware was controlled by Zeiss LSM software. Image stacks were acquired at 2 μm intervals using a 40 × (NA 0.8) water immersion objective. All experiments were performed at room temperature (20–23°C) keeping all confocal imaging parameters constant between experiment e.g., laser power, pinhole, detector, sensitivity.

Neomycin and BSO Treatment, Tissue Fixation, and Immunostaining

In order to reduce cellular GSH, cochlear explants were treated with 200 μM buthionine sulfoximine (BSO, Sigma-Aldrich, UK) for 16–18 h. BSO is an irreversible inhibitor of gamma-glutamylcysteine synthetase (Drew and Miners, 1984; Sun et al., 2005). At the end of the BSO treatment the explants were loaded with MCB and MCB-GSH fluorescence data were collected as described above. In separate ototoxicity experiments, BSO pre-treated and untreated control explants were incubated with 1 mM neomycin (Sigma-Aldrich, UK) for 3 or 6 h at 23–25°C, prior to fixation with 4% paraformaldehyde in 0.1 M phosphate buffer solution (PBS, pH 7.2) for 30–40 min. The tissue was rinsed three times with PBS and then incubated in blocking solution (PBS/0.5% TritonX-100 with 10% secondary host antibody serum) for 2 h, prior to incubation with either a polyclonal or monoclonal anti-myosin VIIA primary antibody (1:1000, Proteus and 1:250 Developmental Studies Hybridoma Bank, Iowa respectively) in blocking solution overnight at 4°C. Samples were then washed in PBS and incubated for 2 h at room temperature with 4′,6′-diamidino-2-phenylindole (DAPI 1 μM), Alexa Fluor 647 phalloidin (33 nM) and goat anti-rabbit-Atto488 or goat anti-mouse-Atto488 secondary antibodies in blocking solution. After labeling, the explants were rinsed three times with PBS and imaged using a Zeiss 510NLO upright confocal microscope.

Image Analysis and Statistics

Images were analyzed offline using IQ software (Andor, UK). The mean MCB-GSH fluorescence intensity was quantified by selecting regions of interest (ROI size 8.4 μm^2) over the different cell types in the organ of Corti in single image planes XY. Care was taken to ensure that ROIs were placed within the boundaries of individual cells and for each image file (from an individual N experiment) the following cells were sampled: 3–5 inner hair cells, 12–15 outer hair cells, 4–6 pillar cells, and 4–6 inner sulcus cells. The mean background intensity was measured from regions devoid of cells from within the same image stacks using 4 different ROIs. All mean intensity values from the ROIs were exported to Excel. The background values were subtracted from the measured MCB-GSH values within each data set. The images were not manipulated in any way and measurements were made from single planes. Ratios were calculated from the absolute measurements from individual cells after background subtraction. Unless indicated data are presented as the mean ± SEM and the statistical tests used are either Student's paired *t*-tests, with significance set at $p < 0.05$ or ANOVA with *post-hoc* Tukey-Kramer's, with significance set at $p < 0.05$.

Results

Cellular GSH Expression in the organ of Corti during Cochlear Maturation and Aging in the Mouse

To evaluate the GSH content of cochlear cells at different ages we used an acute whole auditory bulla preparation from mice in combination with live-imaging. In this preparation a window is made in the cochlear bone, providing optical access to the sensory epithelium, the organ of Corti, *in situ*, at all ages. The preparation maintains the native architecture of the tissue and important cell-cell interactions and causes minimal damage to the organ of Corti (**Figure 1**). Acutely explanted bullae were incubated with monochlorobimane (MCB) which forms a fluorescent adduct with reduced GSH. At steady state this fluorescence is proportional to the cellular GSH content. Live images of MCB-GSH fluorescence were acquired using multiphoton imaging in bullae from mice of different ages ranging from an immature stage prior to hearing onset (P4–6), at hearing onset (P14–16), in young adults (P33–47) and in ~1 year old mice (**Figures 2A–D**). The GSH distribution varied across the different cell types in the organ of Corti with the most obvious differences being between supporting cells and hair cells, consistent with our recent work in neonatal cochlear explants (Blacker et al., 2014). With increasing age, we observed an increase in GSH content in hair cells, with the inner hair cells showing the most obvious increase relative to surrounding cells. Quantification of GSH-MCB fluorescence across a number of different bullae preparations at each age revealed a trend for increased GSH content in outer and inner hair cells with maturation followed by a reduction after 1 year, but we note that these changes did not reach significance. GSH levels in the inner sulcus cells were quite stable across the four ages tested, with mean absolute levels of 194 ± 55, 102 ± 63, 155 ± 72, and 129 ± 88 at P4–6, P14–P16, adult and 1 year old respectively. A potential source of variation comes from loading and optical access in the bullae thus by calculating the GSH ratio between cells within the same bullae the inter-preparation variability in loading is reduced. We first calculated intensity ratios between the hair cells and the inner sulcus supporting cells in the same preparations for all the different ages. The GSH content ratio between the inner hair cell and inner sulcus cell increased from more than two fold between the P15 animals and the adult animals (**Figure 2E**). We also calculated ratios between the inner and outer hair cells and in adult animals we found that inner hair cells had approximately twice the level of GSH compared to outer hair cells. Finally we calculated the ratio between pillar cells (another supporting cell type) and the inner sulcus cells and found no significant changes across ages.

Cellular GSH Content in organ of Corti Explant Cultures

Longer term experiments are not possible in the adult auditory bulla preparation since the hair cells do not survive over longer periods and also we were limited to accessing the upper middle to apical turns of the cochlea. Therefore, in order to assess the effects of ototoxins such as aminoglycosides we switched to using explant cultures from P4–P6 mice. The explant cultures maintain the cellular arrangement of the organ of Corti such that they are comparable with that seen in the acute bullae at that age (see **Figures 1A, 3A; Figures 2A, 3B**). We assessed the GSH content of cochlear cells in this experimental preparation by incubating the immature explants with MCB using the same methodology as described for the bullae preparation. There were no significant differences in GSH expression between cell types when measured

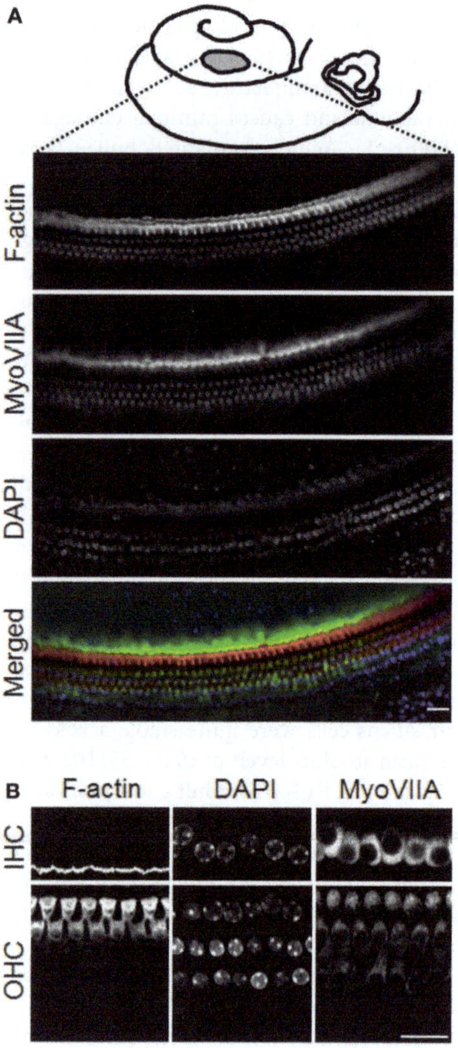

FIGURE 1 | Hair cell status in the *ex vivo* auditory bulla preparation. **(A)** Schematic diagram showing the position of the opening made in the mid to apical turn of the mouse cochlea. Lower planes, confocal optical slices showing inner and outer hair cells labeled with phalloidin (for F-actin, red), DAPI (nuclei, blue) and immunolabeled for myosin VIIA (MyoVIIA, green), and a color merge of the different channels. **(B)** Higher magnification images of inner (IHC) and outer hair cells (OHC). Scale bars: **(A)** 20 μm, **(B)** 20 μm.

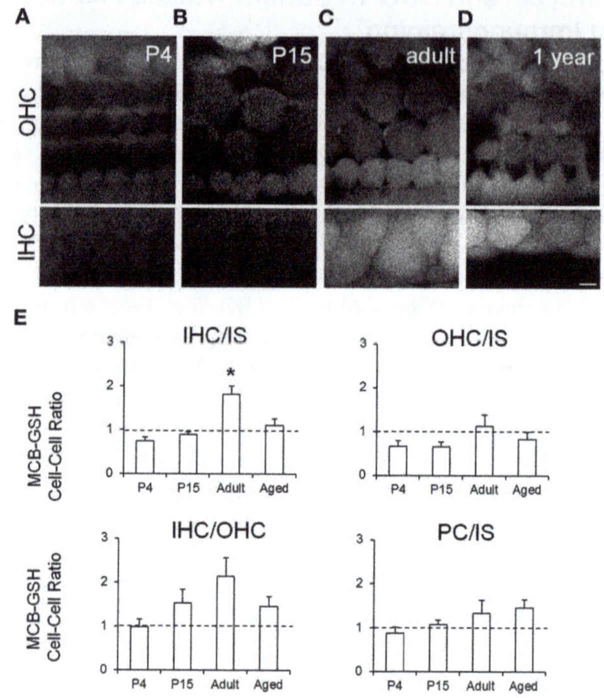

FIGURE 2 | Live imaging and quantification of MCB-GSH staining in the organ of Corti in auditory bulla explant preparations from mice at different stages of hearing development. Higher fluorescence intensities indicate greater cellular GSH content. Representative multiphoton single image planes from **(A)** P4 mice; **(B)** P15 mice; **(C)** adult mice (P30), and **(D)** ~1 year old (aged) mice. Scale bar: 5 μm. **(E)** MCB-GSH fluorescence quantification in OHCs, IHCs, inner sulcus cells (IS) and pillar cells (PC). Ratio values were quantified for hair cells and the IS cells (IHC/IS, OHC/IS), between the two hair cell types (IHC/OHC) and between two supporting cell types (PC/IS). Data are presented as mean ± SEM; $n = 4$ (P4–P6); $n = 5$ (P14–P16); $n = 6$ (P33–P41); $n = 5$ (P357–P424) ANOVA Tukey-Kramer's test.; $^{*}p < 0.05$.

in the explant cultures compared to acute bullae preparations from the same age mice (**Figures 2A, 3B**). In the explant cultures we were able to image almost the whole length of the cochlea. There are known differences in susceptibility to ototoxins and to noise damage between the basal (high frequency) and apical (low frequency) ends of the cochlea. Therefore, we compared GSH content in cells from the basal and apical turns (**Figure 3B**). A complete analysis of GSH content in all of the cell types in the of organ of Corti: Claudius cells (CL), Hensen's cells (HN), outer hair cells (OHC), DC, outer pillars (OP), inner pillars (IP), inner hair cells (IHC), and inner sulcus supporting cells (IS) revealed that although cells exhibit different absolute MCB-GSH fluorescence intensity values there were no significant differences in GSH content in cells of the same type from the apical vs. basal turns (**Figure 3C**). To compare GSH levels between cells we also obtained data by ratioing values within data sets, as we did for the *ex vivo* bulla preparations. This analysis also failed to show any significant differences between apical and basal coil cells (**Figure 3D**). During these experiments we did observe GSH content within the actin-rich hair cell stereocilia in both the explant cultures and in the acute bullae preparations (Supplementary Figure 2).

The Role of GSH in Neomycin Toxicity

Hair cells do not survive in the *ex vivo* whole bullae preparations from adult mice for longer than ~12 h. However, the hair cells in cochlear explant cultures from immature mice are viable for many days allowing us to address whether reducing cellular GSH levels enhanced neomycin-induced hair cell toxicity. Cellular GSH concentration was reduced by incubating cochlear explants in buthionine sulfoximine (BSO) for 18 h. After the BSO treatment, GSH content was evaluated in each cell type in cochlear explant cultures. GSH was reduced by between 65 and 85% across the different cell types with inner hair cells showing the least reduction and outer hair cells the greatest

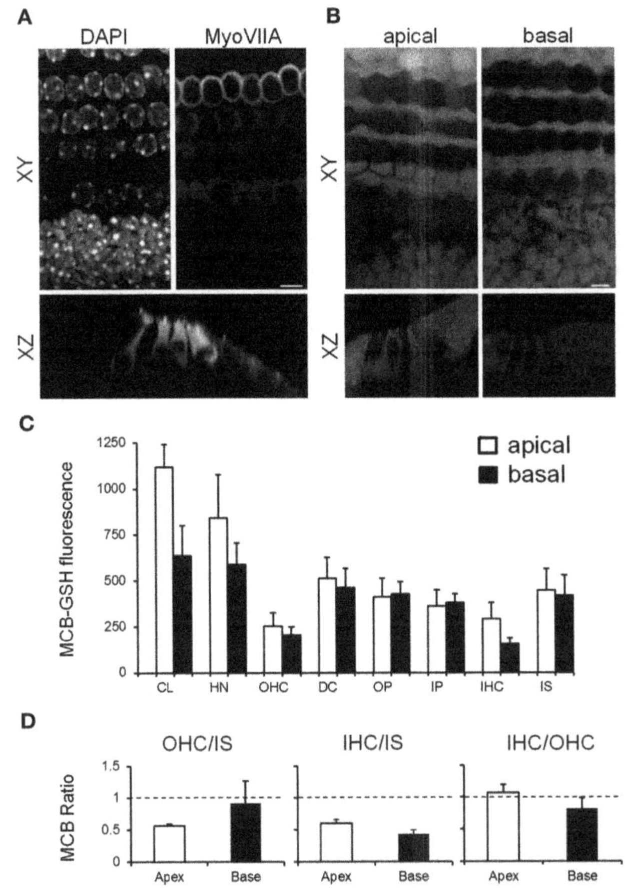

FIGURE 3 | Characterization of GSH content in cochlear explant cultures from P4–P6 mice (A) Confocal images from cultures fixed and immunolabeled with MyoVIIA and DAPI, showing MyoVIIA-positive inner (lower row) and outer hair cells (upper three rows) in XY and XZ profiles. (B) Multiphoton images from MCB loaded live cochlear cultures showing the relative GSH content in the apical and basal cochlear coil coils. Scale bar: 5 μm. **(C)** Quantification of GSH content in the apical and basal cochlear turns. Absolute values measure in apical (white bars) vs. basal (black bars) turn cochlear cells: CL, HN, OHCs, DC, OP, IP, IHCs, and IS cells. **(D)** Average ratio values between cells within data sets for OHCs/IS, IHCs/IS, and IHC/OHC. Data presented are mean ± SEM; $n = 3$–6 different cochlear explants from different animals for apical and basal cells.

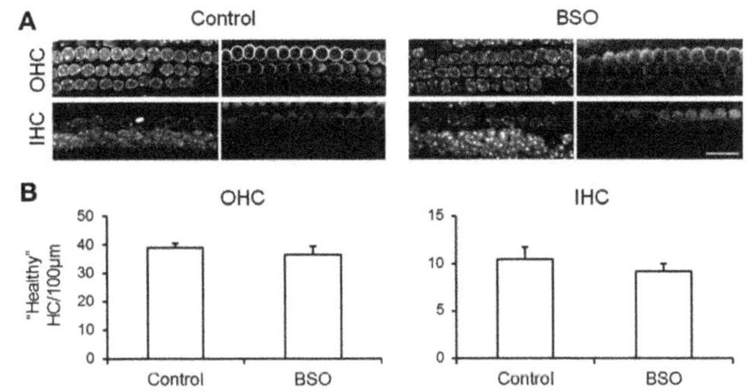

FIGURE 4 | Depletion of cellular GSH using BSO does not cause hair cell death. (A) Confocal images of the OHC and IHC regions in control and BSO-treated cochlear cultures immunolabeled with MyoVIIA (right panels) and stained with DAPI (left panels). **(B)** Quantification of "healthy" hair cells in control and BSO-treated samples per 100 μm length of the cochlea. Cells were considered to be healthy if they exhibited normal chromatin and were positive for MyoVIIA. Data are presented as mean ± SEM. N for control (8) and BSO-treated (9). Student's *t*-test, revealed no statistical differences. Scale bar: 20 μm.

(Supplementary Figure 3). Untreated control and BSO-treated explants were immunostained with a hair cell antibody (myosin VIIA) along with markers for chromatin (DAPI) and for F-actin (phalloidin). Counts of healthy hair cells were made on the basis of positive myosin VIIA staining combined with a healthy nucleus and these revealed that BSO treatment alone for 18 h does not result in hair cell death over this time period (**Figure 4**). In subsequent experiments, explants (control or BSO-treated) were then subjected to neomycin-treatment for 3 or 6 h (**Figure 5**). There was a ~50% reduction in the number of healthy hair cells from control levels (10 inner hair cells and 39 outer hair cells per 100 μm length of the cochlea) at both 3 and 6 h, with the latter showing the greatest reduction (compare **Figures 4, 5**). However, we did not observe any significant difference in the numbers of healthy hair cells after neomycin treatment between explants in which GSH had or had not been depleted by BSO-treatment (**Figure 5**).

Discussion

In this study, we evaluated cellular GSH distribution in organ of Corti cells at different ages, from P5 to ~1 year old animals, using an *ex vivo* whole auditory bulla preparation. A window was opened in the apical region to allow optical access to the cells and for the MCB loading that was used to assess GSH content. Using live multiphoton imaging we determined cellular GSH concentrations in individual cells, overcoming some limitations of biochemical and histological approaches to measuring GSH in intact cells and tissue (Sun et al., 2006). For example, previous studies showed that tissue fixation, when using antibodies to measure GSH, lead to potential alterations in GSH status (Hjelle et al., 1994). Here, using our loading conditions the MCB reaction was at steady state, and thus our measurements of the fluorescent MCB-GSH product reflect cellular GSH levels. We note that we have not attempted to determine GSH levels in subcellular compartments in the present experiments.

The *ex vivo* whole auditory bulla preparation has been used previously both in guinea pigs (Mammano and Ashmore, 1993) and in mice (Tiede et al., 2007, 2009). It is a useful approach to study the organ of Corti in a native but *ex vivo* context. Here we first characterized the hair cell status in this preparation using the expression of the hair cell marker myosin VIIA and assessed the stereocilial bundles using phalloidin. These same assays were applied after MCB assessment of cellular GSH content to confirm the normal cellular status of all the preparations used in this study.

GSH is one of the most important cellular antioxidants. GSH is distributed in mitochondrial, cytosolic and ER pools where it maintains exogenous antioxidants such as vitamins C

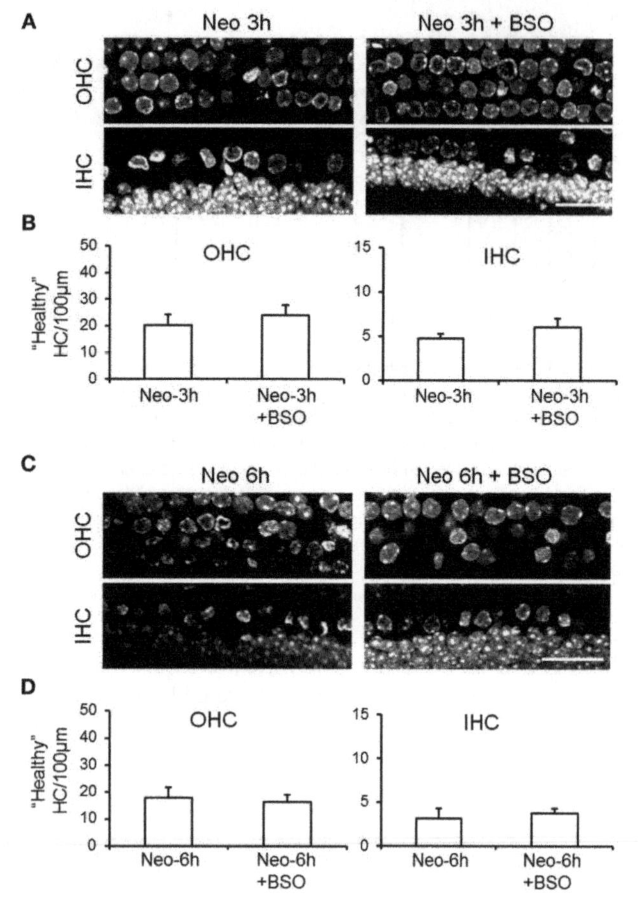

FIGURE 5 | Depletion of cellular GSH does not enhance neomycin induced-hair cell death. (A) Examples of confocal images of DAPI-stained OHC and IHC in cochlear explant cultures treated with neomycin for 3 h compared with those that had been pre-incubated with BSO for 18 h to deplete GSH before neomycin treatment. **(B)** Quantification of "healthy" hair cells per 100 μm length in control or BSO-treated cultures exposed to neomycin for 3 h. **(C)** As above for **(A)** except that neomycin cultures were fixed after 6 h exposure to neomycin. **(D)** Quantification of "healthy" hair cells per 100 μm length in control or BSO-treated cultures exposed to neomycin for 6 h. Data are presented as mean ± SEM. N for Neo-3h (7), Neo-3h+BSO (7), Neo-6h (6) Neo-6h+BSO (8). Student's *t*-test's revealed no significant differences. Scale bar: 20 μm.

and E, peroxide and glutaredoxins in their reduced and active forms. Alterations in cellular GSH have been linked to variety of neurodegenerative diseases such as Parkinson's, Alzheimer's, Huntington's, amyotrophic lateral sclerosis and others (Schulz et al., 2000; Wilson and Shaw, 2007). Moreover, a low level of GSH results in cellular vulnerability toward oxidative stress products, especially in neurons (Murphy et al., 1990; Bolaños et al., 1995; Dringen et al., 1999).

GSH is the major free radical scavenger in the brain, and it has found at higher levels in glial cells compared to the neurons (Keelan et al., 2001). Here we observed a similar difference in the relative GSH content between supporting cells and hair cells in the immature organ of Corti. This finding is consistent with our previous data from the neonatal cochlea which also indicated a higher concentration of enzyme-bound NADPH in pillar cells compared to OHCs (Blacker et al., 2014). It is important to note that NADPH is the co-factor involved to restore GSSG to GSH (Ying, 2008). A potential analogy between supporting cells and glial cells has been proposed by a number of studies (Lahne and Gale, 2008; Monzack and Cunningham, 2013; Mellado Lagarde et al., 2014) and, for the most part, the data herein provide additional support for this suggestion. Whether supporting cells might provide GSH for the hair cells, as has been proposed for glial cells and neurons, remains to be determined. However, here we show that there is an increase in inner hair cell GSH content from the immature stage to when the hearing system is fully functional in the young adult animal. Thus, in the adult, the ratio of cellular GSH levels in inner hair cells compared to supporting cell is reversed. Interestingly, the GSH content of outer hair cells did not increase significantly during this maturation period, although we note that the ratio of inner to outer hair cell GSH content also did not change significantly, indicating perhaps, that the outer hair cell GSH content does increase with age but that the change is more discrete than observed in inner hair cells. By 1 year of age, the GSH content in inner hair cells relative to the supporting cells is reduced. The C57BL/6 mice used in the present study exhibit early onset hearing loss and this may influence these results. However, our measurements were made at the apical end of the cochlea (<10 kHz frequency region) where both the hair cell and the hearing loss is relatively minimal at 12 months (Spongr et al., 1997). A reduction in GSH content with aging has been indicated in HPLC studies on auditory nerves from 3 and 24 months old rats, where it was reduced by as much as 86% (Lautermann et al., 1997). In addition and by association, mitochondrial SOD2 protein expression is reduced by 50% and the levels of glutathione-conjugated proteins (potential indicators of oxidative stress) increased three fold in cochleae from aged mice compared to young animals (Jiang et al., 2007).

GSH content in hair cells isolated from the guinea pig cochlea was measured using MCB (Sha et al., 2001). In that study it was noted that longer outer hair cells, presumed to be from more apical turns, had a greater GSH content than shorter outer hair cells from the basal coils. Unfortunately no direct comparison with inner hair cells was made although it was noted that inner hair cells were considered to be healthier after the isolation procedure, consistent with a higher GSH level and a resistance to cellular stress. The latter observation could also simply have been due to the dissociation procedure being less traumatic for inner hair cells compared to outer hair cells. Previous measurements of GSH in cochlear explants from neonatal rats indicated that there are cell to cell differences (Blacker et al., 2014). Here we show measurements made in the adult cochlea that reveal higher expression of cellular GSH in inner hair cells compared to outer hair cells and also that this enhanced GSH expression appears to develop during cochlear maturation. Higher GSH levels compared to outer hair cells could explain the comparative resistance of inner hair cells to ototoxic agents and to noise trauma.

GSH levels have been strongly implicated in providing a protective role in the cochlea and our data showing raised cellular

GSH in inner hair cells correlates with this assertion. Food deprivation results in a reduction in endogenous GSH and has been correlated with enhanced auditory dysfunction (Hoffman et al., 1987) and supplementation with glutathione monoethyl ester has been shown to ameliorate noise-induced hearing loss in animals on a low protein diet (Ohinata et al., 2000). GSH also slowed the progression of gentamicin ototoxicity when applied as a co-therapy along with the aminoglycoside *in vivo* (Garetz et al., 1994). Further support for an important role for GSH in protecting the cochlea from trauma or toxicity comes from GSH peroxidase (Gpx1) knock out mice that exhibit loss of hair cells and also spiral ganglion neurons in the basal cochlear turn. When those mice were subjected to noise trauma they exhibited increased hearing loss compared to wild-type controls (Ohlemiller et al., 2000). Thus, part of the data presented herein along with a number of other papers have implicated GSH in providing protection from various types of auditory stress. A reduction of ROS generation within hair cells themselves has been suggested although rarely tested directly.

Here we evaluated the role and potential importance of cellular GSH during aminoglycoside ototoxicity. We performed these longer term experiments in cochlear explant cultures from postnatal day 4 to 6 mice. Explants were pre-treated with BSO for 18 h in order to deplete GSH and depletion was confirmed by MCB labeling. After 18 h of BSO-treatment explants were then challenged with 1 mM neomycin for 3 or 6 h. Compared to controls not treated with BSO, there was no significance difference in hair cell survival or death with either 3 or 6 h of neomycin exposure. If anything, we identified a trend for hair cell survival in the BSO-treated explants at the earlier 3 h time point, which was not present after 6 h treatment. The simplest explanation for these data is that ROS production is not as major a determinant of aminoglycoside-induced hair cell death as has been suggested. A number of reports have begun to indicate that mechanisms other than ROS generation may be critical in promoting cell death during ototoxicity. Recent work has indicated that aminoglycosides may block cytoplasmic ribosomal activity (Francis et al., 2013) rather than targeting mitochondria, and this would be consistent with ROS playing a less significant role in hair cell death. Moreover, recent experiments undertaken in live zebrafish have shown that the endoplasmic reticulum (ER) is the primary target of aminoglycosides rather than mitochondria and that ER to mitochondrial transfer of Ca^{2+} may well be responsible for catastrophic mitochondrial depolarization (Esterberg et al., 2013, 2014). Such mitochondrial depolarizations have, in the past, been suggested to result from ROS generation but those data argue strongly against that. Whether ROS contribute to the effects on the ER that have been described in zebrafish hair cells remains to be determined.

An alternative explanation for the lack of effect of GSH depletion on neomycin-induced hair cell death describe here, is that when cellular GSH is reduced, other free radical scavenging systems take over so that that GSH depletion does not cause any additional hair cell death. Although this is possible, we predict that we should still have observed some effect of the GSH depletion in these experiments. A further investigation into potential regulation of other cellular antioxidants present in sensory hair cells is warranted.

In summary, using live imaging to measure cellular GSH levels we observe increased cellular GSH in inner hair cells compared to outer hair cells, but also higher levels in supporting cells compared to the outer hair cells. These data are consistent with the enhanced sensitivity of outer hair cells compared to inner hair cells with various types of cellular stress, from noise, ototoxic drugs to aging. However, when we tested the role that cellular GSH plays during neomycin-induced hair cell death we were unable to provide positive data in support of GSH-dependent protection. Further work is required to determine whether other ROS scavenging systems are able to provide sufficient buffering to cover for the lack of GSH in our experimental condition or whether we need to consider that ROS play a lesser role in aminoglycoside-induced hair cell death than has been previously suggested.

Acknowledgments

We thank Piotr Sirko for the help with the bullae preparations. This work was funded by Action On Hearing Loss through an International Grant (ref: G52 to JEG) and a Pauline Ashley award (to PM) and also by a Conselho Nacional de Desenvolvimento Cientifico e Tecnológico (CNPq) fellowship (249335/2013-1 to PM).

References

Balaban, R. S., Nemoto, S., and Finkel, T. (2005). Mitochondria, Oxidants, and Aging. *Cell* 120, 483–495. doi: 10.1016/j.cell.2005.02.001

Blacker, T. S., Mann, Z. F., Gale, J. E., Ziegler, M., Bain, A. J., Szabadkai, G., et al. (2014). Separating NADH and NADPH fluorescence in live cells and tissues using FLIM. *Nat. Commun.* 5:3936. doi: 10.1038/ncomms4936

Bolaños, J. P., Heales, S. J. R., Land, J. M., and Clark, J. B. (1995). Effect of Peroxynitrite on the mitochondrial respiratory chain: differential Susceptibility of Neurones and Astrocytes in primary culture. *J. Neurochem.* 64, 1965–1972. doi: 10.1046/j.1471-4159.1995.64051965.x

Clerici, W. J., Hensley, K., DiMartino, D. L., and Butterfield, D. A. (1996). Direct detection of ototoxicant-induced reactive oxygen species generation in cochlear explants. *Hear. Res.* 98, 116–124. doi: 10.1016/0378-5955(96)00075-5

Dehne, N., Lautermann, J., ten Cate, W. J. F., Rauen, U., and de Groot, H. (2000). *In vitro* effects of hydrogen peroxide on the cochlear neurosensory epithelium of the guinea pig. *Hear. Res.* 143, 162–170. doi: 10.1016/S0378-5955(00)00036-8

Drew, R., and Miners, J. O. (1984). The effects of buthionine sulphoximine (BSO) on glutathione depletion and xenobiotic biotransformation. *Biochem. Pharmacol.* 33, 2989–2994. doi: 10.1016/0006-2952(84)90598-7

Dringen, R., Kussmaul, L., Gutterer, J. M., Hirrlinger, J., and Hamprecht, B. (1999). The Glutathione system of peroxide detoxification is less efficient in neurons

Esterberg, R., Hailey, D., Rubel, E., and Raible, D. (2014). ER-mitochondrial calcium flow underlies vulnerability of mechanosensory hair cells to damage. *J. Neurosci.* 34, 9703–9719. doi: 10.1523/JNEUROSCI.0281-14.2014

Forge, A., and Schacht, J. (2000). Aminoglycoside antibiotics. *Audiol. Neurootol.* 5, 3–22. doi: 10.1159/000013861

Francis, S. P., Katz, J., Fanning, K. D., Harris, K. A., Nicholas, B. D., Lacy, M., et al. (2013). A novel role of cytosolic protein synthesis inhibition in aminoglycoside ototoxicity. *J. Neurosci.* 33, 3079–3093. doi: 10.1523/JNEUROSCI.3430-12.2013

Garetz, S. L., Altschuler, R. A., and Schacht, J. (1994). Attenuation of gentamicin ototoxicity by glutathione in the guinea pig *in vivo*. *Hear. Res.* 77, 81–87. doi: 10.1016/0378-5955(94)90255-0

Gutteridge, J. M. C., and Halliwell, B. (2000). Free radicals and antioxidants in the Year 2000: a Historical look to the future. *Ann. N.Y. Acad. Sci.* 899, 136–147. doi: 10.1111/j.1749-6632.2000.tb06182.x

Hjelle, O. P., Chaudhry, F. A., and Ottersen, O. P. (1994). Antisera to glutathione: characterization and immunocytochemical application to the rat cerebellum. *Eur. J. Neurosci.* 6, 793–804. doi: 10.1111/j.1460-9568.1994.tb00990.x

Hoffman, D. W., Whitworth, C. A., Jones, K. L., and Rybak, L. P. (1987). Nutritional status, glutathione levels, and ototoxicity of loop diuretics and aminoglycoside antibiotics. *Hear. Res.* 31, 217–222. doi: 10.1016/0378-5955(87)90190-0

Hwang, C., Sinskey, A., and Lodish, H. (1992). Oxidized redox state of glutathione in the endoplasmic reticulum. *Science* 257, 1496–1502.

Jiang, H., Talaska, A. E., Schacht, J., and Sha, S.-H. (2007). Oxidative imbalance in the aging inner ear. *Neurobiol. Aging* 28, 1605–1612. doi: 10.1016/j.neurobiolaging.2006.06.025

Keelan, J., Allen, N. J., Antcliffe, D., Pal, S., and Duchen, M. R. (2001). Quantitative imaging of glutathione in hippocampal neurons and glia in culture using monochlorobimane. *J. Neurosci. Res.* 66, 873–884. doi: 10.1002/jnr.10085

Lahne, M., and Gale, J. E. (2008). Damage-induced activation of ERK1/2 in Cochlear supporting cells is a hair cell death-promoting signal that depends on extracellular ATP and calcium. *J. Neurosci.* 28, 4918–4928. doi: 10.1523/JNEUROSCI.4914-07.2008

Lautermann, J., Crann, S. A., McLaren, J., and Schacht, J. (1997). Glutathione-dependent antioxidant systems in the mammalian inner ear: effects of aging, ototoxic drugs and noise. *Hear. Res.* 114, 75–82. doi: 10.1016/S0378-5955(97)00154-8

Lautermann, J., McLaren, J., and Schacht, J. (1995). Glutathione protection against gentamicin ototoxicity depends on nutritional status. *Hear. Res.* 86, 15–24. doi: 10.1016/0378-5955(95)00049-A

Lu, S. (1999). Regulation of hepatic glutathione synthesis: current concepts and controversies. *FASEB J.* 13, 1169–1183.

Mammano, F., and Ashmore, J. (1993). Reverse transduction measured in the isolated cochlea by laser Michelson interferometry. *Nature* 365, 838–841.

McFadden, S. L., Ding, D., Burkard, R. F., Jiang, H., Reaume, A. G., Flood, D. G., et al. (1999a). Cu/Zn SOD deficiency potentiates hearing loss and cochlear pathology in aged 129,CD-1 mice. *J. Comp. Neurol.* 413, 101–112. doi: 10.1002/(sici)1096-9861(19991011)413:1<101::aid-cne7>3.0.co;2-l

McFadden, S. L., Ding, D., Reaume, A. G., Flood, D. G., and Salvi, R. J. (1999b). Age-related cochlear hair cell loss is enhanced in mice lacking copper/zinc superoxide dismutase. *Neurobiol. Aging* 20, 1–8. doi: 10.1016/S0197-4580(99)00018-4

Meister, A. (1983). Selective modification of glutathione metabolism. *Science* 220, 472–477.

Mellado Lagarde, M. M., Wan, G., Zhang, L. L., Gigliello, A. R., McInnis, J. J., Zhang, Y., et al. (2014). Spontaneous regeneration of cochlear supporting cells after neonatal ablation ensures hearing in the adult mouse. *Proc. Natl. Acad. Sci. U.S.A.* 111, 16919–16924. doi: 10.1073/pnas.1408064111

Monzack, E. L., and Cunningham, L. L. (2013). Lead roles for supporting actors: critical functions of inner ear supporting cells. *Hear. Res.* 303, 20–29. doi: 10.1016/j.heares.2013.01.008

Murphy, T. H., Schnaar, R. L., and Coyle, J. T. (1990). Immature cortical neurons are uniquely sensitive to glutamate toxicity by inhibition of cystine uptake. *FASEB J.* 4, 1624–1633.

Ohinata, Y., Yamasoba, T., Schacht, J., and Miller, J. M. (2000). Glutathione limits noise-induced hearing loss. *Hear. Res.* 146, 28–34. doi: 10.1016/S0378-5955(00)00096-4

Ohlemiller, K. K., McFadden, S. L., Ding, D.-L., Lear, P. M., and Ho, Y.-S. (2000). Targeted mutation of the gene for cellular Glutathione Peroxidase (Gpx1) increases noise-induced hearing loss in mice. *J. Assoc. Res. Otolaryngol.* 1, 243–254. doi: 10.1007/s101620010043

Pierson, M. G., and Gray, B. H. (1982). Superoxide dismutase activity in the cochlea. *Hear. Res.* 6, 141–151. doi: 10.1016/0378-5955(82)90050-8

Priuska, E. M., and Schacht, J. (1995). Formation of free radicals by gentamicin and iron and evidence for an iron/gentamicin complex. *Biochem. Pharmacol.* 50, 1749–1752. doi: 10.1016/0006-2952(95)02160-4

Quirk, W. S., Shivapuja, B. G., Schwimmer, C. L., and Seidman, M. D. (1994). Lipid peroxidation inhibitor attenuates noise-induced temporary threshold shifts. *Hear. Res.* 74, 217–220. doi: 10.1016/0378-5955(94)90189-9

Schulz, J. B., Lindenau, J., Seyfried, J., and Dichgans, J. (2000). Glutathione, oxidative stress and neurodegeneration. *Eur. J. Biochem.* 267, 4904–4911. doi: 10.1046/j.1432-1327.2000.01595.x

Sha, S.-H., Taylor, R., Forge, A., and Schacht, J. (2001). Differential vulnerability of basal and apical hair cells is based on intrinsic susceptibility to free radicals. *Hear. Res.* 155, 1–8. doi: 10.1016/S0378-5955(01)00224-6

Spongr, V. P., Flood, D. G., Frisina, R. D., and Salvi, R. J. (1997). Quantitative measures of hair cell loss in CBA and C57BL/6 mice throughout their life spans. *J. Acoust. Soc. Am.* 101, 3546–3553. doi: 10.1121/1.418315

Sun, X., Erb, H., and Murphy, T. H. (2005). Coordinate regulation of glutathione metabolism in astrocytes by Nrf2. *Biochem. Biophys. Res. Commun.* 326, 371–377. doi: 10.1016/j.bbrc.2004.11.031

Sun, X., Shih, A. Y., Johannssen, H. C., Erb, H., Li, P., and Murphy, T. H. (2006). Two-photon imaging of glutathione levels in intact brain indicates enhanced redox buffering in developing neurons and cells at the cerebrospinal fluid and blood-brain interface. *J. Biol. Chem.* 281, 17420–17431. doi: 10.1074/jbc.M601567200

Tiede, L., Nichols, M. G., Beisel, K., Rocha-Sanchez, S. M., and Hallworth, R. (2007). Determination of hair cell metabolic state in isolated cochlear preparations by two-photon microscopy. *J. Biomed. Opt.* 12:021004. doi: 10.1117/1.2714777

Tiede, L., Steyger, P. S., Nichols, M. G., and Hallworth, R. (2009). Metabolic imaging of the organ of corti—A window on cochlea bioenergetics. *Brain Res.* 1277, 37–41. doi: 10.1016/j.brainres.2009.02.052

Wilson, J. M. B., and Shaw, C. A. (2007). Late appearance of glutamate transporter defects in a murine model of ALS–parkinsonism dementia complex. *Neurochem. Int.* 50, 1067–1077. doi: 10.1016/j.neuint.2006.09.017

Yamane, H., Nakai, Y., Takayama, M., Iguchi, H., Nakagawa, T., and Kojima, A. (1995). Appearance of free radicals in the guinea pig inner ear after noise-induced acoustic trauma. *Eur. Arch. Otorhinolaryngol.* 252, 504–508. doi: 10.1007/BF02114761

Ying, W. (2008). NAD /NADH and NADP /NADPH in cellular functions and cell death: regulation and biological consequences. *Antioxid. Redox Signal.* 10, 180–206. doi: 10.1089/ars.2007.1672

11

The deafness gene DFNA5 induces programmed cell death through mitochondria and MAPK-related pathways

Sofie Van Rossom [1,2], *Ken Op de Beeck* [1], *Vesna Hristovska* [2], *Joris Winderickx* [2]* and *Guy Van Camp* [1]*

[1] Department of Biomedical Sciences, Center of Medical Genetics, University of Antwerp, Antwerp, Belgium, [2] Functional Biology, Department of Biology, KU Leuven, Heverlee, Belgium

Edited by:
Andy Groves,
Baylor College of Medicine, USA

Reviewed by:
Jochen Schacht,
University of Michigan, USA
Michael Anne Gratton,
Saint Louis University, USA

***Correspondence:**
Joris Winderickx,
Functional Biology, Department of Biology, KU Leuven, Kasteelpark Arenberg 31 Box 2433, 3001 Leuven-Heverlee, Belgium
joris.winderickx@bio.kuleuven.be;
Guy Van Camp,
Department of Biomedical Sciences, Center of Medical Genetics, University of Antwerp, Universiteitsplein 1, 2610 Wilrijk-Antwerp, Belgium
guy.vancamp@uantwerpen.be

Cell death exists in many different forms. Some are accidental, but most of them have some kind of regulation and are called programmed cell death. Programmed cell death (PCD) is a very diverse and complex mechanism and must be tightly regulated. This study investigated PCD induced by *DFNA5*, a gene responsible for autosomal dominant hearing loss (HL) and a tumor suppressor gene (TSG) involved in frequent forms of cancer. Mutations in *DFNA5* lead to exon 8 skipping and result in HL in several families. Expression of mutant DFNA5, a cDNA construct where exon 8 is deleted, was linked to PCD both in human cell lines and in *Saccharomyces cerevisiae*. To further investigate the cell death mechanism induced by mutant DFNA5, we performed a microarray study in both models. We used wild-type *DFNA5*, which does not induce cell death, as a reference. Our data showed that the yeast pathways related to mitochondrial ATP-coupled electron transport chain, oxidative phosphorylation and energy metabolism were up-regulated, while in human cell lines, MAP kinase-related activity was up-regulated. Inhibition of this pathway was able to partially attenuate the resulting cell death induced by mutant DFNA5 in human cell lines. In yeast, the association with mitochondria was demonstrated by up-regulation of several cytochrome c oxidase (COX) genes involved in the cellular oxidative stress production. Both models show a down-regulation of protein sorting- and folding-related mechanisms suggesting an additional role for the endoplasmic reticulum (ER). The exact relationship between ER and mitochondria in DFNA5-induced cell death remains unknown at this moment, but these results suggest a potential link between the two.

Keywords: hearing loss, programmed cell death, oxidative stress, mitochondria, MAPK, DFNA5

Introduction

Cell death is a fundamental process of all organisms and inherent to life. The role of programmed cell death (PCD) in the pathology of hearing loss (HL) has been well studied and seems to play a prominent role, especially in the development of the vertebrate inner ear and in the morphogenesis of the semicircular canals (Fekete et al., 1997; Nishikori et al., 1999; Leon et al., 2004). Several genes related to PCD-induced HL have been identified and many of these are related to the mitochondria (Estivill et al., 1998; Jacobs et al., 2005; Ding et al., 2013). Mitochondria are key players during PCD and dysfunction of the mitochondria has been linked to the pathogenesis of many diseases, including HL. Mitochondria are the main producers of cellular ATP due to oxidative phosphorylation. However, this process also generates reactive oxygen species (ROS) (Raha and Robinson, 2000). Due to the mitochondrial production of ROS, the reduced DNA repair capacity and the close proximity of mtDNA to ROS generation sites, mtDNA (mitochondrial DNA) is very susceptible to mutations. Enhanced oxidative stress will have detrimental effects on cellular health and plays a major role during aging, mutagenesis, and cell death (Gredilla and Barja, 2005; Maynard et al., 2009; Gredilla et al., 2010).

Due to the relative slow speech perception detoriation, it is assumed that DFNA5-related HL is due to cochlear dysfunction. The cochlea seems to be highly susceptible to the detrimental effects of mitochondrial damage due to the post-mitotic character of its sensory epithelium (Sha et al., 2001).

It is estimated that in the Caucasian population at least 5% of the post-lingual non-syndromic HL is due to mutations in the mtDNA (Estivill et al., 1998; Jacobs et al., 2005). Most mutations in mtDNA affect the mitochondrial *MTRNR1* and the *MTTS1* genes encoding respectively a mitochondrial 12S rRNA and a $tRNA^{Ser}$. Mutations in these mitochondrial genes lead to variable clinical severity of HL due to impaired mitochondrial tRNA metabolism and protein synthesis (Casano et al., 1999; Fischel-Ghodsian, 1999; Jin et al., 2007; Ding et al., 2013; Dowlati et al., 2013). Also many of the nuclear DNA mutations leading to HL are related to mitochondrial dysfunction and PCD. These include genes such as *OPA1*, *TIMM8A*, *SMAC/DIABLO*, *MPV17*, *PDSS1*, *BCS1L*, *SUCLA2*, *C10ORF2*, *COX10*, *PLOG1*, and *RRM2B* (Roesch et al., 2002; Antonicka et al., 2003; Payne et al., 2004; Mollet et al., 2007; Cheng et al., 2011; Meyer Zum Gottesberge et al., 2012; Luo et al., 2013). These genes contribute to various fundamental mitochondrial aspects, such as mitochondrial protein transport, mitochondrial fragmentation, and oxidative phosphorylation. Mutations in these genes are thought to induce mitochondrial stress and trigger cell death in the cochlea leading to HL. The explanation for the tissue specific effect of these genes leading to more prominent cell death in the cochlea and the hair cells remains unknown at this moment.

In addition to the genes directly associated with the mitochondria, two other genes related to apoptosis, a specific form of PCD, have been linked with hearing loss. *MSBR3*, a gene encoding a methionine sulfoxide reductase, is associated with caspase-3 activity. This can initiate apoptosis, eventually leading to degeneration of the inner hair cells and recessive non-syndromic HL (Ahmed et al., 2011). Overexpression of the *TJP2* gene, due to a genomic duplication, altered the expression of several apoptotic genes, inducing a dominant non-syndromic form of HL (Walsh et al., 2010).

From these examples, it is clear that a prominent association exists between (mitochondria-related) PCD and non-syndromic HL. Many forms of HL, such as age-related hearing impairment (ARHI), noise-induced hearing loss (NIHL), monogenic forms of HL and ototoxicity, have been associated with dysfunctional mitochondria and PCD, underscoring the importance and the need to further investigate the role of PCD in the pathogenesis of deafness (Casano et al., 1999; Sha et al., 2009; Someya et al., 2009; Liu et al., 2010; Chen et al., 2012).

One of the monogenic deafness genes that is related to PCD is *DFNA5*. *DFNA5* was originally identified as a gene responsible for an autosomal dominant form of HL in a Dutch family (Van Laer et al., 1998). Today, eight families with mutations in *DFNA5* (mut*DFNA5*) associated with HL have been identified. The phenotype of the HL is very similar with the exception of the age-of-onset which varies from 15 to 50 years old. The HL is symmetric and starts in the high frequencies, but spreads to the lower frequencies in a later stage. Four of the eight mutations differ at the genomic level, but they all result in skipping of exon 8, yielding an immature truncated protein (Yu et al., 2003; Bischoff et al., 2004; Cheng et al., 2007; Park et al., 2010; Nishio et al., 2014). The structure of DFNA5 is unknown at this moment, but hydrophobic cluster analysis revealed that DFNA5 consists of two regions, domain A and domain B, connected by a hinge region (Op de Beeck et al., 2011). Mutations in *DFNA5* result in a truncated protein lacking the last part of domain B due to a premature stop codon. This premature stop codon is caused by skipping of exon 8 as a result of the different genomic mutations in DFNA5 present in the families. Op de Beeck et al. (2011) have also demonstrated that only the first part, domain A, present in both wild-type and mutDFNA5, is sufficient to induce cell death after transfection in human cell lines. Domain B did not have any cell death inducing capacity. This led to the hypothesis that domain B will normally shield this cell death-inducing domain A to avoid inappropriate activation of domain A. Due to the partial lack of domain B in mutDFNA5, this shielding may not be possible, leading to a constitutive activation of mutDFNA5 (Op de Beeck et al., 2011).

In addition to HL, wild-type *DFNA5* (wt*DFNA5*) has also been correlated with several forms of cancer, such as breast, colorectal, hepatocellular, and gastric cancer. Endogenous *DFNA5* is epigenetically silenced by hypermethylation in cancer cells resulting in a decreased *DFNA5* expression level. Based on these findings, it is hypothesized that *DFNA5* is a tumor suppressor gene (TSG) (Akino et al., 2007; Kim et al., 2008a,b; Wang et al., 2013).

The function of DFNA5 remained unknown for a long time, but previous functional studies by Op de Beeck et al. (2011) revealed that DFNA5 induces a growth defect in mut*DFNA5*-transfected HEK293T cells, as well as other cells, leading to PCD (Op de Beeck et al., 2011). The cell death-inducing capacity of DFNA5 was not only restricted to human cell lines, but was also observed in the yeast model *Saccharomyces cerevisiae* (Van Rossom et al., 2012). This inspired us to use these two different model organisms to further elucidate the mechanisms related to *DFNA5*.

The *Saccharomyces cerevisiae* yeast model has several advantages as a model organism compared to human cell lines. The rapid growth, inexpensive media and the relatively easy genetic modifications, made the budding yeast *Saccharomyces cerevisiae* a valuable model to unravel regulators of different human pathologies (reviewed in Winderickx et al., 2008). Thirty percent of known genes involved in human diseases have an ortholog in yeast and due to this high degree of conservation, yeast is very suitable for fundamental research to identify core regulators of diverse signaling mechanisms (Foury, 1997). This was demonstrated in particular for mechanisms related to PCD where numerous yeast homologs of human genes related to cell death have been identified to play a common role (Wissing et al., 2004; Buttner et al., 2007; Madeo et al., 2009). The conservation of PCD mechanisms has been confirmed for DFNA5-related PCD in a previous study using the budding yeast *Saccharomyces cerevisiae* (Van Rossom et al., 2012). This study demonstrated the value of yeast to unravel PCD mechanisms-related to human genes. Transformation of mutant *DFNA5* (mut*DFNA5*) in yeast led to the induction of PCD. Several mitochondrial proteins, such as Fis1, Por1, Aac1 and Aac3, were shown to be involved. Moreover, mutDFNA5 was found to co-localize with a mitochondrial marker protein (Westermann and Neupert, 2000). These former observations established a role for mitochondria in DFNA5-related cell death in yeast and demonstrated the value of yeast as a model organism to unravel DFNA5-related (mitochondrial) HL.

In the current study, we performed a transcriptomic analysis and confirmed the significance of mitochondria in *DFNA5*-induced cell death in *Saccharomyces cerevisiae*. Additionally, Gene Ontology (GO) analysis suggested a role for the endoplasmic reticulum (ER). The latter observation was not only present in *Saccharomyces cerevisiae*, but was also confirmed in human cell lines. Furthermore, we show that the MAPK pathways, namely the induction of the extracellular signal regulated kinase (ERK) and c-Jun N-terminal kinase (JNK), are activated upon mut*DFNA5* transfection in human cell lines. Our data suggest the presence of a cellular adaptive response related to mitochondria, MAPK pathways and potentially for the ER. The exact correlation between those processes and DFNA5 remains unclear but further study will lead to a better understanding of DFNA5-induced cell death mechanisms and to HL-related to mitochondrial damage in general.

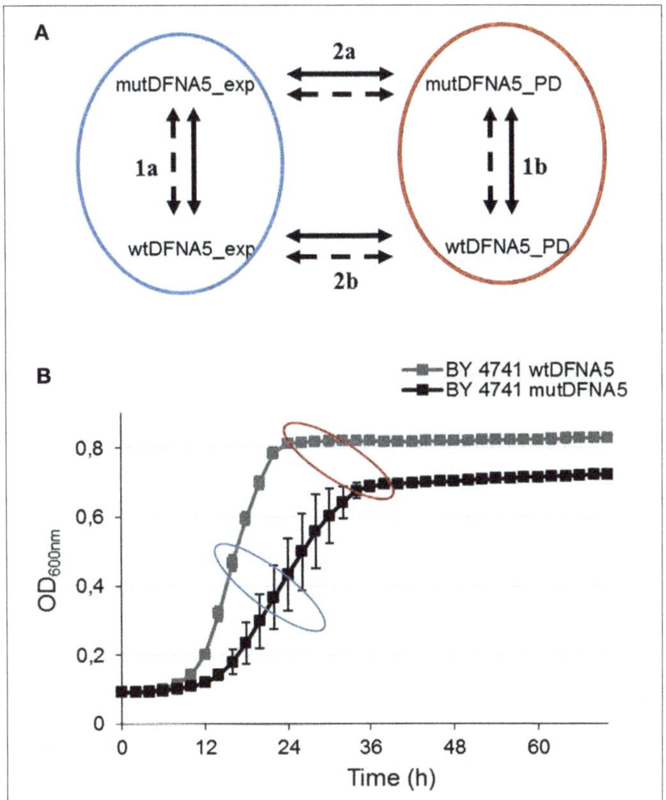

FIGURE 1 | Yeast microarray design. (A) Illustration of the different comparisons that were made between the RNA samples. RNA was collected from yeast strains transformed with either wt*DFNA5* or mut*DFNA5* at two different time-points. The bold and dashed lines represent the color flip of each RNA sample. **(B)** Growth profile of the *Saccharomyces cerevisiae* BY4741 background strain transformed with either wt*DFNA5* (gray squares) or mut*DFNA5* (black squares). The blue and red ellipse illustrate respectively the mid-exponential and post-diauxic time-points when RNA was collected.

Material and Methods

Yeast

Yeast Strains and Growth Conditions

In this study, we used the BY4741 (MATa his3Δ1 leu2Δ0 met15Δ0 ura3Δ0) wild-type strain (Brachmann et al., 1998). Full-length cDNA of either wt*DFNA5* or mut*DFNA5* was isolated and amplified as previously described (Gregan et al., 2003). Amplified products were ligated into yeast pYX212 plasmid containing an HA-marker (Clontech, Mountain View, CA, USA) using *EcoRI* and *BamHI* restriction sites. All constructs were verified by bidirectional sequencing on an ABI genetic analyser 3130 × l (AppliedBiosystems, FosterCity, CA, USA).

Yeast strains were grown at 30°C in selective medium containing 2% glucose (SD-URA). Fifty milliliter yeast cultures, transformed with either wt*DFNA5* or mut*DFNA5*, were harvested in mid-exponential phase ($OD_{600nm} = 3.5 - 4.2$) and at the post-diauxic shift ($OD_{600nm} = 7.4 - 8.4$) (**Figure 1**). Standard transformation techniques were applied for these transformations (Gietz et al., 1992).

RNA Extraction Yeast

RNA was collected from yeast at mid-exponential phase and just after the post-diauxic shift using RNA pure kit following the manufactures instructions (GenHunter® Corporation, Nashville, TN, USA). All steps were performed in duplo at 4°C to avoid RNA degradation. This resulted in eight different RNA samples: mid-exponential wt*DFNA5*, (WT_E1 and WT_E2), mid-exponential mut*DFNA5* (Mut_E1 and Mut_E2), post-diauxic wt*DFNA5* (WT_S1 and WT_S2), and post-diauxic mut*DFNA5* (Mut_S1 and Mut_S2) (**Figure 1**).

Microarray Design and Analysis

Microarray experiments were performed at the VIB Nucleomics Core (www.nucleomics.be). Before labeling, RNA concentration and purity were determined spectrophotometrically using the Nanodrop ND-1000 (Nanodrop Technologies). RNA integrity was assessed using a Bioanalyzer 2100 (Agilent). Per sample, an amount of 1 μg of total RNA spiked with 10 viral polyA transcript controls (Agilent, Santa Clara, CA, USA) was converted to double stranded cDNA in a reverse transcription reaction. Subsequently, the samples were converted to antisense cRNA, amplified and labeled with Cyanine 3-CTP (Cy3) or Cyanine 5-CTP (Cy5) in an *in vitro* transcription reaction according to the manufacturer's protocol (Agilent, Santa Clara, CA, USA). A mixture of purified and labeled cRNA (Cy3 label: 5 pmol; Cy5 label: 3.5 pmol) was hybridized on Agilent Yeastv2 arrays followed by washing, according to the manufacturer's procedures. To assess the raw probe signal intensities, arrays were scanned using the Agilent DNA MicroArray Scanner and probe signals were quantified using Agilent's Feature Extractor software (version 10.5.1.1).

In total four different comparisons were made. Each comparison was done in duplo by a color flip. The different comparisons are shown in **Figure 1A**. Gene expressions of strains transformed with wt*DFNA5* were compared to strains transformed with mut*DFNA5*, both in mid-exponential phase (comparison 1a) and at the post-diauxic shift (comparison 1b). Additionally, comparisons were made between the mid-exponential and the post-diauxic shift of either wt*DFNA5*-(comparison 2b) or mut*DFNA5*-(comparison 2a) transformed cells.

Analysis of the microarray data was performed using the R package LIMMA (http://www.bioconductor.org) (Gentleman et al., 2004). Fold changes were computed using raw Cy3 and Cy5 intensities values provided by Agilent's Feature Extractor software (version 10.5.1.1) and loess normalization and background correction were performed to determine the log2-ratios per array. Differential expression was assessed via the moderated t-statistic, described in (Smyth, 2004). To control the false discovery rate, multiple testing correction was performed. This generated four differentially expressed gene lists. All the (raw) data files have been completely uploaded to the gene expression omnibus and have been stored under accession number GSE70169.

HEK293T Cells

Cell Culture and Growth Conditions

The microarray experiments in human cell lines were performed using Human Embryonic Kidney 293T cells (HEK293T). HEK293T cells were subcultured in 60 mm dishes at a density of 2×10^6 cells in Dulbecco's modified Eagle's medium containing 4500 mg/L glucose supplemented with 10% (v/v) fetal calf serum, 100 U/ml penicillin, 100 µg/ml streptomycin, and 2 mM L-glutamine. Overnight cultures were transfected with either control (empty EGFP vector), wt*DFNA5* or mut*DFNA5* using lipofectamine. Six hours post transfection, cells were harvested using Triple-x reagent for RNA extraction. All products for human cell line cultures were obtained from Invitrogen (San Diego, CA, USA). Full-length cDNA of either wt*DFNA5* or mut*DFNA5* was isolated and amplified as previously described (Gregan et al., 2003).

RNA Extraction

An RNeasy mini kit was used for RNA extraction from transfected HEK293T cells (Qiagen, Hilden, Germany) at different time-points. For the microarray experiment, RNA was extracted 12 h post-transfection. For the gene analysis by real time rtPCR, RNA was extracted at either 3, 6, 12, 15, 18, 20, or 24 h post-transfection. For the microarray experiment, the integrity of the resulting RNA was checked on an automated Experion electrophoresis system (Biorad, Hercules, CA, USA).

Microarray Design and Analysis

The "Totalprep RNA Amplification" kit was used to amplify the RNA samples (Illumina, Ambion, Austin, TX, USA). Doublestranded-cDNA was generated from the mRNA fractions followed by an *in vitro* transcription reaction which produced cRNA strands containing biotin-UTP nucleotides. Seven Hundred Fifty nano gram of the resulting cRNA samples were hybridized to an Illumina human HT12v3 beadchip (Illumina, San Diego, CA, USA).

Six independent biological replicates were used for either wt*DFNA5*- or mut*DFNA5*-transfected HEK293T cells and loaded on the chip. Overnight hybridization at 58°C was followed by washing and streptavidin-Cy3 dye labeling (Amersham, Buckinghamshire, England). An Illumina Iscan equipped with Iscan control software was used to measure the intensity values and XY coordinates for every probe on the array. The resulting data files were then analyzed using the R package "Beadarray v1.14.0" (Dunning et al., 2007) followed by a quality control and quantile normalization. LIMMA v3.2.1 was used for the further analysis of the normalized intensity values to determine the differentially expressed genes (Smyth, 2004).

All the (raw) data files have been completely uploaded to the gene expression omnibus and have been stored under accession number GSE70169.

Real Time rtPCR

To confirm the results obtained from the microarray data in HEK293T cells, gene expression was studied in human HEK293T cell lines using Power SYBR Green RNA-to CT 1 Step Kit (Invitrogen, San Diego, CA, USA). Each reaction mixture contained 200 nM final primer concentration (primer pairs are shown in Supplemental Data Table 1) and 30 ng RNA template. All reactions were performed in triplicate on a LightCycler 480 system (Roche, Basel, Switzerland) and resulting data were analyzed by Qbase plus (Biogazelle, Ghent, Belgium). Three housekeeping genes were used each time as a reference, namely *GAPDH*, *RPL13A*, and *YWHAZ*.

Western Blot Analysis

For western blotting, cells were lysed using RIPA buffer (25 mM Tris-HCl (pH 7.6), 150 mM NaCl, 1% NP-40, 1% sodium deoxycholate, 0.1% SDS) (Pierce, Rockford, IL, USA) containing a PhosSTOP Phosphatase Inhibitor Cocktail Tablet (Roche), an EDTA-free protease tablet and 10 µl (25 units/µl) benzonase (70746-4 Novagen®, Merck Millipore, Darmstadt, Germany). Transfected HEK293T cells were lysed for 20′ at 4°C and centrifugated at 2000 g at 4°C to obtain protein lysates.

Proteins were electrophoretically separated and blotted onto a nitrocellulose membrane (Whatman, Kent, UK). This membrane was blocked for 1 h in 5% non-fat dry milk and afterwards incubated overnight (4°C) in one of the following primary antibodies: anti-phospho-SAPK/JNK (Thr183/Tyr185, #4668), anti-phospho-p44/42 (ERK1/2, #4370), anti-SAPK/JNK (#9252), anti-p44/42 (ERK1/2, #9102) (Cell Signaling Technologies, MA, USA), or anti-β-Actin (A5316, Sigma Aldrich, MO, USA). After washing, the membranes were incubated with either a secondary goat anti-rabbit (ab6721, Abcam, Cambridge, UK) or sheep anti-mouse (NA931, GE Healthcare, Buckingmersham, UK) antibody. Finally, the corresponding proteins were visualized using Enhanced ChemiLuminescence Western Blotting Substrate (Thermo Scientific, IL, USA).

MAPK Inhibition

The SP600125 JNK inhibitor was used to inhibit the MAPK pathway. Twelve hours post-transfection, HEK293T cells were incubated with 25 μM for 12 h. Next, cells were collected and viability was measured by flow cytometry (CyflowML, Partec, Germany) using propidium iodide as a cell death marker.

Gene Ontology Analysis

In addition to the determination of the differentially expressed genes, GO analysis was performed in order to identify enriched GO annotations. We used an open-source application, the Ontologizer, as a tool to statistically analyse the high-throughput data (Ashburner et al., 2000). A standard method for statistics, the "Term-for-Term analysis," was used followed by Benjamini-Hochberg correction for multiple testing (Hochberg and Benjamini, 1990; Tavazoie et al., 1999). Differentially expressed genes with a corrected *p*-value below 0.05 and a log2 (fold change) of 1.5 and 0.5 in yeast and human cell lines respectively, were selected for this analysis.

Results

To study the biological pathways of cell death induced by *DFNA5* in *S. cerevisiae*, we performed a transcriptomic study. RNA samples were collected in duplo in the mid-exponential phase and at the post-diauxic shift of yeast cells transformed with either wt*DFNA5* of mut*DFNA5*. **Figure 1** shows all the comparisons studied between the different RNA samples (comparisons are labeled 1a, 1b, 2a, and 2b). Analysis of the microarray data was performed using the LIMMA package provided in R and generated four lists of differentially expressed genes. For the GO-enriched term analysis, the cut-off for adjusted *p*-values of differentially expressed genes was set to 0.05 and the cut-off of the log2 (fold change) was respectively set to 1.5 and 0.5 for yeast and human cell lines.

Investigation of the differentially expressed genes in mid-exponential phase (comparison 1a) revealed no significantly up- or down-regulated genes. Therefore, this comparison was excluded and only comparisons 1b, 2a, and 2b (shown in **Figure 1**) will be taken into account and described.

Mitochondria-Related Processes are Up-Regulated in mutDFNA5 in Post-Diauxic Shift

Comparison of the differentially expressed genes (adjusted $p < 0.05$) in the post-diauxic shift (1b) resulted in 451 significantly up-regulated genes when expressing mut*DFNA5* and using wt*DFNA5* as a reference. The top 34 differentially up-regulated genes at the post-diauxic shift are shown in **Table 1**. Differentially expressed genes with a log2 (fold change) equal or higher than 1.5 were selected for GO-enriched annotations, generating 85 significantly up-regulated genes, which resulted in 65 significantly up-regulated enriched GO terms.

Analysis of the biological, cellular, and molecular GO annotations confirmed the role of the mitochondria in mut*DFNA5*-induced cell death (Supplemental Data Table 2, indicated in bold). Analysis of the GO annotations revealed that the molecular cytochrome-c oxidase activity (GO: 0004129) related process was the most significantly up-regulated mitochondrial process. Further down the list, several biological, molecular and cellular GO processes related to mitochondrial mechanisms, such as mitochondrial ATP synthesis-coupled electron transport (GO:0042775), aerobic respiration (GO:0009060), the mitochondrial respiratory chain (GO:0005746), mitochondrial respiratory chain complex IV (GO:0005751), and oxidative phosphorylation (GO:0006119) were significantly up-regulated suggesting mitochondrial dysfunction (Supplemental Data Table 2).

Next we compared the identified GO terms with the list containing the highest differentially up-regulated genes generated by the R package LIMMA to evaluate the resemblances (**Table 1**). As shown in **Table 1**, several mitochondrial genes related to these GO processes were indeed present in the list, including *COX/1/2/3* and *AI5_ALPHA* (**Table 1**, bold). COX1/2/3 are three main subunits of cytochrome c oxidase, the terminal enzyme of the mitochondrial electron transport chain, encoded by the mitochondrial genome. The electron transport chain is part of mitochondrial oxidative phosphorylation providing most of the cellular ATP (Srinivasan and Avadhani, 2012). *AI5_ALPHA* is an endonuclease encoding a mobile intron of the *COXI* gene (Moran et al., 1992; Seraphin et al., 1992). Up-regulation of the main *COX* genes suggests enhanced COX activity, which has been associated with increased oxidative stress (Singh et al., 2009; Srinivasan and Avadhani, 2012). Previous data indeed demonstrated a change in redox homeostasis due to mut*DFNA5* expression in yeast (Van Rossom et al., 2012). The same study also showed increased oxidative stress measured by a dihydroethidium bromide staining (DHE). Moreover, preliminary experiments in human cell lines confirmed this and also revealed enhanced oxidative stress measured by a DHE staining (unpublished results).

In addition, two other groups of significantly enriched GO annotations could be distinguished, namely GO annotations related to catabolic and metabolic energy processes, such as oligosaccharide catabolic process (GO:0009313) or maltose catabolic processes (GO:0000025), and mechanisms related to transporter activity, such as cation (GO:0008324) and several sugar (GO:0005353 for example) transmembrane activities (Supplemental Data Table 2, respectively underlined and indicated in blue). Consistent with the previous results, comparison of these processes with the highest differentially up-regulated genes in **Table 1** confirmed these identified GO terms (**Table 1**). Different maltose and sucrose genes like *MAL12*, *MAL32*, and *SUC2*, and transmembrane transporter genes like *HXT4/7* were present in the list (**Table 1**).

TABLE 1 | Top 34 of the differentially up-regulated genes upon transfection of mut*DFNA5* in yeast at the post-diauxic shift.

Gene name	LogFC	AveExpr	adj.p.val	Gene name	LogFC	AveExpr	adj.p.val
MAL12	4.16	9.08	0.04	YOL047C	2.39	10.40	0.01
COX3	4.13	7.46	< 0.01	Q0297	2.38	7.24	0.01
MAL32	3.91	8.19	0.04	MND1	2.27	7.03	0.01
ANB1	3.60	9.59	0.01	VAR1	2.23	4.18	0.02
SLZ1	3.08	6.38	< 0.01	YPL141C	2.22	9.49	0.01
PRM7	3.07	11.62	0.01	HXT4	2.22	13.42	0.05
YPR077C	3.05	9.44	< 0.01	YNR034W-A	2.20	13.88	0.02
PRM7	3.04	11.01	0.01	YDR034W-B	2.17	9.17	0.02
HXT7	3.02	14.80	0.03	**COX2**	2.16	6.19	0.01
YDR374C	2.94	6.69	0.02	OLI1	2.15	15.96	< 0.01
YPL014W	2.89	8.59	0.02	YBL065W	2.15	6.87	0.01
AI5_ALPHA	2.89	10.49	0.04	SPR28	2.13	7.20	< 0.01
RTA1	2.83	7.90	< 0.01	**COX1**	2.12	7.77	0.01
YPR078C	2.65	7.06	< 0.01	DRE2	2.05	12.58	0.01
YLR194C	2.45	13.79	0.01	YKR075C	2.01	13.64	< 0.01
SUC2	2.44	11.79	0.04	YJL218W	2.00	6.92	0.04
SPO20	2.43	9.06	0.01	YLR338W	1.95	7.52	0.01

LogFC, logarithm of fold change, up-regulation in mutDFNA5 yeast samples using wtDFNA5 as a reference; adj.p.value, p-value adjusted for multiple hypothesis testing. Genes involved in processes related to the COX activity are indicated in bold.

These results revealed an important role for mitochondria-related processes in mut*DFNA5* transformed yeast cells in the post-diauxic shift.

Processes Associated with Glycolysis are Down-Regulated in *mutDFNA5* at Post-Diauxic Shift

To investigate the significantly down-regulated processes and genes in the post-diauxic shift between wtDFNA5 and mutDFNA5, we used the same method as described in Section Mitochondria-related Processes are Up-regulated in mutDFNA5 in Post-diauxic Shift. This revealed 585 significantly down-regulated genes in cells expressing mut*DFNA5* as compared to those expressing wt*DFNA5* (adjusted $p < 0.05$). The top 34 highest differentially down-regulated genes are shown in **Table 2**.

The significantly down-regulated biological GO annotations can be divided in two main groups (Supplemental Data Table 3). One group is related to ribosomal processes and hence translation such as cytosolic ribosome (GO:0022626) and the positive regulation of translation fidelity (GO:0045903) (Supplemental Data Table 3, indicated in bold). This down-regulation is probably due to the fact that yeast is entering the post-diauxic shift and that mutDFNA5 has a growth defect compared to wtDFNA5. Hence, this is probably not due to mut*DFNA5* expression. The second group was correlated with the biosynthesis and metabolism of glucose (GO:0006007), monosaccharide (GO:0046365) and glycolysis (GO:0006096).

Again, we compared the identified GO terms using the list containing the highest differentially down-regulated genes generated by the R package LIMMA to evaluate the resemblances (**Table 2**). As expected, this list contained several components associated with the glycolysis and several protein components of the small and large ribosomal subunit.

Interestingly, the list also contained several genes such as *TPI, TDH2/3, PGK1,* and *CDC19*, which are all enzymes playing a role in either the glycolytic or the pentose phosphate pathway (PPP) (**Table 2** indicated in bold). *CDC19* is the yeast homolog of the human pyruvate kinase (PK) gene. Down-regulation of PK has been correlated with the activation of the PPP and the redirection of the metabolic flux from glycolysis to PPP both in human cell lines and in yeast (Ralser et al., 2007; Christofk et al., 2008; Anastasiou et al., 2011). This will enhance the anti-oxidant response and hence increase the tolerance for oxidative stress (Ralser et al., 2007; Gruning et al., 2011; Kruger et al., 2011). The down-regulation of genes involved in glycolysis and the PPP could suggest a link with oxidative stress providing a protection mechanism for mut*DFNA5*-transformed yeast cells.

Induction of ER-Related Processes upon mutDFNA5 Expression in Yeast

In addition to the comparison of mut*DFNA5* and wt*DFNA5* in the post-diauxic shift, the modifications between mid-exponential phase and at the post-diauxic shift were investigated separately both in mut*DFNA5*-(comparison 2a **Figure 1**) and wt*DFNA5*-(comparison 2b **Figure 1**) transformed yeast cells. As both wtDFNA5 and mutDFNA5 cells demonstrated differentially expressed genes in exponential phase compared to post-diauxic shift, we expected the presence of many significantly up- or down regulated genes related to the post-diauxic shift but not solely due to mut*DFNA5* expression. Therefore, genes which were differentially expressed at the post-diauxic shift upon mut*DFNA5* transformation, but do not show any differences upon wt*DFNA5* expression in post-diauxic phase, are potentially related to mut*DFNA5*-associated processes. These were assigned as mut*DFNA5*-related changes not associated with the post-diauxic shift in yeast.

TABLE 2 | Top 34 of the differentially down-regulated genes upon transfection of mut*DFNA5* in yeast at the post-diauxic shift.

Gene name	LogFC	AveExpr	adj.p.val	Gene name	LogFC	AveExpr	adj.p.val
ENO2	−3.00	16.12	0.01	ERG25	−1.77	14.05	0.05
SSA2	−2.68	14.66	0.01	YNR021W	−1.74	11.30	< 0.01
VHT1	−2.54	13.48	0.02	YBT1	−1.73	12.67	0.05
DET1	−2.44	16.33	0.01	KAP122	−1.71	9.48	< 0.01
RPS22A	−2.44	14.70	< 0.01	**CDC19**	−1.71	16.94	0.02
PGK1	−2.39	16.90	0.01	YDR509W	−1.70	6.06	< 0.01
TDH3	−2.30	15.32	0.01	RPS9B	−1.67	15.08	< 0.01
TPI1	−2.06	17.08	0.01	GNP1	−1.64	12.19	0.01
PDC1	−2.05	16.95	0.03	FTR1	−1.61	13.04	0.04
TDH2	−2.02	14.26	0.01	GPD1	−1.61	13.24	0.05
YHR140W	−1.95	8.34	0.03	RPL16B	−1.61	15.38	0.01
TOS4	−1.94	10.23	0.05	YGR266W	−1.61	9.17	0.03
YRO2	−1.91	14.89	0.03	RPA43	−1.60	10.54	< 0.01
FBA1	−1.91	17.14	0.01	ARC1	−1.59	13.85	0.01
RPL9A	−1.90	14.27	0.03	PGI1	−1.58	16.09	0.03
RPL22A	−1.86	14.33	0.01	RPL18B	−1.57	9.61	0.01
URA7	−1.83	12.90	< 0.01	SPE3	−1.56	12.70	0.01

LogFC, logarithm of fold change, down-regulation in mutDFNA5 yeast samples using wtDFNA5 as a reference; adj.p.value, p-value adjusted for multiple hypothesis testing. Genes involved in processes related to the glycolysis or the pentose phosphate pathways are indicated in bold.

Genes with an adjusted *p*-value below 0.05 and a log2 (fold change) above 1.5 were selected for GO analysis. The GO-enriched processes significantly associated with up-regulated genes were very similar between comparison 2a and 2b and were associated with translation. GO-enriched terms significantly associated with down-regulated genes were related to ribosomes and RNA and were present both in wt*DFNA5*- and in mut*DFNA5*-transformed yeast cells. These processes were probably due to the shift to respiration and not in particular related to mut*DFNA5* (data not shown). However, three main classes could be distinguished at the post-diauxic shift. Two of them were more prominent in mut*DFNA5*-transformed yeast cells. One class was related to the biosynthesis and the metabolism of lipids (GO:0008610), such as (ergo)sterols (GO:0016126), (phyto)steroids (GO:0006694), and fatty acids (GO:0006633) (Supplemental Data Table 4, indicated in bold). The other group was associated with the ER (GO:0005783), such as the ER membrane (GO:0005789) and protein targeting to ER (GO: 0045047) (Supplemental Data Table 4, processes are underlined).

The third group which could be distinguished was related to the cytoskeleton (GO:0005856) and was more pronounced in wt*DFNA5*-transformed yeast cells. Cellularly enriched GO terms such as the microtubule cytoskeleton (GO:0015630) and the microtubule organizing center (GO:0005815) were present in this list (Supplemental Data Table 5, indicated in bold).

Association of DFNA5 with the MAPK-Related Mechanisms in HEK293T Cells

To further elucidate the *DFNA5*-related pathways, a microarray experiment was performed in human HEK293T cells. As described previously, mut*DFNA5* induced a growth defect in transfected HEK293T cells compared to wt*DFNA5* and control (cells transfected with an empty vector) (Op de Beeck et al., 2011). These cell death events were evident from 9 h post-transfection and peaked at 12 h (data not shown). Therefore RNA samples of HEK293T cells were collected 12 h post-transfection. A transcriptomic analysis was performed on HEK293T cells transfected with either wt*DFNA5* or mut*DFNA5*. Six biological replicates of every RNA sample were collected although one wt*DFNA5*-transfected sample did not survive quality control. Subsequent analyses, using wt*DFNA5* as a reference, were therefore performed on five wt*DFNA5*- vs. six mut*DFNA5*-transfected samples. Analysis using "Beadarray" and "LIMMA" packages available in R identified 228 significantly up- and 222 significantly down-regulated genes after correction for multiple hypothesis testing ($p < 0.05$). In addition to individual gene expression, GO analysis was performed to determine the biologically, cellularly, and molecularly enriched GO annotations linked to the differentially expressed genes.

Table 3 shows the top 34 of the significantly up-regulated genes. It contains several genes related to the MAPK pathway such as *EGR1/2, FOSB,* and*JUNB* (indicated in bold). Interestingly, this list also contained the *PMAIP1* gene. *PMAIP1* encodes a BH3-only protein belonging to the BCL2 protein family, a family of important regulators of apoptotic cell death related to the mitochondria. The top 34 highest down-regulated genes are shown in **Table 4** and contains several genes related to protein folding such as *HSPA6, ATF3,* and *CTH* (indicated in bold, **Table 4**).

Subsequent GO analysis of the biological annotations revealed, in addition to the more general development processes,

TABLE 3 | Top 34 of the significantly up-regulated genes in mut*DFNA5* transfected HEK293T cells.

Gene symbol	logFC	AveExpr	adj.p.val	Gene symbol	logFC	AveExpr	adj.p.val
ZCCHC12	2.63	12.07	<0.01	**PMAIP1 (2750367)**	1.00	10.76	<0.01
ETV5	1.88	9.11	<0.01	ETV4	0.99	7.71	<0.01
LOC387763	1.86	10.00	<0.01	SPRY2	0.97	9.96	<0.01
EGR1	1.83	11.82	<0.01	**PMAIP1 (6020598)**	0.96	9.30	<0.01
ARC	1.61	8.76	<0.01	CCNA1	0.94	7.60	<0.01
FOSB	1.58	8.85	<0.01	TRIM9	0.92	10.00	<0.01
KCTD12	1.40	10.32	<0.01	MAFF	0.90	7.95	<0.01
JUNB	1.40	9.09	<0.01	FAM84B	0.90	12.04	<0.01
ADAMTS1	1.24	9.88	<0.01	EPHA2	0.89	7.98	<0.01
EGR2	1.19	8.12	<0.01	CYP1B1	0.88	8.52	<0.01
FOS	1.18	10.17	<0.01	NDRG1	0.87	9.54	<0.01
CITED1	1.16	11.66	<0.01	SERTAD1	0.85	10.14	<0.01
MAFB	1.12	9.32	<0.01	MCL1	0.81	10.20	<0.01
GPR3	1.07	8.29	<0.01	SPRY4	0.81	7.66	<0.01
TNFRSF12A	1.06	9.77	<0.01	VGF	0.79	8.30	<0.01
TRIB1	1.04	11.60	<0.01	NEFM	0.79	11.58	<0.01
ANXA1	1.03	8.98	<0.01	GEM	0.79	7.88	<0.01

LogFC, logarithm of fold change, down-regulation in mutDFNA5 yeast samples using wtDFNA5 as a reference; adj.p.value, p-value adjusted for multiple hypothesis testing. The array address of the specific splice variant on the microarray is provided between parentheses. Genes involved in processes related to either the MAPK pathway, cAMP response or the mitochondria are indicated in bold.

TABLE 4 | Top 34 of the highest significantly down-regulated genes in mut*DFNA5* transfected HEK293T cells.

Gene symbol	logFC	AveExpr	adj.p.val	Gene symbol	logFC	AveExpr	adj.p.val
HSPA6 (160092)	−1.54	10.49	<0.01	HRK	−0.64	8.82	<0.01
DDIT4	−1.26	10.18	<0.01	C5orf13	−0.64	9.27	<0.01
CLEC2D	−0.97	9.47	<0.01	LRAP	−0.63	13.23	<0.01
ZNF256	−0.91	9.10	<0.01	CLEC2D	−0.61	14.72	<0.01
TDP1	−0.87	10.90	<0.01	GUSBL1	−0.60	10.04	<0.01
LRP5L	−0.84	8.76	<0.01	DTL	−0.60	10.17	<0.01
CTH (60138)	−0.80	10.40	<0.01	ZSCAN16	−0.58	8.66	<0.01
SNORD15B	−0.78	8.76	<0.01	**CTH (1470576)**	−0.58	8.75	<0.01
C17orf48	−0.76	8.45	<0.01	LOC654194	−0.58	13.17	<0.01
LOC389816	−0.73	8.57	<0.01	SNORD68	−0.58	10.17	<0.01
HSPA6 (1710553)	−0.71	9.28	<0.01	ZNF205	−0.57	7.83	<0.01
ZMAT3	−0.70	12.59	<0.01	ZNF416	−0.57	8.56	<0.01
PMS2L3	−0.67	8.69	<0.01	LRRC26	−0.57	8.19	<0.01
PCDHGA9	−0.66	7.61	<0.01	Hs.537645	−0.57	7.54	<0.01
CTH (6220504)	−0.65	8.29	<0.01	**ATF3 (4780128)**	−0.56	11.95	<0.01
C3orf34	−0.64	12.64	<0.01	ACOT2	−0.55	9.15	<0.01
FANCE	−0.64	9.35	<0.01	PCK2	−0.55	9.22	<0.01

LogFC, logarithm of fold change, down-regulation in mutDFNA5 yeast samples using wtDFNA5 as a reference; adj.p.value, p-value adjusted for multiple hypothesis testing. The array address of the specific splice variant on the microarray is provided between parentheses. Genes involved in processes related to protein folding are indicated in bold.

the up-regulation of the MAPK pathway (GO:0043407) and the cAMP response (GO:0051591) (Supplemental Data Table 6, indicated in bold). The response to protein folding (GO:0006986) and to topologically incorrect protein (GO:0035966) were the only two significantly down-regulated processes and both were related to protein folding (Supplemental Data Table 7). The most important genes that are involved in these processes were *HSPA6*, a heat shock protein and several chaperones proteins, such as *DNAJB1* and *DNAJB2*.

These results demonstrate the association of mut*DFNA5*-induced cell death with the MAPK pathways. The identification of processes related to protein folding supports the results in yeast in which GO terms related to protein folding and the ER were significantly associated with mutDFNA5.

Validation of the MAPK Role in DFNA5-Related Cell Death in HEK293T Cells

The data generated by the transcriptomic analysis in HEK293T cells were validated by real-time rtPCR of newly collected RNA samples. *EGR1* and *FOSB* gene expression was investigated on different time-points ranging from 3 to 72 h post-transfection. As shown in **Figure 2**, significantly up-regulated *EGR1* and *FOSB* gene expression was observed in cells transfected with mut*DFNA5* from 12 to 18 h post transfection ($p < 0.05$) (**Figure 2**). Hence the data generated by the transcriptomic analyses were indeed confirmed by real time rtPCR as demonstrated by up-regulation of genes related to the MAPK pathway.

After confirmation by real time rtPCR, the significance of the activated MAPK pathway was further validated by two independent experiments. To investigate the significance of the MAPK pathway, we wondered whether inhibition of the MAPK pathway would attenuate this mutDFNA5-induced growth defect.

Therefore, a specific JNK inhibitor, namely SP600125, was added, followed by a viability assay to determine the effect on cell survival. Different concentrations of the JNK inhibitor SP600125 were used to measure viability by flow cytometry (CyFlow ML, Partec, Germany) and these results were compared to untreated mut*DFNA5*-transfected HEK293T cells. Overnight treatment of the cells with different concentrations of SP600125 did not have any major effect on transfection efficiency, but significantly increased the viability of mut*DFNA5*-transfected cells. Although, addition of 12.5 and 25 μM SP600125 both significantly increased the viability with a *p*-value of 0.020 and 0.004 respectively SP600125 had the greatest effect with a concentration of 25 μM SP600125 since the viability was raised from 31.93 to 51.00% (**Figure 3**).

Next, to evaluate the effect of MAPK up-regulation on protein level, different MAPK proteins were studied by western blotting. There are three main MAPK pathways in human cell lines represented by the ERK, JNK, and p38 MAPK branch. Consistent with the results obtained by real time rtPCR and the viability assay, activation of the MAPK pathway proteins was also demonstrated by western blotting. Total protein lysates were collected from HEK293T cells 12 h post-transfection. Three phosphorylated (activated) and non-phosphorylated (not activated) proteins of the MAPK pathway were studied using six different antibodies. No differences were seen in the expression level of non-phosphorylated ERK and JNK (**Figure 4A**). Activation of JNK and to a minor extent of ERK (p42/p44) was seen upon mut*DFNA5* transfection compared to control and wt*DFNA5* (**Figure 4B**). The expression of p38 was also evaluated but no difference in protein expression was observed between mutDFNA5 compared to wtDFNA5 and control (data not shown). β-Actin was used as a loading control.

These results suggest that DFNA5 induces PCD mediated through activation of the MAPK pathways. Addition of a MAPK inhibitor partially attenuated the mutDFNA5-induced growth defect identifying the MAPK pathway as an early event in mutDFNA5-associated cell death.

Comparison of the Yeast Microarray Results with the Gene Expression in Human Cell Lines

In order to study the significance of the yeast results, a comparison was made between the two microarray experiments. Human homologs of the significantly up- and down-regulated yeast genes at the post-diauxic shift (comparison 1b) were identified using Ensemble Biomart. Of the 451 significantly up- and 585 significantly down-regulated yeast genes, respectively 296 and 647 human homologs were identified. These specific human homologs were analyzed using the R package LIMMA, which generated a new list of human genes. The FC cut-off of the resulting gene list was set to FC 1.2, resulting in 16 up- and 14 down-regulated human genes (Supplemental Tables 8A,B). *TM7SF2, UCP2,* and *VPS33B*, three down-regulated human genes, were selected to verify the yeast results in human cell lines using real-time rtPCR. *UCP2* and *VPS33B* were evaluated because they were the two most down-regulated genes present in

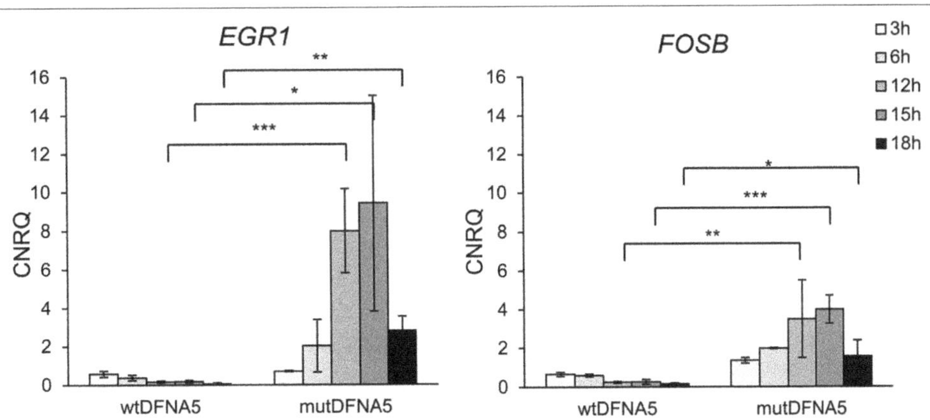

FIGURE 2 | Increased *EGR1* and *FOSB* gene expression in mut*DFNA5*-transfected HEK293T cells. RNA samples were collected from HEK293T cells transfected with either wt*DFNA5* or mut*DFNA5* and gene expression was measured by real-time rtPCR. Significantly increased expression was seen in mut*DFNA5* at 12 h [p(egr1) = 0.000; p(fosB) = 0.006], 15 h [p(egr1) = 0.017; p(fosB) = 0.000] and 18 h [p(egr1) = 0.004; p(fosB) = 0.026] post-transfection. *$p < 0.05$; **$p < 0.01$; ***$p < 0.001$. CNRQ, calibrated normalized relative quantities.

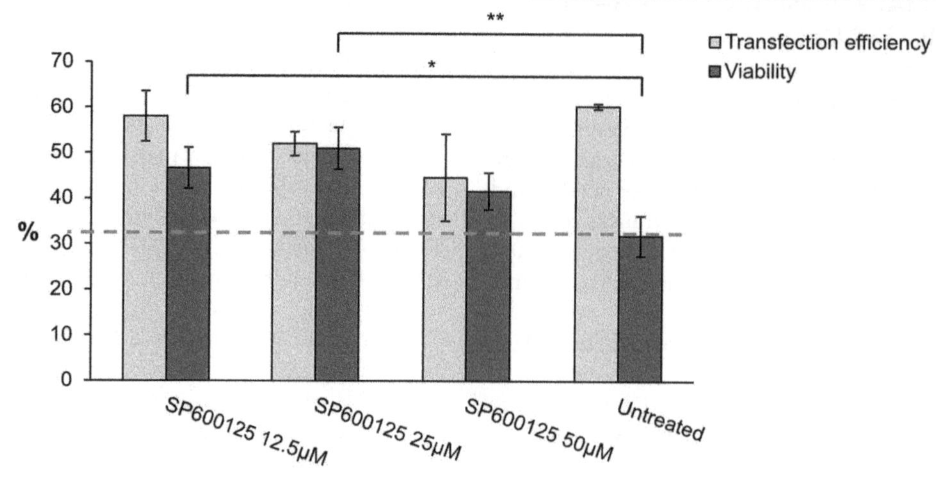

FIGURE 3 | MAPK inhibitor effect on mut*DFNA5* transfected HEK293T cells. Mut*DFNA5*-transfected HEK293T cells were pretreated with different amounts of SP600125 (JNK inhibitor). Cell viability was measured and compared to untreated mut*DFNA5*-transfected HEK293T cells. $^{*}p < 0.05$; $^{**}p < 0.01$.

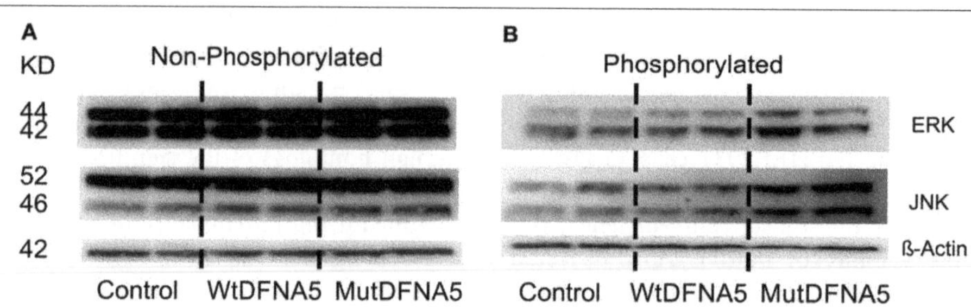

FIGURE 4 | Activation of the MAPK pathway by mutDFNA5. (A) Western blot analysis of non- phosphorylated ERK (p42/p42) and JNK. No differences were seen in protein expression level of ERK and JNK between control, wtDFNA5 and mutDFNA5 transfected HEK293T cells. **(B)** Western blot analysis of phosphorylated, activated ERK (p42/p42) and JNK. Increased expression of JNK and to a lesser extent of ERK was seen in mutDFNA5 transfected HEK293T cells as compared to wtDFNA5 and control.

the list. UCP2, an uncoupling protein, is a mitochondrial carrier located at the mitochondrial inner membrane. Suppression of UCP2 has been linked to increased ROS production (Deng et al., 2012; Dando et al., 2013) and lifespan regulation (Andrews and Horvath, 2009; Andrews, 2010). The Vacuolar protein sorting 33 homolog (VPS33B) gene is involved in intracellular vesicle Golgi-to-lysosome transport (Pevsner et al., 1996; Lo et al., 2005). *TM7SF2* was selected based on its function in relation to the yeast results. TM7SF2 is a transmembrane protein present in the ER and associated with biosynthesis of cholesterol. In addition to its role in cholesterol synthesis, TM7SF2 appears to be involved in the inflammatory response upon cellular stress (Holmer et al., 1998; Bennati et al., 2006; Schiavoni et al., 2010; Bellezza et al., 2013).

To verify the yeast results in human cell lines, RNA was collected from HEK293T cells transfected with either wt*DFNA5* or mut*DFNA5* at different time-points starting at 12 h after transfection as this was the time-point of the human microarray experiment. The *TM7SF2, UCP2,* and *VPS33B* genes had a fold change of respectively 1.23, 1.31, and 1.27 on the microarray. Real-time rtPCR on RNA samples 12 h post-transfection confirmed these microarray results as all three genes were down-regulated in mut*DFNA5* compared to wt*DFNA5* (**Figure 5A**) with fold changes comparable to the microarray (respectively 1.35, 1.48, and 1.59). Although not significantly, these three genes were down-regulated in HEK293T cells at 12 h after transfection (**Figure 5A**). The down-regulation was still present at 20 h, peaked at 24 h after transfection and was even significant for TM7SF2 (p:0.01) and UCP2 (p:0.07) at respectively 20 h and 24 h after transfection (**Figure 5B**). Due to this down-regulation, we can conclude that there are some similarities between the yeast and the HEK293T microarray. Differences are seen when looking at the individual genes, but upon study of the different pathways a role for processes related to protein folding were seen in both model systems.

Discussion

This study further investigated the biological effects induced by *DFNA5* expression in *Saccharomyces cerevisiae* and in human HEK293T cells. A previous study in human cell lines revealed that mut*DFNA5* is a cell death-inducing gene (Op de Beeck et al., 2011). As described previously (Van Rossom et al., 2012), transformation of mut*DFNA5* in yeast resulted in a growth defect

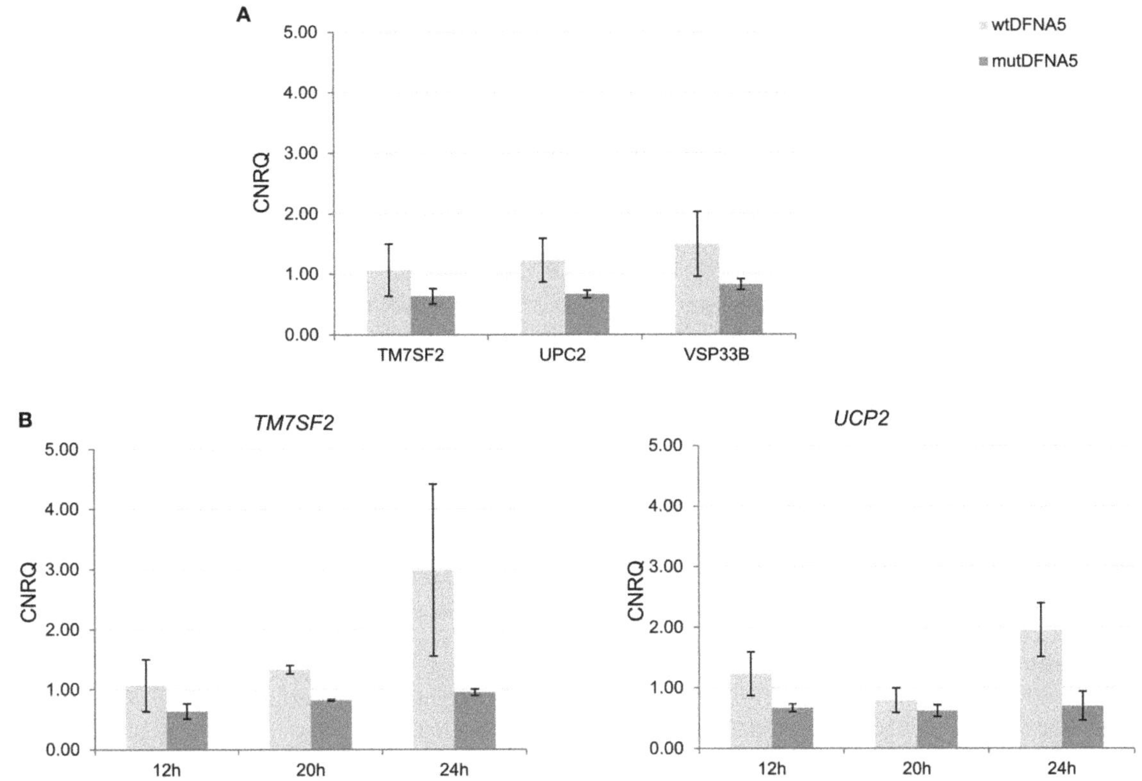

FIGURE 5 | Validation of the yeast microarray by real-time rtPCR in HEK293T cells. (A) Gene expression 12 h post-transfection in human HEK293T cells of three selected genes. **(B)** Gene expression 12, 20, and 24 h post-transfection with either wt*DFNA5* or mutant *DFNA5*. *UCP2*, uncoupling protein 2 (mitochondrial, proton carrier); *TM7SF2*, transmembrane 7 superfamily member 2; *VPS33B*, vacuolar protein sorting 33 homolog. Light gray, wt*DFNA5*; Dark gray, mut*DFNA5*. $^*p < 0.05$. CNRQ, calibrated normalized relative quantities.

associated with four different mitochondria-related proteins. This study was the first to establish a possible link between the mitochondria and DFNA5. In addition, the 2012 study observed that the protein quality control system, responsible for correct protein folding and degradation, had problems coping with mutDFNA5. A failing protein quality control system could indicate the presence of ER stress, as the ER can be involved in protein folding and degradation.

This study confirmed the involvement of mitochondria-related processes upon expression of mut*DFNA5* in *Saccharomyces cerevisiae*, especially the ATP-coupled electron transport. Several genes related to either the glycolysis and the PPP were significantly down-regulated upon mut*DFNA5* transformation in yeast. Furthermore, we show that the JNK and ERK MAPK pathways are activated *in vitro* after transfection of mut*DFNA5* in HEK293T cells and that inhibition of this pathway is able to partially attenuate the resulting cell death. Additionally, this study also revealed an association of GO annotations related to the ER and protein folding in both model organisms.

Oxidative Stress and Hearing Loss

The up-regulation of different cytochrome c oxidase (*COX*) genes revealed a potential association of the mutDFNA5-related cell death mechanisms with oxidative stress in yeast. Increased oxidative stress was already demonstrated in yeast (Van Rossom et al., 2012) and was later confirmed in human cell lines (unpublished results). Enhanced COX activity has indeed been associated with increased oxidative stress (Singh et al., 2009; Srinivasan and Avadhani, 2012). COX is the rate limiting enzyme of respiration which regulates the bio-energetic status of the cell. Dependent on the cellular energetic requirements, the COX activity can be rapidly adapted. The ratio of ATP/ADP is one of the regulators of the COX activity. High ADP levels or ATP utilization will increase the enzyme activity and stimulate the respiration (Napiwotzki and Kadenbach, 1998; Arnold and Kadenbach, 1999). Activation of the COX activity could result in higher oxidative stress generated at the mitochondria.

Additionally, the correlation of mutDFNA5 with several genes of the PPP can also be linked to oxidative stress in yeast as the PPP plays a major role in the anti-oxidant response. Reduced expression of *CDC19*, the yeast homolog of PK, and of *TPI* has been correlated with the activation of the PPP and the redirection of the metabolic flux from glycolysis to PPP both in human cell lines and in yeast (Christofk et al., 2008; Gruning et al., 2011, 2014). This study revealed reduced gene expression of both *TPI* and *CDC19*, indicating a shift in redox sensing in eukaryotes mediating a fast response to oxidative stress. Activation of the PPP is correlated with the inhibition of ROS accumulation and enhancement of the anti-oxidant response upon shift from fermentation to respiration. PPP activation will enhance the anti-oxidant response and hence increase the tolerance for oxidative stress (Ralser et al., 2007; Gruning et al., 2011; Kruger et al., 2011). These data clearly demonstrate a change in redox homeostasis due to mut*DFNA5* expression which was shown previously in yeast (Van Rossom et al., 2012).

Furthermore, enhanced oxidative stress is often related to a failing protein quality control system (Davies, 2001; Shang et al., 2001; Bender et al., 2010, 2011; Shang and Taylor, 2011). This possibility was already suggested by the proteolytic degradation previously seen upon wt*DFNA5* transformation, but which was absent in mut*DFNA5*-transformed yeast cells (Van Rossom et al., 2012). MutDFNA5 seemed to escape this quality control system, in contrast to wtDFNA5 which was subject to the normal clearance system. Moreover, the authors suggested a possible link between protein degradation and the mitochondria in mutDFNA5-induced cell death as yeast seemed to have problems with proper mutDFNA5 protein turnover. The same link was confirmed in both model organisms used in the current study.

Role of ER Stress in the Pathology of Hearing Loss

The increase in mitochondrial metabolism seen in this study and the decrease of protein folding processes, can also be explained by the presence of cellular ER stress leading to an unfolded protein response. Mitochondria and ER form an interconnected network which is important for several biological processes mediating an adaptive response under various cellular stress conditions (De Brito and Scorrano, 2010; Marchi et al., 2014). The association between mutDFNA5 and the GO terms related to lipid metabolism, protein targeting to ER and the ER membrane, suggest the presence of ER stress (Schroder, 2008). Mitochondria depend on the ER for the import of several proteins and lipids and for Ca^{2+} exchange involved in cell death and mitochondrial metabolism (Sauner and Levy, 1971; Zecchini et al., 2007; Stiban et al., 2008; Wiel et al., 2014). Enhanced Ca^{2+} supply will increase ATP production and mitochondrial respiration, processes which were indeed both up-regulated at the post-diauxic shift upon mut*DFNA5* expression. Prolonged enhancement however will eventually have a detrimental effect on the mitochondria.

Despite limited knowledge correlating mutDFNA5 with ER stress, a correlation has been established between ER stress and certain causes of HL. Ototoxicity (HL due to the use of pharmaceuticals such as aminoglycoside antibiotics and platinum-based chemotherapeutics) was shown to be correlated with ER stress-dependent pathways. Certain pain relievers, contributing to tinnitus and progressive bilateral sensorineural HL, were shown to induce ROS overproduction, altered ER morphology and changes in ER stress markers, such as CHOP (Kalinec et al., 2014).

Taken together, the previous observation of the importance of the mitochondria in mutDFNA5-related cell death and the known correlation between the ER and the mitochondria points to a potential role for the ER in DFNA5-induced cell death. The failing of the protein quality control system in mutDFNA5 suggests the involvement of the ER, but this remains unclear at this moment and needs to be further investigated in the future.

Contribution of the Mitochondria in MAPK-Related Cell Death

In addition to the mitochondria, the MAPK pathways seem to play a prominent role in mutDFNA5-induced cell death in HEK293T cells. The link between the mitochondria and MAPK in DFNA5-related cell death is unknown at this moment, but several mitochondria-MAPK correlations have been described. It is known that MAPK pathways can be induced by ROS production generated by the mitochondria (Chambers and Lograsso, 2011). As increased oxidative stress has been shown in an earlier study in yeast and in human cell lines (unpublished results), this can provide a direct link between these two processes. This could suggest that ROS activates the MAPK pathway and hence lays up-stream of the MAPK pathway in DFNA5-induced cell death. However, we showed in this study that a specific MAPK inhibitor was able to attenuate the cell death and we have unpublished results showing that several anti-oxidants did not inhibit DFNA5-induced cell death. This implies that ROS is either a secondary event not directly causing cell death, or that the activation of MAPK is an early event in the cell death process, up-stream of ROS production. Furthermore, comparison of yeast and the human microarray results identified *UCP2*, a gene associated with the mitochondria, which showed reduced gene expression in *mutDFNA5* compared to *wtDFNA5*. Interestingly, mitochondrial stress has been linked to the down-regulation of *UCP2* by activation of the MAPK pathway and of JNK activation in particular (Emre et al., 2007; Selimovic et al., 2008). *UCP2* reduction was an early event required for the amplification of the activated MAPK pathway enabling mitochondrial ROS production (Emre et al., 2007; Basu Ball et al, 2011). This down-regulation enables mitochondrial ROS production providing the amplification loop stimulating the MAPK pathway. UCP2 can therefore provide the link between MAPK and the mitochondria, regulating the ROS production, a feature deregulated in both model organisms.

However, we did not observe an up-regulation of MAPK-related pathways in yeast. This could be explained by the differences in timing between the experiments. For human cell lines, the experiment was performed 12 h post-transfection, while yeast RNA was collected at the post-diauxic shift.

In conclusion, this study confirms the role of the mitochondria in mutDFNA5-induced toxicity in yeast. Additionally, it shows that mutDFNA5-induced cell death is mediated by the MAPK pathway, especially through the ERK and the JNK branch. Inhibition of this pathway could significantly enhance the cell viability of mut*DFNA5*-transfected HEK293T cells which suggests the importance of this signaling cascade for DFNA5. How the MAPK pathways perform their role in cell death and the connection with DFNA5-related mechanisms remains uncertain at this moment but is a good starting for future studies. Future studies further unraveling the DFNA5-induced cell death mechanism are important as they may lead to new insights in the involvement of mitochondria in HL and have the potential to lead to new future therapies.

Acknowledgments

This investigation was supported by grants from FWO-Vlaanderen to Guy Van Camp, IWT-Vlaanderen, the KU Leuven Research Fund (KU Leuven-BOF) and KU Leuven R&D to Joris Winderickx, and the Flemisch Society Alzheimer's Research (SAO). We are grateful to IWT-Vlaanderen for a fellowship to Sofie Van Rossom and to FWO-Vlaanderen for fellowships. This study was supported by funding from the Belgian Science Policy Office Interuniversity Attraction Poles (BELSPO-IAP) programme through the project IAP P7/43-BeMGI.

References

Ahmed, Z. M., Yousaf, R., Lee, B. C., Khan, S. N., Lee, S., Lee, K., et al. (2011). Functional null mutations of MSRB3 encoding methionine sulfoxide reductase are associated with human deafness DFNB74. *Am. J. Hum. Genet.* 88, 19–29. doi: 10.1016/j.ajhg.2010.11.010

Akino, K., Toyota, M., Suzuki, H., Imai, T., Maruyama, R., Kusano, M., et al. (2007). Identification of DFNA5 as a target of epigenetic inactivation in gastric cancer. *Cancer Sci.* 98, 88–95. doi: 10.1111/j.1349-7006.2006.00351.x

Anastasiou, D., Poulogiannis, G., Asara, J. M., Boxer, M. B., Jiang, J. K., Shen, M., et al. (2011). Inhibition of pyruvate kinase M2 by reactive oxygen species contributes to cellular antioxidant responses. *Science* 334, 1278–1283. doi: 10.1126/science.1211485

Andrews, Z. B. (2010). Uncoupling protein-2 and the potential link between metabolism and longevity. *Curr. Aging Sci.* 3, 102–112. doi: 10.2174/1874609811003020102

Andrews, Z. B., and Horvath, T. L. (2009). Uncoupling protein-2 regulates lifespan in mice. *Am. J. Physiol. Endocrinol. Metab.* 296, E621–E627. doi: 10.1152/ajpendo.90903.2008

Antonicka, H., Leary, S. C., Guercin, G. H., Agar, J. N., Horvath, R., Kennaway, N. G., et al. (2003). Mutations in COX10 result in a defect in mitochondrial heme A biosynthesis and account for multiple, early-onset clinical phenotypes associated with isolated COX deficiency. *Hum. Mol. Genet.* 12, 2693–2702. doi: 10.1093/hmg/ddg284

Arnold, S., and Kadenbach, B. (1999). The intramitochondrial ATP/ADP-ratio controls cytochrome c oxidase activity allosterically. *FEBS Lett.* 443, 105–108. doi: 10.1016/S0014-5793(98)01694-9

Ashburner, M., Ball, C. A., Blake, J. A., Botstein, D., Butler, H., Cherry, J. M., et al. (2000). Gene ontology: tool for the unification of biology. The Gene Ontology Consortium. *Nat. Genet.* 25, 25–29. doi: 10.1038/75556

Basu Ball, W., Kar, S., Mukherjee, M., Chande, A. G., Mukhopadhyaya, R., and Das, P. K. (2011). Uncoupling protein 2 negatively regulates mitochondrial reactive oxygen species generation and induces phosphatase-mediated anti-inflammatory response in experimental visceral leishmaniasis. *J. Immunol.* 187, 1322–1332. doi: 10.4049/jimmunol.1004237

Bellezza, I., Roberti, R., Gatticchi, L., del Sordo, R., Rambotti, M. G., Marchetti, M. C., et al. (2013). A novel role for Tm7sf2 gene in regulating TNFalpha expression. *PLoS ONE* 8:e68017. doi: 10.1371/journal.pone.0068017

Bender, T., Leidhold, C., Ruppert, T., Franken, S., and Voos, W. (2010). The role of protein quality control in mitochondrial protein homeostasis under oxidative stress. *Proteomics* 10, 1426–1443. doi: 10.1002/pmic.200800619

Bender, T., Lewrenz, I., Franken, S., Baitzel, C., and Voos, W. (2011). Mitochondrial enzymes are protected from stress-induced aggregation by mitochondrial chaperones and the Pim1/LON protease. *Mol. Biol. Cell* 22, 541–554. doi: 10.1091/mbc.E10-08-0718

Bennati, A. M., Castelli, M., Della Fazia, M. A., Beccari, T., Caruso, D., Servillo, G., et al. (2006). Sterol dependent regulation of human TM7SF2 gene expression: role of the encoded 3beta-hydroxysterol Delta14-reductase in human cholesterol biosynthesis. *Biochim. Biophys. Acta* 1761, 677–685. doi: 10.1016/j.bbalip.2006.05.004

Bischoff, A. M., Luijendijk, M. W., Huygen, P. L., van Duijnhoven, G., De Leenheer, E. M., Oudesluijs, G. G., et al. (2004). A novel mutation identified in the DFNA5 gene in a Dutch family: a clinical and genetic evaluation. *Audiol. Neurootol.* 9, 34–46. doi: 10.1159/000074185

Brachmann, C. B., Davies, A., Cost, G. J., Caputo, E., Li, J., Hieter, P., et al. (1998). Designer deletion strains derived from *Saccharomyces cerevisiae* S288C: a useful set of strains and plasmids for PCR-mediated gene disruption and other applications. *Yeast* 14, 115–132.

Buttner, S., Eisenberg, T., Carmona-Gutierrez, D., Ruli, D., Knauer, H., Ruckenstuhl, C., et al. (2007). Endonuclease G regulates budding yeast life and death. *Mol. Cell* 25, 233–246. doi: 10.1016/j.molcel.2006.12.021

Casano, R. A., Johnson, D. F., Bykhovskaya, Y., Torricelli, F., Bigozzi, M., and Fischel-Ghodsian, N. (1999). Inherited susceptibility to aminoglycoside ototoxicity: genetic heterogeneity and clinical implications. *Am. J. Otolaryngol.* 20, 151–156. doi: 10.1016/S0196-0709(99)90062-5

Chambers, J. W., and Lograsso, P. V. (2011). Mitochondrial c-Jun N-terminal kinase (JNK) signaling initiates physiological changes resulting in amplification of reactive oxygen species generation. *J. Biol. Chem.* 286, 16052–16062. doi: 10.1074/jbc.M111.223602

Chen, F. Q., Zheng, H. W., Hill, K., and Sha, S. H. (2012). Traumatic noise activates Rho-family GTPases through transient cellular energy depletion. *J. Neurosci.* 32, 12421–12430. doi: 10.1523/JNEUROSCI.6381-11.2012

Cheng, J., Han, D. Y., Dai, P., Sun, H. J., Tao, R., Sun, Q., et al. (2007). A novel DFNA5 mutation, IVS8+4 A>G, in the splice donor site of intron 8 causes late-onset non-syndromic hearing loss in a Chinese family. *Clin. Genet.* 72, 471–477. doi: 10.1111/j.1399-0004.2007.00889.x

Cheng, J., Zhu, Y., He, S., Lu, Y., Chen, J., Han, B., et al. (2011). Functional mutation of SMAC/DIABLO, encoding a mitochondrial proapoptotic protein, causes human progressive hearing loss DFNA64. *Am. J. Hum. Genet.* 89, 56–66. doi: 10.1016/j.ajhg.2011.05.027

Christofk, H. R., Vander Heiden, M. G., Harris, M. H., Ramanathan, A., Gerszten, R. E., Wei, R., et al. (2008). The M2 splice isoform of pyruvate kinase is important for cancer metabolism and tumour growth. *Nature* 452, 230–233. doi: 10.1038/nature06734

Dando, I., Fiorini, C., Pozza, E. D., Padroni, C., Costanzo, C., Palmieri, M., et al. (2013). UCP2 inhibition triggers ROS-dependent nuclear translocation of GAPDH and autophagic cell death in pancreatic adenocarcinoma cells. *Biochim. Biophys. Acta* 1833, 672–679. doi: 10.1016/j.bbamcr.2012.10.028

Davies, K. J. (2001). Degradation of oxidized proteins by the 20S proteasome. *Biochimie* 83, 301–310. doi: 10.1016/S0300-9084(01)01250-0

De Brito, O. M., and Scorrano, L. (2010). An intimate liaison: spatial organization of the endoplasmic reticulum-mitochondria relationship. *EMBO J.* 29, 2715–2723. doi: 10.1038/emboj.2010.177

Deng, S., Yang, Y., Han, Y., Li, X., Wang, X., Li, X., et al. (2012). UCP2 inhibits ROS-mediated apoptosis in A549 under hypoxic conditions. *PLoS ONE* 7:e30714. doi: 10.1371/journal.pone.0030714

Ding, Y., Leng, J., Fan, F., Xia, B., and Xu, P. (2013). The role of mitochondrial DNA mutations in hearing loss. *Biochem. Genet.* 51, 588–602. doi: 10.1007/s10528-013-9589-6

Dowlati, M. A., Derakhshandeh-Peykar, P., Houshmand, M., Farhadi, M., Shojaei, A., Fallah, M., et al. (2013). Novel nucleotide changes in mutational analysis of mitochondrial 12SrRNA gene in patients with nonsyndromic and aminoglycoside-induced hearing loss. *Mol. Biol. Rep.* 40, 2689–2695. doi: 10.1007/s11033-012-2355-8

Dunning, M. J., Smith, M. L., Ritchie, M. E., and Tavare, S. (2007). beadarray: R classes and methods for Illumina bead-based data. *Bioinformatics* 23, 2183–2184. doi: 10.1093/bioinformatics/btm311

Emre, Y., Hurtaud, C., Nubel, T., Criscuolo, F., Ricquier, D., and Cassard-Doulcier, A. M. (2007). Mitochondria contribute to LPS-induced MAPK activation via uncoupling protein UCP2 in macrophages. *Biochem. J.* 402, 271–278. doi: 10.1042/BJ20061430

Estivill, X., Govea, N., Barcelo, E., Badenas, C., Romero, E., Moral, L., et al. (1998). Familial progressive sensorineural deafness is mainly due to the mtDNA A1555G mutation and is enhanced by treatment of aminoglycosides. *Am. J. Hum. Genet.* 62, 27–35. doi: 10.1086/301676

Fekete, D. M., Homburger, S. A., Waring, M. T., Riedl, A. E., and Garcia, L. F. (1997). Involvement of programmed cell death in morphogenesis of the vertebrate inner ear. *Development* 124, 2451–2461.

Fischel-Ghodsian, N. (1999). Genetic factors in aminoglycoside toxicity. *Ann. N.Y. Acad. Sci.* 884, 99–109. doi: 10.1111/j.1749-6632.1999.tb08639.x

Foury, F. (1997). Human genetic diseases: a cross-talk between man and yeast. *Gene* 195, 1–10. doi: 10.1016/S0378-1119(97)00140-6

Gentleman, R. C., Carey, V. J., Bates, D. M., Bolstad, B., Dettling, M., Dudoit, S., et al. (2004). Bioconductor: open software development for computational biology and bioinformatics. *Genome Biol.* 5:R80. doi: 10.1186/gb-2004-5-10-r80

Gietz, D., St Jean, A., Woods, R. A., and Schiestl, R. H. (1992). Improved method for high efficiency transformation of intact yeast cells. *Nucleic Acids Res.* 20:1425. doi: 10.1093/nar/20.6.1425

Gredilla, R., and Barja, G. (2005). Minireview: the role of oxidative stress in relation to caloric restriction and longevity. *Endocrinology* 146, 3713–3717. doi: 10.1210/en.2005-0378

Gredilla, R., Bohr, V. A., and Stevnsner, T. (2010). Mitochondrial DNA repair and association with aging—An update. *Exp. Gerontol.* 45, 478–488. doi: 10.1016/j.exger.2010.01.017

Gregan, J., Van Laer, L., Lieto, L. D., Van Camp, G., and Kearsey, S. E. (2003). A yeast model for the study of human DFNA5, a gene mutated in nonsyndromic hearing impairment. *Biochim. Biophys. Acta* 1638, 179–186. doi: 10.1016/S0925-4439(03)00083-8

Gruning, N. M., Du, D., Keller, M. A., Luisi, B. F., and Ralser, M. (2014). Inhibition of triosephosphate isomerase by phosphoenolpyruvate in the feedback-regulation of glycolysis. *Open Biol.* 4:130232. doi: 10.1098/rsob.130232

Gruning, N. M., Rinnerthaler, M., Bluemlein, K., Mulleder, M., Wamelink, M. M., Lehrach, H., et al. (2011). Pyruvate kinase triggers a metabolic feedback loop that controls redox metabolism in respiring cells. *Cell Metab.* 14, 415–427. doi: 10.1016/j.cmet.2011.06.017

Hochberg, Y., and Benjamini, Y. (1990). More powerful procedures for multiple significance testing. *Stat. Med.* 9, 811–818. doi: 10.1002/sim.4780090710

Holmer, L., Pezhman, A., and Worman, H. J. (1998). The human lamin B receptor/sterol reductase multigene family. *Genomics* 54, 469–476. doi: 10.1006/geno.1998.5615

Jacobs, H. T., Hutchin, T. P., Kappi, T., Gillies, G., Minkkinen, K., Walker, J., et al. (2005). Mitochondrial DNA mutations in patients with postlingual, nonsyndromic hearing impairment. *Eur. J. Hum. Genet.* 13, 26–33. doi: 10.1038/sj.ejhg.5201250

Jin, L., Yang, A., Zhu, Y., Zhao, J., Wang, X., Yang, L., et al. (2007). Mitochondrial tRNASer(UCN) gene is the hot spot for mutations associated with aminoglycoside-induced and non-syndromic hearing loss. *Biochem. Biophys. Res. Commun.* 361, 133–139. doi: 10.1016/j.bbrc.2007.06.171

Kalinec, G. M., Thein, P., Parsa, A., Yorgason, J., Luxford, W., Urrutia, R., et al. (2014). Acetaminophen and NAPQI are toxic to auditory cells via oxidative and endoplasmic reticulum stress-dependent pathways. *Hear. Res.* 313, 26–37. doi: 10.1016/j.heares.2014.04.007

Kim, M. S., Chang, X., Yamashita, K., Nagpal, J. K., Baek, J. H., Wu, G., et al. (2008a). Aberrant promoter methylation and tumor suppressive activity of the DFNA5 gene in colorectal carcinoma. *Oncogene* 27, 3624–3634. doi: 10.1038/sj.onc.1211021

Kim, M. S., Lebron, C., Nagpal, J. K., Chae, Y. K., Chang, X., Huang, Y., et al. (2008b). Methylation of the DFNA5 increases risk of lymph node metastasis in human breast cancer. *Biochem. Biophys. Res. Commun.* 370, 38–43. doi: 10.1016/j.bbrc.2008.03.026

Kruger, A., Gruning, N. M., Wamelink, M. M., Kerick, M., Kirpy, A., Parkhomchuk, D., et al. (2011). The pentose phosphate pathway is a metabolic redox sensor and regulates transcription during the antioxidant response. *Antioxid. Redox Signal.* 15, 311–324. doi: 10.1089/ars.2010.3797

Leon, Y., Sanchez-Galiano, S., and Gorospe, I. (2004). Programmed cell death in the development of the vertebrate inner ear. *Apoptosis* 9, 255–264. doi: 10.1023/B:APPT.0000025802.07676.a5

Liu, Y. M., Li, X. D., Guo, X., Liu, B., Lin, A. H., Ding, Y. L., et al. (2010). SOD2 V16A SNP in the mitochondrial targeting sequence is associated with noise induced hearing loss in Chinese workers. *Dis. Markers* 28, 137–147. doi: 10.1155/2010/753073

Lo, B., Li, L., Gissen, P., Christensen, H., Mckiernan, P. J., Ye, C., et al. (2005). Requirement of VPS33B, a member of the Sec1/Munc18 protein family, in megakaryocyte and platelet alpha-granule biogenesis. *Blood* 106, 4159–4166. doi: 10.1182/blood-2005-04-1356

Luo, L. F., Hou, C. C., and Yang, W. X. (2013). Nuclear factors: roles related to mitochondrial deafness. *Gene* 520, 79–89. doi: 10.1016/j.gene.2013.03.041

Madeo, F., Carmona-Gutierrez, D., Ring, J., Büttner, S., Eisenberg, T., and Kroemer, G. (2009). Caspase-dependent and caspase-independent cell death pathways in yeast. *Biochem. Biophys. Res. Commun.* 382, 227–231. doi: 10.1016/j.bbrc.2009.02.117

Marchi, S., Patergnani, S., and Pinton, P. (2014). The endoplasmic reticulum-mitochondria connection: one touch, multiple functions. *Biochim. Biophys. Acta* 1837, 461–469. doi: 10.1016/j.bbabio.2013.10.015

Maynard, S., Schurman, S. H., Harboe, C., de Souza-Pinto, N. C., and Bohr, V. A. (2009). Base excision repair of oxidative DNA damage and association with cancer and aging. *Carcinogenesis* 30, 2–10. doi: 10.1093/carcin/bgn250

Meyer Zum Gottesberge, A. M., Massing, T., and Hansen, S. (2012). Missing mitochondrial Mpv17 gene function induces tissue-specific cell-death pathway in the degenerating inner ear. *Cell Tissue Res.* 347, 343–356. doi: 10.1007/s00441-012-1326-7

Mollet, J., Giurgea, I., Schlemmer, D., Dallner, G., Chretien, D., Delahodde, A., et al. (2007). Prenyldiphosphate synthase, subunit 1 (PDSS1) and OH-benzoate polyprenyltransferase (COQ2) mutations in ubiquinone deficiency and oxidative phosphorylation disorders. *J. Clin. Invest.* 117, 765–772. doi: 10.1172/JCI29089

Moran, J. V., Wernette, C. M., Mecklenburg, K. L., Butow, R. A., and Perlman, P. S. (1992). Intron 5 alpha of the COXI gene of yeast mitochondrial DNA is a mobile group I intron. *Nucleic Acids Res.* 20, 4069–4076. doi: 10.1093/nar/20.15.4069

Napiwotzki, J., and Kadenbach, B. (1998). Extramitochondrial ATP/ADP-ratios regulate cytochrome c oxidase activity via binding to the cytosolic domain of subunit IV. *Biol. Chem.* 379, 335–339. doi: 10.1515/bchm.1998.379.3.335

Nishikori, T., Hatta, T., Kawauchi, H., and Otani, H. (1999). Apoptosis during inner ear development in human and mouse embryos: an analysis by computer-assisted three-dimensional reconstruction. *Anat. Embryol.* 200, 19–26. doi: 10.1007/s004290050255

Nishio, A., Noguchi, Y., Sato, T., Naruse, T. K., Kimura, A., Takagi, A., et al. (2014). A DFNA5 mutation identified in Japanese families with autosomal dominant hereditary hearing loss. *Ann. Hum. Genet.* 78, 83–91. doi: 10.1111/ahg.12053

Op de Beeck, K., Van Camp, G., Thys, S., Cools, N., Callebaut, I., Vrijens, K., et al. (2011). The DFNA5 gene, responsible for hearing loss and involved in cancer, encodes a novel apoptosis-inducing protein. *Eur. J. Hum. Genet.* 19, 965–973. doi: 10.1038/ejhg.2011.63

Park, H. J., Cho, H. J., Baek, J. I., Ben-Yosef, T., Kwon, T. J., Griffith, A. J., et al. (2010). Evidence for a founder mutation causing DFNA5 hearing loss in East Asians. *J. Hum. Genet.* 55, 59–62. doi: 10.1038/jhg.2009.114

Payne, M., Yang, Z., Katz, B. J., Warner, J. E., Weight, C. J., Zhao, Y., et al. (2004). Dominant optic atrophy, sensorineural hearing loss, ptosis, and ophthalmoplegia: a syndrome caused by a missense mutation in OPA1. *Am. J. Ophthalmol.* 138, 749–755. doi: 10.1016/j.ajo.2004.06.011

Pevsner, J., Hsu, S. C., Hyde, P. S., and Scheller, R. H. (1996). Mammalian homologues of yeast vacuolar protein sorting (vps) genes implicated in Golgi-to-lysosome trafficking. *Gene* 183, 7–14. doi: 10.1016/S0378-1119(96)00367-8

Raha, S., and Robinson, B. H. (2000). Mitochondria, oxygen free radicals, disease and ageing. *Trends Biochem. Sci.* 25, 502–508. doi: 10.1016/S0968-0004(00)01674-1

Ralser, M., Wamelink, M. M., Kowald, A., Gerisch, B., Heeren, G., Struys, E. A., et al. (2007). Dynamic rerouting of the carbohydrate flux is key to counteracting oxidative stress. *J. Biol.* 6, 10. doi: 10.1186/jbiol61

Roesch, K., Curran, S. P., Tranebjaerg, L., and Koehler, C. M. (2002). Human deafness dystonia syndrome is caused by a defect in assembly of the DDP1/TIMM8a-TIMM13 complex. *Hum. Mol. Genet.* 11, 477–486. doi: 10.1093/hmg/11.5.477

Sauner, M. T., and Levy, M. (1971). Study of the transfer of phospholipids from the endoplasmic reticulum to the outer and inner mitochondrial membranes. *J. Lipid Res.* 12, 71–75.

Schiavoni, G., Bennati, A. M., Castelli, M., Fazia, M. A., Beccari, T., Servillo, G., et al. (2010). Activation of TM7SF2 promoter by SREBP-2 depends on a new sterol regulatory element, a GC-box, and an inverted CCAAT-box. *Biochim. Biophys. Acta* 1801, 587–592. doi: 10.1016/j.bbalip.2010.01.013

Schroder, M. (2008). Endoplasmic reticulum stress responses. *Cell. Mol. Life Sci.* 65, 862–894. doi: 10.1007/s00018-007-7383-5

Selimovic, D., Hassan, M., Haikel, Y., and Hengge, U. R. (2008). Taxol-induced mitochondrial stress in melanoma cells is mediated by activation of c-Jun N-terminal kinase (JNK) and p38 pathways via uncoupling protein 2. *Cell. Signal.* 20, 311–322. doi: 10.1016/j.cellsig.2007.10.015

Seraphin, B., Faye, G., Hatat, D., and Jacq, C. (1992). The yeast mitochondrial intron aI5 alpha: associated endonuclease activity and *in vivo* mobility. *Gene* 113, 1–8. doi: 10.1016/0378-1119(92)90663-A

Sha, S. H., Chen, F. Q., and Schacht, J. (2009). Activation of cell death pathways in the inner ear of the aging CBA/J mouse. *Hear. Res.* 254, 92–99. doi: 10.1016/j.heares.2009.04.019

Sha, S. H., Taylor, R., Forge, A., and Schacht, J. (2001). Differential vulnerability of basal and apical hair cells is based on intrinsic susceptibility to free radicals. *Hear. Res.* 155, 1–8. doi: 10.1016/S0378-5955(01)00224-6

Shang, F., Nowell, T. R. Jr., and Taylor, A. (2001). Removal of oxidatively damaged proteins from lens cells by the ubiquitin-proteasome pathway. *Exp. Eye Res.* 73, 229–238. doi: 10.1006/exer.2001.1029

Shang, F., and Taylor, A. (2011). Ubiquitin-proteasome pathway and cellular responses to oxidative stress. *Free Radic. Biol. Med.* 51, 5–16. doi: 10.1016/j.freeradbiomed.2011.03.031

Singh, S., Misiak, M., Beyer, C., and Arnold, S. (2009). Cytochrome c oxidase isoform IV-2 is involved in 3-nitropropionic acid-induced toxicity in striatal astrocytes. *Glia* 57, 1480–1491. doi: 10.1002/glia.20864

Smyth, G. K. (2004). Linear models and empirical bayes methods for assessing differential expression in microarray experiments. *Stat. Appl. Genet. Mol. Biol.* 3:3. doi: 10.2202/1544-6115.1027

Someya, S., Xu, J., Kondo, K., Ding, D., Salvi, R. J., Yamasoba, T., et al. (2009). Age-related hearing loss in C57BL/6J mice is mediated by Bak-dependent mitochondrial apoptosis. *Proc. Natl. Acad. Sci. U.S.A.* 106, 19432–19437. doi: 10.1073/pnas.0908786106

Srinivasan, S., and Avadhani, N. G. (2012). Cytochrome c oxidase dysfunction in oxidative stress. *Free Radic. Biol. Med.* 53, 1252–1263. doi: 10.1016/j.freeradbiomed.2012.07.021

Stiban, J., Caputo, L., and Colombini, M. (2008). Ceramide synthesis in the endoplasmic reticulum can permeabilize mitochondria to proapoptotic proteins. *J. Lipid Res.* 49, 625–634. doi: 10.1194/jlr.M700480-JLR200

Tavazoie, S., Hughes, J. D., Campbell, M. J., Cho, R. J., and Church, G. M. (1999). Systematic determination of genetic network architecture. *Nat. Genet.* 22, 281–285. doi: 10.1038/10343

Van Laer, L., Huizing, E. H., Verstreken, M., van Zuijlen, D., Wauters, J. G., Bossuyt, P. J., et al. (1998). Nonsyndromic hearing impairment is associated with a mutation in DFNA5. *Nat. Genet.* 20, 194–197. doi: 10.1038/2503

Van Rossom, S., Op de Beeck, K., Franssens, V., Swinnen, E., Schepers, A., Ghillebert, R., et al. (2012). The splicing mutant of the human tumor suppressor protein DFNA5 induces programmed cell death when expressed in the yeast *Saccharomyces cerevisiae*. *Front. Oncol.* 2:77. doi: 10.3389/fonc.2012.00077

Walsh, T., Pierce, S. B., Lenz, D. R., Brownstein, Z., Dagan-Rosenfeld, O., Shahin, H., et al. (2010). Genomic duplication and overexpression of TJP2/ZO-2 leads to altered expression of apoptosis genes in progressive nonsyndromic hearing loss DFNA51. *Am. J. Hum. Genet.* 87, 101–109. doi: 10.1016/j.ajhg.2010.05.011

Wang, C. J., Tang, L., Shen, D. W., Wang, C., Yuan, Q. Y., Gao, W., et al. (2013). The expression and regulation of DFNA5 in human hepatocellular carcinoma DFNA5 in hepatocellular carcinoma. *Mol. Biol. Rep.* 40, 6525–6531. doi: 10.1007/s11033-013-2581-8

Westermann, B., and Neupert, W. (2000). Mitochondria-targeted green fluorescent proteins: convenient tools for the study of organelle biogenesis in *Saccharomyces cerevisiae*. *Yeast* 16, 1421–1427. doi: 10.1002/1097-0061(200011)16:15<1421::AID-YEA624>3.0.CO;2-U

Wiel, C., Lallet-Daher, H., Gitenay, D., Gras, B., Le Calve, B., Augert, A., et al. (2014). Endoplasmic reticulum calcium release through ITPR2 channels leads to mitochondrial calcium accumulation and senescence. *Nat. Commun.* 5, 3792. doi: 10.1038/ncomms4792

Winderickx, J., Delay, C., De Vos, A., Klinger, H., Pellens, K., Vanhelmont, T., et al. (2008). Protein folding diseases and neurodegeneration: lessons learned from yeast. *Biochim. Biophys. Acta* 1783, 1381–1395. doi: 10.1016/j.bbamcr.2008.01.020

Wissing, S., Ludovico, P., Herker, E., Buttner, S., Engelhardt, S. M., Decker, T., et al. (2004). An AIF orthologue regulates apoptosis in yeast. *J. Cell Biol.* 166, 969–974. doi: 10.1083/jcb.200404138

Yu, C., Meng, X., Zhang, S., Zhao, G., Hu, L., and Kong, X. (2003). A 3-nucleotide deletion in the polypyrimidine tract of intron 7 of the DFNA5 gene causes nonsyndromic hearing impairment in a Chinese family. *Genomics* 82, 575–579. doi: 10.1016/S0888-7543(03)00175-7

Zecchini, E., Siviero, R., Giorgi, C., Rizzuto, R., and Pinton, P. (2007). Mitochondrial calcium signalling: message of life and death. *Ital. J. Biochem.* 56, 235–242.

12

Spontaneous hair cell regeneration is prevented by increased Notch signaling in supporting cells

Melissa M. McGovern[1], Luyi Zhou[1], Michelle R. Randle[1] and Brandon C. Cox[1,2]*

[1] Department of Pharmacology, School of Medicine, Southern Illinois University, Springfield, IL, United States, [2] Department of Surgery, Division of Otolaryngology, School of Medicine, Southern Illinois University, Springfield, IL, United States

Edited by:
Brad Walters,
University of Mississippi Medical Center, United States

Reviewed by:
Byron Haney Hartman,
Stanford University, United States
Amy Kiernan,
University of Rochester, United States

***Correspondence:**
Brandon C. Cox
bcox@siumed.edu

During embryonic development, differentiation of cochlear progenitor cells into hair cells (HCs) or supporting cells (SCs) is partially controlled through Notch signaling. Many studies have shown that inhibition of Notch signaling allows SCs to convert into HCs in both normal and drug damaged neonatal mouse cochleae. This mechanism is also implicated during HC regeneration in non-mammalian vertebrates; however, the mechanism of spontaneous HC regeneration in the neonatal mouse cochlea is less understood. While inhibition of Notch signaling can force SCs to convert into HCs and increase the number of regenerated HCs, it is currently unknown whether this pathway is involved in spontaneous HC regeneration observed *in vivo*. Therefore, we investigated the role of Notch signaling during the spontaneous HC regeneration process using *Atoh1-CreER*^{TM}*::Rosa26*$^{loxP-stop-loxP-DTA/+}$ mice injected with tamoxifen at postnatal day (P) 0 and P1 to ablate HCs and stimulate spontaneous HC regeneration. Expression changes of genes in the Notch pathway were measured using immunostaining and *in situ* hybridization, with most changes observed in the apical one-third of the cochlea where the majority of HC regeneration occurs. Expression of the Notch target genes *Hes1, Hes5, Hey1, HeyL*, and *Jagged1* were decreased. To investigate whether reduction of Notch signaling is involved in the spontaneous HC regeneration process, we overexpressed the *Notch1 intracellular fragment (N1ICD)* in cochlear SCs and other non-sensory epithelial cells in the context of HC damage. Specifically, *Atoh1-CreER*^{TM}*::Rosa26*$^{loxP-stop-loxP-DTA/+}$*::Sox10*^{rtTA}*::TetO-LacZ::TetO-N1ICD* mice were injected with tamoxifen at P0/P1 to stimulate spontaneous HC regeneration and given doxycycline from P0–P7 to induce expression of *N1ICD* as well as *LacZ* for fate-mapping. We observed a 92% reduction in the number of fate-mapped regenerated HCs in mice with *N1ICD* overexpression compared to controls with HC damage but no manipulation of Notch signaling. Therefore, we conclude that increased Notch signaling prevents spontaneous HC regeneration from occurring in the neonatal mouse cochlea. Understanding which components of the Notch pathway regulates regenerative plasticity in the neonatal mouse cochlea will inform investigations focused on stimulating HC regeneration in mature cochlea and eventually in humans to treat hearing loss.

Keywords: hair cell regeneration, cochlea, Notch, CreER, Tet-On, *NICD*

INTRODUCTION

Hearing loss, one of the most prevalent conditions in the world, can result from multiple etiologies such as aging, viral infection, or exposure to noise or ototoxic drugs. In those born with normal hearing, death of sound-sensing hair cells (HCs) located within the cochlea is the most common source of hearing impairment. The mature mammalian cochlea does not regenerate HCs after damage, thus hearing loss is permanent (Bohne, 1976; Hawkins et al., 1976; Oesterle et al., 2008). However, in non-mammalian vertebrates, including birds, fish, and amphibians, the inner ear responds to damage by regenerating lost HCs throughout the life of the animal (reviewed in Bermingham-McDonogh and Rubel, 2003; Stone and Cotanche, 2007). Several studies have suggested that the Notch signaling pathway is involved in the HC regeneration process in non-mammals (reviewed in Stone and Cotanche, 2007; Brignull et al., 2009).

The Notch pathway uses membrane bound ligands and receptors expressed on adjacent cells to generate a mosaic pattern of cell types. In the mammalian cochlea, HCs and neighboring supporting cells (SCs) develop from the same pool of progenitor cells through a Notch-mediated process. As progenitor cells take a HC fate, they begin to express the Notch ligands Delta-like ligand 1 (Dll1), Delta-like ligand 3 (Dll3), and Jagged2 (Jag2) (Lanford et al., 1999, 2000; Morrison et al., 1999; Kiernan et al., 2005; Brooker et al., 2006; Hartman et al., 2007). These ligands signal to neighboring progenitor cells through Notch receptors which inhibits them from becoming HCs and instructs a SC fate (Lanford et al., 2000; Zheng et al., 2000; Zine et al., 2001; Murata et al., 2006; Hayashi et al., 2008; Doetzlhofer et al., 2009). A recent study reported limited down-regulation of Notch target genes after HC damage in the neonatal mouse cochlea (Korrapati et al., 2013). However, inhibition of the Notch signaling pathway, using pharmacological agents or genetically modified mouse models, in the late embryonic and early postnatal cochlea has the consistent effect of inducing the conversion of SCs into HCs either in the undamaged cochlea (Yamamoto et al., 2006; Doetzlhofer et al., 2009; Li et al., 2015; Maass et al., 2015) or after HC loss (Korrapati et al., 2013; Mizutari et al., 2013; Bramhall et al., 2014; Hu et al., 2016). Therefore, active Notch signaling in SCs plays an important role in maintaining their cell fate in the neonatal cochlea.

Recently, several groups have demonstrated that the immature murine cochlea has the capacity to spontaneously regenerate HCs during the first postnatal week (Bramhall et al., 2014; Cox et al., 2014; Hu et al., 2016) and loss of Notch signaling has been shown to increase the degree of HC regeneration over that which occurs spontaneously in HC damaged cochlear explants (Korrapati et al., 2013; Bramhall et al., 2014; Hu et al., 2016). While these results demonstrate that SCs can be forced to convert into HCs through inhibition of the Notch pathway, it is unclear whether the Notch signaling pathway is involved in the mechanism of spontaneous HC regeneration. To address this question, we first investigated changes in Notch signaling during the spontaneous HC regeneration process in the neonatal mouse cochlea and found that the expression of the Notch target genes *Hes1*, *Hes5*, *Hey1*, *HeyL*, and *Jagged1* (*Jag1*) were decreased. Next, to determine whether the spontaneous HC regeneration process is inhibited by sustained Notch signaling, we combined HC damage with overexpression of the *Notch1 intracellular domain* (*N1ICD*) in SCs and other non-sensory epithelial cells and measured the effect on spontaneous HC regeneration. This model showed a 92% reduction in the number of spontaneously regenerated HCs and suggests that weakened Notch signaling contributes to SC plasticity which underlies spontaneous HC regeneration.

MATERIALS AND METHODS

Animals

Plp-CreER^{T2} mice (Jax stock #5975, Doerflinger et al., 2003), *Rosa26*$^{loxP-stop-loxP-DTA}$ mice (Jax stock #6331, Ivanova et al., 2005), *Rosa26*$^{loxP-stop-loxP-tdTomato}$ mice (also called Ai14, Jax stock #7914, Madisen et al., 2010), and *TetO-LacZ* mice (Jax stock #2621, Furth et al., 1994), were obtained from The Jackson Laboratory (Bar Harbor, ME). *Atoh1-CreER*^{TM} mice (Chow et al., 2006) were provided by Dr. Suzanne Baker (St. Jude Children's Hospital, Memphis, TN, United States); *Hes5*^{LacZ} mice (Imayoshi et al., 2010) were provided by Dr. Ryoichiro Kageyama (Kyoto University, Kyoto, Japan); *Sox10*^{rtTA} mice (Ludwig et al., 2004; Walters and Zuo, 2015) were provided by Dr. Michael Wegner (Erlangen University, Erlangen, Germany); and *TetO-N1ICD* mice (Stanger et al., 2005) were provided by Dr. Ben Stranger (University of Pennsylvania, Philadelphia, PA, United States). Genotyping for all mouse lines was performed by Transnetyx, Inc. (Cordova, TN, United States). Mice of both genders were used in all studies and all animal work was performed in accordance with approved animal protocols from the Institutional Animal Care and Use Committee at Southern Illinois University School of Medicine.

Substances Given to Animals

To induce CreER recombination for either HC death or tdTomato expression, tamoxifen (Sigma-Aldrich, St. Louis, MO, United States) was dissolved in 100% corn oil and injected intraperitoneally (IP) at 3 mg/40 g on either postnatal day (P) 0, or both P0 and P1. To induce *LacZ* and *N1ICD* overexpression in cochlear SCs and other non-sensory epithelial cells, doxycycline (100 mg/kg, IP, Fisher, Hampton, NH, United States) was injected at P1 (~6 h after the second tamoxifen injection) as well as administered in the food (2000 mg/kg, Envigo, Huntingdon, United Kingdom) to the nursing mother for the duration of the experiment.

Real-Time qPCR

Quantification of gene expression was conducted using real time quantitative polymerase chain reaction (qPCR). Neonatal pups were euthanized under isoflurane anesthesia (Henry Schein, Melville, NY, United States) and cochleae were collected from P7 animals, flash frozen in either liquid nitrogen or a dry ice slurry, and then stored at −80°C. Isolation of total RNA was conducted using tri-reagent (Fisher, Hampton, NH, United States), and precipitated with isopropanol (Acros Organics, Geel, Belgium) at −20°C overnight followed by purification with DNAse treatment (cat #AM1906, Fisher, Hampton, NH, United States) and reprecipitated using sodium acetate (Fisher, Hampton, NH, United States). Once total RNA was isolated, the concentration was measured using a Nanodrop 2000 (Fisher, Hampton, NH, United States) followed by reverse transcription into cDNA using Thermo Scientific Maxima First Strand cDNA synthesis kit (cat #K1641, Fisher, Hampton, NH, United States) and stored at −20°C. The expression level of selected genes was measured from cDNA by qPCR using Sybr Green (cat #K0391, Fisher, Hampton, NH, United States) and a CFX Connect Optics Module (Bio-Rad, Hercules, CA, United States). Comparison of gene expression among samples was conducted using the Pfaffl method which is a modified version of the delta-delta Ct equation that takes into account the efficiency of each primer set (Pfaffl, 2001). Gene expression was normalized to a housekeeping gene (Rpl19), which has been used previously for qPCR experiments in cochlear tissue (Basch et al., 2011; Korrapati et al., 2013; Wan et al., 2014; Maass et al., 2016). Data are expressed as fold change from control. **Table 1** lists the primer sets used for each gene that was investigated and each primer set was tested for specificity with a reverse transcriptase-negative control to ensure they did not detect genomic DNA.

Immunostaining

Neonatal pups were euthanized under isoflurane anesthesia and cochleae were collected and post-fixed in 4% paraformaldehyde (Polysciences, Inc., Warrington, PA, United States) for ∼2 h at room temperature (RT). The samples were then transferred to 10 mM Phosphate Buffered Saline (PBS, Sigma, St. Louis, MO, United States) and stored at 4°C. Following whole mount dissection, cochleae were cut into 3 turns of equal length and placed into a 48 well plate for immunostaining as free floating tissue. Samples were blocked and permeabilized at RT for 1 h with a solution of Normal Horse Serum or Normal Goat Serum (10%, NHS, or NGS, Vector Labs, Burlingame, CA, United States), Bovine Serum Albumin (1%, BSA, Fisher, Hampton, NH, United States), and Triton-X-100 (1%, Sigma, St. Louis, MO, United States) in 10 mM PBS prior to the application of the primary antibodies. Primary antibodies were diluted in a solution of 10 mM PBS containing NHS or NGS (5%), BSA (1%), and Triton-X-100 (0.1%) and incubated overnight at 4°C or 37°C. The following primary antibodies were used: chicken anti-β-galactosidase (β-gal, 1:500, cat#ab9361, Abcam, Cambridge, United Kingdom), goat anti-Jagl (1:500, cat#sc6011, Santa Cruz Biotechnology, Dallas, TX, United States), rabbit anti-myosin VIIa (1:200, cat#25-6790, Proteus Biosciences, Ramona, CA, United States), rabbit anti-S100a1 (1:1000, cat#ab868, Abcam, Cambridge, United Kingdom), and goat anti-Sox2 (1:400, cat#sc-17320, Santa Cruz Biotechnology, Dallas, TX, United States). The next day, samples were washed three times with 10 mM PBS for 5 min each at RT. Alexa fluor-conjugated secondary antibodies (Life Technologies, Waltham, MA, United States) were diluted 1:1000 in a solution of NHS or NGS (5%), BSA (1%), and Triton-X-100 (0.1%) in 10 mM PBS and incubated for ∼3 h in the dark at RT. Following the secondary antibodies, samples were washed three times for 5 min each in 10 mM PBS followed by a 20-min incubation with Hoechst (1:2000, Fisher, Hampton, NH, United States) and three more, 5-min washes in 10 mM PBS at RT. Following immunofluorescent labeling, samples were mounted on slides in Prolong Gold (Fisher, Hampton, NH, United States).

Additionally, chicken anti-β-gal antibodies produced excessive background and therefore to increase the signal to noise ratio, signal enhancer (enough volume to cover each sample, cat#R37107, Thermo Fisher Scientific, Hampton, NH, United States) was applied at RT for 30 min followed by three 5-min PBS washes prior to the blocking/permeabilization step. A low pH antigen unmasking solution (AUM, cat#H-3300, Vector Labs, Burlingame, CA, United States) was beneficial to increase antibody binding to the epitope for the anti-Jagl antibodies. For this step, samples were incubated in a hybridization oven at 95°C for 45 min with a 1:100 dilution of the AUM solution in ddH_2O followed by three 5-min washes in 10 mM PBS prior to blocking/permeabilization.

Imaging was conducted using a Leica SP5 or a Zeiss LSM 800 confocal microscope and images were processed with LAS-lite (Leica, Wetzlar, Germany) or Zen Blue lite (Zeiss, Oberkochen, Germany) software.

In Situ Hybridization

Probes were prepared by transfecting plasmids containing the full-length mouse cDNA sequences for *Hes1* (Accession: BC051428, Clone ID: 6478994, Dharmacon, Inc., Lafayette, CO, United States), *Hes5* (Accession: BC103539, Clone ID: 40039948, Dharmacon, Inc., Lafayette, CO, United States), *Hey1* (Accession: BC086635, Clone ID: 6809680, Dharmacon, Inc., Lafayette, CO, United States), and *HeyL* (Accession: BC130263, Clone ID: 40142873, Dharmacon, Inc., Lafayette, CO, United States) into competent *Escherichia coli* cells (Fisher, Hampton, NH, United States) and incubating for 1 h at 37°C before spreading the cells on an agar plate containing the appropriate selection marker and incubating overnight. Once a clone was selected, it was inoculated with the appropriate selection antibiotic

TABLE 1 | Primer sets used for qPCR of Notch effector genes.

Gene	Forward primer	Reverse primer	Reference
Hes1	TCAACACGACACCGGACAAAC	ATGCCGGGAGCTATCTTTCTT	Chonko et al., 2013
Hes5	GCACCAGCCCAACTCCAA	GGCGAAGGCTTTGCTGTGT	White et al., 2006
Hey1	CACTGCAGGAGGGAAAGGTTAT	CCCCAAACTCCGATAGTCCAT	Korrapati et al., 2013
HeyL	GCGCAGAGGGATCATAGAGAA	TCGCAATTCAGAAAGGCTACTG	Korrapati et al., 2013
N1ICD	GACAACTCCTACCTCTGCTTATGCC	TTACTGTTGCACTCGTTGACCTCG	Yamamoto et al., 2006

and incubated overnight in 250 ml of media containing the selection marker at 37°C, after which cells were centrifuged and the supernatant was decanted. The cells were processed with a ZymoPURE plasmid maxiprep kit (cat#D4202, Zymo Research, Irvine, CA, United States) to isolate the plasmid DNA. Concentration was measured on a Nanodrop 2000 (Fisher, Hampton, NH, United States) and the plasmids were linearized and cleaned up with phenol::chloroform::isoamyl alcohol (Fisher, Hampton, NH, United States). Plasmids were sequenced by GenScript (Piscataway, NJ, United States) and each sequence was entered into BLAST (NCBI, Bethesda, MD, United States) to determine their correspondence to the endogenous mouse mRNA sequence (*Hes1* = 97.4% homology, *Hes5* = 100% homology, *Hey1* = 99.9% homology, and *HeyL* = 99.5% homology). Then the probes were digoxigenin-labeled (DIG; cat# 286 036 910, Roche, Indianapolis, IN, United States) through *in vitro* transcription and cut into ~300 bp pieces though a mild alkaline bath to facilitate interaction with the endogenous RNA.

Cochleae were fixed in RNase free 4% paraformaldehyde (PFA; Polysciences, Inc., Warrington, PA, United States) for ~2 h at RT or overnight at 4°C. Following fixation, cochleae were dissected and dehydrated in a graded methanol series (Fisher, Hampton, NH, United States) for 5 min in each concentration [25, 50, 75, and 100% diluted in RNase free 10 mM PBS with 0.1% Tween-20 (PTw) (Sigma, St. Louis, MO, United States)]. Samples were rehydrated through a reverse graded methanol series and transferred to RNase free 2 ml tubes. Samples were washed three times for 5 min each in RNase free PTw at RT. Next, samples were digested for 15 min at RT with 10 μg/ml proteinase K (Fisher, Hampton, NH, United States) in PTw then incubated with 4% PFA containing 0.2% glutaraldehyde (Sigma, St. Louis, MO, United States) for 20 min to halt the digestion. Then samples were again washed twice with RNase free PTw for 5 min each. Next, hybridization buffer [50% formamide (Sigma St. Louis, MO, United States), 1.5× saline-sodium citrate (SSC, Sigma, St. Louis, MO, United States), pH adjusted to 4.5 with citric acid (Sigma, St. Louis, MO, United States), 50 μg/ml yeast tRNA (Sigma, St. Louis MO, United States), 100 μg/ml heparin (Sigma, St. Louis, MO, United States), 0.2% Tween-20 (Sigma, St. Louis, MO, United States), 0.5% CHAPS (3-[(3-Cholamidopropyl)dimethylammonio]-1-propanesulfonate hydrate Sigma, St. Louis, MO, United States), and 5mM EDTA pH 8.0, (Millipore, Billerica, MA, United States)] was added to each sample and incubated at 60°C for 3 h followed by the addition of the DIG-labeled riboprobe to the hybridization buffer at a concentration of 0.5 μg/ml (*Hes5*) or 1 μg/ml (*Hes1*, *Hey1*, and *HeyL*) and incubated at 60°C overnight.

The following day, samples were rinsed twice (~1 min each) with hybridization buffer and washed twice (30 min each) with hybridization buffer at 60°C. Samples were then washed with a 1:1 mixture of hybridization buffer and 1X MABT [maleic acid buffer containing Tween-20, 5X stock concentration of 500 mM maleic acid (Sigma, St. Louis, MO, United States), 744 mM NaCl (Sigma, St. Louis, MO, United States), 44 mM Tween-20 (Sigma, St. Louis, MO, United States) and ddH_2O and pH adjusted with Tris Base (Roche, Indianapolis, IN, United States) to ~7.5] for 20 min at 60°C. Samples were then rinsed three times (~1 min each) with 1X MABT and washed twice (30 min each) with 1X MABT at RT. Samples were blocked with 1X MABT containing 20% sheep serum (Sigma, St. Louis, MO, United States) and 2% Boehringer blocking reagent (Sigma, St. Louis, MO, United States) for 3 h at RT. Next the samples were incubated overnight at 4°C with anti-digoxigenin antibodies (cat#11093274910, Sigma, St. Louis, MO, United States) in 1X MABT at a final concentration of 1:2000.

The following day, samples were rinsed three times (~1 min each) with 1X MABT and then washed three times (1 h each) with 1X MABT at RT followed by an overnight wash at 4°C. Samples were then washed twice with alkaline phosphatase buffer [100 mM Tris (Sigma, St. Louis, MO, United States) pH 9.5, 50 mM $MgCl_2$ (Fisher, Hampton, NH, United States), 100 mM NaCl (Sigma, St. Louis, MO, United States), and 0.1% Tween-20 (Sigma, St. Louis, MO, United States)] for 1 h each and then processed with 4.5 μl/ml nitro-blue tetrazolium (Sigma, St. Louis, MO, United States) and 3.5 μl/ml 5-bromo-4-chloro-3′-indolyphosphate (Sigma, St. Louis, MO, United States) in alkaline phosphatase buffer in the dark between 2 and 20 h. Samples were then washed twice in alkaline phosphatase buffer (5 min each), washed three times in PTw (1 h each), and fixed in 4% PFA for 30 min. Samples were then cleared in 60% glycerol overnight and mounted on slides in 100% glycerol (Fisher, Hampton, NH, United States) and imaged with a Neurolucida system (MicroBrightField, Inc., United States) integrated with a Zeiss AxioImager M2 microscope (Carl Zeiss Microscopy, Germany) or an Olympus IX70 microscope (Olympus Corporation, Waltham, MA, United States). All *in situ* experiments were performed with matched experimental and control samples from the same litter run in parallel.

Quantification and Statistical Analysis

For quantification of Sox2-positive and Hes5-LacZ-positive cells, images were taken from two representative regions in the apical turn of the cochlea and cells in either a 150 μm or 200 μm region per image were quantified and averaged for each sample. Positive expression of LacZ was determined by the overlap of LacZ labeling and nuclear staining with Hoechst once antibody background was reduced using the imaging software. The same trained examiner counted images for both control and experimental samples to make sure that the same threshold for positive staining was maintained. To quantify the amount of HC regeneration (LacZ-positive HCs) in the model where *N1ICD* was overexpressed, images of the entire cochlea were taken using tile scan with z-series. Each cochlea was measured and divided into six equal sections as previously described (McGovern et al., 2017). For quantification of HCs in cochlea overexpressing *N1ICD*, 200 μm regions were selected from two representative images per cochlear turn and total HCs were quantified and averaged. All data are presented as mean ± standard error of the mean (SEM). Data was analyzed using a one- or two-way ANOVA or a Student's *t*-test with Graphpad Prism 6.02 (Graphpad Software Inc., La Jolla, CA, United States).

RESULTS

Hes5 Expression Is Reduced During Spontaneous HC Regeneration

Because the majority of spontaneously regenerated HCs are formed in the apical turn of the cochlea (Cox et al., 2014), we investigated gene changes in this region at the cellular level. We first measured changes in the expression of *Hes5*, a direct inhibitor of HC fate that is a well-known target of active Notch signaling (Mulvaney and Dabdoub, 2012; Abdolazimi et al., 2016). *Hes5* is expressed in many SC subtypes during the first postnatal week including Deiters' cells, outer pillar cells, inner phalangeal cells, border cells, and some cells of the greater epithelial ridge (GER) (**Figures 1A–C,G–I,M–O, 2B–B''',D–D''',F–F'''**; Lanford et al., 2000; Zine et al., 2001; Hartman et al., 2009; Cox et al., 2014; Maass et al., 2015). To quantify the number of cells that express *Hes5*, we used the $Hes5^{LacZ}$ reporter line which has *LacZ* knocked into the endogenous *Hes5* locus and therefore is a faithful representation of endogenous *Hes5* expression (Imayoshi et al., 2010). Others have shown that β-galactosidase (β-gal), transcribed by the *LacZ* gene, continues to be expressed ~1 day after mRNA of the endogenous gene becomes undetectable (Morrison et al., 1999). Therefore, we used $Hes5^{LacZ}$ mice to approximate the window when cells lose *Hes5* expression. $Atoh1\text{-}CreER^{TM}::Rosa26^{loxP-stop-loxP-DTA}$ mice (hereinafter referred to as *Atoh1-DTA* mice) were bred with $Hes5^{LacZ}$ mice and injected with tamoxifen (3 mg/40 g, IP) on both P0 and P1 to induce HC ablation and initiate spontaneous HC regeneration. Samples were analyzed at P2, P4, and P6, which was previously established as the window of spontaneous HC regeneration seen in the neonatal mouse cochlea (Cox et al., 2014). We quantified the number of cells that expressed Hes5-LacZ as well as the number of SC and immature HC nuclei using anti-Sox2 antibodies. Significantly fewer Hes5-LacZ-positive cells were detected in the $Atoh1\text{-}DTA::Hes5^{LacZ}$ cochlea at P2 (216.1 ± 12.3 vs. 107.3 ± 19.1; $p < 0.001$; $N = 3$) and P4 (185.6 ± 13.3 vs. 115.5 ± 14.1; $p < 0.01$ as determined by a two-way ANOVA with a Tukey's *post hoc* test; $N = 3$) compared to control samples that lacked either the $Atoh1\text{-}CreER^{TM}$ or $Rosa26^{DTA}$ allele (**Figures 1A–L,S**). However, there was no difference observed in Hes5-LacZ expression at P6 (140.1 ± 11.6 vs. 120.3 ± 7.3; $N = 4$; **Figures 1M–S**). There were also no differences in the number of Sox2-positive cells after HC damage at any age (**Figures 1B,E,H,K,N,Q,S**) suggesting that as a whole, the Sox2-positive cell population is not reduced.

Differences among SC subtypes have previously been documented (Lanford et al., 2000; Doetzlhofer et al., 2009; Yu et al., 2010; Taylor et al., 2012; Lagarde et al., 2013; Maass et al., 2016), which may indicate that not all SC subtypes maintain plasticity postnatally. Furthermore, loss of *Hes5* at embryonic ages has been implicated in the formation of supernumerary outer HCs, but not inner HCs (Zine et al., 2001). We therefore sought to investigate changes in *Hes5* expression within discrete SC subpopulations. To divide the SC subtypes into two groups, we used pillar and Deiters' cells as a landmark. *S100a1* is a calcium binding protein that is expressed in the cytoplasm and nucleus of pillar and Deiters' cells within the neonatal cochlea (White et al., 2006; Buckiová and Syka, 2009). Therefore, combining anti-S100a1 antibodies with anti-Sox2 and anti-β-gal antibodies allowed us to tease apart two groups of SC subpopulations: (1) pillar cells and Deiters' cells which are labeled by S100a1, and (2) inner phalangeal and border cells which are $Hes5^{LacZ}$-positive/Sox2-positive cells located medial to S100a1 labeling (**Figures 2A–B''',D–D''',F–F'''**). Because $Hes5^{LacZ}$ is also expressed in the cells of the GER, the medial border of inner phalangeal and border cells was established for quantification by measuring the width of tdTomato expression medial to inner pillar cells in $Plp\text{-}CreER^{T2}::Rosa26^{loxP-stop-loxP-tdTomato}$ mice injected with tamoxifen (3 mg/40 g, IP) at P0, which has previously been shown to target inner phalangeal and border cells, but not the GER (**Supplementary Figures S1A–C**; Doerflinger et al., 2003; Gómez-Casati et al., 2010; Cox et al., 2012; Mellado Lagarde et al., 2014; McGovern et al., 2017).

After HC damage and regeneration was induced in $Atoh1\text{-}DTA::Hes5^{LacZ}$ mice by tamoxifen injection at P0 and P1, there was a significant decrease in the number of Hes5-LacZ-positive pillar and Deiters' cells detected at P2 (113.1 ± 3.8 vs. 63.6 ± 5.1, $p < 0.01$, $N = 4$), P4 (104.4 ± 1.5 vs. 42.1 ± 5.7, $p < 0.001$, $N = 4\text{-}5$), and P6 (98.6 ± 2.4 vs. 25.3 ± 4.4, $p < 0.001$, $N = 4$) compared to control cochleae which lacked either the $Atoh1\text{-}CreER^{TM}$ or $Rosa26^{DTA}$ allele (**Figures 2B–H**). Of note, the number of Sox2-positive cells within this population did not decrease until P4 (140.2 ± 3.1 vs. 98.1 ± 11.5, $p < 0.001$; $N = 4\text{-}5$) and was also decreased at P6 (130.3 ± 2.7 vs. 75.0 ± 6.0, $p < 0.0001$; $N = 4$; **Figures 2B–H**). Additionally, there was an increase in the number of Sox2-positive/Hes5-LacZ-negative pillar and Deiters' cells at P2 (39.0 ± 1.6 vs. 102.2 ± 21.9, $p < 0.001$; $N = 4$; **Figures 2B–H**), suggesting that *Hes5* is downregulated in these SCs, but the cells are still alive. In contrast, neither the number of *Hes5*-LacZ-positive cells, nor the number of Sox2-positive cells within the inner phalangeal and border cells region were significantly altered from control samples (**Figures 2B–G''',I**), suggesting that weakened Notch signaling is limited to pillar and Deiters' cells during the HC regeneration process.

Reduced Expression of Notch Effectors *Hes1, Hes5, Hey1,* and *HeyL* Was Observed During Spontaneous HC Regeneration

Further changes in the expression of Notch target genes were investigated using *in situ* hybridization. *Atoh1-DTA* mice as well as littermate controls, which lacked the $Atoh1\text{-}CreER^{TM}$ or $Rosa26^{DTA}$ allele, were injected with tamoxifen (3 mg/40 g, IP) on P0 and P1 to induce HC damage as well as spontaneous HC regeneration. Samples were collected and analyzed at P4 using probes that target *Hes1*, *Hes5*, *Hey1*, and *HeyL*. Paired samples from the same litter (control and *Atoh1-DTA*) were processed in parallel where each solution, as well as each incubation time, was identical. Comparisons were only made between the one experimental and the one control sample that were processed together. Staining intensity in the sensory

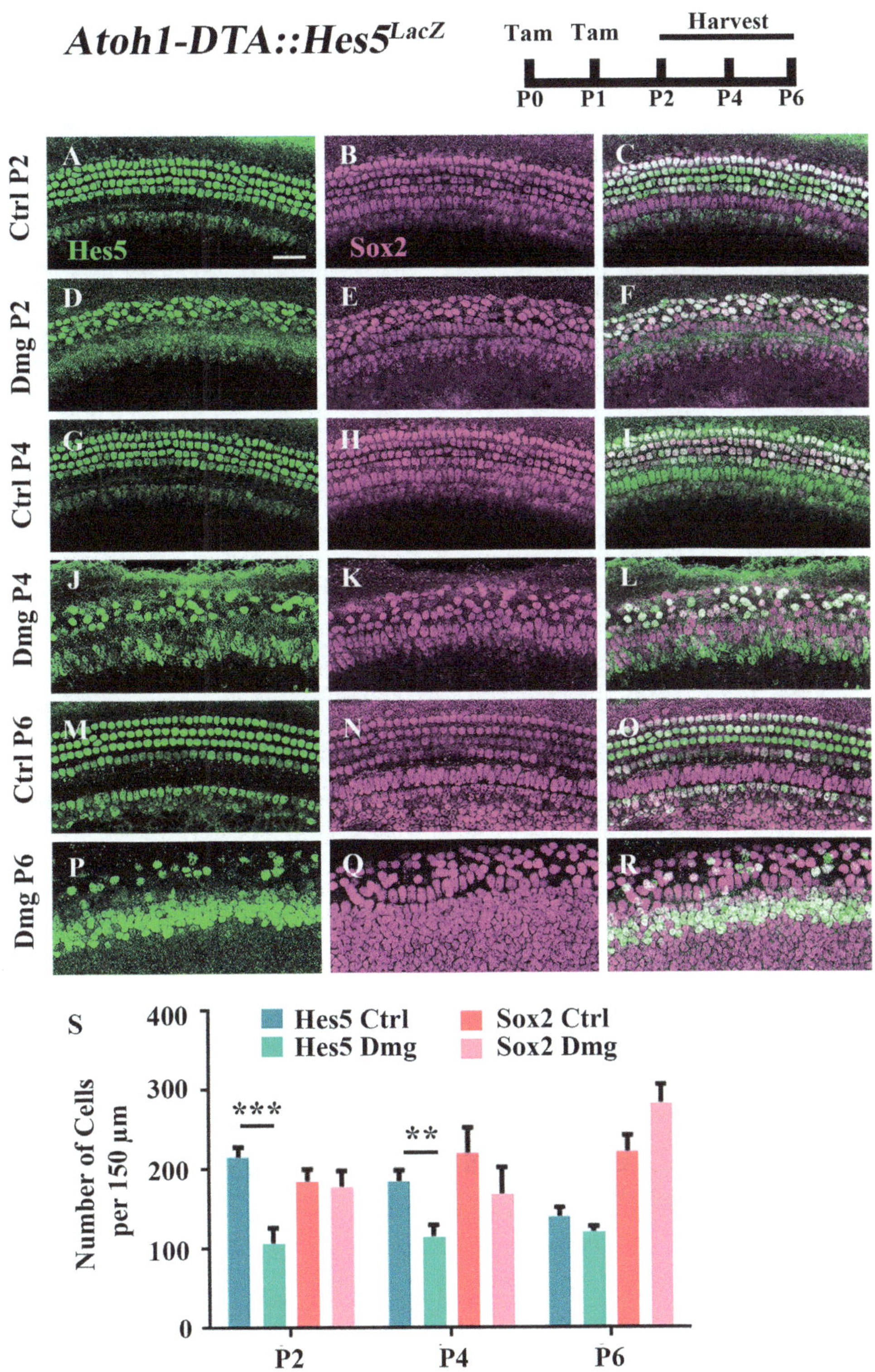

FIGURE 1 | Hes5-LacZ-positive cells, but not Sox2-positive cells, are reduced during the spontaneous HC regeneration process. *Atoh1-DTA::Hes5^{LacZ}* mice were injected with tamoxifen (Tam) at P0–P1 to induce HC death and spontaneous HC regeneration and cochleae were collected at P2, P4, and P6. **(A–R)** Representative confocal slice images with anti-β-gal antibodies to detect Hes5-LacZ expression (green) and anti-Sox2 antibodies to label all SC nuclei (magenta). **(A–C, G–I, M–O)** Images are taken from P2, P4, or P6 control samples, respectively. Scale bar = 25 μm. **(S)** Fewer Hes5-LacZ-positive cells were detected in HC damaged samples at P2 and P4, but not P6. There was no significant difference in the number of Sox2-positive cells in the *Atoh1-DTA::Hes5^{LacZ}* cochlea after HC damage compared to undamaged controls. $^{**}p < 0.01$, $^{***}p < 0.001$, as determined by a two-way ANOVA with a Sidak's *post hoc* test. $N = 3–5$.

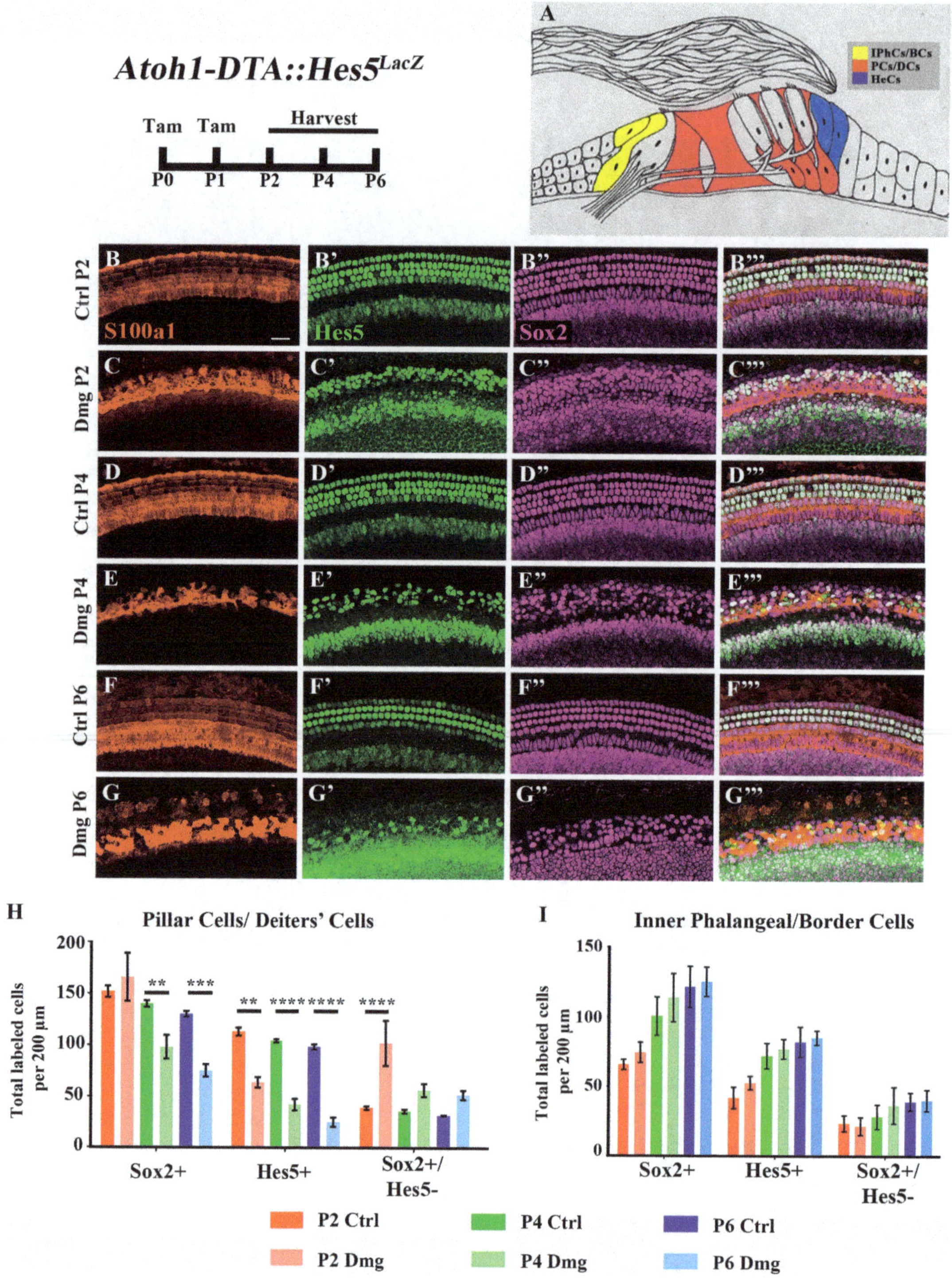

FIGURE 2 | Hes5-LacZ-positive cells are reduced in lateral SCs, but not medial SCs. **(A)** Pillar and Deiters' cells (red, PCs/DCs) are labeled with S100a1 and inner phalangeal/border cells (yellow, IPhCs/BCs) lie medial to the S100a1 expressing region. Hensen cells (blue, HeCs) express Sox2 and border the lateral edge of the S100a1 region, but do not have Hes5 expression. **(B–G''')** *Atoh1-DTA::Hes5*^{LacZ} mice were injected with tamoxifen (Tam) at P0–P1 to induce HC death and spontaneous HC regeneration and cochleae were collected at P2, P4, or P6. Representative confocal slice images with anti-βgal antibodies to detect Hes5-LacZ expression (green), anti-Sox2 antibodies to label all SC nuclei (magenta), and anti-S100a1 antibodies to label the cytoplasm of PCs/DCs (red). Scale bar = 25 µm **(H)** In the PCs/DCs region, fewer Sox2-positive cells were detected at P4 and P6 after HC damage, while a decreased number of Hes5-LacZ-positive cells were detected at all three ages. Only at P2 were there significantly more Sox2-positive/Hes5-LacZ-negative cells detected. **(I)** There was no significant change in the number of Sox2-positive, Hes5-LacZ-positive, or Sox2-positive/Hes5-LacZ-negative cells in the IPhCs/BCs region. $^{**}p < 0.01$, $^{***}p < 0.001$, $^{****}p < 0.0001$ as determined by a two-way ANOVA with a Tukey's or Sidak's *post hoc* test. $N = 4–5$.

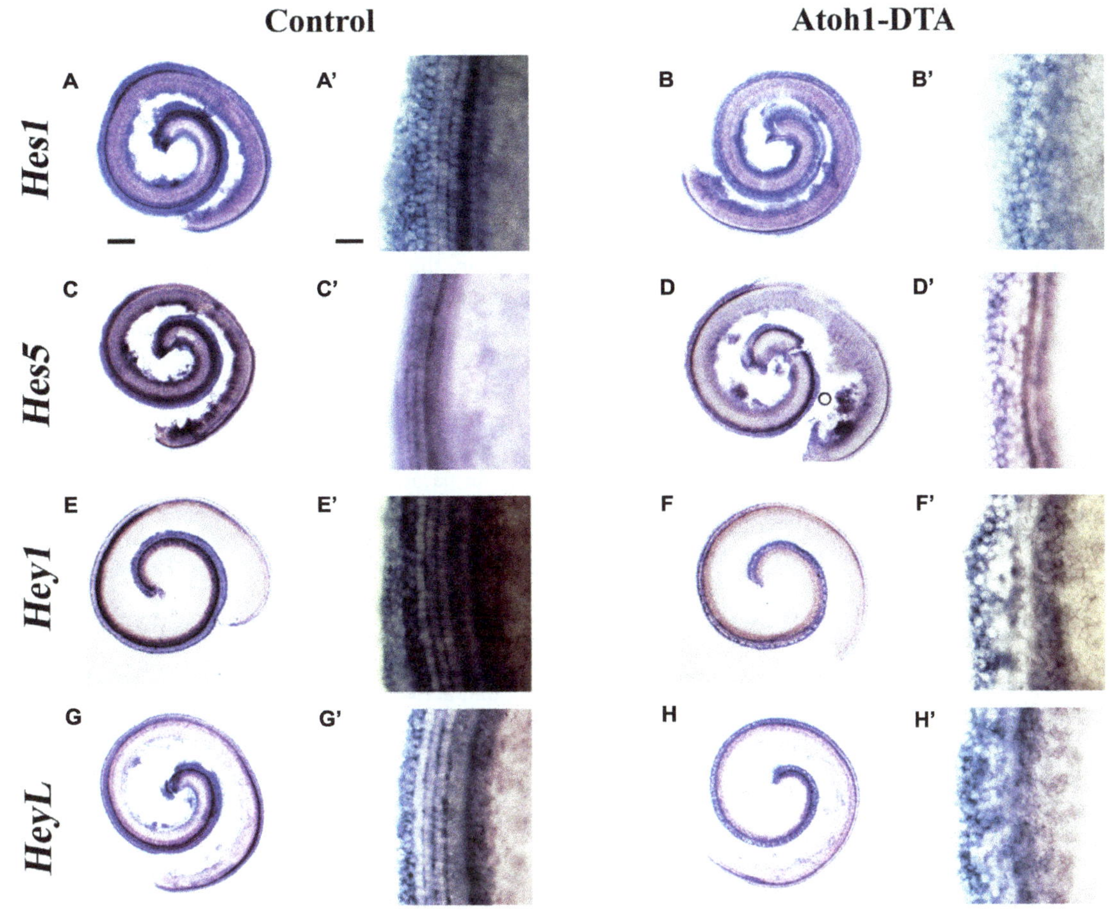

I

Gene	Number of Paired Samples with Decreased Expression	Number of Paired Samples with No Change	Number of Paired Samples with Increased Expression
Hes1	4	0	0
Hes5	4	2	1
Hey1	3	0	1
HeyL	4	0	1

FIGURE 3 | *Hes1*, *Hes5*, *Hey1*, and *HeyL* are decreased during spontaneous HC regeneration. **(A–B')** *Hes1*, **(C–D')** *Hes5*, **(E–F')** *Hey1*, and **(G–H')** *HeyL* transcripts were investigated during spontaneous HC regeneration using *in situ* hybridization. Low magnification images show the whole cochlea and high magnification images were taken from the apical turn where the majority of spontaneous HC regeneration occurs. Control cochlea **(A,A',C,C',E,E',G,G')** as well as *Atoh1-DTA* **(B,B',D,D',F,F',H,H')** littermates were injected with tamoxifen (Tam) at P0 and P1 to induce HC damage and spontaneous HC regeneration. Samples were collected at P4 and incubated with probes to label mRNA of Notch downstream effectors. Paired samples from the same litter (control and *Atoh1-DTA*) were processed in parallel and comparisons were only made between the paired samples. While there was some variability in the results obtained among experiments **(I)**, the majority of experiments showed decreased gene expression for all four Notch effectors in *Atoh1-DTA* cochleae compared to control. Scale bar for **(A,B,C,D,E,F,G,H)** = 200 μm, Scale bar for **(A',B',C',D',E',F',G',H')** = 20 μm. *N* = 4–7.

region (low magnification images in **Figures 3A,B,C,D,E,F,G,H**) and at the HC level (high magnification images taken in the apical turn, **Figures 3A',B',C',D',E',F',G',H'**) was compared between the paired control and experimental samples to determine increased or decreased expression. Expression of *Hes1* was consistently decreased in *Atoh1-DTA* samples compared to controls (**Figure 3A–B',I**, *N* = 4), while variable results were obtained for the other tested genes. For *Hes5*, four out of seven samples showed decreased expression, while one showed increased expression and two showed no change in expression (**Figures 3C–D',I**). *Hey1* expression was also variable with three samples showing decreased expression and one sample showing increased expression (**Figures 3E–F',I**). For *HeyL*, four samples showed decreased expression, while one showed increased expression (**Figures 3G–H',I**). SC-to-HC conversion is a dynamic and non-synchronous process that occurs throughout the first postnatal week (Cox et al., 2014); the variability of individual gene changes we observed may depend on the stage of SC conversion into HCs at the time of analysis. Nevertheless, because the majority of the samples showed decreased expression of Notch effectors, we conclude that loss of HCs in the neonatal mouse cochlea caused a modest decrease in Notch signaling in neighboring SCs.

The Notch Ligand and Target Gene *Jag1* Is Reduced During Spontaneous HC Regeneration

The Notch ligand *Jag1* is expressed by neonatal SCs and is also a downstream target of Notch activation (Daudet and Lewis, 2005; Murata et al., 2009). Therefore, it can be used as an indicator of active Notch signaling. Early in development *Jag1* mediates lateral induction, establishing the progenitor pool from which all HCs and SCs differentiate (Brooker et al., 2006; Kiernan et al., 2006; Murata et al., 2009). However, its function during and after HC differentiation is not well understood, yet it is expressed throughout the organ of Corti from the cells of the GER to the 3rd row of Deiters' cells (**Figures 4A–C,G–I,M–O**; Oesterle et al., 2008). We investigated changes in *Jag1* in the context of HC loss and spontaneous HC regeneration as an additional way to assess changes in the Notch signaling pathway. Specifically, *Atoh1-DTA* mice were injected with tamoxifen (3 mg/40 g, IP) at P0 and P1 to induce HC ablation thus initiating spontaneous HC regeneration. Samples were collected at P2, P4, and P6 and immunolabeled with antibodies against S100a1 and Jag1. Because Jag1 is a membrane bound protein, we could not determine which neighboring cells expressed Jag1 and therefore quantitative analysis was not performed. However, qualitative analysis of *Atoh1-DTA* cochleae showed that Jag1 labeling was reduced in the lateral region of the organ of Corti, where outer pillar cells and Deiters' cells are located, yet maintained in medial SCs, including inner pillar cells, inner phalangeal/border cells, and the cells of the GER (**Figures 4D–F,J–L,P–R**). In contrast, Jag1 labeling was consistent in all SCs throughout the width of organ of Corti in control mice (**Figures 4A–C,G–I,M–O**). These data confirm the results obtained using the $Hes5^{LacZ}$ reporter mice and demonstrate that Notch signaling is reduced in some SC subtypes, but not others, during spontaneous HC regeneration.

Overexpression of *N1ICD* Caused Increased Notch Activity in the Neonatal Cochlea

While immunostaining and *in situ* hybridization results suggest a modest decrease in Notch signaling during spontaneous HC regeneration, it is currently unknown whether Notch signaling is involved in the mechanism of spontaneous HC regeneration or if it is simply correlated. To investigate this question more directly, we induced overexpression of *N1ICD* in SCs and other non-sensory epithelial cells (all other cells within the organ of Corti except for HCs and tympanic border cells, hereinafter referred to as non-HCs) in the context of HC damage and quantified the number of regenerated HCs using fate-mapping. This was achieved by combining CreER/loxP and Tet-on genetically modified mouse systems to modify gene expression in adjacent cell populations.

To ensure feasibility of using these two inducible systems in adjacent groups of cells without cross-reaction, dual reporter expression was investigated in *Atoh1-CreER*^{TM} :: *Rosa26*$^{loxP-stop-loxP-tdTomato}$ :: *Sox10*^{rtTA} :: *TetO-LacZ* mice. tdTomato expression was induced with tamoxifen injection (3 mg/40 g, IP) at P0 and P1, while LacZ expression was induced by administering doxycycline to the nursing mother in the food (2000 mg/kg) from P0–P7, as well as a single injection (100 mg/kg) to each pup at P1. Samples were analyzed at P7. As expected, tdTomato expression was only detected in HCs, while LacZ expression was observed in SCs and non-HCs (**Figures 5A–G**). We also observed variability in the intensity of LacZ expression cell to cell, which was similar to the previously described pattern using the same doxycycline induction paradigm in *Sox10*^{rtTA}::*TetO-LacZ* mice (Walters and Zuo, 2015).

To investigate whether downregulation of Notch signaling plays a role in spontaneous HC regeneration, we used *Sox10*^{rtTA}::*TetO-LacZ*::*TetO-N1ICD* mice to overexpress *N1ICD* as well as *LacZ* to fate-map cells. Therefore, in this mouse model, *Sox10*^{rtTA} must activate two Tet-on alleles simultaneously. To verify that active Notch signaling was achieved in our model and that the presence of the *TetO-LacZ* allele did not affect the level of Notch activation, we measured *N1ICD* expression levels using qPCR. Specifically, *Sox10*^{rtTA}-negative, *Sox10*^{rtTA}::*TetO-N1ICD*, and *Sox10*^{rtTA}::*TetO-LacZ*::*TetO-N1ICD* mice were administered doxycycline, both in the diet to the nursing mother (2000 mg/kg), as well as a single injection to the pups (100 mg/kg, IP) at P1. RNA was extracted from samples collected at P7 and *N1ICD* expression was analyzed with qPCR. Of note, the primers used for *N1ICD* detection recognize both the endogenous and transgenic transcripts and data is expressed as fold change relative to the *Sox10*^{rtTA}-negative control. In both *Sox10*^{rtTA}::*TetO-N1ICD* and *Sox10*^{rtTA}::*TetO-LacZ*::*TetO-N1ICD* groups, *N1ICD* was increased 5 to 6-fold (6.4 $\pm$ 0.9-fold for *Sox10*^{rtTA}::*TetO-N1ICD*, $p < 0.001$, $N = 10$ and 5.7 $\pm$ 0.8-fold for *Sox10*^{rtTA}::*TetO-LacZ*::*TetO-N1ICD*, $p < 0.001$, $N = 10$ compared to *Sox10*^{rtTA}-negative samples; as determined by a one-way ANOVA with a Tukey's *post hoc* test, **Figure 6A**). There was no difference in the expression level of *N1ICD* between *Sox10*^{rtTA}::*TetO-N1ICD* and *Sox10*^{rtTA}::*TetO-LacZ*::*TetO-N1ICD* samples, indicating that the addition of the *TetO-LacZ* allele did not interfere with increased Notch activity induced by the *TetO-N1ICD* allele.

To further confirm increased Notch activity in our model, we used qPCR to investigate the expression level of Notch target genes, *Hes1*, *Hes5*, *Hey1*, and *HeyL*. All Notch effector genes were increased 2 to 13-fold in *Sox10*^{rtTA}::*TetO-LacZ*::*TetO-N1ICD* cochleae compared to *Sox10*^{rtTA}-negative controls (*Hes1* increased 2.6 $\pm$ 0.1-fold, $p < 0.0001$, $N = 10$; *Hes5* increased 12.7 $\pm$ 1.2-fold, $p < 0.0001$, $N = 10$; *Hey1* increased 2.4 $\pm$ 0.2-fold, $p < 0.0001$, $N = 10$; and *HeyL* increased 7.5 $\pm$ 0.7-fold, $p < 0.0001$, $N = 10$ compared to *Sox10*^{rtTA}-negative controls as determined by a Student's t-test for each gene; **Figure 6B**). Therefore, we conclude that Notch signaling was increased by *N1ICD* overexpression in our model.

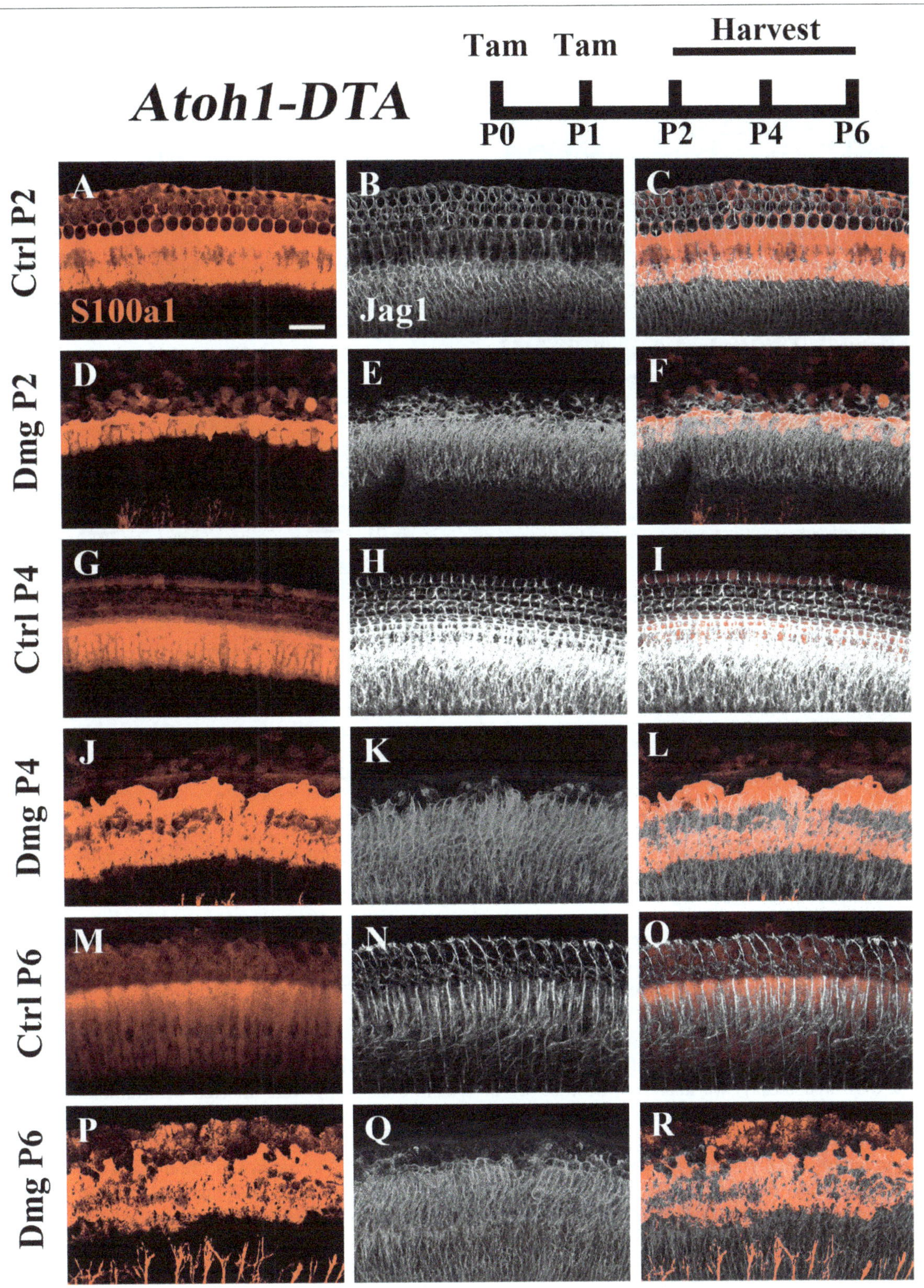

FIGURE 4 | Jag1 labeling is reduced in lateral, but not medial, SCs during spontaneous HC regeneration. *Atoh1-DTA* mice were injected with tamoxifen (Tam) at P0–P1 to induce HC death and spontaneous HC regeneration and cochleae were collected at P2, P4, or P6. **(A,R)** Representative maximum projection images with anti-Jag1 antibodies to detect Jag1 expression (white) and anti-S100a1 (red) antibodies to mark the pillar and Deiters' cells region. After HC damage, both S100a1 and Jag1 labeling was reduced in the outer pillar and Deiters' cell region, while expression is maintained in medial SCs **(D–F,J–L,P–R)** and in all SCs in control samples **(A–C,G–I,M–O)**. Scale bar = 25 μm. *N* = 3.

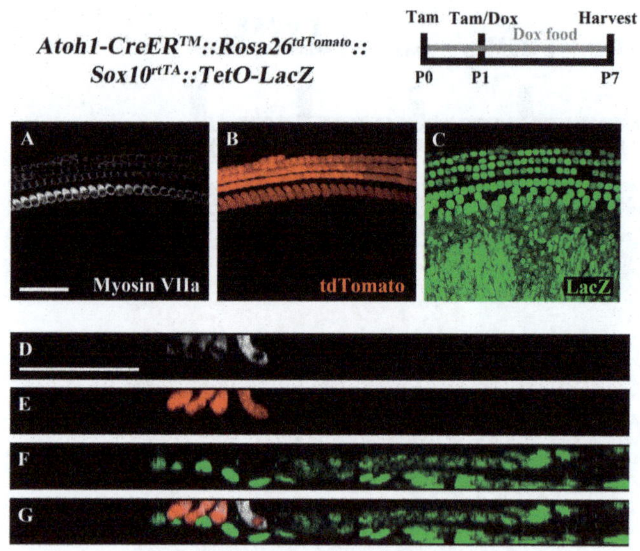

FIGURE 5 | The combination of CreER/loxP and Tet-On genetic systems allow gene manipulation in distinct cell types without cross-reactivity. *Atoh1-CreER^{TM}::Rosa26$^{loxP-stop-loxP-tdTomato}$::Sox10^{rtTA}::TetO-LacZ* mice were injected with tamoxifen (Tam) at P0 and P1 to induce tdTomato expression. Doxycycline (Dox) was administered to nursing mother in the diet and each pup received a dox injection at P1 to induce LacZ expression. Cochleae were collected at P7 and stained with antibodies against myosin VIIa (white) to label HCs and β-gal (green) to label LacZ-positive cells. **(A–C)** Representative confocal slice images show expression of endogenous tdTomato fluorescence (red) detected in HCs similar to Cox et al. (2014). β-gal expression (green) was detected in SCs and other non-HCs similar to Walters and Zuo (2015). **(D–G)** Optical cross-sections showing expression of tdTomato in HCs and β-gal in SCs and all non-HCs. Scale bar = 50 μm. *N* = 3.

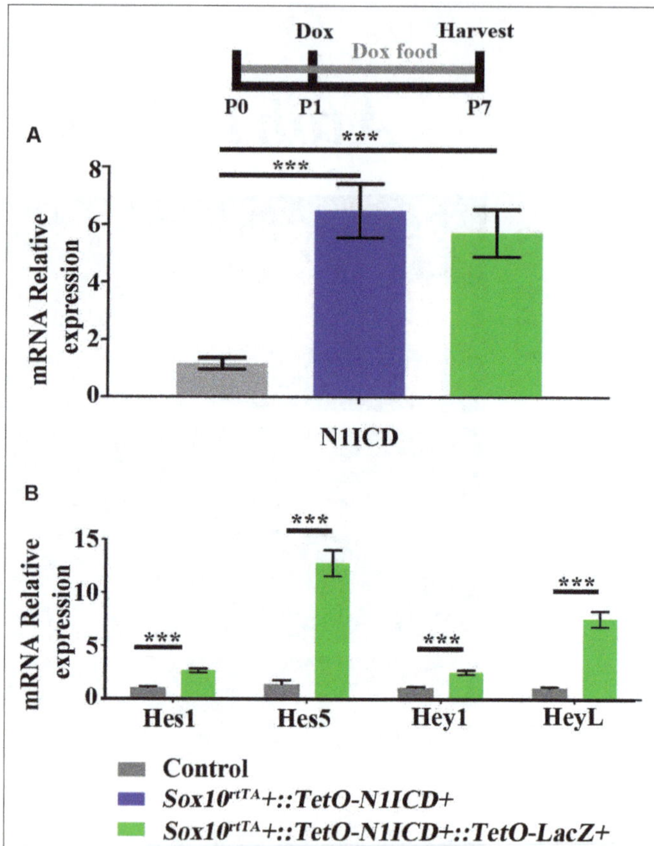

FIGURE 6 | Increased expression of *N1ICD* driven by *Sox10^{rtTA}* leads to increased expression of Notch downstream effectors. *Sox10^{rtTA}*-negative, *Sox10^{rtTA}::TetO-N1ICD,* and *Sox10^{rtTA}::TetO-LacZ::TetO-N1ICD* mice were administered doxycycline (Dox), in the diet to nursing mother, as well as an injection to each pup at P1. Cochleae were frozen at P7 and mRNA transcripts were measured. **(A)** *N1ICD* expression was increased in *Sox10^{rtTA}::TetO-N1ICD,* and *Sox10^{rtTA}::TetO-LacZ::TetO-N1ICD* cochlea, compared to *Sox10^{rtTA}*-negative controls. There was no difference in the expression of *N1ICD* when *TetO-LacZ* was also present. **(B)** Expression level of Notch effectors *Hes1, Hes5, Hey1*, and *HeyL* were increased in *Sox10^{rtTA}::TetO-LacZ::TetO-N1ICD* cochlea, compared to *Sox10^{rtTA}*-negative controls. $^{***}p < 0.001$ as determined by a one-way ANOVA with a Dunnett's *post hoc* test or a Student's *t*-test. *N* = 10.

Spontaneous HC Regeneration Is Reduced When the *N1ICD* Is Overexpressed in SCs and Other Non-HCs

To investigate whether spontaneous HC regeneration could be prevented by increased Notch signaling, we overexpressed *N1ICD* in SCs and other non-HCs in the context of HC damage using *Atoh1-DTA::Sox10^{rtTA}::TetO-LacZ::TetO-N1ICD* mice. The effect of increased Notch signaling on spontaneous HC regeneration was investigated by quantifying the number of fate-mapped SCs. Specifically, we analyzed the number of LacZ-positive HCs in each of four groups. First, to verify the expression pattern of *Sox10^{rtTA}* in a normal neonatal cochlea, the number of LacZ-positive HCs was quantified in *Sox10^{rtTA}::TetO-LacZ* mice. Second, to determine the number of spontaneously regenerated HCs that occur naturally in the neonatal mouse cochlea after HC loss at birth, we quantified LacZ-positive HCs in *Atoh1-DTA::Sox10^{rtTA}::TetO-LacZ* mice. Third, to determine the effect of *N1ICD* overexpression in SCs and other non-HCs in the neonatal mouse cochlea, LacZ-positive HCs were quantified in *Sox10^{rtTA}::TetO-LacZ::TetO-N1ICD* mice. Finally, to investigate whether overexpression of *N1ICD* in SCs and other non-HCs will prevent spontaneous HC regeneration from occurring, we quantified LacZ-positive HCs in *Atoh1-DTA::Sox10^{rtTA}::TetO-LacZ::TetO-N1ICD* mice. Mice from each group were injected with tamoxifen (3 mg/kg, IP) at P0 and P1 to induce HC damage. *N1ICD* and *LacZ* expression were induced through administration of doxycycline given both in the food (2000 mg/kg) to the nursing mother, as well as one doxycycline injection (100 mg/kg, IP) given to the pups at P1, ~6 h after tamoxifen injection. Samples were collected at P7 and processed for immunostaining with antibodies against myosin VIIa, Sox2, and β-gal.

As expected from previous work (Walters and Zuo, 2015), *LacZ* expression in *Sox10^{rtTA}::TetO-LacZ* mice was observed in SCs and other non-HCs within the P7 cochlea. We also observed 2.0 ± 2.0 LacZ-positive HCs in the very apical tip (**Figures 7Q,R**, *N* = 4). There was no significant change in LacZ-positive HCs when *N1ICD* was overexpressed without HC damage in

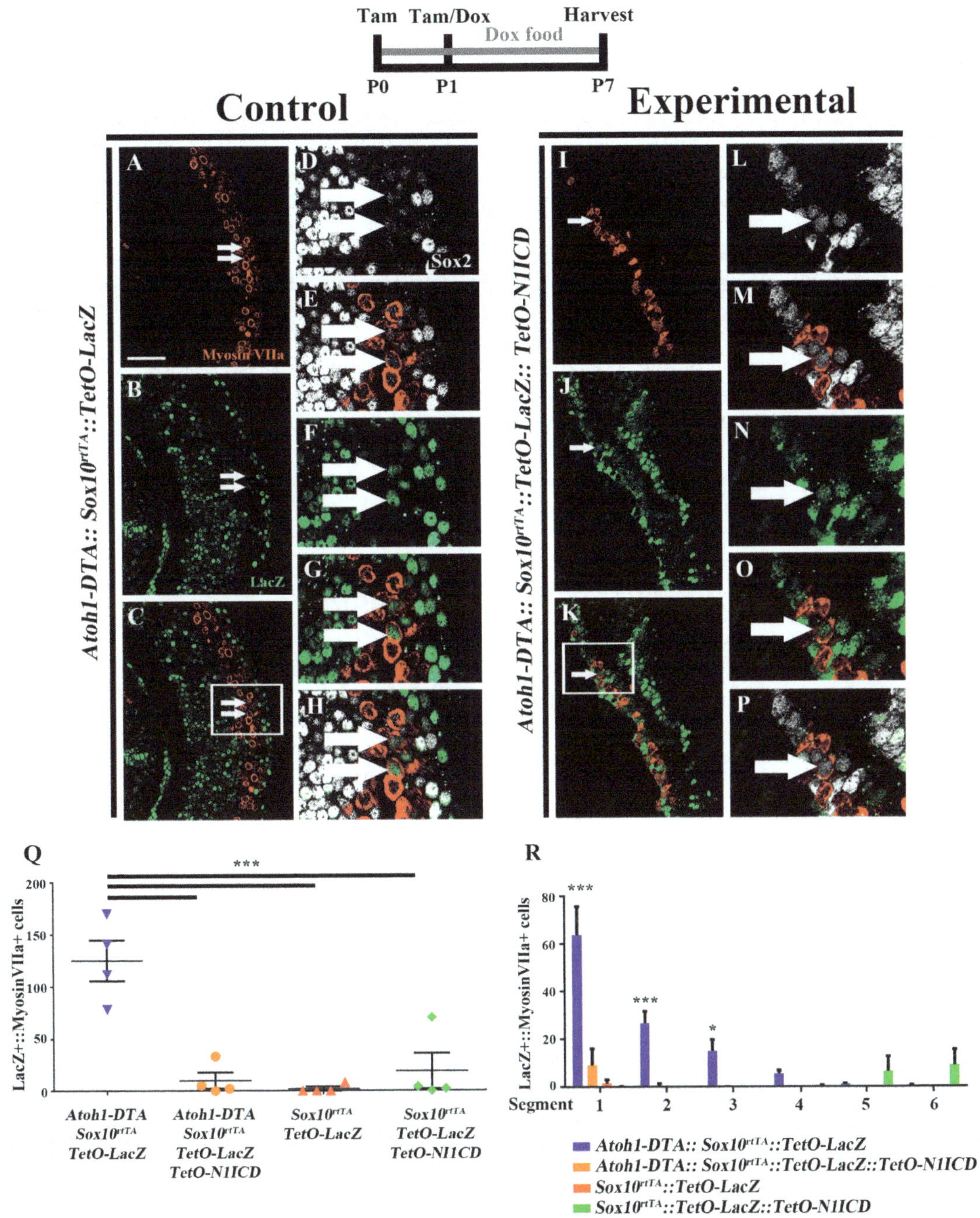

FIGURE 7 | Fewer spontaneously regenerated HCs were observed in the presence of *N1ICD* overexpression. Representative confocal slice images taken from the apical turn of the cochlea of **(A–H)** *Atoh1-DTA::Sox10^{rtTA}::TetO-LacZ* and **(I–P)** *Atoh1-DTA::Sox10^{rtTA}::TetO-LacZ::TetO-N1ICD* mice that were injected with tamoxifen (Tam) at P0/P1 to induce CreER-mediated HC loss and induce spontaneous HC regeneration, as well as administered doxycycline (Dox) in the diet to nursing mother with a dox injection given to pups at P1 to induce expression of *N1ICD* and the *LacZ* reporter in SCs and all non-HCs. Cochlea were collected at P7 and stained with antibodies against myosin VIIa (red), Sox2 (white), and β-gal (green). Fewer fate-mapped regenerated HCs (LacZ-positive/myosin VIIa-positive cells, white arrows) were observed when *N1ICD* was overexpressed in combination with HC damage compared to samples with HC damage and normal Notch signaling. **(D–H,L–P)** High magnification images from boxes in **(C,K)** showing LacZ-positive/Sox2-positive/myosin VIIa-positive regenerated HCs. Scale bar = 25 μm. **(Q)** Quantification of LacZ-positive HCs from the images presented in **(A–P)** and the two additional controls. Comparison of the number of LacZ-positive HCs between the group with spontaneous HC regeneration and normal Notch signaling (blue, *Atoh1-DTA::Sox10^{rtTA}::TetO-LacZ* mice) and the experimental group with *N1ICD* overexpression as well as HC damage (orange, *Atoh1-DTA::Sox10^{rtTA}::TetO-LacZ::TetO-N1ICD)*, showed a ~92% decrease in the number of LacZ-positive, regenerated HCs. **(R)** LacZ-positive HCs after HC damage with physiological Notch signaling (blue, *Atoh1-DTA::Sox10^{rtTA}::TetO-LacZ*) decreased in an apical to basal gradient while LacZ-positive HCs were only detected in the base when *N1ICD* was overexpressed without HC damage (green, *Sox10^{rtTA}::TetO-LacZ::TetO-N1ICD*) mice. Segment 1 is the most apical region and segment 6 is the most basal. N = 3–4. *$p < 0.05$, ***$p < 0.001$ as determined by a two-way ANOVA with a Tukey's *post hoc* test. N = 4.

Sox10^{rtTA}*::TetO-LacZ::TetO-N1ICD* mice (19.0 ± 17.2, compared to *Sox10*^{rtTA}*::TetO-LacZ* controls, $N = 4$, $p = 0.8$ as determined by a one-way ANOVA with a Tukey's *post hoc* test; **Figure 7Q**). However, we observed disorganization of HCs (**Supplementary Figures S2A,G**) as well as an expansion of Sox2 expression both medial and lateral to the organ of Corti, (**Supplementary Figures S2A–D,F–I**). Quantification of HCs in *Sox10*^{rtTA}*::TetO-LacZ::TetO-N1ICD* mice showed that there was no difference in the number of HCs compared to *Sox10*^{rtTA}*::TetO-LacZ* mice (91.0 ± 2.5 compared to 88.7 ± 5.9 per 200 μm, $p = 0.5$ as determined by a Student's *t*-test, **Supplementary Figure S2E**) and therefore this phenotype likely did not affect spontaneous HC regeneration observed in our study.

When LacZ was used for fate-mapping during spontaneous HC regeneration, significantly more LacZ-positive HCs were detected in *Atoh1-DTA::Sox10*^{rtTA}*::TetO-LacZ* mice than in *Sox10*^{rtTA}*::TetO-LacZ* controls (125.3 ± 19.7 compared to 2.0 ± 2.0, $p = 0.0002$, $N = 4$, **Figure 7Q**). When *N1ICD* was overexpressed in the context of HC damage (*Atoh1-DTA::Sox10*^{rtTA}*::TetO-LacZ::TetO-N1ICD* mice), there was a 92% reduction in LacZ-positive HCs compared to similar samples without *N1ICD* overexpression (*Atoh1-DTA::Sox10*^{rtTA}*::TetO-LacZ* mice) (10.0 ± 7.7 compared to 125.3 ± 19.7, $p = 0.0003$, $N = 4$, **Figures 7A–Q**). Moreover, the number of LacZ-positive HCs when *N1ICD* was overexpressed and HCs were killed was not significantly different from controls lacking both HC damage and *N1ICD* overexpression (*Sox10*^{rtTA}*::TetO-LacZ* samples) (10.0 ± 7.7 compared to 2.0 ± 2.0, $p = 0.9$) or *N1ICD* overexpression alone (*Sox10rtTA::TetO-LacZ::TetO-N1ICD* samples) (10.0 ± 7.7 compared to 19.0 ± 17.0, $p = 0.9$ as determined by a one-way ANOVA with a Tukey's *post hoc* test; **Figure 7Q**). Therefore, we conclude that overexpression of *N1ICD* prevented the majority of spontaneous HC regeneration from occurring. Of note, we observed an expansion of Sox2 expressing cells in *Atoh1-DTA::Sox10*^{rtTA}*::TetO-LacZ::TetO-N1ICD* mice, similar to what we observed in *Sox10*^{rtTA}*::TetO-LacZ::TetO-N1ICD* controls (**Supplementary Figures S2F–M**).

We wanted to better understand the location of fate-mapped, spontaneously regenerated HCs in our samples because the majority of spontaneous HC regeneration is known to occur in the apical third of the neonatal cochlea (Cox et al., 2014) and because Notch signaling decreases in a basal to apical gradient during the first postnatal week (Maass et al., 2015). Therefore, the whole cochlea was imaged, measured, and divided into six equal segments from apex to base as previously described (McGovern et al., 2017) and the total number of LacZ-positive/myosin VIIa-positive HCs within each segment was quantified. The majority of fate-mapped, spontaneously regenerated HCs (from *Atoh1-DTA::Sox10*^{rtTA}*::TetO-LacZ* mice) were found in the two most apical segments (63.8 ± 12.0 in segment 1 and 26.8 ± 4.9 in segment 2) and this declined in an apical to basal gradient (15.4 ± 4.8 in segment 3, 5.6 ± 1.4 in segment 4, 1.2 ± 0.3 in segment 5, and 0.4 ± 0.4 in segment 6, $r^2 = 0.66$. $p < 0.0001$ **Figure 7R**), similar to the previous report (Cox et al., 2014). In one *Sox10*^{rtTA}*::TetO-LacZ::TetO-N1ICD* sample that did not have HC damage, we observed 67 LacZ-positive HCs in the two basal segments, but no LacZ-positive HCs were detected in the middle or apical segments of the cochlea where the majority of HC regeneration was observed (**Figure 7R**). The other three *Sox10*^{rtTA}*::TetO-LacZ::TetO-N1ICD* samples had no LacZ-positive HCs. Therefore, the LacZ-positive HCs observed in *N1ICD* overexpressing controls did not interfere with the quantification of fate-mapped, spontaneously regenerated HCs predominantly observed in the apical turn of the cochlea. When *N1ICD* was overexpressed along with HC damage, the fate-mapped regenerated HCs in the *Atoh1-DTA::Sox10*^{rtTA}*::TetO-LacZ::TetO-N1ICD* mice were all located within the first two apical segments (**Figure 7R**), similar to the control with spontaneous HC regeneration and no manipulation of Notch (*Atoh1-DTA::Sox10*^{rtTA}*::TetO-LacZ* mice). This illustrates that the regenerative capacity of SCs is correlated to the basal to apical changes in the Notch signaling pathway. Our data show weakened Notch signaling during the spontaneous HC regeneration process, as well as the suppression of HC regeneration by increased Notch activity. Taken together, this suggests that Notch signaling plays a role in the ability of SCs to spontaneously convert into, thus regenerate, HCs.

DISCUSSION

This study investigated the role of Notch signaling during spontaneous HC regeneration within the neonatal mouse cochlea *in vivo*. After HC damage and during the window of spontaneous HC regeneration, we observed a modest decrease in Notch signaling, as evidenced by decreased expression of the Notch target genes *Hes1, Hes5, Hey1, HeyL,* and *Jag1* using immunostaining or *in situ* hybridization. These changes suggest that Notch signaling is weakened in SCs after HC loss occurs and may allow their conversion into HCs. To investigate this further, we increased Notch signaling in SCs and other non-HCs by overexpressing *N1ICD* during the window of spontaneous HC regeneration. In samples with increased Notch signaling, there was a 92% reduction in the number of spontaneously regenerated HCs, suggesting that Notch signaling plays a role in spontaneous HC regeneration.

The Expression of *Hes1*, *Hes5*, *Hey1*, and *HeyL* Were Reduced During the Window of Spontaneous HC Regeneration

Using *in situ* hybridization and a *Hes5*^{LacZ} knockin reporter line, we discovered that the expression of *Hes1, Hes5, Hey1,* and *HeyL* was reduced after HC loss and during the spontaneous HC regeneration process. Both *Hes1* and *Hes5* directly inhibit a HC fate by inhibiting the expression of *Atoh1*, a transcription factor that is necessary for HC differentiation (Zheng et al., 2000; Mulvaney and Dabdoub, 2012; Abdolazimi et al., 2016). Previously, Korrapati et al. (2013) found that HC damage after gentamicin treatment *in vitro* leads to downregulation of *Hes5*, but no other Notch-related genes expressed in SCs. However, no HC regeneration was observed in this model until Notch signaling was inhibited with a γ-secretase inhibitor, which caused decreased expression of all Notch downstream effectors. This suggests that reduction of *Hes5* signaling alone is insufficient to induce spontaneous HC regeneration, however, when reduced expression is expanded to additional Notch effectors, regeneration is possible. In support, overexpression of *Hes1* is able to inhibit the production of ectopic HCs in the GER that were created by ectopic expression of *Atoh1*. This indicates that *Hes1* is also a direct inhibitor of HC fate (Zheng et al., 2000). Furthermore, combined loss of *Hes1*, *Hes5*, and *Hey1* during late embryonic development [embryonic day (E) 18.5] caused increased outer HCs with disorganized pillar and Deiters' cells (Tateya et al., 2011). Unfortunately, less is known about the function of the Notch effector *HeyL* in cochlear development, however, it is expressed around the time of HC differentiation and is linked to neuronal differentiation in other systems (Doetzlhofer et al., 2009; Jalali et al., 2011). Therefore, combined reduction of *Hes1, Hes5*, and *Hey1*, and possibly *HeyL*, observed in our study are correlated with the ability of SCs to spontaneously regenerate HCs in the neonatal mouse cochlea, thus supporting our conclusion that weakened Notch signaling allows SC-to-HC conversion and plays a role in spontaneous HC regeneration.

Jag1 Is Reduced During the Spontaneous HC Regeneration Process

In the developing cochlea, *Jag1* is initially expressed throughout the sensory epithelium, then restricted to SCs, with expression in all SC subtypes from the GER to the 3rd row of Deiters' cells at neonatal ages and in adulthood (Morrison et al., 1999; Daudet and Lewis, 2005; Oesterle et al., 2008; Murata et al., 2009). However, its function during and after HC differentiation is not well understood. Furthermore, *Jag1* is both a Notch ligand as well as a Notch target gene (Daudet and Lewis, 2005; Murata et al., 2006) and as such, reduced expression of this gene can indicate loss of Notch signaling. Consistent with results from the *Hes5^{LacZ}* reporter and *in situ* hybridization, Jag1 expression was decreased in *Atoh1-DTA* samples in outer pillar and Deiters' cells, the SC subtypes located underneath outer HCs in the lateral compartment of the cochlea. This finding further supports our conclusion that there is a modest decrease in Notch activity in SCs after HC damage and during HC regeneration in the neonatal cochlea.

The Majority of Spontaneous HC Regeneration Is Prevented When *N1ICD* Is Overexpressed in SCs and Other Non-HCs in the Neonatal Mouse Cochlea

Previous work has focused on the effect of induced Notch inhibition via pharmacologic manipulation with γ-secretase inhibitors (Yamamoto et al., 2006; Korrapati et al., 2013; Li et al., 2015) or deletion of Notch receptors or *RBP-J* (Yamamoto et al., 2006; Bramhall et al., 2014; Li et al., 2015). From these studies we know that loss of Notch signaling triggers SC-to-HC conversion, however, while this approach produces new HCs, it applies a blanket reduction in all Notch related genes, as well as potentially affects other signaling pathways that γ-secretase interacts with such as ErbB-4, E-Cadherin, N-Cadherin, EphrinB, and CD44 (Ni et al., 2001; Lammich et al., 2002; Marambaud et al., 2002, 2003; Georgakopoulos et al., 2006). Therefore, it is unclear whether decreased Notch signaling in SCs is part of the molecular mechanism for spontaneous HC regeneration. Our study attempts to address this gap in knowledge by showing that overexpression of *N1ICD* in SCs and other non-HCs causes an increase in Notch signaling and results in a 92% reduction in the number of regenerated HCs. However, the mouse model we used generated supraphysiological levels of Notch activity with *N1ICD* increased 5 to 6-fold and *Hes*/*Hey* genes increased 2 to 13-fold over controls. It is possible that the level of Notch signaling is important in controlling HC and SC fate. In support of this notion, there was one *Atoh1-DTA::Sox10^{rtTA}::TetO-LacZ::TetO-N1ICD* sample with 33 fate-mapped regenerated HCs, while the other three samples that had 0-5 fate-mapped regenerated HCs. While not directly tested, the sample with more regenerated HCs may have had lower expression of *N1ICD* compared to the other three samples, which could have been caused by decreased exposure to doxycycline. Despite the limitation of supraphysiological *N1ICD* and Notch effector levels in our model, data from this study support a role for Notch signaling during the spontaneous HC regeneration process.

Sox10^{rtTA} is a knockin allele that may produce decreased expression of *Sox10* in the neonatal cochlea. It is possible that decreased *Sox10* expression may alter normal spontaneous HC regeneration making it more dependent on Notch signaling and therefore making *N1ICD* overexpression more effective at preventing regeneration. While we cannot rule out this possibility, a previous study showed that *Sox10^{rtTA}* mice do not have a haploinsufficient phenotype in the cochlea (Walters and Zuo, 2015). Yet little is known about the relationship between *Sox10* and Notch signaling, and further research is needed.

Unexpectedly, in the control samples where *N1ICD* was overexpressed without HC damage (*Sox10^{rtTA}::TetO-LacZ::TetO-N1ICD* mice) and in experimental samples (*Atoh1-DTA::Sox10^{rtTA}::TetO-LacZ::TetO-N1ICD* mice), we observed an expansion of the region with Sox2-positive cells both medial and lateral to the organ of Corti. *Sox10^{rtTA}::TetO-LacZ::TetO-N1ICD* controls also had disorganized HCs, but no decrease in HC number. Similar studies were done previously in the embryonic and early neonatal cochlea where *N1ICD* overexpression led to ectopic sensory patches containing both Sox2-positive cells and HCs in non-sensory regions. Yet this was only observed when *N1ICD* was overexpressed prior to E14.5 (Hartman et al., 2010; Pan et al., 2010, 2013; Liu et al., 2012; Campbell et al., 2015). Studies where *N1ICD* overexpression was induced after E14.5 showed no ectopic HCs or Sox2-positive cells (Liu et al., 2012; Pan et al., 2013). These studies demonstrate that *N1ICD* overexpression can induce Sox2 expression and sensory progenitor cells in non-sensory regions, yet there is a temporal limitation for when these cells can respond. Therefore, the increased numbers of Sox2-positive cells we observed when *N1ICD* was overexpressed at P0 was unexpected. We may have overcome temporal limitations by producing supraphysiological levels of *N1ICD* and Notch effectors, but further experiments are needed to confirm this hypothesis. Regardless of the cause, we do not believe expanded Sox2 expression altered the spontaneous HC regeneration process or affected the conclusions of our study since all abnormalities, except HC disorganization, were observed outside the organ of Corti.

Notch signaling changes dynamically in the first week after birth where ligands, receptors, and effectors are downregulated in a basal-to-apical gradient between P0 and P6 (Murata et al., 2006; Hartman et al., 2007; Maass et al., 2015). However, Jag1 is the exception and its expression in SCs continues throughout adulthood (Oesterle et al., 2008). During the first postnatal week, inhibition of Notch signaling using γ-secretase inhibitors has differential effects on SC-to-HC conversion along the basal to apical axis. Notch inhibition at P0 produces a ~200% increase in HCs in the apex compared to only a ~30% increase in the base, while there is no evidence of HC production in any cochlear turn when γ-secretase inhibitors are used at P3 or later (Maass et al., 2015). There are conflicting reports for whether SCs can produce HCs in response to Notch inhibition in the adult cochlea (Batts et al., 2009; Doetzlhofer et al., 2009; Hartman et al., 2009; Mizutari et al., 2013). These data taken together with our results suggest that spontaneous HC regeneration likely occurs when HCs are killed at P0–P1 because SCs, especially those in the apical turn, are still dependent on Notch signaling to maintain their cell fate. As the cochlea matures, it appears that SC fate maintenance becomes uncoupled from Notch signaling, yet the upstream regulators or epigenetic changes that cause downregulation of the Notch pathway, as well as the mechanisms that maintain SC fate after the first postnatal week are unknown.

Nevertheless, while previous studies have shown that increased numbers of regenerated HCs can form when Notch signaling is inhibited (Korrapati et al., 2013; Bramhall et al., 2014; Hu et al., 2016), the findings presented here are the first to demonstrate that the spontaneous HC regeneration process is prevented by increased Notch signaling. This suggests that weakened Notch signaling plays a role in the spontaneous HC regeneration process. Understanding the molecular mechanism of spontaneous HC regeneration is a critical step to understanding why HC regeneration does not occur in the mature cochlea. Additionally, while some Notch effectors, such as *Hes1* and *Hes5*, are well established as inhibitors of HC fate, less is known about the contribution of other effectors on SC-to-HC conversion. The findings presented here will hopefully drive research to identify cellular and molecular changes that occur within the first postnatal week to uncouple Notch signaling and SC fate maintenance. Understanding what assumes control over SC fate in the adult cochlea will potentially lead investigations into therapeutic targets to stimulate HC regeneration in the mature cochlea.

AUTHOR CONTRIBUTIONS

MM designed and performed the experiments, analyzed the data, and wrote the manuscript. LZ and MR performed the experiments, analyzed the data, and contributed to writing the manuscript. BC designed the experiments, analyzed the data, and wrote the manuscript.

FUNDING

This work was supported by the Office of the Assistant Secretary of Defense for Health Affairs (W81XWH-15-1-0475), the Office of Naval Research (N00014-13-1-0569), and the National Institutes of Health (R01 DC014441). The SIUSOM Research Imaging Facility is supported by a grant from the Office of Naval Research (N00014-15-1-2866) and the National Center for Research Resources-Health (S10RR027716).

ACKNOWLEDGMENTS

We thank Kaley Graves from Southern Illinois University School of Medicine for technical assistance, Dr. Bernd Fritzsch from the University of Iowa, and Dr. Andy Wilber from Southern Illinois University School of Medicine for their assistance with *in situ* hybridization experiments. We thank Dr. Andy Groves from Baylor College of Medicine for the critical discussion and assistance with *in situ* hybridization experiments. We are grateful to Dr. Suzanne Baker (St. Jude Children's Research Hospital) for sharing *Atoh1-CreER^{TM}* mice, Dr. Ryoichiro Kageyama (Kyoto University) for sharing *Hes5^{LacZ}* mice, Dr. Michael Wegner (Erlangen University) for sharing *Sox10^{rtTA}* mice, and Dr. Ben Stranger (University of Pennsylvania) for sharing *TetO-N1ICD* mice.

SUPPLEMENTARY MATERIAL

The Supplementary Material for this article can be found online at: https://www.frontiersin.org/articles/10.3389/fncel.2018.00120/full#supplementary-material

FIGURE S1 | Inner phalangeal and border cells labeling by *Plp-CreER^{T2}::Rosa26^{tdTomato}*. **(A–C)** Representative confocal images of *Plp-CreER^{T2}::Rosa26^{tdTomato}* samples injected with tamoxifen (Tam) at P0. tdTomato labeling allowed the measurement of the inner phalangeal and border cell region for quantification of Hes5-LacZ and Sox2 expressing cells in **Figure 2**. This width was 9.6 μm at P2, 13.2 μm at P4, and 16.8 μm at P6. Scale bar = 25 μm.

FIGURE S2 | Expansion of the Sox2-postive region and HC disorganization when *N1ICD* is overexpressed. **(A–D)** Representative confocal images taken from the apical turn of the cochlea from *Sox10^{rtTA}::TetO-LacZ::TetO-N1ICD* mice that were injected with tamoxifen (Tam) at P0/P1 as well as administered doxycycline (Dox) in the diet to nursing mother with a doxycycline injection given to pups at P1 to induce expression of *N1ICD* and the *LacZ* reporter in SCs and other non-HCs. Cochlea were collected at P7 and stained with antibodies against myosin VIIa (red), Sox2 (white), and β-gal (green). While there was disorganization of HCs **(A)**, there was no change in the number of HCs in any of the cochlear turns. (**E**, quantified in a 200 μm region). Scale bar = 25 μm. *N* = 4. **(F–I)** Maximum projection images of *Sox10^{rtTA}::TetO-LacZ* and **(J–M)** *Atoh1-DTA::Sox10^{rtTA}::TetO-LacZ::TetO-N1ICD* apical turns showing expanded Sox2 expression medial and lateral to the organ of Corti. Scale bar = 20 μm.

REFERENCES

Abdolazimi, Y., Stojanova, Z., and Segil, N. (2016). Selection of cell fate in the organ of Corti involves the integration of Hes/Hey signaling at the Atoh1 promoter. *Development* 143, 841–850. doi: 10.1242/dev.129320

Basch, M. L., Ohyama, T., Segil, N., and Groves, A. K. (2011). Canonical Notch signaling is not necessary for prosensory induction in the mouse cochlea: insights from a conditional mutant of RBPj. *J. Neurosci.* 31, 8046–8058. doi: 10.1523/JNEUROSCI.6671-10.2011

Batts, S. A., Shoemaker, C. R., and Raphael, Y. (2009). Notch signaling and Hes labeling in the normal and drug-damaged organ of Corti. *Hear. Res.* 249, 15–22. doi: 10.1016/j.heares.2008.12.008

Bermingham-McDonogh, O., and Rubel, E. W. (2003). Hair cell regeneration: winging our way towards a sound future. *Curr. Opin. Neurobiol.* 13, 119–126. doi: 10.1016/S0959-4388(03)00018-7

Bohne, B. A. (1976). Safe level for noise exposure? *Ann. Otol. Rhinol. Laryngol.* 85, 711–724. doi: 10.1177/000348947608500602

Bramhall, N. F., Shi, F., Arnold, K., Hochedlinger, K., and Edge, A. S. (2014). Lgr5-positive supporting cells generate new hair cells in the postnatal cochlea. *Stem Cell Reports* 2, 311–322. doi: 10.1016/j.stemcr.2014.01.008

Brignull, H. R., Raible, D. W., and Stone, J. S. (2009). Feathers and fins: non-mammalian models for hair cell regeneration. *Brain Res.* 1277, 12–23. doi: 10.1016/j.brainres.2009.02.028

Brooker, R., Hozumi, K., and Lewis, J. (2006). Notch ligands with contrasting functions: jagged1 and Delta1 in the mouse inner ear. *Development* 133, 1277–1286. doi: 10.1242/dev.02284

Buckiová, D., and Syka, J. (2009). Calbindin and S100 protein expression in the developing inner ear in mice. *J. Comp. Neurol.* 513, 469–482. doi: 10.1002/cne.21967

Campbell, D. P., Chrysostomou, E., and Doetzlhofer, A. (2015). Canonical Notch signaling plays an instructive role in auditory supporting cell development. *Sci. Rep.* 6:19484. doi: 10.1038/srep19484

Chonko, K. T., Jahan, I., Stone, J., Wright, M. C., Fujiyama, T., Hoshino, M., et al. (2013). Atoh1 directs hair cell differentiation and survival in the late embryonic mouse inner ear. *Dev. Biol.* 381, 401–410. doi: 10.1016/j.ydbio.2013.06.022

Chow, L. M., Tian, Y., Weber, T., Corbett, M., Zuo, J., and Baker, S. J. (2006). Inducible Cre recombinase activity in mouse cerebellar granule cell precursors and inner ear hair cells. *Dev. Dyn.* 235, 2991–2998. doi: 10.1002/dvdy.20948

Cox, B. C., Chai, R., Lenoir, A., Liu, Z., Zhang, L., Nguyen, D.-H., et al. (2014). Spontaneous hair cell regeneration in the neonatal mouse cochlea in vivo. *Development* 141, 816–829. doi: 10.1242/dev.103036

Cox, B. C., Liu, Z., Lagarde, M. M., and Zuo, J. (2012). Conditional gene expression in the mouse inner ear using cre-loxP. *J. Assoc. Res. Otolaryngol.* 13, 295–322. doi: 10.1007/s10162-012-0324-5

Daudet, N., and Lewis, J. (2005). Two contrasting roles for Notch activity in chick inner ear development: specification of prosensory patches and lateral inhibition of hair-cell differentiation. *Development* 132, 541–551. doi: 10.1242/dev.01589

Doerflinger, N., Macklin, W., and Popko, B. (2003). Inducible site-specific recombination in myelinating cells. *Genesis* 35, 63–72. doi: 10.1002/gene.10154/full

Doetzlhofer, A., Basch, M. L., Ohyama, T., Gessler, M., Groves, A. K., and Segil, N. (2009). Hey2 regulation by FGF provides a notch-independent mechanism for maintaining pillar cell fate in the organ of Corti. *Dev. Cell* 16, 58–69. doi: 10.1016/j.devcel.2008.11.008

Furth, P. A., Onget, L. S., Bögert, H., Grusst, P., Gossen, M., Kistner, A., et al. (1994). Temporal control of gene expression in transgenic mice by a tetracycline-responsive promoter. *Biochemistry* 91, 9302–9306. doi: 10.1073/pnas.91.20.9302

Georgakopoulos, A., Litterst, C., Ghersi, E., Baki, L., Xu, C. J., Serban, G., et al. (2006). Metalloproteinase/presenilin1 processing of ephrinB regulates EphB-induced Src phosphorylation and signaling. *EMBO J.* 25, 1242–1252. doi: 10.1038/sj.emboj.7601031

Gómez-Casati, M. M., Murtie, J., Taylor, B., and Corfas, G. (2010). Cell-specific inducible gene recombination in postnatal inner ear supporting cells and glia. *J. Assoc. Res. Otolaryngol.* 11, 19–26. doi: 10.1007/s10162-009-0191-x

Hartman, B. H., Basak, O., Nelson, B. R., Taylor, V., Bermingham-Mcdonogh, O., and Reh, T. A. (2009). Hes5 expression in the postnatal and adult mouse inner ear and the drug-damaged cochlea. *J. Assoc. Res. Otolaryngol.* 10, 321–340. doi: 10.1007/s10162-009-0162-2

Hartman, B. H., Hayashi, T., Nelson, B. R., Bermingham-McDonogh, O., and Reh, T. (2007). Dll3 is expressed in developing hair cells in the mammalian cochlea. *Dev. Dyn.* 236, 2875–2883. doi: 10.1002/dvdy.21307

Hartman, B. H., Reh, T. A., and Bermingham-McDonogh, O. (2010). Notch signaling specifies prosensory domains via lateral induction in the developing mammalian inner ear. *Proc. Natl. Acad. Sci. U.S.A.*107, 15792–15797. doi: 10.1073/pnas.1002827107

Hawkins, J. E., Johnsson, L. G., Stebbins, W. C., Moody, D. B., and Coombs, S. L. (1976). Hearing loss and cochlear pathology in monkeys after noise exposure. *Acta Otolaryngol.* 81, 337–343. doi: 10.3109/00016487609119971

Hayashi, T., Kokubo, H., Hartman, B. H., Ray, C. A., Reh, T. A., and Bermingham-McDonogh, O. (2008). Hesr1 and Hesr2 may act as early effectors of Notch signaling in the developing cochlea. *Dev. Biol.* 316, 87–99. doi: 10.1016/j.ydbio.2008.01.006

Hu, L., Lu, J., Chiang, H., Wu, H., Edge, A. S., and Shi, F. (2016). Diphtheria toxin-induced cell death triggers Wnt-dependent hair cell regeneration in neonatal mice. *J. Neurosci.* 36, 9479–9489. doi: 10.1523/JNEUROSCI.2447-15.2016

Imayoshi, I., Sakamoto, M., Yamaguchi, M., Mori, K., and Kageyama, R. (2010). Essential roles of notch signaling in maintenance of neural stem cells in developing and adult brains. *J. Neurosci.* 30, 3489–3498. doi: 10.1523/JNEUROSCI.4987-09.2010

Ivanova, A., Signore, M., Caro, N., Greene, N. D., Copp, A. J., and Martinez-Barbera, J. P. (2005). In vivo genetic ablation by Cre-mediated expression of diphtheria toxin fragment A. *Genesis* 43, 129–135. doi: 10.1002/gene.20162

Jalali, A., Bassuk, A. G., Kan, L., Israsena, N., Mukhopadhyay, A., McGuire, T., et al. (2011). HeyL promotes neuronal differentiation of neural progenitor cells. *J. Neurosci. Res.* 89, 299–309. doi: 10.1002/jnr.22562

Kiernan, A. E., Cordes, R., Kopan, R., Gossler, A., and Gridley, T. (2005). The Notch ligands DLL1 and JAG2 act synergistically to regulate hair cell development in the mammalian inner ear. *Development* 132, 4353–4362. doi: 10.1242/dev.02002

Kiernan, A. E., Xu, J., and Gridley, T. (2006). The notch ligand JAG1 is required for sensory progenitor development in the mammalian inner ear. *PLoS Genet.* 2:e4. doi: 10.1371/journal.pgen.0020004

Korrapati, S., Roux, I., Glowatzki, E., and Doetzlhofer, A. (2013). Notch signaling limits supporting cell plasticity in the hair cell-damaged early postnatal murine cochlea. *PLoS One* 8:e73276. doi: 10.1371/journal.pone.0073276

Lagarde, M. M., Cox, B. C., Fang, J., Taylor, R., Forge, A., and Zuo, J. (2013). Selective ablation of pillar and deiters' cells severely affects cochlear postnatal development and hearing in mice. *J. Neurosci.* 33, 1564–1576. doi: 10.1523/JNEUROSCI.3088-12.2013

Lammich, S., Okochi, M., Takeda, M., Kaether, C., Capell, A., Zimmer, A. K., et al. (2002). Presenilin-dependent intramembrane proteolysis of CD44 leads to the liberation of its intracellular domain and the secretion of an Aβ-like peptide. *J. Biol. Chem.* 277, 44754–44759. doi: 10.1074/jbc.M206872200

Lanford, P. J., Lan, Y., Jiang, R., Lindsell, C., Weinmaster, G., Gridley, T., et al. (1999). Notch signalling pathway mediates hair cell development in mammalian cochlea. *Nature* 21, 289–292. doi: 10.1038/6804

Lanford, P. J., Shailam, R., Norton, C. R., Ridley, T., and Kelley, M. W. (2000). Expression of Math1 and HES5 in the cochleae of wildtype and Jag2 mutant mice. *J. Assoc. Res. Otolaryngol.* 1, 161–171. doi: 10.1007/s101620010023

Li, W., Wu, J., Yang, J., Sun, S., Chai, R., Chen, Z.-Y., et al. (2015). Notch inhibition induces mitotically generated hair cells in mammalian cochleae via activating the Wnt pathway. *Proc. Natl. Acad. Sci. U.S.A.* 112, 166–171. doi: 10.1073/pnas.1415901112

Liu, Z., Owen, T., Fang, J., and Zuo, J. (2012). Overactivation of notch1 signaling induces ectopic hair cells in the mouse inner ear in an age-dependent manner. *PLoS One* 7:e34123. doi: 10.1371/journal.pone.0034123

Ludwig, A., Schlierf, B., Schardt, A., Nave, K. A., and Wegner, M. (2004). Sox10-rtTA mouse line for tetracycline-inducible expression of transgenes in neural crest cells and oligodendrocytes. *Genesis* 40, 171–175. doi: 10.1002/gene.20083

Maass, J. C., Gu, R., Basch, M. L., Waldhaus, J., Lopez, E. M., Xia, A., et al. (2015). Changes in the regulation of the Notch signaling pathway are temporally correlated with regenerative failure in the mouse cochlea. *Front. Cell. Neurosci.* 9:110. doi: 10.3389/fncel.2015.00110

Maass, J. C., Gu, R., Cai, T., Wan, Y. W., Cantellano, S. C., Asprer, J. S. T., et al. (2016). Transcriptomic analysis of mouse cochlear supporting cell maturation reveals large-scale changes in Notch responsiveness prior to the onset of hearing. *PLoS One* 11:e0167286. doi: 10.1371/journal.pone.0167286

Madisen, L., Zwingman, T. A., Sunkin, S. M., Oh, S. W., Zariwala, H. A., Gu, H., et al. (2010). A robust and high-throughput Cre reporting and characterization system for the whole mouse brain. *Nat. Neurosci.* 13, 133–140. doi: 10.1038/nn.2467

Marambaud, P., Shioi, J., Serban, G., Georgakopoulos, A., Sarner, S., Nagy, V., et al. (2002). A presenilin-1/γ-secretase cleavage releases the E-cadherin intracellular domain and regulates disassembly of adherens junctions. *EMBO J.* 21, 1948–1956. doi: 10.1093/emboj/21.8.1948

Marambaud, P., Wen, P. H., Dutt, A., Shioi, J., Takashima, A., Siman, R., et al. (2003). A CBP binding transcriptional repressor produced by the PS1/is an element of-cleavage of N-cadherin is inhibited by PS1FAD mutations. *Cell* 114, 635–645. doi: 10.1016/j.cell.2003.08.008

McGovern, M. M., Brancheck, J., Grant, A. C., Graves, K. A., and Cox, B. C. (2017). Quantitative analysis of supporting cell subtype labeling among creer lines in the neonatal mouse cochlea. *J. Assoc. Res. Otolaryngol.* 18, 227–245. doi: 10.1007/s10162-016-0598-0

Mellado Lagarde, M. M., Wan, G., Zhang, L., Gigliello, A. R., McInnis, J. J., Zhang, Y., et al. (2014). Spontaneous regeneration of cochlear supporting cells after neonatal ablation ensures hearing in the adult mouse. *Proc. Natl. Acad. Sci. U.S.A.* 111, 16919–16924. doi: 10.1073/pnas.1408064111

Mizutari, K., Fujioka, M., Hosoya, M., Bramhall, N., Okano, H. J., Okano, H., et al. (2013). Notch inhibition induces cochlear hair cell regeneration and recovery of hearing after acoustic trauma. *Neuron* 77, 58–69. doi: 10.1016/j.neuron.2012.10.032

Morrison, A., Hodgetts, C., Gossler, A., Hrabé De Angelis, M., and Lewis, J. (1999). Expression of delta1 and serrate1 (Jagged 1) in the mouse inner ear. *Mech. Dev.* 84, 169–172. doi: 10.1016/S0925-4773(99)00066-0

Mulvaney, J., and Dabdoub, A. (2012). Atoh1, an essential transcription factor in neurogenesis and intestinal and inner ear development: function, regulation, and context dependency. *J. Assoc. Res. Otolaryngol.* 13, 281–293. doi: 10.1007/s10162-012-0317-4

Murata, J., Ohtsuka, T., Tokunaga, A., Nishiike, S., Inohara, H., Okano, H., et al. (2009). Notch-Hes1 pathway contributes to the cochlear prosensory formation potentially through the transcriptional down-regulation of p27Kip1. *J. Neurosci. Res.* 87, 3521–3534. doi: 10.1002/jnr.22169

Murata, J., Tokunaga, A., Okano, H., and Kubo, T. (2006). Mapping of Notch activation during cochlear development in mice: implications for determination of prosensory domain and cell fate diversification. *J. Comp. Neurol.* 497, 502–518. doi: 10.1002/cne.20997

Ni, C., Murphy, M., Golde, T., and Carpenter, G. (2001). gamma -secretase cleavage and nuclear localization of ErbB-4 receptor tyrosine kinase. *Science* 294, 2179–2181. doi: 10.1126/science.1065412

Pan, W., Jin, Y., Chen, J., Rottier, R. J., Steel, K. P., and Kiernan, A. E. (2013). Ectopic expression of activated notch or SOX2 reveals similar and unique roles in the development of the sensory cell progenitors in the mammalian inner ear. *J. Neurosci.* 33, 16146–16157. doi: 10.1523/JNEUROSCI.3150-12.2013

Oesterle, E. C., Campbell, S., Taylor, R. R., Forge, A., and Hume, C. R. (2008). Sox2 and Jagged1 expression in normal and drug-damaged adult mouse inner ear. *J. Assoc. Res. Otolaryngol.* 9, 65–89. doi: 10.1007/s10162-007-0106-7

Pan, W., Jin, Y., Stanger, B., Kiernan, A. E., and Martin, G. (2010). Notch signaling is required for the generation of hair cells and supporting cells in the mammalian inner ear. *Proc. Natl. Acad. Sci. U.S.A.* 107, 15798–15803. doi: 10.1073/pnas.1003089107

Pfaffl, M. (2001). A new mathematical model for relative quantification in real-time RT–PCR. *Nucleic Acids Res.* 29, 16–21. doi: 10.1093/nar/29.9.e45

Stanger, B. Z., Datar, R., Murtaugh, L. C., and Melton, D. A. (2005). Direct regulation of intestinal fate by Notch. *Proc. Natl. Acad. Sci. U.S.A.* 102, 12443–12448. doi: 10.1073/pnas.0505690102

Stone, J. S., and Cotanche, D. A. (2007). Hair cell regeneration in the avian auditory epithelium. *Int. J. Dev. Biol.* 51, 633–647. doi: 10.1387/ijdb.072408js

Tateya, T., Imayoshi, I., Tateya, I., Ito, J., and Kageyama, R. (2011). Cooperative functions of Hes/Hey genes in auditory hair cell and supporting cell development. *Dev. Biol.* 352, 329–340. doi: 10.1016/j.ydbio.2011.01.038

Taylor, R. R., Jagger, D. J., and Forge, A. (2012). Defining the cellular environment in the organ of Corti following extensive hair cell loss: a basis for future sensory cell replacement in the cochlea. *PLoS One* 7:e30577. doi: 10.1371/journal.pone.0030577

Walters, B. J., and Zuo, J. (2015). A Sox10rtTA/+ mouse line allows for inducible gene expression in the auditory and balance organs of the inner ear. *J. Assoc. Res. Otolaryngol.* 16, 331–345. doi: 10.1007/s10162-015-0517-9

Wan, G., Gómez-Casati, M. E., Gigliello, A. R., Charles Liberman, M., and Corfas, G. (2014). Neurotrophin-3 regulates ribbon synapse density in the cochlea and induces synapse regeneration after acoustic trauma. *elife* 3:e03564. doi: 10.7554/eLife.03564

White, P. M., Doetzlhofer, A., Lee, Y. S., Groves, A. K., and Segil, N. (2006). Mammalian cochlear supporting cells can divide and trans-differentiate into hair cells. *Nature* 441, 984–987. doi: 10.1038/nature04849

Yamamoto, N., Tanigaki, K., Tsuji, M., Yabe, D., Ito, J., and Honjo, T. (2006). Inhibition of Notch/RBP-J signaling induces hair cell formation in neonate mouse cochleas. *J. Mol. Med.* 84, 37–45. doi: 10.1007/s00109-005-0706-9

Yu, Y., Weber, T., Yamashita, T., Liu, Z., Valentine, M. B., Cox, B. C., et al. (2010). In vivo proliferation of postmitotic cochlear supporting cells by acute ablation of the retinoblastoma protein in neonatal mice. *J. Neurosci.* 30, 5927–5936. doi: 10.1523/JNEUROSCI.5989-09.2010

Zheng, J. L., Shou, J., Guillemot, F., Kageyama, R., and Gao, W. Q. (2000). Hes1 is a negative regulator of inner ear hair cell differentiation. *Development* 127, 4551–4560.

Zine, A., Aubert, A., Qiu, J., Therianos, S., Guillemot, F., Kageyama, R., et al. (2001). Hes1 and Hes5 activities are required for the normal development of the hair cells in the mammalian inner ear. *J. Neurosci.* 21, 4712–4720. doi: 10.1523/JNEUROSCI.21-13-04712.2001

13

Hair cell damage recruited Lgr5-expressing cells are hair cell progenitors in neonatal mouse utricle

*Jinchao Lin *, Xiaodong Zhang, Fengfang Wu and Weinian Lin*

Department of Otolaryngology-Head and Neck Surgery, Quanzhou First Hospital Affiliated to Fujian Medical University, Quanzhou, Fujian, China

Edited by:
Allison B. Coffin,
Washington State University, USA

Reviewed by:
Byron Haney Hartman,
Stanford University, USA
Mingliang Tang,
Chinese Academy of Sciences, China

***Correspondence:**
Jinchao Lin, Department of Otolaryngology-Head and Neck Surgery, Quanzhou First Hospital Affiliated to Fujian Medical University, 250 Dong Street, Quanzhou 362000, Fujian, China
jclin1234@163.com

Damage-activated stem/progenitor cells play important roles in regenerating lost cells and in tissue repair. Previous studies reported that the mouse utricle has limited hair cell regeneration ability after hair cell ablation. However, the potential progenitor cell population regenerating new hair cells remains undiscovered. In this study, we first found that Lgr5, a Wnt target gene that is not usually expressed in the neonatal mouse utricle, can be activated by 24 h neomycin treatment in a sub-population of supporting cells in the striolar region of the neonatal mouse utricle. Lineage tracing demonstrated that these Lgr5-positive supporting cells could regenerate new hair cells in explant culture. We isolated the damage-activated Lgr5-positive cells with flow cytometry and found that these Lgr5-positive supporting cells could regenerate hair cells *in vitro*, and self-renew to form spheres, which maintained the capacity to differentiate into hair cells over seven generations of passages. Our results suggest that damage-activated Lgr5-positive supporting cells act as hair cell progenitors in the neonatal mouse utricle, which may help to uncover a potential route to regenerate hair cell in mammals.

Keywords: hair cell, Lgr5, progenitor cells, regeneration, utricle

Introduction

Hair cells are the mechanosensory cells in the inner ear that are responsible for hearing, balance, and body orientation. The utricle, which is a vestibular organ, requires these mechanosensory hair cells to detect linear acceleration. The mammalian cochlea also requires these sensory hair cells to detect auditory information. Previous studies showed that in birds, both the basilar papilla and the utricle have the ability to regenerate lost hair cells (Corwin and Cotanche, 1988; Jørgensen and Mathiesen, 1988; Ryals and Rubel, 1988; Roberson et al., 1992; Weisleder and Rubel, 1993). However, the mature mammalian cochlea lacks the ability to regenerate new hair cells, and only the neonatal mammalian cochlea has a very limited capacity to self-renew hair cells (Chai et al., 2012; Shi et al., 2012, 2013; Cox et al., 2014). In contrast, the mature mammalian utricle has the ability to replace a portion of lost hair cells through regeneration. Recently, multiple studies reported that spontaneous hair cell regeneration occurs in the mouse utricle after hair cell damage and that hair cell numbers continue to increase after birth (Forge et al., 1993; Warchol et al., 1993; Rubel et al., 1995; Lambert et al., 1997; Oesterle et al., 2003; Kawamoto et al., 2009; Lin et al., 2011; Burns et al., 2012a; Golub et al., 2012). Utricle supporting cells have been demonstrated as a reliable source to regenerate hair cells via both direct differentiation and mitotic division (Lin et al., 2011; Burns et al., 2012a,b; Golub et al., 2012). However, identity of the sub-population of supporting cells contributing to the newly regenerated hair cells remains unclear. In the mouse utricle, the striolar region mainly contains the type I hair cells and the extra-striolar region mainly contains the type II hair cells (Dechesne and Thomasset, 1988; Dechesne et al., 1988; Desai et al., 2005), however, the difference of the supporting cells in these two regions remains largely unknown.

In rapid proliferating tissues like the integumentary and intestinal systems, adult stem cells are capable of self-renewing. Following tissue injury, these endogenous stem cells are activated to initiate the self-repair system and to regenerate lost cells (Tumbar et al., 2004; Barker et al., 2007; Jaks et al., 2008; Lim et al., 2013). In organs with low levels of proliferation, such as the liver and pancreas, there are no adult stem cells in the absence of tissue damage. However upon tissue injury, the damage recruited Lgr5-positive stem cells are activated to regenerate the lost cells (Huch et al., 2013a,b). Similar to the liver and pancreas, the utricle is also an organ with little proliferation and limited regeneration ability after damage. Previous studies have reported that after damage, the spontaneously regenerated hair cells come from supporting cells (Li et al., 2003; Oshima et al., 2007; Lin et al., 2011; Burns et al., 2012a; Golub et al., 2012), however, the source of the progenitor cell population responsible for regenerating hair cells in the mammalian utricle has not been identified.

Previous studies reported that Wnt signaling plays important roles in tissue repair (Logan and Nusse, 2004). Lgr5 is a Wnt downstream target gene that acts as a stem cell marker in rapidly proliferating organs, such as integumentary tissue and intestine (Barker et al., 2007; Jaks et al., 2008), as well as in organs with little proliferation, such as the liver and pancreas, (Huch et al., 2013a,b). In the cochlea, recent studies showed that Lgr5 is expressed in a subpopulation of supporting cells, including the third Deiters' cells, inner pillar cells, inner phalangeal cells and greater epithelial ridge (GER) cells. Lgr5-expressing cells in the cochlea can regenerate hair cells both *in vivo* and *in vitro*, thus acting as a hair cell progenitor in the mouse cochlea (Chai et al., 2011, 2012; Shi et al., 2012, 2013; Bramhall et al., 2014). In neonatal cochlea, these Lgr5-expressing progenitor cells also have the ability to regenerate new hair cells via either direct differentiation or mitotic division after hair cell loss (Cox et al., 2014). However, the roles of Lgr5 and Lgr5-expressing cells after damage in the utricle remain unknown.

In this study, we report the activation of Lgr5 expression in a subset of supporting cells in the striolar region of neonatal utricle after neomycin induced hair cell loss, and use linage tracing to demonstrate that these Lgr5-positive cells can regenerate new hair cells. Furthermore, we found that when isolated by flow cytometry, these Lgr5-positive cells could regenerate hair cells *in vitro*, and self-renew to form spheres. Together, we concluded that the damage activated Lgr5-expressing cells are hair cell progenitors in the neonatal mouse utricle.

Materials and Methods

Animals

We used Lgr5-EGFP-CreERT2 (Jackson Laboratory, Stock 008875) mice to detect Lgr5 expression, and Lgr5-EGFP-CreERT2 and ROSA26R-tdTomato (Jackson Laboratory, Stock 007908) mice to trace the lineage of Lgr5-expressing progenitor cells. Mice were housed with open access to food and water. For culture experiments, mice were killed by CO_2 inhalation followed by decapitation. This study was carried out in strict accordance with the recommendations in the Guide for the Care and Use of Laboratory Animals of the National Institutes of Health. The protocol was approved by the Committee on the Ethics of Animal Experiments of Quanzhou First Hospital Affiliated to Fujian Medical University. The IACUC committee members at Quanzhou First Hospital Affiliated to Fujian Medical University approved this study. All surgery was performed under sodium pentobarbital anesthesia, and all efforts were made to minimize suffering.

Whole Organ Cultures

Temporal bones were isolated from P1 mice and placed in ice cold HBSS (Sigma). The otoconia and the otoconial membranes were removed, utricles were isolated using Dumont fine forceps and cultured free-floating in a 96-well plate containing 100 μl of DMEM/F12 (Invitrogen) with 1% N2 (Invitrogen), 2% B27 (Invitrogen), bFGF (1 ng/ml; Sigma), IGF-1 (50 ng/ml; Sigma), EGF (20 ng/ml; Sigma), heparin sulfate (50 ng/ml; Sigma), and ampicillin (50 ng/ml; Sigma) at 37°C with 95% air/5% CO_2. Each well contained one utricle. To damage hair cells, 1mM neomycin (Sigma) was added to the culture medium for 24 h. To activate the Cre for lineage tracing, 4OH-tamoxifen (800 nM, Sigma) was added to the culture medium. The culture medium was changed daily. For all whole organ culture experiments, we only used one utricle per mouse; n values represent the number of animals. For each experiment, at least 3 mice were used.

Genotyping and qRT-PCR

Transgenic mice were genotyped using genomic DNA from tail tips by adding 100 μl 50 mM NaOH, incubated at 98°C for 20–40 min, followed by the addition of 10 μl 1 M HCl. The genotyping primers were as follows: Lgr5: wild-type (F) CTGCTCTCTGCTCCCAGTCT; (R) ATACCCCATCCCTT TTGAGC; mutant (R) GAACTTCAGGGTCAGCTTGC; td-Tomato: wild-type (F) AAGGGAGCTGCAGTGGAGT; (R) CC GAAAATCTGTGGGAAGTC; mutant (F) GGCATTAAAGC AGCGTATC; (R) CTGTTCCTGTACGGCATGG.

For quantitative reverse transcriptase polymerase chain reaction (qRT-PCR), total RNA was extracted from isolated utricles using TRIzol (Invitrogen), followed by cDNA synthesis using the GoScript™ Reverse Transcription System (Promega, A5001). qRT-PCR reactions were performed with GoTaq® qPCR Master Mix (Promega, A6001) on a 7500HT Fast Real-Time PCR System (Applied Biosystems). Each qPCR reaction was carried out in triplicate and the relative quantification of gene expression analyzed using the $^{\Delta\Delta}C_T$ method with the housekeeping gene β-actin as the endogenous reference.

Primer pairs were designed using Primer3 software. Lgr5 (F) CCTACTCGAAGACTTACCCAGT; (R) GCATTGGGG TGAATGATAGCA-3; Sox2 (F) GCGGAGTGGAAACTTTT GTCC; (R) CGGGAAGCGTGTACTTATCCTT; Brn3.1 (F) CG ACGCCACCTACCATACC; (R) CCCTGATGTACCGCGTG AT-3′; Jagged1 (F) TCAAACGTGAGAGTGTCTAACG; (R) CC GGGCCGAAGAGATTTCTG; β-actin (F) GGCTGTATTCCC CTCCATCG; (R) CCAGTTGGTAACAATGCCATGT.

Cell Counting

For whole organ culture experiments, we randomly took 2 representative pictures from the striolar region or extra-striolar regions for analyses. When we took the pictures, Lgr5-EGFP and tdTomato expression was used as a reference to define the striolar region. For cell counting, we either counted the number of hair cells in representative pictures and normalized to undamaged control to get the hair cell percentage (for example, **Figures 1E, 2G**); or counted Lgr5+ supporting cell number in representative pictures and normalized to total Sox2+ supporting cells to get the Lgr5+ supporting cell percentage (for example, **Figure 1F**); or counted the total tdTomato+ or myosin7a/tdTomato double positive cell number per utricle (for example, **Figures 2H,I**). For all experiments, n values represent the number of mice.

Isolation of Lgr5-Expressing Cells by Flow Cytometry

20–30 utricles from Lgr5-EGFP-CreERT2 mice were cultured with 1 mM Neomycin for 24 h and recovered for 24 h and then trypsinized at 37°C for 10 min and mechanically dissociated in PBS with 2% fetal bovine serum (FBS, Invitrogen), DNAse (10 units/ml, Qiagen) and EDTA (2 mM, Sigma). The cells were filtered through a cell strainer (40 μm diameter) prior to sorting. The dissociated cells were sorted on a BD FACS AriaIII (BD Biosciences) using the channel for GFP, and positive fractions were collected.

Culture of Sorted Cells

Florescence Activated Cell Sorting (FACS) isolated Lgr5-expressing cells (20 cells/ul, 2000 cells per well) were plated on a laminin-coated dish and cultured for 10 d in DMEM/F12 with 2% B27, 1% N2, EGF, bFGF, IGF-1 and heparan sulfate (same as whole organ culture). Cells that had not attached were removed 1 d after plating. To label dividing cells, EdU (1.0 μM; Invitrogen) was added to the culture medium. The cells were fixed and stained for EDU and hair cell marker Myosin7a after 10 d of culture.

Sphere Formation and Differentiation

Two hundred FACS-isolated Lgr5-expressing cells were cultured to form spheres in 96 well ultra-low attachment plates (Costar) with a density of 2 cells/μl for 5 d in DMEM/F12 medium (Invitrogen) with 1% N2 and 2% B27, EGF, bFGF, IGF-1 and heparin sulfate. The spheres were collected every 5 d, mechanically dissociated with a 25 G needle (BD Labware) and re-seeded in fresh medium. For differentiation, spheres were plated on a laminin-coated dish and cultured for 5 d in DMEM/F12.

Histological Methods

Proteins were detected in whole-mount utricles using standard immunofluorescence labeling methods. Utricles were fixed with 4% PFA (Sigma) for 1 h at room temperature, rinsed with PBS for 3 times, and incubated for 1 h in blocking solution (2% bovine serum albumin, 5% normal goat serum, 0.5% Triton X-100). Utricles were incubated overnight at 4°C with one of the following primary antibodies diluted 1/100–1/1000 in blocking solution: rabbit anti-myosin VIIa (1:1000, Proteus Biosciences), Sox2 (1:400; Santa Cruz Biotechnology). Secondary antibodies, conjugated to Alexa Fluor 488, 594, or 647 and diluted 1/500, were purchased from Invitrogen. To label cell nuclei, organs were soaked in 4′, 6-diamidino-2-phenylindole (DAPI) (Sigma) at 1 μg/ml for 10 min. Images were acquired using confocal microscopy (Zeiss LSM710) and analyzed with Image J (NIH) and Photoshop CS4 (Adobe Systems).

Statistical Analyses

Throughout the text and in graphs, data are expressed as mean ± SD. The immunohistochemical data was analyzed using Student's *t*-test when comparing two groups or by one-way ANOVA followed by Dunnett's Multiple Comparisons Test when comparing more than two groups. Values of $p < 0.05$ were considered statistically significant.

Results

Activation of Lgr5 Expression in a Subset of Supporting Cells in the Striolar Region After Hair Cell Damage

Lgr5 has been reported as a stem cell marker in a variety of organs, including intestine, liver, pancreas and hair follicles (Barker et al., 2007, 2010; Jaks et al., 2008; Huch et al., 2013a,b). In this study, we explored the expression of Lgr5 using the Lgr5-EGFP-CreERT2 mice, where GFP is under the control of the Lgr5 locus. In the mouse utricle, similar to the liver (Huch et al., 2013b), we found Lgr5 expression is not detectable at P1 plus 1 day *in vitro* (DIV; **Figures 1A,C**). However, when we cultured the P1 utricle from Lgr5-EGFP-CreERT2 mice and treated it with 1 mM neomycin for 24 h, we found the treatment significantly damaged the hair cell both in striolar and extra-striolar region (**Figure 1E**), and Lgr5 expression was robustly activated specifically in a subset of supporting cells in the striolar region (**Figures 1B,D**). Quantification data suggested 25.2 ± 7.3% of striolar supporting cells were Lgr5-GFP-positive ($n = 3$), and no hair cells were observed to be GFP-positive ($n = 3$) (**Figure 1F**). qPCR experiments confirmed that the expression of Lgr5 is undetectable at P1 in the absence of neomycin, and has been robustly activated following neomycin induced hair cell damage ($n = 3$) (**Figure 1G**). Interestingly, we found that during embryonic development, Lgr5 was also mainly expressed in a subset of supporting cells in the striolar region (Sup-**Figures 1A–D**). This result suggested that during development the expression of Lgr5 was rapidly down-regulated and became undetectable after birth. Compared to P1 Lgr5 expression after damage, the Lgr5 expression at E17.5 was restricted to the striolar

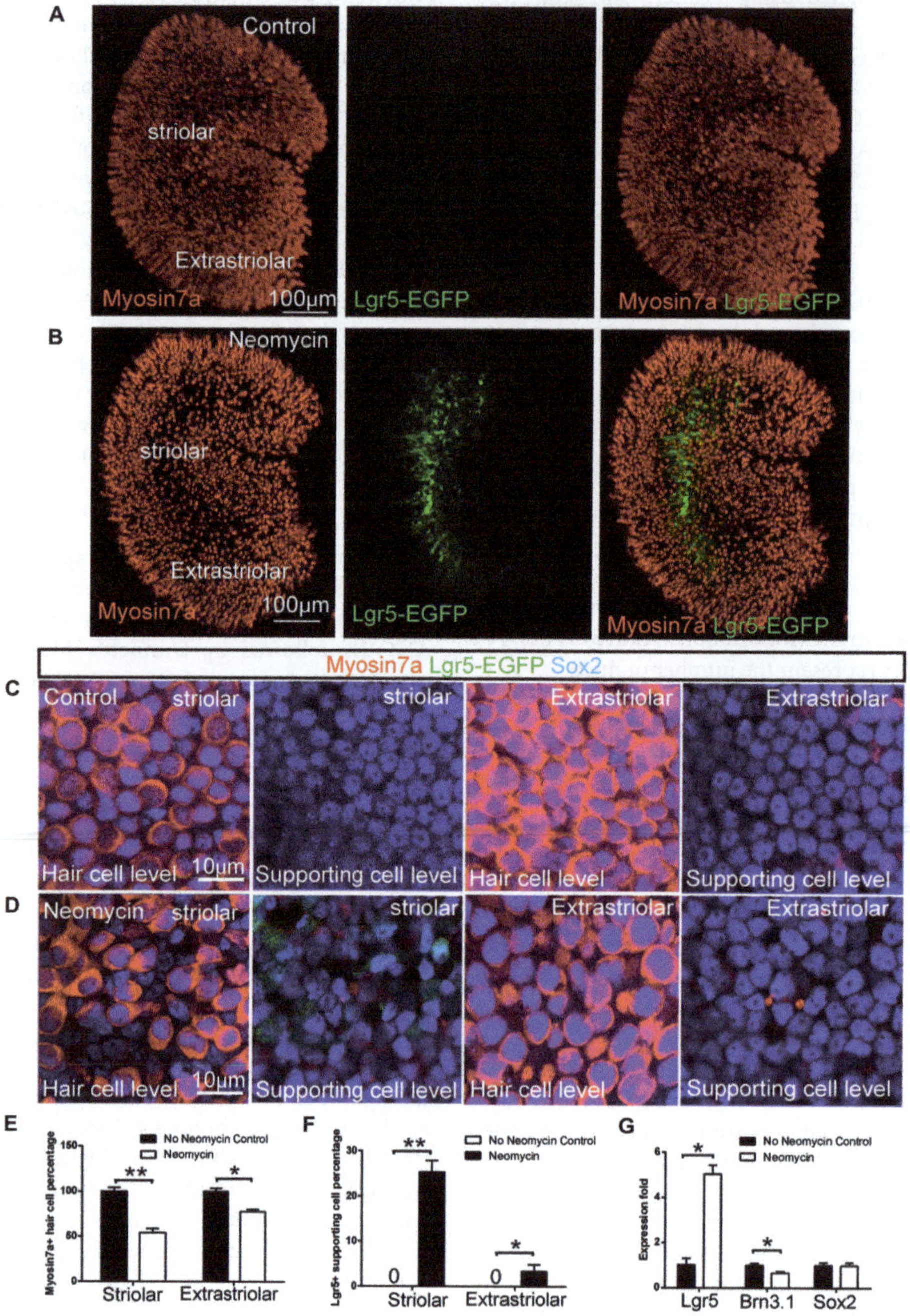

FIGURE 1 | Neomycin-induced hair cell damage activated Lgr5 expression in mouse utricles. (A) In Lgr5-EGFP-CreERT2 control utricles without damage, no Lgr5-EGFP expression was detected at P1. **(B)** In contrast, in Lgr5-EGFP-CreERT2 utricles with neomycin damage, many Lgr5-EGFP-positive supporting cells were detected in the striolar region. **(C)** High magnification picture showed there was no Lgr5-EGFP expression in both striolar and extra-striolar region in control utricle without damage. **(D)** In Lgr5-EGFP-CreERT2 utricle withs neomycin damage, Lgr5-EGFP was mainly expressed in a subset of supporting cells in the striolar region. **(E)** Quantification and comparison of Myosin7a-positive hair cell in the striolar and extra-striolar region of utricles with or without neomycin damage. **(F)** Quantification and comparison of Lgr5-EGFP-positive supporting cell in the striolar and extra-striolar region of utricles with or without neomycin damage. **(G)** Quantitative PCR showed that neomycin treatment significantly increased the expression level of Lgr5 and slightly decreased the expression level of the hair cell marker Brn3.1 as compared to control utricles. $^{*}p < 0.05$, $^{**}p < 0.01$, $n = 3$ mice in **(E–G)**. Scale Bars: **(A,B)**: 100 μm; **(C,D)**: 10 μm.

region and mainly in the supporting cells; however at E17.5 there was also very low expression of Lgr5 in some of the hair cells, while in P1 utricle after damage, there was no Lgr5 expression in hair cells.

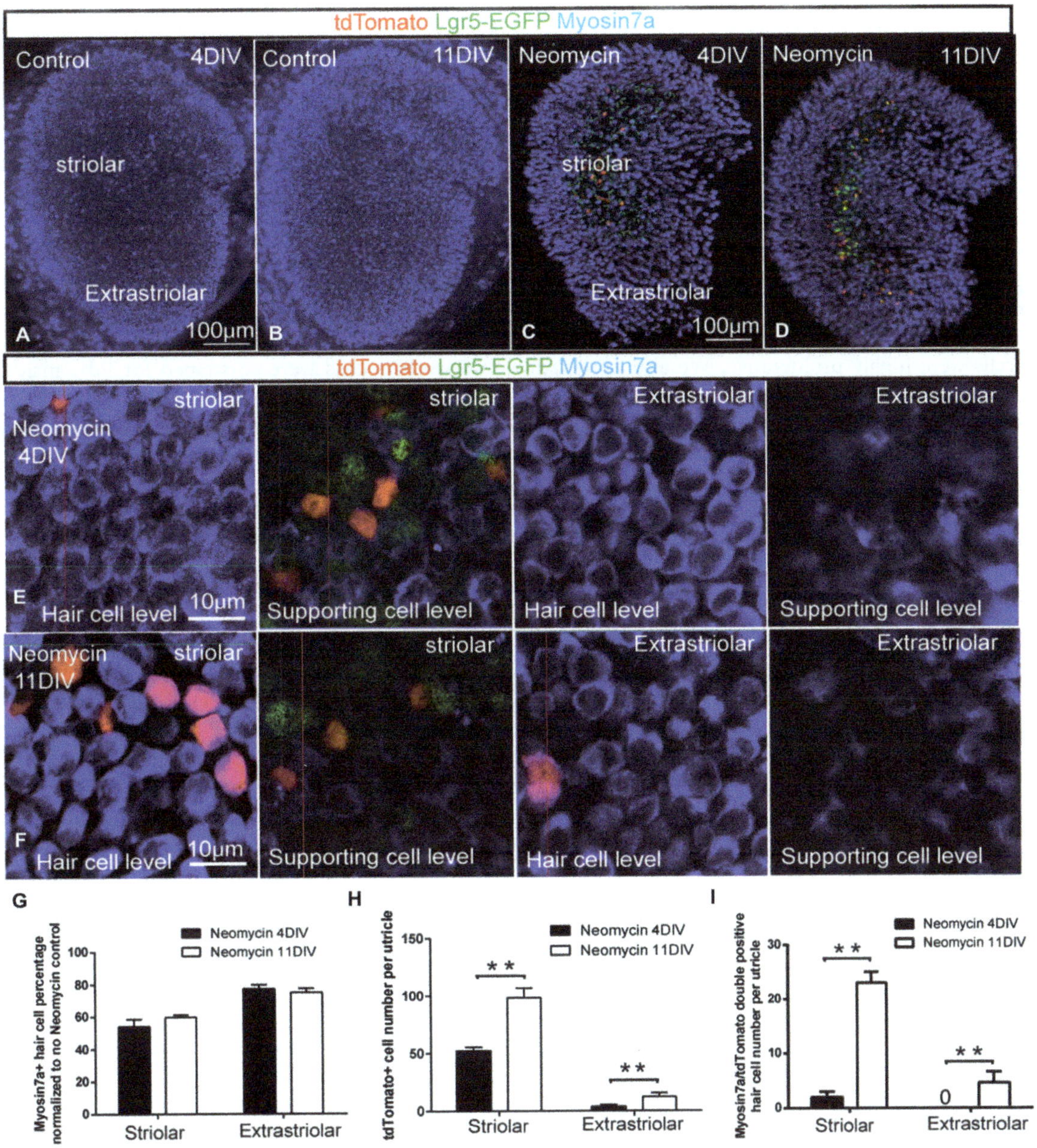

FIGURE 2 | Damage-activated Lgr5-positive cells generated hair cells in whole organ culture. (A–B) In Lgr5-EGFP-CreERT2 control utricles, there was no Lgr5-GFP expression and no tdTomato reporter expression after 4 or 11 days in culture. **(C)** In Lgr5-EGFP-CreERT2 utricles with neomycin damage, tdTomato reporter expression was detected mostly in the supporting cells in the striolar region at 4 days in culture. **(D)** At 11 days in culture, the total number of tdTomato-positive cells was increased and tdTomato reporter expression was also detected in Myo7a-positive hair cells. **(E)** High magnification picture showed most of the tdTomato-positive cells were supporting cells in the striolar region at 4 days in culture. **(F)** High magnification picture showed significant numbers of tdTomato-positive cells were hair cells in the striolar region at 11 days in culture. **(G)** The total hair cell number was not significantly increased from 4 days to 11 days in culture. **(H)** The total tdTomato-positive cell number was significantly increased from 4 to 11 days in culture. **(I)** The myosin7a and tdTomato double positive hair cells number was significantly increased from 4 to 11 days in culture. $^{**}p < 0.01$, $n = 3$ mice in **(G–I)**. Scale Bars: **(A–D)**: 100 µm; **(E,F)**: 10 µm.

Damage Activated Lgr5-Positive Cells Generated Hair Cells in Whole Organ Culture

Previous studies reported that Lgr5-positive cells in the cochlea have the ability to regenerate hair cells (Chai et al., 2012; Shi et al., 2012). To ask whether the damage activated Lgr5-positive supporting cells in the utricle could regenerate hair cells, we crossed Lgr5-EGFP-CreERT2 mice with ROSA26R-tdTomato reporter mice in which a floxed STOP cassette prevents transcription of a downstream red fluorescent protein (tdTomato). Utricles were dissected from P1 double transgenic mice, and treated with 1 mM neomycin for 24 h (1 DIV) to damage the hair cells. In control samples without neomycin treatment, there was neither Lgr5-GFP expression nor tdTomato reporter expression (n = 3) (**Figures 2A,B**). After neomycin treatment, 800 nM 4OH-tamoxifen was administrated for 72 h to activate the Cre for lineage tracing the Lgr5-positive cells (4 DIV). When utricle tissues were examined at 4 DIV, tdTomato reporter expression was almost only observed in a subset of supporting cells in the striolar region, and very few hair cells were found to be tdTomato positive (n = 3) (**Figures 2C,E,I**). When the lineage tracing was extended to 11 DIV, we found the total number of tdTomato-positive cells was significantly increased (n = 3) (**Figure 2H**), suggesting these lineage traced Lgr5-positive cells were highly proliferative. We also observed significant number of hair cell marker myosin7a and tdTomato double positive hair cells (n = 3) (**Figures 2D,F,I**), indicating that these new regenerated hair cells were indeed derived from Lgr5-positive supporting cells. However, the total hair cell number in the striolar region only slightly increased and was not statistically significant (P = 0.13, n = 3) (**Figure 2G**). Of the GFP-positive supporting cells, only a small population has been lineage traced with tdTomato, presumably due to the low efficiency of 4OH-tamoxifen in culture and the incomplete labeling of tdTomato reporters by Lgr5-EGFP-CreERT2 mouse (Barker et al., 2007).

FACS Isolated Lgr5-Positive Cell Divided and Generated Hair Cells in Cell Culture

Next we tested whether the damage-activated Lgr5-expressing supporting cells could act as hair cell progenitors to divide and differentiate into hair cells, when isolated by FACS. In this experiment, we first cultured the P1 utricles from Lgr5-EGFP-CreERT2 mice with 1 mM neomycin for 24 h, then allowed recovery for 24 h, followed by purifying the GFP-positive cells by FACS. We found that 6.02% of the cells were GFP-positive (n = 3) (**Figure 3A**). 96.6 ± 5.1% of Lgr5-positive supporting cells sorted by flow cytometry were also GFP positive (n = 3), and isolated Lgr5-positive supporting cells showed no staining of the hair cell marker myosin7a (0.0 ± 0.0%, n = 3) (**Figure 3B**). However, almost all of the Lgr5-positive cells displayed the supporting cell marker Sox2 (96.7 ± 4.8%, n = 3) (**Figure 3C**). qPCR data also demonstrated that the GFP-positive cells had significantly higher Lgr5 expression level, as well as expression of the supporting cell markers Jagged1 and Sox2, and significantly lower expression of the hair cell marker Brn3.1, compared with the GFP-negative cells (n = 3) (**Figure 3D**).

Next, we cultured the damage activated Lgr5-positive cells with a density of 20 cells/μl for 10 days and found that these damage-activated Lgr5-positive supporting cells formed colonies (more than 5 cells) that expressed myosin7a (**Figure 3E**). After 10 days in culture, 2000 Lgr5-positive supporting cells generated 31.6 ± 2.8 colonies, among which 38.5 ± 3.9% colonies contained myosin7a-positive hair cells (arrow). These colonies contained a total number of 87.1 ± 15.7 myosin7a-positive hair cells, indicating that the hair cells resided in the colonies might be generated via mitotic regeneration (arrow) (n = 3) (**Figures 3E,G**). Moreover, 2000 Lgr5-positive supporting cells also generated around 182.5 ± 34.2 myosin7a-positive hair cells (arrow head) outside of the colonies, indicating these hair cells resided separately might be generated via direct differentiation (arrow head) (n = 3) (**Figures 3E,H**). In contrast, 2000 Lgr5-negative cells generated 20.2 ± 3.9 colonies, with only 1.2 ± 1.7 colonies containing myosin7a-positive hair cells. Only 4.7 ± 4.2 myosin7a-positive hair cells were generated within colonies, and 26.9 ± 13.5 myosin7a-positive hair cells resided outside the colonies (**Figures 3F–H**).

We next added 1.0 μM EdU to the culture medium from day 3 to day 5 to label dividing cells, and found evidence of proliferation in damage-activated Lgr5-positive supporting cells (**Figure 3I**). 8.2 ± 1.9% and 1.2 ± 0.9% of the myosin7a-positive hair cells were co-stained for EdU inside and outside of the colonies, respectively (**Figures 3I,J**). In contrast, Lgr5-negative cells also proliferated as indicated by EdU incorporation but no myosin7a/EdU double positive hair cells were observed (**Figure 3J**).

FACS Isolated Lgr5-Positive Cell Self-Renew to Form Spheres and Could be Passaged for 7 Generations

To assess the potential of damage-activated Lgr5-positive supporting cells to self-renew and expand the colony, we used a sphere assay to examine Lgr5-positive cells isolated from cultured utricles. As described above, we first sorted the damage activated Lgr5-positive supporting cells with FACS, then cultured 200 isolated cells to form spheres with a density of 2 cells/μl in ultra-low attachment plates. In the first generation, the sphere number derived from damage-activated Lgr5-positive cells was only slightly higher than the Lgr5-negative cells. However, from the second to the fifth generation, the Lgr5-positive cells formed significantly more spheres than the Lgr5-negative cells (**Figures 4A–C**). Multiple passages suggested that spheres derived from Lgr5-positive cells expanded significantly more rapidly than from Lgr5-negative cells (**Figure 4C**). From the sixth generation on, there were no spheres formed in the Lgr5-negative group and the total number of spheres started to decrease in the Lgr5-positive group, therefore we only passaged the spheres to the seventh generation. When we measured the size of the spheres, we found Lgr5-positive cells formed smaller and more homogenous spheres than Lgr5-negative cells in the first four generations (**Figure 4D**). When we compared multiple generations, we found the size of spheres also increased with the passage number (**Figure 4D**).

Spheres Derived from Lgr5-Positive Cells Maintained the Capacity to Differentiate into Hair Cells

To determine if the passaged spheres derived from damage activated Lgr5-positive supporting cells still maintained the ability to differentiate into hair cells, we collected the spheres from different generations and differentiated the spheres for 5 days. For the first generation of spheres, we found that on the first day of the differentiation the spheres from both damage-activated Lgr5-positive cells and Lgr5-negative cells contained

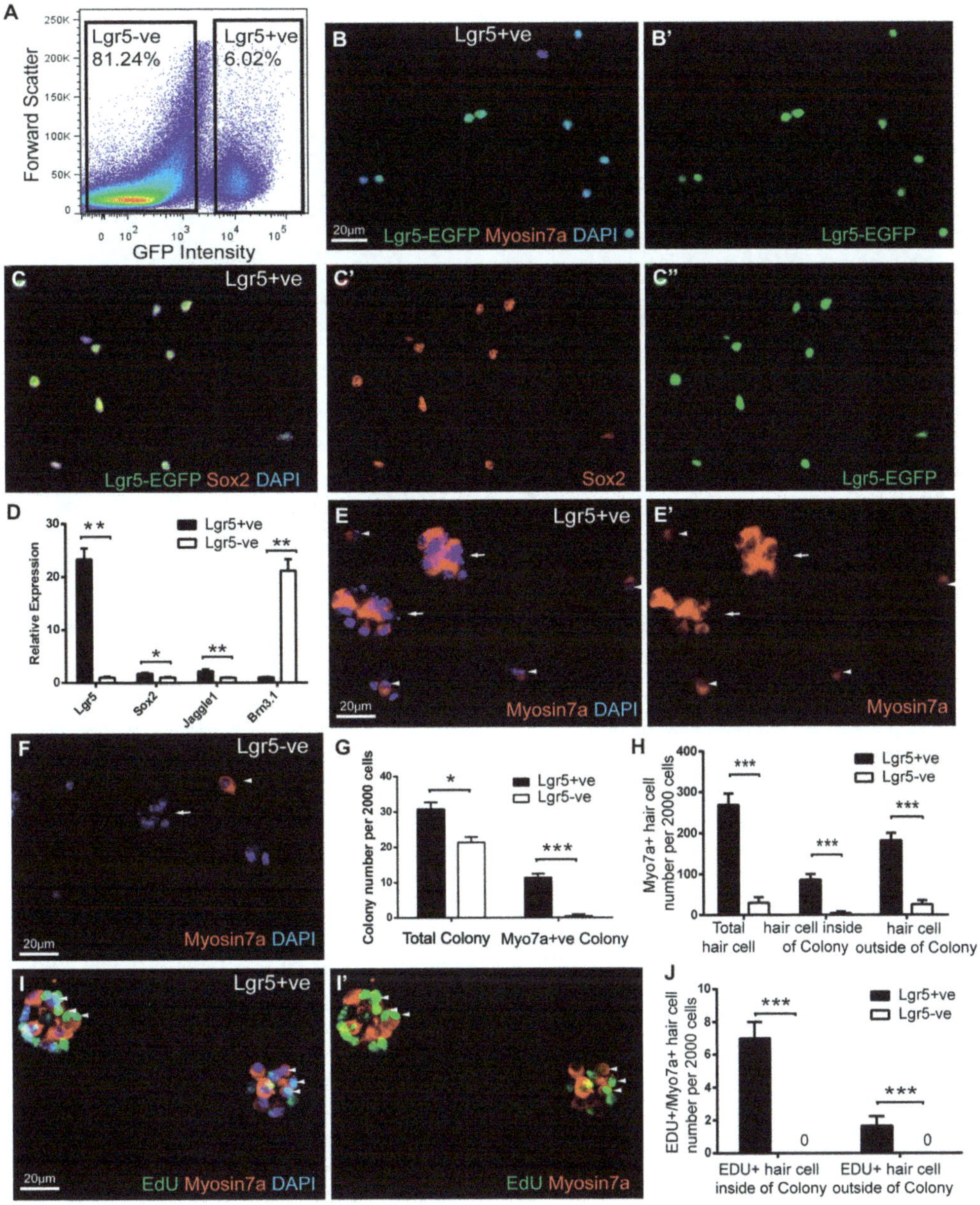

FIGURE 3 | FACS isolated Lgr5-positive cell divided and generated hair cells in culture. (A) Lgr5-GFP-positive and Lgr5-GFP-negative cells were isolated using FACS. **(B,C)** Immunostaining showed that among the FACS isolated Lgr5-EGFP-positive cells, 96.6% were GFP-positive, 96.7% were Sox2-positive, and none were Myo7a-positive. **(D)** Quantitative PCR showed that FACS isolated Lgr5-EGFP-positive cells had significantly higher Lgr5 expression, slightly higher Sox2 and Jagged1 expression, and significantly lower Brn3.1 expression compared to the Lgr5-EGFP-negative cells. **(E,F)** FACS isolated Lgr5-EGFP-positive cells generated significantly more colonies and Myo7a-positive cells than Lgr5-EGFP-negative cells. **(G)** Quantification of colony number generated from Lgr5-EGFP-positive and Lgr5-EGFP-negative cells. **(H)** Quantification of Myo7a-positive hair cells generated from Lgr5-EGFP-positive and Lgr5-EGFP-negative cells. **(I)** FACS isolated Lgr5-EGFP-positive cells mitotically generated hair cells in cell culture. **(J)** Quantification of EDU/Myo7a double positive hair cell number generated from Lgr5-EGFP-positive and Lgr5-EGFP-negative cells. $^{*}p < 0.05$, $^{**}p < 0.01$, $^{***}p < 0.001$, $n = 3$ in **(D,G,H,J)**. Scale Bars: 20 μm.

no myosin7a-positive hair cell (**Figures 5A,B**), but almost all the spheres were positive for the supporting cell marker Sox2 (**Figure 5D**). Upon 5 days of differentiation, the spheres derived from Lgr5-positive cells generated significantly more myosin7a-positive hair cells than the Lgr5-negative cells (6.7 ± 3.5 vs. 0.4 ± 0.5 myosin7a-positive hair cells in Lgr5-positive and Lgr5-negative cells, respectively) (**Figures 5C,E,F**).

After multiple generations of passages, we found that from the first to the fourth generation there was no significant difference in the number of differentiated hair cells per sphere (**Figure 5C**),

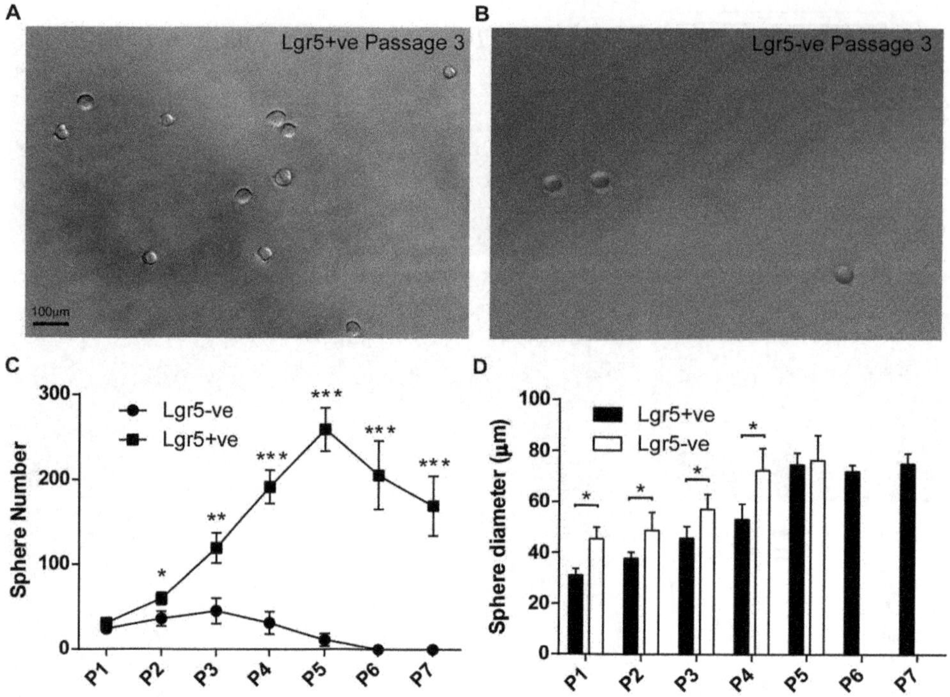

FIGURE 4 | FACS isolated Lgr5-positive cells self-renew to form spheres. (A,B) FACS isolated Lgr5-EGFP-positive cells generated significantly more spheres than Lgr5-EGFP-negative cells. **(C)** Quantification of sphere number generated from FACS isolated Lgr5-EGFP-positive and Lgr5-EGFP-negative cells over seven generations. **(D)** Quantification of sphere size generated from FACS isolated Lgr5-EGFP-positive and Lgr5-EGFP-negative cells over seven generations. $^{*}p < 0.05$, $^{**}p < 0.01$, $^{***}p < 0.001$, $n = 3$ in **(C,D)**. Scale Bars: 100 μm.

suggesting that hair cell regeneration ability remained robust in the early sphere generations. Although the number of differentiated hair cells per sphere decreased from the fifth to the seventh generations, the seventh generation of spheres derived from damage-activated Lgr5-positive supporting cells still generated 3.2 ± 2.6 hair cells per sphere, suggesting that the seventh generation of sphere still maintained the capacity to differentiate into hair cells (**Figures 5C,G**).

Discussion

In birds, both the basilar papilla and the utricle have been reported to maintain hair cell regeneration capacity (Corwin and Cotanche, 1988; Jørgensen and Mathiesen, 1988; Ryals and Rubel, 1988; Roberson et al., 1992; Weisleder and Rubel, 1993). Supporting cells in the mammalian cochlea and utricle share evolutionarily conserved marker genes and signaling pathways with those supporting cells in birds, which act as hair cell progenitors. In the mature mammalian cochlea, hair cells and supporting cells are quiescent and the mature mammalian cochlea does not regenerate hair cell spontaneously, thus severe hair cell loss leads to permanent hearing loss (Bermingham-McDonogh and Rubel, 2003; Brigande and Heller, 2009). The mammalian vestibular system still maintains a limited ability to regenerate lost hair cells (Forge et al., 1993; Warchol et al., 1993; Rubel et al., 1995; Lambert et al., 1997; Oesterle et al., 2003; Kawamoto et al., 2009; Lin et al., 2011; Burns et al., 2012a; Golub et al., 2012), therefore, the mammalian utricle could serve as a useful model to study hair cell regeneration. Multiple studies reported that utricular supporting cells have the capacity to replenish lost hair cells via both direct differentiation and mitotic division (Lin et al., 2011; Burns et al., 2012a,b; Golub et al., 2012). However, the clearly defined progenitor cell population in the mammalian utricle has not been identified. In this study, we demonstrate that in the mouse utricle, the Lgr5 expression was activated in a specific subset of striolar supporting cells after neomycin-induced hair cell loss. These damaged-activated Lgr5-positive supporting cells exhibit progenitor cell properties and have the ability to regenerate lost hair cells. Previous studies reported that the hair cell types in the striolar and extra-striolar region are different: type I hair cells are mainly located in the striolar region, while type II hair cells are mainly located in the extra-striolar region (Dechesne and Thomasset, 1988; Dechesne et al., 1988; Desai et al., 2005). In 2012, Burns found that in adult utricle, newly arising hair cells are mainly located in the peripheral edge and striola, and after hair cell ablation mitotic regeneration of hair cells was observed in the striola (Burns et al., 2012a,b). In our study, we found the damage-activated Lgr5-positive supporting cells are also restricted to the striolar region, suggesting the striolar and extra-striolar supporting cells are two distinct populations with different properties. Interestingly, the damage-activated Lgr5-positive supporting cells only cover around 25% of the whole supporting cell population in the striolar region, which

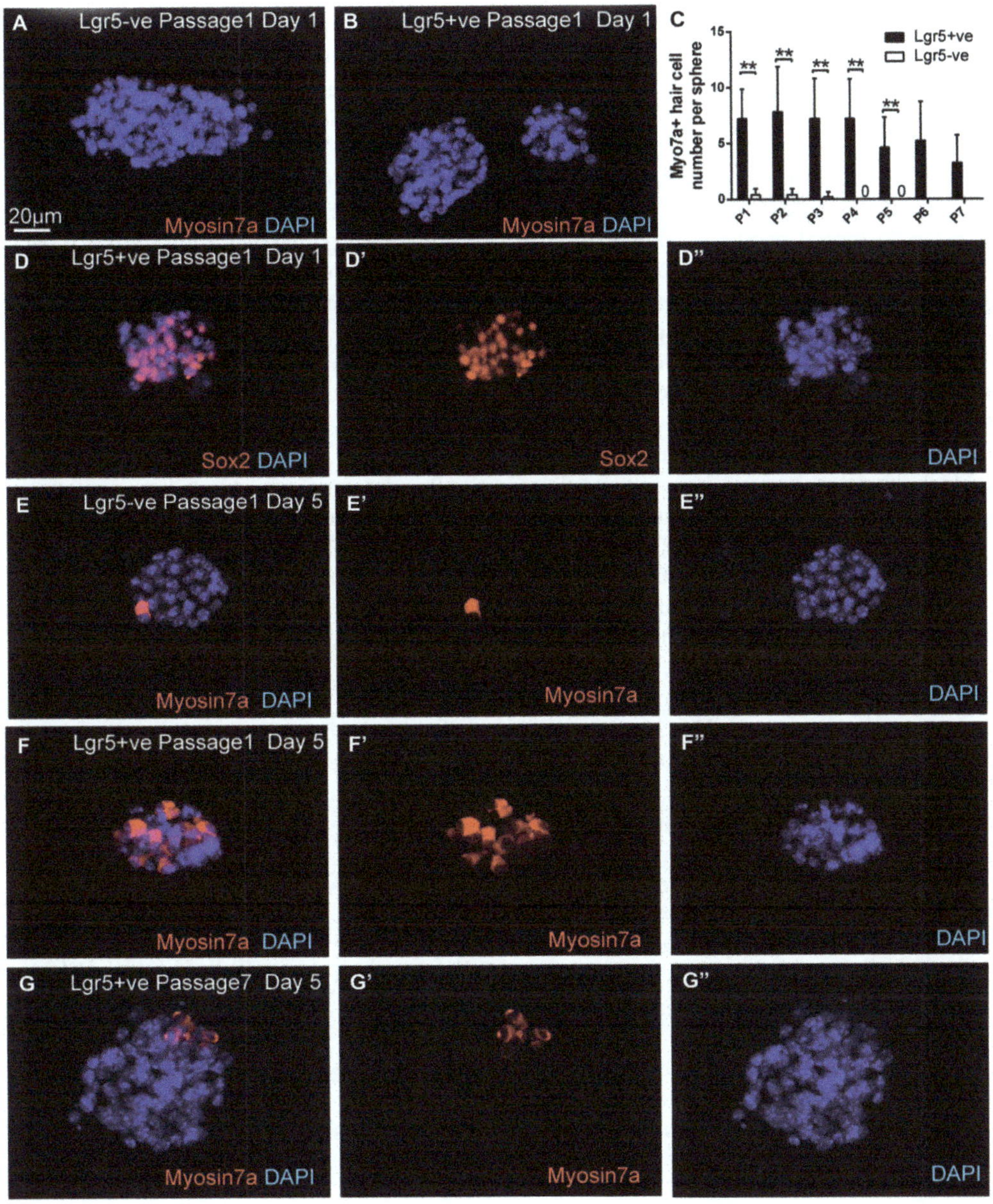

FIGURE 5 | Spheres derived from Lgr5-positive cells maintained the capacity to differentiate into hair cells. (A,B) The spheres derived from both Lgr5-EGFP-positive and Lgr5-EGFP-negative cells contained no Myo7a-positive hair cells at the first day of differentiation **(C)** Quantification of Myo7a-positive hair cell number per sphere generated from Lgr5-EGFP-positive and Lgr5-EGFP-negative cells over seven generations. **(D)** At the first day of differentiation, the majority of the spheres were Sox2-positive. **(E,F)** The sphere derived from Lgr5-EGFP-positive cells generated significantly more Myo7a-positive hair cells than the one derived from Lgr5-EGFP-negative cells. **(G)** The sphere derived from Lgr5-EGFP-positive cells maintained the capacity to generate Myo7a-positive hair cells after seven passages. $^{**}p < 0.01$, $n = 3$ in **(C)**. Scale Bars: 20 μm.

also indicates that striolar supporting cells do not consist of a single population but may contain several subpopulations with distinct functions. It will be interesting to further investigate the different functions of supporting cell subpopulations in the future. More interestingly, we found that at E17.5, Lgr5 was also mainly expressed in a subset of supporting cells in the striolar region, and this expression pattern is similar to the Lgr5 expression after hair cell damage at P1, which indicates that in the postnatal stages, the damage-activated expression of Lgr5 in striolar supporting cells may be partially a recapitulation of developmental mechanisms. Further study will be performed to investigate the detailed mechanism.

Previous reports showed that after hair cell ablation, utricular supporting cells have the ability to regenerate lost hair cells (Burns et al., 2012a,b; Golub et al., 2012). Compared to Sox2, which is widely expressed in all supporting cells, Lgr5 is limited to a subpopulation of the striolar supporting cells. This suggests that this subset of supporting cells with progenitor cell properties is restricted as in non-mammalian vertebrates, in which a small subset of supporting cell population regenerates lost hair cells by proliferation followed by trans-differentiation (Stone and Cotanche, 2007).

Recent studies showed that after tissue damage, the Wnt signaling pathway is activated as a self-repair system and plays key roles in tissue repair in several organs including the liver and pancreas (Minear et al., 2010; Huch et al., 2013a,b). Lgr5, a downstream target gene of Wnt signaling, was first described as a stem cell marker in the intestine, where Lgr5-expressing cells are precursors for all cells in the intestinal crypts (Barker et al., 2007). Deletion of Lgr5 in the intestine leads to the rapid and complete loss of intestinal crypts (de Lau et al., 2011). By far, Lgr5 has been demonstrated as the stem cell marker in multiple organs, including the stomach, hair follicles, liver, pancreas and cochlea (Barker et al., 2007, 2010; Jaks et al., 2008; Chai et al., 2012; Shi et al., 2012, 2013; Huch et al., 2013a,b). Recently, damage recruited Lgr5-positive cells have also been demonstrated as stem cells that can form organoids containing all mature cell types in regeneration-inactive organs such as the liver and pancreas (Huch et al., 2013a,b). In this study, our data indicated that in the utricle, another regeneration-inactive organ, damage recruited Lgr5-positive cells exhibit progenitor cell properties and are capable of regenerating hair cells.

In the mammalian cochlea and utricle, there is little or no detectable proliferation of postnatal cells in the sensory epithelium. However, when supporting cells were isolated they could self-renew to form spheres with the ability to regenerate hair cells *in vitro* (White et al., 2006; Oshima et al., 2007, 2009; Jeon et al., 2011; Sinkkonen et al., 2011), although it was unclear which cell population could proliferate. A recent study showed that Lgr5-positive cells in the cochlea could self-renew to form spheres, with these spheres giving rise to hair cells derived from Lgr5-positive supporting cells (Shi et al., 2012). In the present study, our results showed that FACS sorted damage-activated Lgr5-positive supporting cell have significantly higher sphere formation capacity compared to Lgr5-negative cells. The spheres derived from Lgr5-positive cells were smaller and more homogenous solid spheres, whereas the spheres derived from Lgr5-negative cells were larger and more hollow. When we collected spheres for differentiation, our data showed that the spheres derived from Lgr5-positive cells generated significantly more hair cells than the spheres derived from Lgr5-negative cells, indicating that damage-activated Lgr5-positive supporting cells were enriched in the population of hair cell progenitors in the utricle. After seven passages, spheres derived from Lgr5-positive cells still maintained the capacity for differentiation into hair cells. However, we cannot rule out the possibility that other progenitor cell population in the utricle could contribute to regenerate hair cells after sphere formation.

In summary, we report here that neomycin-induced hair cell loss activates Lgr5 expression in a subpopulation of striolar supporting cells in the utricle. These damage recruited Lgr5-positive supporting cells act as hair cell progenitors both *ex vivo* and *in vitro*. These Lgr5-positive cells could self-renew to form spheres, which maintained the capacity to differentiate into hair cells over seven generation of passages. Therefore, we demonstrated that damage-recruited Lgr5-positive supporting cells could act as hair cell progenitors in neonatal mouse utricle, and serve as candidate therapeutic targets for hair cell regeneration in mammals.

Author Contributions

Conceived and designed experiments: JL. Provided reagents: JL. Performed experiments: JL, XZ, FW, WL. Analyzed the data: JL, XZ, FW, WL. Wrote the paper: JL, XZ, FW, WL.

Acknowledgments

This work was supported by Quanzhou Sci and Tech Key Project (2012Z21).

References

Barker, N., Huch, M., Kujala, P., van de Wetering, M., Snippert, H. J., van Es, J. H., et al. (2010). Lgr5(+ve) stem cells drive self-renewal in the stomach and build long-lived gastric units *in vitro*. *Cell Stem Cell* 6, 25–36. doi: 10.1016/j.stem.2009.11.013

Barker, N., van Es, J. H., Kuipers, J., Kujala, P., van den Born, M., Cozijnsen, M., et al. (2007). Identification of stem cells in small intestine and colon by marker gene Lgr5. *Nature* 449, 1003–1007. doi: 10.1038/nature06196

Bermingham-McDonogh, O., and Rubel, E. W. (2003). Hair cell regeneration: winging our way towards a sound future. *Curr. Opin. Neurobiol.* 13, 119–126. doi: 10.1016/s0959-4388(03)00018-7

Bramhall, N. F., Shi, F., Arnold, K., Hochedlinger, K., and Edge, A. S. (2014). Lgr5-positive supporting cells generate new hair cells in the postnatal cochlea. *Stem Cell Rep* 2, 311–322. doi: 10.1016/j.stemcr.2014.01.008

Brigande, J. V., and Heller, S. (2009). Quo vadis, hair cell regeneration? *Nat. Neurosci.* 12, 679–685. doi: 10.1038/nn.2311

Burns, J. C., Cox, B. C., Thiede, B. R., Zuo, J., and Corwin, J. T. (2012a). In vivo proliferative regeneration of balance hair cells in newborn mice. *J. Neurosci.* 32, 6570–6577. doi: 10.1523/JNEUROSCI.6274-11.2012

Burns, J. C., On, D., Baker, W., Collado, M. S., and Corwin, J. T. (2012b). Over half the hair cells in the mouse utricle first appear after birth, with significant numbers originating from early postnatal mitotic production in peripheral and striolar growth zones. *J. Assoc. Res. Otolaryngol.* 13, 609–627. doi: 10.1007/s10162-012-0337-0

Chai, R., Kuo, B., Wang, T., Liaw, E. J., Xia, A., Jan, T. A., et al. (2012). Wnt signaling induces proliferation of sensory precursors in the postnatal mouse cochlea. *Proc. Natl. Acad. Sci. U S A* 109, 8167–8172. doi: 10.1073/pnas.1202774109

Chai, R., Xia, A., Wang, T., Jan, T. A., Hayashi, T., Bermingham-McDonogh, O., et al. (2011). Dynamic expression of Lgr5, a Wnt target gene, in the developing and mature mouse cochlea. *J. Assoc. Res. Otolaryngol.* 12, 455–469. doi: 10.1007/s10162-011-0267-2

Corwin, J. T., and Cotanche, D. A. (1988). Regeneration of sensory hair cells after acoustic trauma. *Science* 240, 1772–1774. doi: 10.1126/science.3381100

Cox, B. C., Chai, R., Lenoir, A., Liu, Z., Zhang, L., Nguyen, D., et al. (2014). Spontaneous hair cell regeneration in the neonatal mouse cochlea *in vivo Development* 141, 816–829. doi: 10.1242/dev.103036

Dechesne, C. J., and Thomasset, M. (1988). Calbindin (CaBP 28 kDa) appearance and distribution during development of the mouse inner ear. *Brain Res.* 468, 233–242. doi: 10.1016/0165-3806(88)90135-6

Dechesne, C. J., Thomasset, M., Brehier, A., and Sans, A. (1988). Calbindin (CaBP 28 kDa) localization in the peripheral vestibular system of various vertebrates. *Hear. Res.* 33, 273–278. doi: 10.1016/0378-5955(88)90157-8

de Lau, W., Barker, N., Low, T. Y., Koo, B. K., Li, V. S., Teunissen, H., et al. (2011). Lgr5 homologues associate with Wnt receptors and mediate R-spondin signalling. *Nature* 476, 293–297. doi: 10.1038/nature10337

Desai, S. S., Zeh, C., and Lysakowski, A. (2005). Comparative morphology of rodent vestibular periphery. I. Saccular and utricular maculae. *J. Neurophysiol.* 93, 251–266. doi: 10.1152/jn.00746.2003

Forge, A., Li, L., Corwin, J. T., and Nevill, G. (1993). Ultrastructural evidence for hair cell regeneration in the mammalian inner ear. *Science* 259, 1616–1619. doi: 10.1126/science.8456284

Golub, J. S., Tong, L., Ngyuen, T. B., Hume, C. R., Palmiter, R. D., Rubel, E. W., et al. (2012). Hair cell replacement in adult mouse utricles after targeted ablation of hair cells with diphtheria toxin. *J. Neurosci.* 32, 15093–15105. doi: 10.1523/JNEUROSCI.1709-12.2012

Huch, M., Bonfanti, P., Boj, S. F., Sato, T., Loomans, C. J., van de Wetering, M., et al. (2013a). Unlimited *in vitro* expansion of adult bi-potent pancreas progenitors through the Lgr5/R-spondin axis. *EMBO J.* 32, 2708–2721. doi: 10.1038/emboj.2013.204

Huch, M., Dorrell, C., Boj, S. F., van Es, J. H., Li, V. S., van de Wetering, M., et al. (2013b). *In vitro* expansion of single Lgr5+ liver stem cells induced by Wnt-driven regeneration. *Nature* 494, 247–250. doi: 10.1038/nature11826

Jaks, V., Barker, N., Kasper, M., Van Es, J. H., Snippert, H. J., Clevers, H., et al. (2008). Lgr5 marks cycling, yet long-lived, hair follicle stem cells. *Nat. Genet.* 40, 1291–1299. doi: 10.1038/ng.239

Jeon, S. J., Fujioka, M., Kim, S. C., and Edge, A. S. (2011). Notch signaling alters sensory or neuronal cell fate specification of inner ear stem cells. *J. Neurosci.* 31, 8351–8358. doi: 10.1523/JNEUROSCI.6366-10.2011

Jørgensen, J. M., and Mathiesen, C. (1988). The avian inner ear. Continuous production of hair cells in vestibular sensory organs, but not in the auditory papilla. *Naturwissenschaften* 75, 319–320. doi: 10.1007/bf00367330

Kawamoto, K., Izumikawa, M., Beyer, L. A., Atkin, G. M., and Raphael, Y. (2009). Spontaneous hair cell regeneration in the mouse utricle following gentamicin ototoxicity. *Hear. Res.* 247, 17–26. doi: 10.1016/j.heares.2008.08.010

Lambert, P. R., Gu, R., and Corwin, J. T. (1997). Analysis of small hair bundles in the utricles of mature guinea pigs. *Am. J. Otol.* 18, 637–643.

Li, H., Liu, H., and Heller, S. (2003). Pluripotent stem cells from the adult mouse inner ear. *Nat. Med.* 9, 1293–1299. doi: 10.1038/nm925

Lim, X., Tan, S. H., Koh, W. L., Chau, R. M., Yan, K. S., Kuo, C. J., et al. (2013). Interfollicular epidermal stem cells self-renew via autocrine Wnt signaling. *Science* 342, 1226–1230. doi: 10.1126/science.1239730

Lin, V., Golub, J. S., Nguyen, T. B., Hume, C. R., Oesterle, E. C., and Stone, J. S. (2011). Inhibition of Notch activity promotes nonmitotic regeneration of hair cells in the adult mouse utricles. *J. Neurosci.* 31, 15329–15339. doi: 10.1523/JNEUROSCI.2057-11.2011

Logan, C. Y., and Nusse, R. (2004). The Wnt signaling pathway in development and disease. *Annu. Rev. Cell Dev. Biol.* 20, 781–810. doi: 10.1146/annurev.cellbio.20.010403.113126

Minear, S., Leucht, P., Jiang, J., Liu, B., Zeng, A., Fuerer, C., et al. (2010). Wnt proteins promote bone regeneration. *Sci. Transl. Med.* 2:29ra30. doi: 10.1126/scitranslmed.3000231

Oesterle, E. C., Cunningham, D. E., Westrum, L. E., and Rubel, E. W. (2003). Ultrastructural analysis of [3H]thymidine-labeled cells in the rat utricular macula. *J. Comp. Neurol.* 463, 177–195. doi: 10.1002/cne.10756

Oshima, K., Grimm, C. M., Corrales, C. E., Senn, P., Martinez Monedero, R., Géléoc, G. S., et al. (2007). Differential distribution of stem cells in the auditory and vestibular organs of the inner ear. *J. Assoc. Res. Otolaryngol.* 8, 18–31. doi: 10.1007/s10162-006-0058-3

Oshima, K., Senn, P., and Heller, S. (2009). Isolation of sphere-forming stem cells from the mouse inner ear. *Methods Mol. Biol.* 493, 141–162. doi: 10.1007/978-1-59745-523-7_9

Roberson, D. F., Weisleder, P., Bohrer, P. S., and Rubel, E. W. (1992). Ongoing production of sensory cells in the vestibular epithelium of the chick. *Hear. Res.* 57, 166–174. doi: 10.1016/0378-5955(92)90149-h

Rubel, E. W., Dew, L. A., and Roberson, D. W. (1995). Mammalian vestibular hair cell regeneration. *Science* 267, 701–707. doi: 10.1126/science.7839150

Ryals, B. M., and Rubel, E. W. (1988). Hair cell regeneration after acoustic trauma in adult Coturnix quail. *Science* 240, 1774–1776. doi: 10.1126/science.3381101

Shi, F., Hu, L., and Edge, A. S. (2013). Generation of hair cells in neonatal mice by beta-catenin overexpression in Lgr5-positive cochlear progenitors. *Proc. Natl. Acad. Sci. U S A* 110, 13851–13856. doi: 10.1073/pnas.1219952110

Shi, F., Kempfle, J. S., and Edge, A. S. (2012). Wnt-responsive lgr5-expressing stem cells are hair cell progenitors in the cochlea. *J. Neurosci.* 32, 9639–9648. doi: 10.1523/JNEUROSCI.1064-12.2012

Sinkkonen, S. T., Chai, R., Jan, T. A., Hartman, B. H., Laske, R. D., Gahlen, F., et al. (2011). Intrinsic regenerative potential of murine cochlear supporting cells. *Sci.* 1:26. doi: 10.1038/srep00026

Stone, J. S., and Cotanche, D. A. (2007). Hair cell regeneration in the avian auditory epithelium. *Int. J. Dev. Biol.* 51, 633–647. doi: 10.1387/ijdb.072408js

Tumbar, T., Guasch, G., Greco, V., Blanpain, C., Lowry, W. E., Rendl, M., et al. (2004). Defining the epithelial stem cell niche in skin. *Science* 303, 359–363. doi: 10.1126/science.1092436

Warchol, M. E., Lambert, P. R., Goldstein, B. J., Forge, A., and Corwin, J. T. (1993). Regenerative proliferation in inner ear sensory epithelia from adult guinea pigs and humans. *Science* 259, 1619–1622. doi: 10.1126/science.8456285

Weisleder, P., and Rubel, E. W. (1993). Hair cell regeneration after streptomycin toxicity in the avian vestibular epithelium. *J. Comp. Neurol.* 331, 97–110. doi: 10.1002/cne.903310106

White, P. M., Doetzlhofer, A., Lee, Y. S., Groves, A. K., and Segil, N. (2006). Mammalian cochlear supporting cells can divide and trans-differentiate into hair cells. *Nature* 441, 984–987. doi: 10.1038/nature04849

14

Role of calcium-sensing receptor in mechanotransducer-channel-mediated Ca^{2+} influx in hair cells of zebrafish larvae

*Li-Yih Lin[1], Ya-Hsin Yeh[1], Giun-Yi Hung[1,2,3], Chia-Hao Lin[4,5], Pung-Pung Hwang[4] and Jiun-Lin Horng[5]**

[1] Department of Life Science, National Taiwan Normal University, Taipei, Taiwan, [2] Department of Pediatrics, Taipei Veterans General Hospital, Taipei, Taiwan, [3] Department of Pediatrics, Faculty of Medicine, National Yang-Ming University, Taipei, Taiwan, [4] Institute of Cellular and Organismic Biology, Academia Sinica, Taipei, Taiwan, [5] Department of Anatomy and Cell Biology, School of Medicine, College of Medicine, Taipei Medical University, Taipei, Taiwan

Edited by:
*Youji Wang,
Shanghai Ocean University, China*

Reviewed by:
*Zhongmin Lu,
University of Miami, United States
Katie Kindt,
National Institutes of Health (NIH),
United States*

***Correspondence:**
*Jiun-Lin Horng
jlhorng@tmu.edu.tw*

The calcium-sensing receptor (CaSR) is an extracellular Ca^{2+} sensor that plays a critical role in maintaining Ca^{2+} homeostasis in several organs, including the parathyroid gland and kidneys. In this study, through *in situ* hybridization, the expression of CaSR mRNA was found in the neuromasts of zebrafish larvae. Immunohistochemistry further demonstrated that the CaSR protein was present in neuromast hair cell stereocilia and basolateral membranes. Based on the expression and subcellular localization of the CaSR in hair cells, we hypothesized that the CaSR is expressed in zebrafish lateral-line hair cells to regulate mechanotransducer (MET)-channel-mediated Ca^{2+} entry. Using the scanning ion-selective electrode technique, MET-channel-mediated Ca^{2+} influx at the stereocilia of hair cells was measured in intact larvae. Ca^{2+} influx was suppressed after larvae were pretreated with a CaSR activator (R-568) or high-Ca^{2+} (HCa) medium. Gene knockdown by using morpholino oligonucleotides decreased CaSR expression in hair cells and eliminated the effects of R-568 and HCa on Ca^{2+} influx. In addition, we found that treatment with R-568 attenuated neomycin-induced hair cell death. This study is the first to demonstrate that the CaSR is involved in mechanotransduction in zebrafish hair cells.

Keywords: calcium-sensing receptor, hair cell, mechanotransducer channel, zebrafish, scanning ion-selective electrode technique

INTRODUCTION

The calcium-sensing receptor (CaSR), a G-protein-coupled receptor, is activated by extracellular Ca^{2+} to regulate Ca^{2+} absorption and Ca^{2+} homeostasis in several organs, including the kidneys, intestines, bone, and parathyroid gland (Brown and MacLeod, 2001; Hofer and Brown, 2003; Smajilovic and Tfelt-Hansen, 2007). In the parathyroid gland, reduced plasma Ca^{2+} levels cause a CaSR-mediated increase in parathyroid hormone (PTH) secretion (Chattopadhyay and Brown, 2006). CaSR-knockout mice displayed highly elevated PTH levels, even when plasma Ca^{2+} levels were considerably elevated, demonstrating the direct effect of the CaSR on PTH secretion (Ho et al., 1995). In the kidneys, CaSR activation inhibits both transcellular and paracellular Ca^{2+} transport in the thick ascending limb (Motoyama and Friedman, 2002). Loss-of-function mutations of the CaSR lead to decreased urinary Ca^{2+} excretion in humans and mice (Brown et al., 1998; Toka et al., 2012). In sum, these findings indicate that the CaSR plays a critical role in regulating Ca^{2+} homeostasis.

The CaSR is also involved in regulating different functions in tissues that are not related to Ca^{2+} homeostasis, such as those in the brain, pancreas, blood vessels, and heart (Smajilovic and Tfelt-Hansen, 2007). In the brain, the CaSR activates several ion channels, including non-selective cation channels (Ye et al., 1996; Chattopadhyay et al., 1999a) and calcium-sensitive K^+ channels (Chattopadhyay et al., 1999b; Ye et al., 2004). Activation of the CaSR opens intermediate-conductance calcium-sensitive K^+ (IKCa) channels in arterial endothelial cells (Weston et al., 2005). By contrast, an *in vitro* study demonstrated that the coexpression of the CaSR with the K^+ channel (Kir4.1 or Kir4.2) in *Xenopus* oocytes inhibits the function of the K^+ channel (Huang et al., 2007). Altogether, these findings suggest that the CaSR can sense extracellular Ca^{2+} and modulate the function of ion channels.

Hair cells in the inner ears of mammals are specialized mechanosensory cells involved in hearing and balance. Apical hair bundles are a special morphological feature of hair cells and consist of stereocilia that contain mechanotransducer (MET) channels (Kazmierczak and Muller, 2012). Deflection of hair bundles opens the MET channel and causes Ca^{2+} and K^+ influx, which activates signal transduction in hair cells. An electrophysiological analysis of isolated hair cells showed that the MET channel is a non-selective cation channel with high Ca^{2+} permeability (Fettiplace, 2009). After entry through the MET channel, Ca^{2+} binds to calmodulin or acts at an unknown intracellular site to drive slow and fast adaptations (Wu et al., 1999; Peng et al., 2016). Moreover, extracellular Ca^{2+} affects the open probability of the MET channel (Ricci and Fettiplace, 1998; Farris et al., 2006; Peng et al., 2016). A study demonstrated that decreasing extracellular Ca^{2+} increased the open probability of the MET channel and amplified the blocking efficacy of aminoglycoside antibiotics (Ricci, 2002). Small organic molecules such as the fluorescent styryl dye FM1-43, which has been used as a marker of hair cell viability (Gale et al., 2001; Meyers et al., 2003; Coffin et al., 2009; Ou et al., 2010), and aminoglycoside antibiotics, which can cause hair cell death (Fettiplace, 2009; Froehlicher et al., 2009), have been found to pass through MET channels.

Ca^{2+} homeostasis is critical for the survival and functioning of hair cells during the detection and transmission of acoustic information. To maintain the intracellular Ca^{2+} concentration, hair cells contain numerous Ca^{2+}-buffering proteins, such as calbindin, calmodulin, and parvalbumin (Hackney et al., 2005). Hair bundles express a plasma membrane Ca^{2+} ATPase pump (PMCA) to extrude Ca^{2+}, which enters through MET channels during stimulation (Dumont et al., 2001). Disruption of intracellular Ca^{2+} homeostasis or mutations of the PMCA gene impair hair cell function and cause hearing loss (Gillespie and Muller, 2009; Bortolozzi et al., 2010). Furthermore, elevated intracellular Ca^{2+} levels have been observed in chick and mouse cochlear explants following exposure to ototoxic agents (Hirose et al., 1999; Matsui et al., 2004). In a study of zebrafish, dying hair cells exhibited a transient increase in intracellular Ca^{2+} after exposure to aminoglycosides (Esterberg et al., 2013). These data suggest that alterations in intracellular Ca^{2+} homeostasis play an essential role in aminoglycoside-induced hair cell death.

Extracellular Ca^{2+} is also crucial for hair cell function (Dumont et al., 2001; Go et al., 2010). Experiments with mouse cochlear cultures showed that elevating the extracellular Ca^{2+} or Mg^{2+} concentration suppressed neomycin-provoked hair cell damage; conversely, decreasing the extracellular Ca^{2+} or Mg^{2+} concentration enhanced the damage (Richardson and Russell, 1991). In zebrafish, increases in either extracellular Ca^{2+} or Mg^{2+} have been found to protect hair cells from neomycin-induced cell death, and the lack of external Ca^{2+} in the medium has been found to led to hair cell death (Coffin et al., 2009; Lin et al., 2013). These findings demonstrate that intra- and extracellular Ca^{2+} is critical for hair cell functioning and survival. However, the mechanism by which hair cells sense environmental Ca^{2+} concentrations and maintain an appropiate internal Ca^{2+} concentration has not yet been determined.

Inner-ear hair cells of mammals are embedded in the temporal bone, whereas zebrafish hair cells are situated in lateral-line neuromasts on the embryonic skin and can be easily observed and investigated (Ghysen and Dambly-Chaudiere, 2007). Neuromasts contain a core of approximately 15 hair cells with a structure and function similar to those of inner-ear hair cells in other vertebrates, including humans (Froehlicher et al., 2009; Ou et al., 2010). Lateral-line hair cells are also sensitive to ototoxic drugs, including aminoglycosides and cisplatin (Ou et al., 2007, 2010; Froehlicher et al., 2009). Therefore, zebrafish is a valuable *in vivo* model for studying vertebrate hair cells (Froehlicher et al., 2009; Ou et al., 2010).

CaSRs have been identified in several teleost fish organs, including the gills, olfactory organ, kidneys, and corpuscles of Stannius (Flanagan et al., 2002; Loretz et al., 2009; Lin et al., 2014). A electrophysiological study of goldfish (*Carassius auratus*) revealed that the signaling activity of the olfactory nerve increased with increasing environmental Ca^{2+} levels, presumably through CaSR activation (Hubbard et al., 2002). In a study of rainbow trout, treatment with CaSR activators stimulated the secretion of stanniocalcin, a hypocalcemic hormone, and decreased Ca^{2+} uptake (Radman et al., 2002). However, the cellular distribution and function of the CaSR in neuromast hair cells have not been investigated.

The scanning ion-selective electrode technique (SIET) has been applied to study the transport of various ions (Na^+, Cl^-, H^+, $NH_4{}^+$, and Ca^{2+}) by skin ionocytes in zebrafish and medaka (*Oryzias latipes*) (Smith et al., 1999; Wu et al., 2010; Shih et al., 2012; Horng et al., 2015). In previous studies, we also applied this non-invasive technique to detect MET-channel-mediated Ca^{2+} entry at zebrafish hair cells (Lin et al., 2013, 2015). In these studies, a Ca^{2+}-selective microelectrode was used to deflect hair bundles and simultaneously record Ca^{2+} flux, and the findings demonstrated that SIET is a sensitive approach for assaying MET channels *in vivo* (Lin et al., 2013, 2015).

In this study, the SIET was used to investigate CaSR function in hair cells of intact zebrafish larvae. We hypothesized that the CaSR is expressed in hair bundles of hair cells, where this protein can sense external Ca^{2+} and regulate Ca^{2+} entry. *In situ* hybridization (ISH) and immunohistochemistry (IHC) were used to determine the localization of CaSR mRNA and protein in hair cells. Morpholino oligonucleotides (MOs) were injected to knock down CaSR protein expression. The results clearly indicate that the addition of external Ca^{2+} and a CaSR activator (R-568) suppressed Ca^{2+} influx at the hair bundles. Furthermore, we found that treatment with R-568 attenuated neomycin-induced hair cell death.

MATERIALS AND METHODS

Zebrafish

Adult zebrafish (*Danio rerio*, AB strain) were reared in circulating dechlorinated tap water at 28°C, with a 14-h light/10-h dark photoperiod. Fertilized eggs were incubated in artificial normal water (NW) containing 0.5 mM NaCl, 0.2 mM $CaSO_4$, 0.2 mM $MgSO_4$, 0.16 mM KH_2PO_4, and 0.16 mM K_2HPO_4 (pH 7.0). The solutions were prepared by adding various salts (Sigma-Aldrich, St. Louis, MO, United States) to double-distilled water. Larvae were not fed, and the NW was changed daily to ensure optimal water quality during the experiments. The experimental protocols were approved by the Taipei Medical University Animal Care and Utilization Committee (Approval No. LAC-2015-0368).

Whole-Mount ISH

For ISH, primers (forward: 5′-AAGACGGGCGATATCCTG CTTGGA-3′; reverse: 5′-TGCTCGATGATGGCAGCCATGGC-3′) were used in polymerase chain reaction (PCR) to obtain DNA fragments of zebrafish *casr* (nucleotides 482–1008; XM_684005). The fragments were then inserted into a pGEM-T Easy vector (Promega, Madison, WI, United States). The inserted fragments were amplified through PCR using T7 and SP6 primers, and the products were used as templates for *in vitro* transcription by using T7 or SP6 RNA polymerase (Roche, Mannheim, Germany) in the presence of digoxigenin (DIG)-UTP (Roche) to synthesize sense (T7) and antisense (SP6) probes. The sizes of 3λ DIG-labeled RNA probes were examined using 1% agarose gels, and probe quality and concentrations were determined using dot blot assays. For the dot blot assays, synthesized probes and standard RNA probes were spotted on a nitrocellulose membrane according to the manufacturer's instructions. After cross-linking and blocking, the membrane was incubated with an alkaline phosphatase-conjugated anti-DIG antibody and stained with nitro blue tetrazolium (NBT) and 5-bromo-4-chloro-3-indolyl phosphate (BCIP) (Roche, Mannheim, Germany).

Zebrafish larvae were anesthetized on ice and fixed with 4% paraformaldehyde in phosphate-buffered saline (PBS; 1.4 mM NaCl, 0.2 mM KCl, 0.1 mM Na_2HPO_4, and 0.002 mM KH_2PO_4; pH 7.4) at 4°C overnight. Samples were subsequently washed with diethylpyrocarbonate-treated PBST (PBS with 0.1% Tween-20) several times (10 min/wash). After washing, samples were first incubated with a hybridization buffer [HyB, 50% formamide, 5× saline-sodium citrate (SSC), and 0.1% Tween 20] at 65°C for 5 min and then with HyB containing 500 μg/mL yeast transfer tRNA at 65°C for 4 h before hybridization. After hybridization with 100 ng/mL DIG-labeled antisense or sense RNA probes overnight, larvae were serially washed with 50% formamide–2× SSC (at 65°C for 20 min), 2× SSC (at 65°C for 10 min), 2× SSC (at 65°C for 10 min), 0.2× SSC (at 65°C for 30 min, twice), and PBST (at room temperature for 10 min). Larvae were then immunoreacted with an alkaline phosphatase-coupled anti-DIG antibody (1:8000) and stained with NBT and BCIP.

Whole-Mount Immunocytochemistry

For immunocytochemical staining of the CaSR, zebrafish larvae were first fixed with 4% paraformaldehyde in PBS for 2 h at 4°C. After fixation, the larvae were briefly rinsed with PBS and were then gradually dehydrated with 100% methanol. Following rehydration with PBS, the larvae were blocked with 3% bovine serum albumin for 1 h. The larvae were then incubated with an rabbit anti-CaSR polyclonal antibody (1:500; Herberger and Loretz, 2013; Kwong et al., 2014) or a rabbit anti-S100 polyclonal antibody (1:250; Dako, Carpinteria, CA, United States) in PBS at 4°C overnight. Subsequently, the larvae were washed with PBS for 20 min and incubated with an Alexa Fluor 488 goat anti-rabbit antibody (1:200; Invitrogen) for 2 h in the dark at room temperature. For double immunocytochemical staining, the larvae were incubated overnight at 4°C with CaSR polyclonal and mouse anti-actin monoclonal antibodies (1:100; Chemicon, Temecula, CA, United States). After washing, samples were incubated with Alexa Fluor 568 goat anti-mouse and Alexa Fluor 488 goat anti-rabbit antibodies for 2 h at room temperature. Images were acquired using an upright microscope (Imager M1, Carl Zeiss, Oberkochen, Germany) or a Leica TCS-SP5 confocal laser scanning microscope (Leica Lasertechnik, Heidelberg, Germany).

Microinjection of Antisense MOs

Morpholino-modified antisense oligonucleotides were purchased from Gene Tools (Philomath, OR, United States). Zebrafish *casr* MO1 (5′-AGTTGGAACCTAATGTGGTCTTCAT-3′; nt −31 to −7; Lin et al., 2014) and *casr* MO2 (5′-ACT TCA GAT GAA ACC TCA TTGCTT C-3′; nt −6 to 19; Kwong et al., 2014) were prepared with sterile water. A standard control MO was provided by Gene Tools; it had no target and no significant biological activity. Following the procedures described in previous studies (Kwong et al., 2014; Lin et al., 2014), the MO solution (4 ng/embryo) containing 0.1% phenol red (as a visual indicator) was injected into zebrafish embryos at the one-to-two-cell stage by using an IM-300 microinjection system (Narishige Scientific Instrument Laboratory, Tokyo, Japan).

Scanning Ion-Selective Electrode Technique (SIET)

The SIET (Faszewski and Kunkel, 2001; Garber et al., 2005) was used to measure Ca^{2+} influx at the apices of neuromasts. Glass capillary tubes (no. TW 150-4 with 1.12- and 1.5-mm inner and outer diameters, respectively; World Precision Instruments, Sarasota, FL, United States) were pulled on a Sutter P-97

Flaming Brown pipette puller (Sutter Instruments, San Rafael, CA, United States) into micropipettes with tip diameters of 3–4 μm. The micropipettes were then baked at 120°C overnight and were coated with dimethyl chlorosilane (Sigma-Aldrich) for 30 min. A Ca^{2+}-selective microelectrode was fabricated as previously described (Garber et al., 2005; Lin et al., 2013). To create a Ca^{2+}-selective microelectrode, the micropipettes were backfilled with a 1-cm column of electrolyte (100 mM $CaCl_2$) and frontloaded with a 20–30-μm column of Ca^{2+} ionophore I cocktail A (Sigma-Aldrich).

Details of the system are provided in our previous studies (Wu et al., 2010; Shih et al., 2012; Lin et al., 2013, 2015; Horng et al., 2015). The ion-selective microelectrode was connected to the main amplifier with a Ag/AgCl wire electrode holder and preamplifier (Applicable Electronics, East Falmouth, MA, United States), and the circuit was completed with a salt bridge (3 M KCl in 3% agarose connected to a Ag/AgCl wire). A step-wise motor-driven three-dimensional (3D) positioner (Applicable Electronics) was attached to an upright microscope (BX-50WI, Olympus, Tokyo, Japan) and was used to oscillate and position the microelectrode. A 10× dry and 60× water-immersion objective lens (working distance: 3.3 mm) were used. The microscope was equipped with a digital camera (ILCE-6300, Sony, Japan) that enabled imaging and recording on a monitor. Automated Scanning Electrode Technique (ASET) software (Science Wares, East Falmouth, MA, United States) was used for data acquisition, preliminary processing, and controlling the 3D electrode positioner. The microelectrode was oscillated with an excursion distance of 10 μm, and a typical cycle was completed in 3–4 s. The voltage measurement recorded nearest to the tissue was subtracted from the measurement recorded at the opposite end of the cycle. This subtraction served as a self-referencing feature of the probe.

Calibration of the Ion-Selective Microelectrode

Before collecting biological data, the efficiency of the Ca^{2+} probe was determined using a method described in a previous study (Garber et al., 2005). The Nernstian properties of each electrode were measured by positioning the Ca^{2+} microelectrode in a series of standard solutions (0.1, 1, 10, and 100 mM $CaCl_2$). Linear regression yielded a Nernstian slope of 30 ± 0.53 ($n = 10$) for Ca^{2+}, which was obtained by plotting the voltage output of the probe against log[Ca^{2+}] values. According to technical documents provided by Sigma, the selectivity coefficients of the Fluka Ca^{2+} ionophore I cocktail A are approximately 1000-times more selective for Ca^{2+} than for Mg^{2+}.

Measurement of Ca^{2+} Flux at Neuromasts

The SIET was performed at room temperature (26–28°C) in a small plastic recording chamber filled with 1 mL of recording medium that contained NW, 300 μM MOPS buffer, and 0.1 mg/L ethyl 3-aminobenzoate methanesulfonate (tricaine, Sigma-Aldrich). The pH of the recording medium was adjusted to 7.0 by NaOH or HCl addition. Before each measurement, an anesthetized 4-day postfertilization (dpf) larva was placed in a 1 mm-wide trench of the chamber and observed through a 60× water-immersion lens. The microelectrode was then placed in the recording medium and was positioned at the apical surface of the larva's L1 neuromast, where stereocilia are located, to record Ca^{2+} activity (Ghysen and Dambly-Chaudiere, 2007; Haehnel et al., 2012). The microelectrode was oscillated orthogonally for 10 μm to deflect the kinocilia and to record Ca^{2+} influx (Lin et al., 2013). The microelectrode was tested in several positions to identify the strongest signal. Ca^{2+} influxes at neuromasts were measured for five to ten replicates, and the median value was employed to calculate ionic fluxes by using ASET software (Applicable Electronics). Briefly, voltage gradients measured using ASET software were converted into concentration (activity) gradients by using the following equation: $\Delta C = C_b \times 10^{(\Delta V/S)} - C_b$. ΔC (measured in $\mu mole \cdot L^{-1} \cdot cm^{-3}$) represents the concentration gradient between the two points. C_b (measured in $\mu mole \cdot L^{-1}$) represents the background ion concentration, which is calculated as the average of the concentration at each point. ΔV (in μV) denotes the voltage gradient obtained from ASET. S indicates the Nernst slope of the electrode. The concentration gradient was subsequently converted into (extracellular) ion flux according to Fick's law of diffusion and using the following equation: $J = D(\Delta C)/\Delta X$. J (in $pmol \cdot cm^{-2} \cdot s^{-1}$) denotes the net flux of the ion. D is the diffusion coefficient, which is 8×10^{-6} $cm^2 \cdot s^{-1}$ for Ca^{2+}. ΔC (in $pmol \cdot cm^{-3}$) represents the concentration gradient. ΔX (in cm) indicates the distance between the two points. The SIET was performed on the L1 neuromasts (Ghysen and Dambly-Chaudiere, 2007; Haehnel et al., 2012) of the posterior lateral lines in zebrafish larvae. Before SIET measurements, larvae were preincubated in drug medium for 30 min. Thereafter, larvae were placed in the drug-free recording medium and Ca^{2+} influxes of L1 neuromasts were measured. One L1 neuromast per larva was examined.

Scanning Electron Microscopy

Embryos were fixed overnight at 4°C in PBS-buffered 4% paraformaldehyde–5% glutaraldehyde. After being rinsed with PBS, specimens were postfixed with 2% osmium tetraoxide in 0.1 M cacodylate buffer for another 2 h. After being rinsed with cacodylate buffer and dehydrated with ethanol, specimens were critical point dried with liquid CO_2 in a K850 critical point drier (Quorum Technologies Ltd., East Grinstead, United Kingdom) and were sputter coated for 3 min with a gold-palladium complex in a vacuum evaporator (IB-2; Hitachi, Ltd., Tokyo, Japan). Coated specimens were examined using scanning electron microscopy (SEM; Hitachi S-2400, Tokyo, Japan). The hair bundle of L1 neuromasts in the posterior lateral lines were observed.

Drug Preparation and Treatment

Neomycin (10 mg/mL, Sigma-Aldrich) was dissolved in NW to a final concentration of 1 or 10 μM (pH 7.0). R-568 (Santa Cruz Biotechnology) was dissolved in DMSO to a stock concentration of 10 mM, and adequate stock was dissolved in NW to final concentrations of 2–16 μM. The final concentration of DMSO in the working solutions was <0.1%. In R-568 experiments, the 0 R-568 treatment group was incubated in medium containing 0.1% DMSO. Larvae were immersed in the drug medium for 30 min. Thereafter, larvae were immersed in the drug-free recording medium and were measured using the SIET. $CaSO_4$ was dissolved in NW to a final concentration of 2 mM to prepare HCa NW. The pH of media was adjusted to 7.0. For hair-cell-counting experiments, larvae were incubated in neomycin for 1 h. For R-568 and neomycin incubation, larvae were preincubated in R-568 for 10 min, followed by incubation in R-568 and neomycin. After treatments, larvae were washed with NW, and hair cells were labeled with rhodamine 123 (Sigma) for 10–15 min or FM1-43 (Molecular Probes) for 2 min. Rhodamine 123 was dissolved in ethanol to a stock concentration of 2.6 mM and then dissolved in NW to a final concentration of 2.6 μM. Similarly, FM1-43 was dissolved in DMSO to a stock concentration of 3 mM and then dissolved in NW to a final concentration of 3 μM. Live larvae were observed under an upright microscope (BX60; Olympus) equipped with a digital camera (Canon 50D). The hair cell numbers of L1 neuromasts in the posterior lateral lines were determined (Ghysen and Dambly-Chaudiere, 2007; Haehnel et al., 2012). One L1 neuromast per larva was examined.

Statistical Analysis

Data are presented as mean ± standard error (SE). Values obtained under each condition were analyzed using one-way analysis of variance (ANOVA), followed by Tukey's pairwise comparisons. Student's unpaired *t*-test (two-tailed) was used for simple comparisons of two means. In all cases, significance was accepted at a level of 0.05. All experiments were repeated for at least three independent trials to confirm results, and representative data from one of the trial are displayed in the figures.

RESULTS

Localization of the CaSR in Neuromast Hair Cells of Zebrafish Larvae

Whole-mount ISH was used to determine the localization of *casr* mRNA in 3-dpf zebrafish larvae. Signals of *casr* mRNA were identified in the lateral-line neuromasts of larvae (arrowheads in **Figure 1A**) and in ionocytes dispersed on the yolk sac skin (white arrows in **Figure 1A**). These signals were not detected in the negative control reacted with the sense probe (**Figure 1B**). Whole-mount IHC was further used to determine

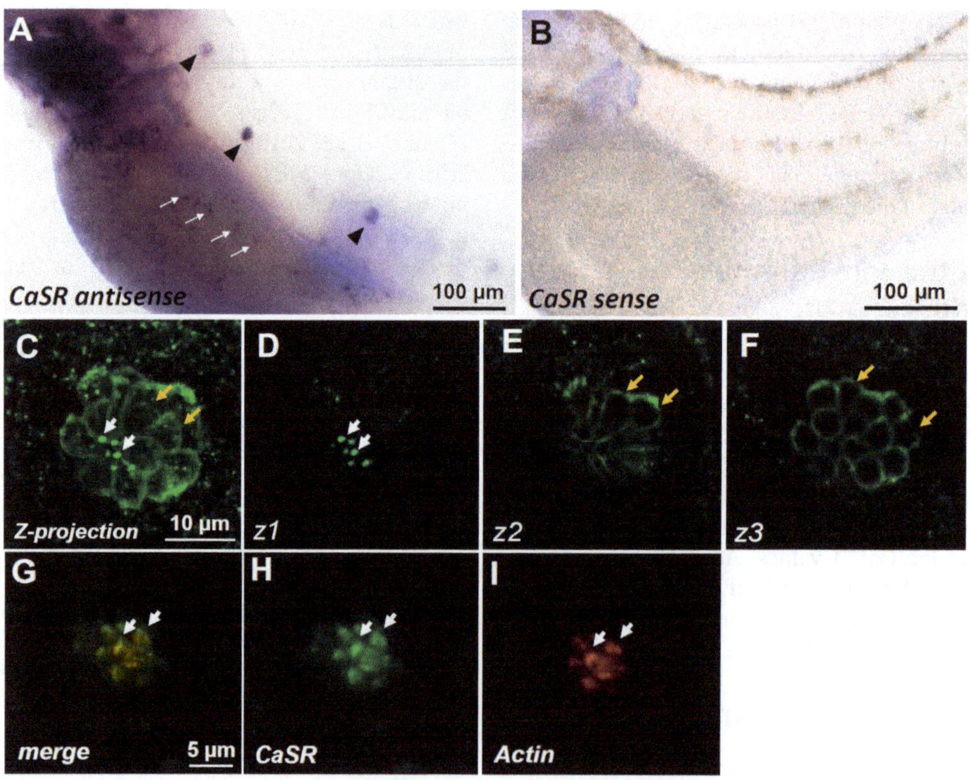

FIGURE 1 | *In situ* hybridization and immunocytochemistry of the Ca^{2+}-sensing receptor (CaSR) in zebrafish larvae. CaSR mRNA was expressed in neuromasts (arrowheads) and ionocytes (arrows) of 3- day-postfertilization (dpf) larvae **(A)**. The sense probe detected no signal in larval skin **(B)**. Confocal images of CaSR antibody-labeled lateral-line neuromasts of 4-dpf larvae (**C**, a Z-projection). Confocal *z*-stacks of the same neuromast revealed that the CaSR was expressed in stereocilia (white arrows in **C,D**) and basolateral membranes (orange arrows in **C,E,F**). Double immunocytochemical labeling of the CaSR **(H)** and actin **(I)** in 4-dpf larvae; the merged image is shown in **(G)**. White arrows indicate the colocalization of both CaSR and actin signals in stereocilia.

the localization of the CaSR protein in 4-dpf larval neuromasts. Confocal microscopic images revealed CaSR signals in the stereocilia (white arrows in **Figures 1C,D**) and basolateral membranes of hair cells (yellow arrows in **Figures 1C,E,F**). Optical sections in various focal planes (z1: at stereocilia; z2: at 3 μm below the stereocilia; z3: at 6 μm below the stereocilia) are, respectively, presented in **Figures 1D–F**. Double IHC was used to identify coexpressed CaSR and actin in hair cell stereocilia (**Figures 1G–I**).

Effects of the CaSR Activator (R-568) on Ca^{2+} Influx at Neuromasts

To investigate the role of the CaSR in Ca^{2+} influx at the apical surface of hair cells, 4-dpf larvae were treated with a CaSR activator (R-568). R-568 has been shown to activate the CaSR in mammalian and fish studies (Greenwood et al., 2009; Lu et al., 2009). Real-time recordings of Ca^{2+} influxes at neuromast hair cells of larvae treated with 0, 2, 4, and 8 μM R-568 are presented in **Figure 2A**. Ca^{2+} influx was detected before the addition of R-568, but the influx gradually declined after the addition of R-568 (arrows in **Figure 2A**). Treatment with 2, 4, and 8 μM R-568, respectively, reduced Ca^{2+} influxes by 37, 66, and 74% (**Figure 2C**). **Figure 2B** presents background fluxes (without larva).

Effect of CaSR Knockdown on Ca^{2+} Influx at Neuromasts

CaSR-specific MOs were used to knock down the protein expression of the CaSR. No obvious difference was observed in the phenotype of CaSR MO-injected zebrafish embryos (CaSR morphants) and control MO-injected embryos (control morphants) or wild-type embryos. CaSR protein expression in 4-dpf morphants was analyzed using IHC. CaSR signals were found in the stereocilia and basolateral membranes of hair cells in wild-type embryos (**Figures 3A,B**) and control morphants (**Figures 3C,D**). The signals were remarkably lower in CaSR morphants (**Figures 3E–H**). SEM was used to examine the L1 hair bundle morphology of neuromasts. No obvious difference was identified in neuromast kinocilia and apical membrane appearance between 4-dpf CaSR morphants and control morphants (**Figures 3I,K,M**). The S100 antibody was used to label neuromast hair cells in zebrafish, and no significant difference was found in the morphology and number of hair cells in the L1 neuromast between 4-dpf control morphants and CaSR morphants (**Figures 3J,L,N,O**).

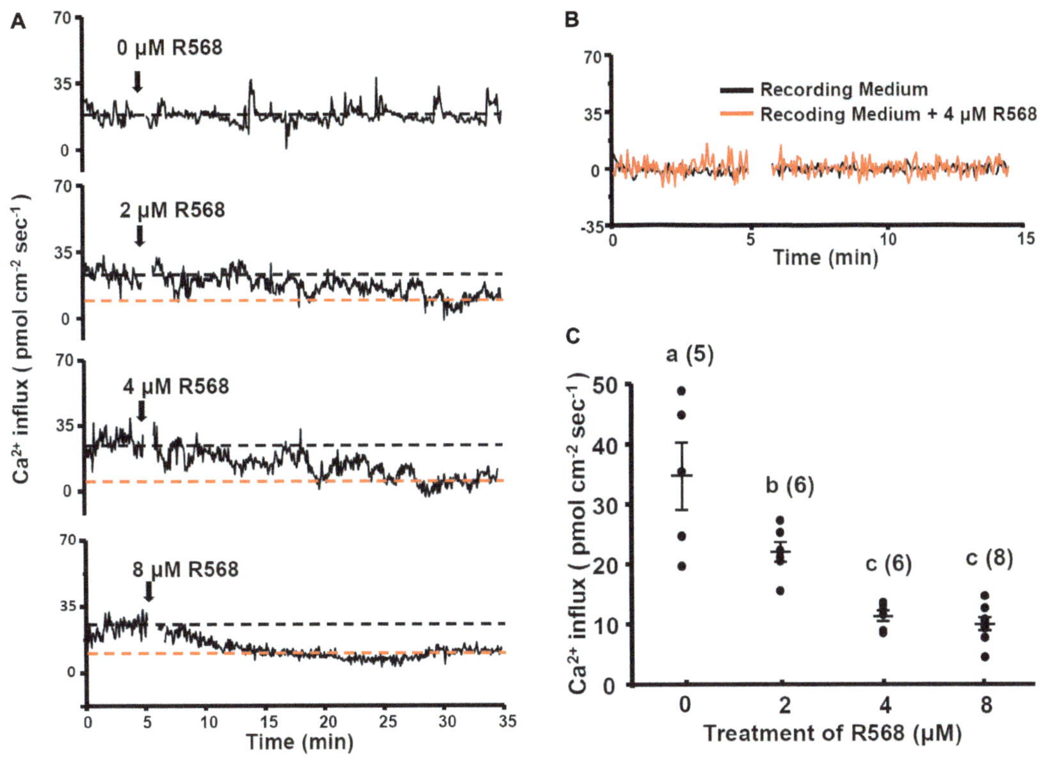

FIGURE 2 | Effect of R-568 on neuromast Ca^{2+} influxes. Sequential recordings of L1 neuromast Ca^{2+} influxes of 4-dpf larvae before and after the addition of 0, 2, 4, and 8 μM R-568 (arrows in **A**). The black dotted line denotes the average Ca^{2+} influx (time: 3–5 min) before the addition of the drug. The red dotted line denotes the average Ca^{2+} influx 30 min after the addition of the drug (time: 30–33 min). **(B)** Illustrates the fluxes of the background signal in recording medium (black line) and the recording medium with R-568 (red line; no fish). **(C)** Larvae were preincubated in normal water with 2, 4, or 8 μM R-568 for 30 min. The larvae were then placed in the normal recording medium without R-568, and Ca^{2+} influxes at L1 neuromasts were recorded. Data are presented as mean ± SE. [a,b,c] indicate significant difference (by one-way ANOVA and Tukey's comparison, $p < 0.05$). Numbers in parentheses are the numbers of neuromasts. One L1 neuromast per larva was examined.

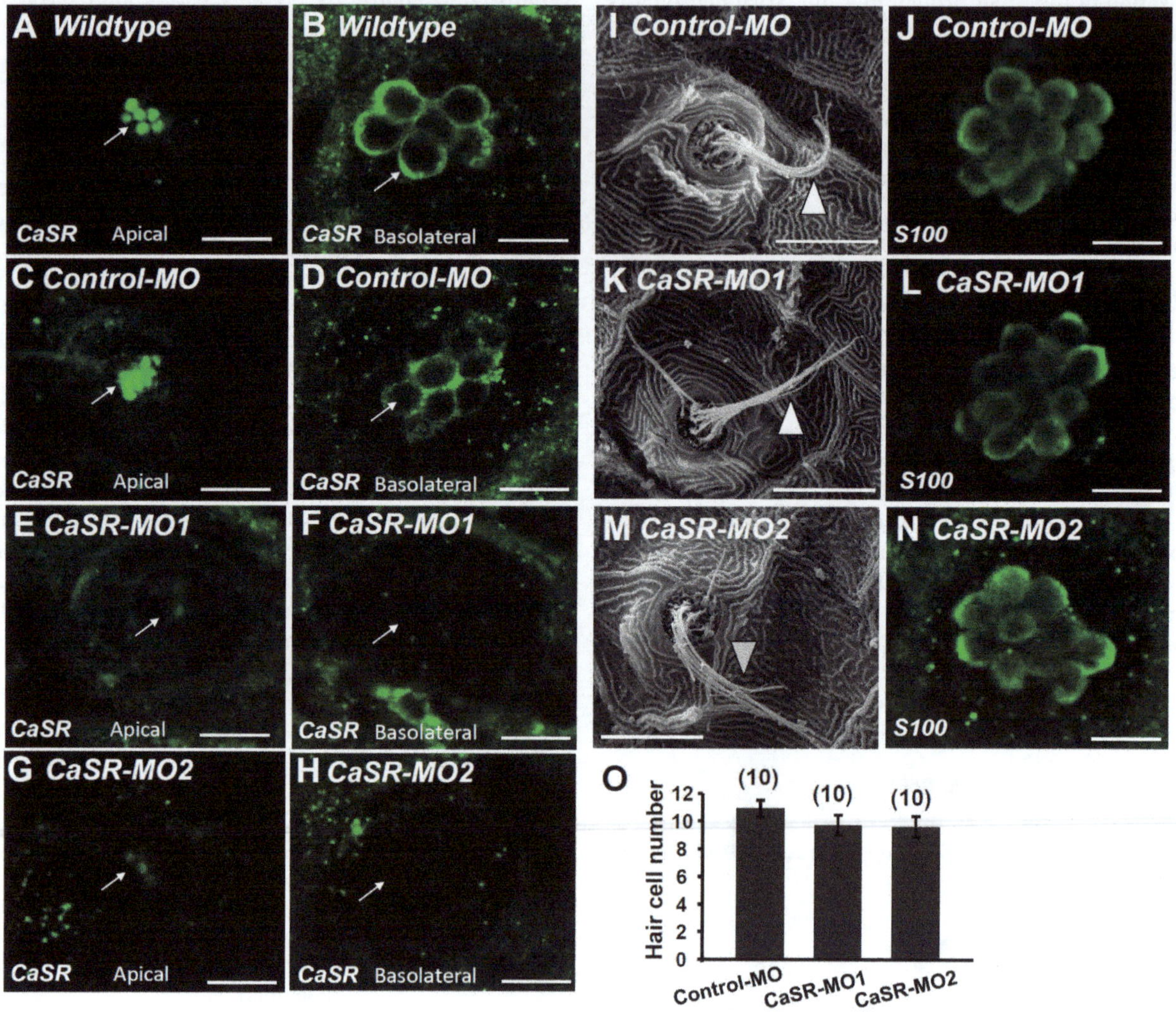

FIGURE 3 | Ca^{2+}-sensing receptor (CaSR) protein expression in neuromast hair cell of CaSR morpholino oligonucleotide (MO) knockdown larvae. Immunocytochemical staining with CaSR antibodies was conducted in 4-dpf wild-type larvae **(A,B)**, control MO-injected larvae (control-MO; **C,D**), and CaSR-MO-injected larvae (CaSR-MO; **E–H**). CaSR signals (green) were detected in the apical (arrows; **A,C**) and basolateral (arrows; **B,D**) membranes of hair cells in wild-type and control-MO larvae. In CaSR-MOs, the CaSR signal was weak in the apical and basolateral membranes **(E–H)**. Scanning electron microscopy images revealed the morphologies of L1 neuromat hair bundles in 4-dpf control-MOs and CaSR-MOs (arrowheads; **I,K,M**). Immunocytochemical staining with S100 antibodies was conducted in 4-dpf control-MOs and CaSR-MOs **(J,L,N)**. The hair cell numbers of L1 neuromasts in the posterior lateral lines were determined **(O)**. Data are presented as mean ± SE. No significant differences were identified (one-way ANOVA and Tukey's comparison, $p < 0.05$). Numbers in parentheses are the numbers of neuromasts. One L1 neuromast per larva was examined.

No significant difference was observed in L1 neuromast Ca^{2+} influxes between 4-dpf CaSR morphants and control morphants. Furthermore, R-568 (2 μM) treatment reduced Ca^{2+} influxes in control morphants, but not in CaSR morphants (**Figure 4**). The results indicate that CaSR knockdown through MOs did not affect Ca^{2+} influxes in hair cells but neutralized the effect of R-568.

Effect of HCa Exposure on Ca^{2+} Influx at Neuromasts

In this experiment, 4-dpf larvae were incubated in HCa water (2 mM Ca^{2+}) for 30 min and were then transferred to the recording medium to measure Ca^{2+} influxes at L1 neuromasts. Similar to R-568 treatment (**Figure 2**), HCa treatment suppressed Ca^{2+} influxes by 47%. Treatment with a combination of HCa and R-568 (2 μM) did not suppress Ca^{2+} influxes more than did HCa treatment alone (**Figure 5A**).

HCa treatment also suppressed Ca^{2+} influxes in control morphants, but not in CaSR morphants (**Figures 5B,C**).

R-568 Attenuated Neomycin-Induced Hair Cell Death

In this experiment, two fluorescent dyes, FM1-43 and rhodamine 123 (Rho-123), were used to label living hair cells in 4-dpf zebrafish larvae (Johnson et al., 1980; Hu, 2007). Exposure of

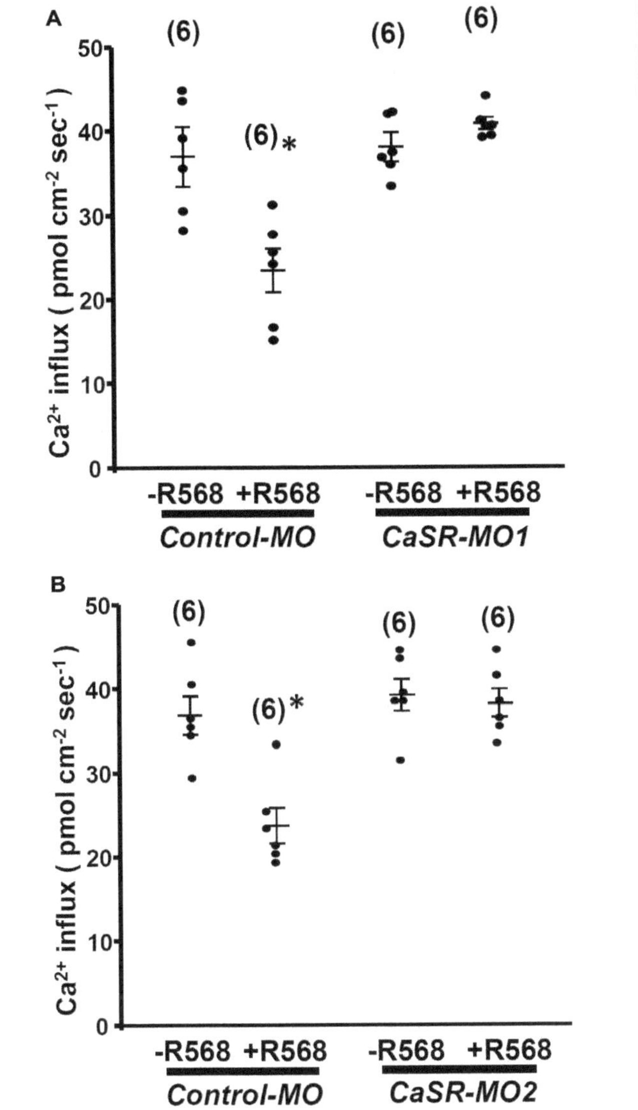

FIGURE 4 | Effect of R-568 on Ca^{2+} influx at neuromasts in Ca^{2+}-sensing receptor (CaSR) morpholino-oligonucleotide (MO)-injected larvae. In 4-dpf control MO-injected larvae (control-MO), treatment with 2 μM R-568 reduced Ca^{2+} influxes at L1 neuromast hair cells. However, treatment with 2 μM R-568 did not alter neuromast hair cell Ca^{2+} influxes in CaSR-MO1- **(A)** or MO2-**(B)** injected larvae. Data are presented as mean ± SE. *Significant difference from the -R-568 group (without R-568; Student's *t*-test, $p < 0.05$). Numbers in parentheses are the numbers of neuromasts. One L1 neuromast per larva was examined.

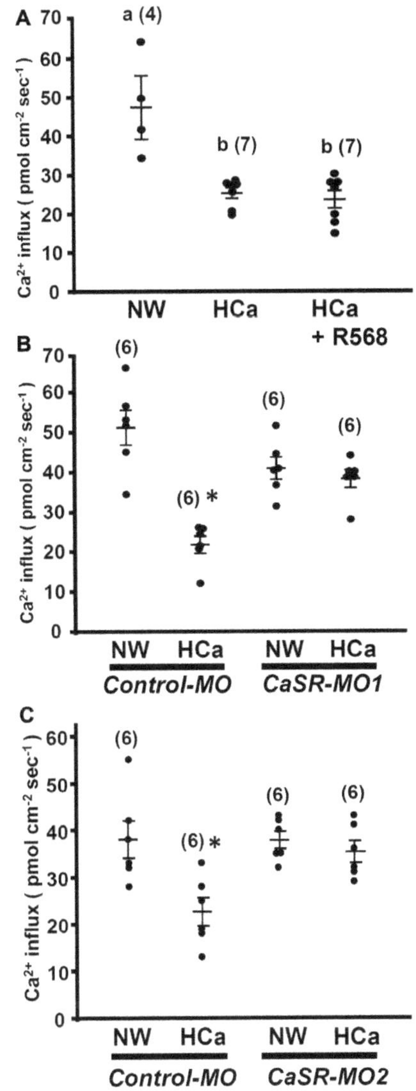

FIGURE 5 | High external Ca^{2+} alters neuromast Ca^{2+} influxes. 4-dpf larvae were preincubated in normal water (NW; 0.2 mM Ca^{2+}) or HCa NW (HCa; 2 mM Ca^{2+}) for 30 min. After preincubation, larvae were placed in normal recording medium, and L1 neuromast Ca^{2+} influxes were recorded. After HCa treatment, neuromast hair cell Ca^{2+} influxes decreased **(A)**. Incubation in HCa medium containing 2 μM R-568 did not suppress Ca^{2+} influx more than HCa treatment alone did **(A)**. In control morpholino oligonucleotide (MO)-injected larvae (control-MO; **B,C**), HCa preincubation decreased Ca^{2+} influx at neuromast hair cells. In Ca^{2+}-sensing receptor (CaSR) MO1- **(B)** and MO2- **(C)** injected larvae, HCa exerted no effect on Ca^{2+} influxes at neuromast hair cells. Data are presented as mean ± SE. A significant difference was found between [a] and [b] (by one-way ANOVA and Tukey's comparison, $p < 0.05$). *Significant difference from the NW group (Student's *t*-test, $p < 0.05$). Numbers in parentheses are the numbers of neuromasts. One L1 neuromast per larva was examined.

larvae to 1 μM neomycin for 1 h decreased the numbers of Rho-123- and FM1-43-labeled L1 neuromast hair cells by 47% and 50%, respectively (**Figure 6**). The treatment of 1 μM neomycin-exposed larva with R-568 at a concentration of 16 μM, but not at lower doses (2, 4, and 8 μM), was found to effectively neutralize the effects of neomycin on hair cells (**Figures 6E,J**). Treatment with 16 μM R-568 alone did not affect the number of hair cells. Treatment with R-568 at a concentration of 16 μM was found to partial neutralize the effects of 10 μM neomycin (**Figure 7J**).

DISCUSSION

The SIET was developed to enable the non-invasive measurement of ion flux in tissues or cells (Garber et al., 2005). Jaffe and Nuccitelli (1974) first developed and applied the "vibrating

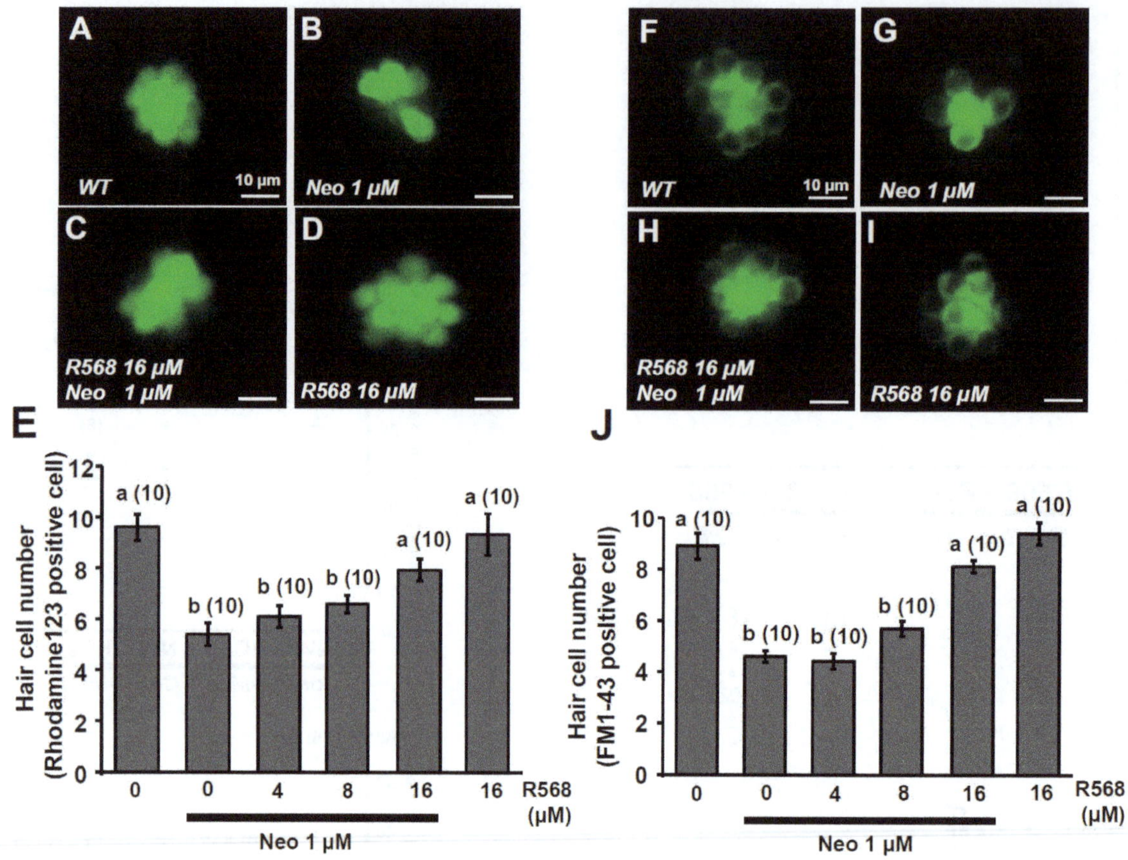

FIGURE 6 | Effect of R-568 on 1 µM neomycin-induced hair cell death. 4-dpf larvae were incubated in 1 µM neomycin media with various levels of R-568 **(E,J)** for 1 h. After treatment, neuromast hair cells were labeled with rhodamine 123 **(A–E)** or FM1-43 **(F–J)**. R-568 at 16 µM neutralized the neuromast hair cell death caused by 1 µM neomycin **(E,J)**. Data are presented as mean ± SE. A significant difference was found between ^{a} and ^{b} (by one-way ANOVA and Tukey's comparison, $p < 0.05$). Numbers in parentheses are the numbers of neuromasts. One L1 neuromast per larva was examined.

probe" or "vibrating voltage probe" technique to biological systems, and the technique was later modified into the SIET (Adlimoghaddam et al., 2014; D'Silva et al., 2017), non-invasive microelectrode ion flux estimation technique (Shabala et al., 2006; Koseki et al., 2012), and the non-invasive micro-test technique. To date, these techniques have been applied to various systems, including plants (Ma et al., 2015; Lei et al., 2017), *Caenorhabditis elegans* (Adlimoghaddam et al., 2014), glioma cells (Hu et al., 2014), *Escherichia coli* (Shabala et al., 2006; Koseki et al., 2012), and mosquito larvae (Boudko et al., 2001; D'Silva et al., 2017). In previous studies, using the non-invasive SIET, we analyzed ion fluxes in intact zebrafish and medaka larvae (Wu et al., 2010; Shih et al., 2012; Lin et al., 2013, 2015; Horng et al., 2015). We also demonstrated that the SIET is suitable for studying hair cells in intact zebrafish larvae (Lin et al., 2013, 2015). The SIET can be used to detect specific ion fluxes at the surface of neuromasts, where hair bundles are located. The "vibrating" feature of the SIET may be used to simultaneously stimulate a hair bundle mechanically and record ion fluxes. Alternative electrophysiological approaches can be used to determine MET channel activity. Measurements of microphonic potential represent the overall voltage response of hair cells but don't reveal the specific types of ion activity involved in mechanotransduction (Olt et al., 2016). Researchers have applied the single-cell patch-clamp technique to measure the basolateral electrical activities of hair cells after removing supporting and mantle cells (Ricci et al., 2013; Olt et al., 2016).

The MO is used for gene knockdown in a range of model animals, including *Xenopus*, zebrafish, sea urchin, and chick. Guidelines for MO use in zebrafish have been published to help researchers distinguish specific phenotypes from off-target effects (Stainier et al., 2017). According to suggestions in the guidelines, we used three MOs (control-MO, UTR MO [MO1], and ATG MO [MO2]) to evaluate the effect of *casr* knockdown in zebrafish embryos. Control MO-injected embryos did not exhibit developmental abnormalities. The doses of MO1 and MO2 used in this study did not result in significant mortality or abnormal behavior in the morphants, and this result is consistent with those of previous studies (Kwong et al., 2014; Lin et al., 2014). The neuromast hair cell morphology of MO1- and MO2-injected morphants was not significantly different from that of control morphants and wild-type embryos (**Figure 3**). CaSR protein expression in *casr* morphants was lower than in control and wild-type embryos, and Ca^{2+} influxes at neuromast hair

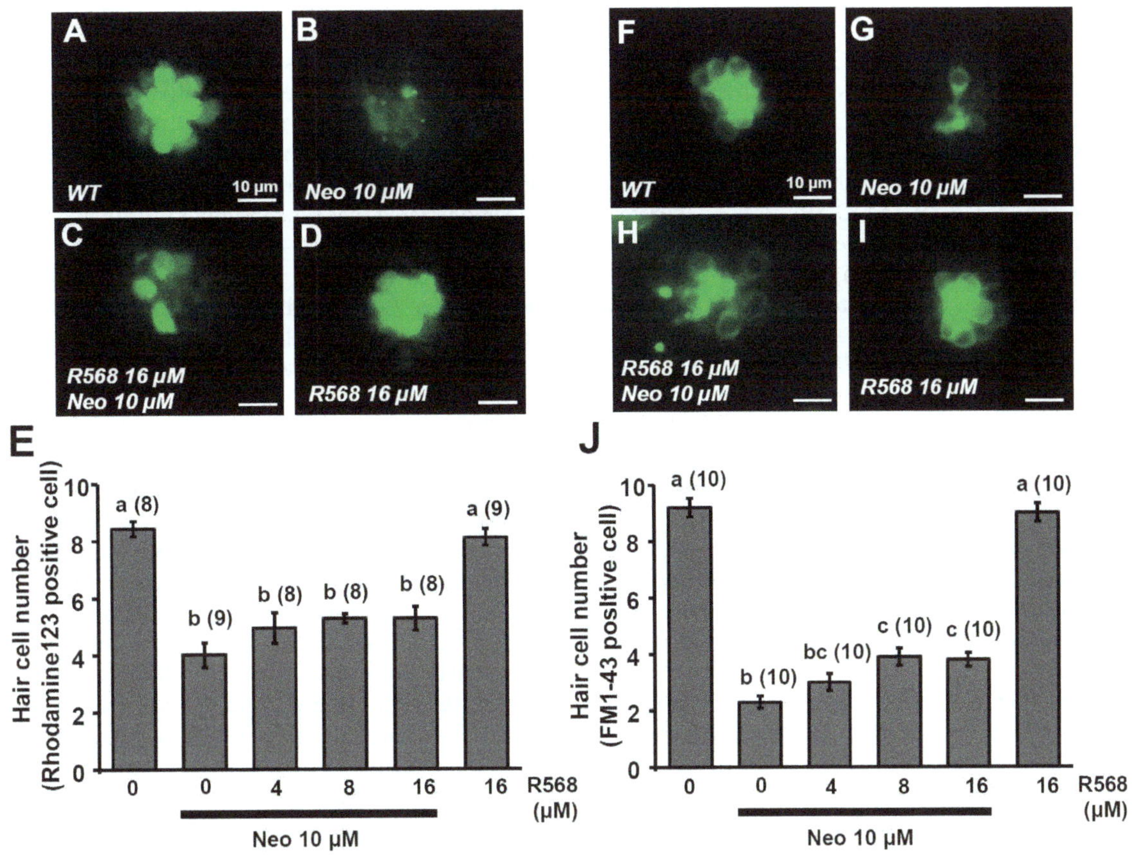

FIGURE 7 | Effect of R-568 on 10 μM neomycin-induced hair cell death. 4-dpf larvae were incubated in 10 μM neomycin media with various levels of R-568 **(E,J)** for 1 h. After incubation, neuromast hair cells were labeled with rhodamine 123 **(A–E)** or FM1-43 **(F–J)**. The addition of 16 μM R-568 partial neutralize the neuromast hair cell death induced by 10 μM neomycin (J). Data are presented as mean ± SE. A significant difference was found between values with superscript letters ([a,b,c]; by one-way ANOVA and Tukey's comparison, $p < 0.05$). Numbers in parentheses are the numbers of neuromasts. One L1 neuromast per larva was examined.

cells was affected by the MOs (**Figures 3–5**). These results demonstrated that the MOs used in this study resulted in minimal off-target effects, and hair cell function was impaired after CaSR knockdown.

The MET channels expressed at the tips of stereocilia are cation-permeable and exhibit high selectivity for Ca^{2+}. Research for MET channel identification has been conducted for more than 20 years, and several candidates have been proposed, including analogs of the epithelial Na^{+} channel, multiple transient receptor potential channels (TRPN, TRPC, and TRPML; Fettiplace and Kim, 2014), and transmembrane channel-like proteins (Fettiplace, 2016). Deflection of a hair bundle tenses the tip link and activates the MET channel. Open MET channels reclose via an initial fast adaptation mechanism followed by a much slower, myosin-based motor process, both of which are driven by Ca^{2+} entry through the channel itself (Holt et al., 2002; Stauffer et al., 2005; Fettiplace and Kim, 2014). A previous study also demonstrated that Ca^{2+} acts as a permeable blocker of the channel, decreasing total MET current (Ricci and Fettiplace, 1998). Ca^{2+} is then exported back to the endolymph by PMCA, which is present in high concentrations in the stereociliary membrane (Fettiplace and Kim, 2014). In a previous study, the alteration of endolymph Ca^{2+} homeostasis and the absence of PMCA2 in various mutants caused the disruption of the MET process and led to deafness (Giacomello et al., 2012).

Zebrafish are exposed to various Ca^{2+} concentrations in their natural environment, from 0.01 mM (soft water) to 3 mM (hard water) (Hoenderop et al., 2005; Pan et al., 2005; Lin and Hwang, 2016; USGS Office of Water Quality, 2017). Studies of fish have indicated strong CaSR expression in gills and the olfactory epithelium (Loretz et al., 2004; Loretz, 2008). CaSR expression at the body surfaces of fish may enable the direct measurement of environmental Ca^{2+} concentrations. Ionocytes in fish gills and embryos proliferate in response to reduced environmental Ca^{2+} concentrations (Uchida et al., 2002; Pan et al., 2005). Extracellular recording from the olfactory bulb of goldfish through electroencephalogram showed that the olfactory system is acutely sensitive to changes in external freshwater Ca^{2+} concentrations (0.05–3 mM; Hubbard et al., 2002). These findings suggest that the CaSR may be involved in the functional regulation of gills and olfactory systems during physiological responses to changes in Ca^{2+} concentrations. Studies of hair cells have found that extracellular Ca^{2+} is critical for MET channel function (Richardson and Russell, 1991; Coffin et al., 2009; Lin et al., 2013). In the present study, we demonstrated CaSR protein expression in hair bundles and suggested that the CaSR senses high environmental Ca^{2+} and reduces Ca^{2+} influx at stereocilia.

The CaSR activation increases PMCA activity in mouse mammary epithelial cells (VanHouten et al., 2007). HEK-293 cells expressing activating CaSR variants show reduced PMCA expression (Ranieri et al., 2013). Hence, PMCA is a potential downstream target of the CaSR. PMCA expression has been observed in rat hair cell stereocilia and basolateral membranes (Chen et al., 2012). In zebrafish, the PMCA mRNA expression pattern recapitulates the GFP expression in the Tg:*atp2b1a*-GFP line (Go et al., 2010). However, no clear evidence has demonstrated that PMCA protein expression occurs in stereocilia. Thus, the speculation that PMCA protein expression occurs in zebrafish stereocilia and is regulated by the CaSR requires further investigation. If PMCA is expressed in the stereocilia of zebrafish hair cells, we cannot exclude the possibility that CaSR activation increases PMCA activity. Thus, the effects we observed in this study may be a combined result of reduced MET-channel-mediated Ca^{2+} influx and increased PMCA-mediated Ca^{2+} efflux. Therefore, the functional roles of the CaSR, PMCA, and MET channels in zebrafish hair cells remain to be determined.

To investigate the function of the CaSR, zebrafish larvae were treated with R-568 or HCa, both of which suppress MET-channel-mediated Ca^{2+} influx in hair cells (**Figures 2, 5**). Treatment with a combination of R-568 and HCa^{2+} did not enhance the inhibition of Ca^{2+} influx, suggesting that the CaSR may mediate the effect of HCa^{2+} on hair cells. In the CaSR morpholino knockdown experiments, the inhibitory effect of R-568 on the MET channel was neutralized (**Figure 4**). The results suggest that R-568 acts through the CaSR rather than through the MET channel, excluding the possibility that R-568 might directly block the MET channel.

Previous studies have indicated that neomycin is taken up by hair cells through the MET channel, leading to cell death (Marcotti et al., 2005; Alharazneh et al., 2011). Blockers of MET channels (curare, quinine, and amiloride) significantly reduce gentamicin uptake and prevent hair cell death (Alharazneh et al., 2011). Low extracellular Ca^{2+} and noise exposure increase the opening probability of MET channels and neomycin uptake, which induce hair cell death (Farris et al., 2006; Coffin et al., 2009; Li and Steyger, 2009). High levels of extracellular Ca^{2+} or Mg^{2+} may decrease the opening probability of MET channels and neomycin uptake, which, in turn, may protect hair cells from neomycin-induced death (Richardson and Russell, 1991; Coffin et al., 2009). In the present study, treatment with 2 μM of a CaSR activator (R-568) significantly suppressed MET-channel-mediated Ca^{2+} influx (**Figure 2**), suggesting that R-568 played a protective role during neomycin treatment. Our data indicate that 16 μM R-568 completely and partially neutralized hair cell death-inducing effects caused by 1 and 10 μM neomycin, respectively (**Figures 6, 7**). Previous studies have found that HCa^{2+} (2 mM) can neutralize damage to hair cells caused by 100 μM neomycin (Coffin et al., 2009; Lin et al., 2013). Our results suggest that CaSR stimulation contributes to a part of the protective effect of HCa^{2+}.

The fluorescent dyes DASPEI (which is used to label mitochondria), YO-PRO1 (which is used to label DNA), and FM1-43 are frequently used to label hair cells (Ou et al., 2010). In the present study, we stained larvae with rhodamine 123, a mitochondrial dye, for the first time. Rhodamine-123-labeled hair cells were distinguishable and countable, and the data were comparable with those for FM1-43 staining. Hence, in this study, we demonstrated that rhodamine 123 is suitable for labeling hair cells.

Previous studies have indicated that activation of the CaSR opens the Ca^{2+}-activated K^+ channel and non-selective cation channel in endothelial cells, neurons, and astrocytoma cells (Ye et al., 1996; Chattopadhyay et al., 1999a,b; Weston et al., 2005). Researchers have suggested that the CaSR regulates K^+ channels and TRPC channels through mitogen-activated protein kinase or the phospholipase C (PLC)-PKC pathway (Ye et al., 2004; Chow et al., 2011; Kong et al., 2012). Another study indicated that CaSR stimulation in HEK293 cells activates both PLC and phosphatidylinositol 4-kinase (PI-4-K) and subsequently Kir currents (Liu et al., 2016). In the present study, activation of the CaSR attenuated MET-channel-mediated Ca^{2+} influx in hair cells. In sum, the findings demonstrate that the CaSR senses extracellular Ca^{2+} and thereafter affects the function of the channels through a direct or indirect pathway.

Ca^{2+} is not the only CaSR agonist. Experiments on parathyroid gland and kidney cells have demonstrated that various divalent (e.g., Mg^{2+} and Sr^{2+}) and trivalent (La^{3+} and Gd^{3+}) cations and aminoglycoside antibiotics (e.g., neomycin) can activate the CaSR (Riccardi and Brown, 2010; Alfadda et al., 2014). Gd^{3+}, La^{3+}, and aminoglycosides are also used as MET channel blockers (Waguespack and Ricci, 2005; Fettiplace, 2009). The data of the present study do not confirm whether neomycin directly acts on the CaSR in neuromast hair cells. Therefore, the functional mechanism of the CaSR in hair cells requires further investigation.

ETHICS STATEMENT

This study was carried out in accordance with the recommendations of 'Taipei Medical University Animal Care and Utilization Committee'. The protocol was approved by the 'Taipei Medical University Animal Care Committee' (Approval No. LAC-2015-0368).

AUTHOR CONTRIBUTIONS

All authors had full access to all the study data and assume responsibility for the integrity of the data and the accuracy of data analysis. L-YL and J-LH: study concept and design, critical revision of the manuscript for intellectual content, funding acquisition, and study supervision. Y-HY and C-HL: acquisition and analysis of data. L-YL, Y-HY, C-HL, and J-LH: interpretation of data. L-YL, G-YH, P-PH, and J-LH: drafted the manuscript. Y-HY, G-YH, and P-PH: administrative, technical, and material support.

FUNDING

This study was supported by grants to J-LH and L-YL from the Ministry of Science and Technology, Taiwan (MOST 104-2311-B-003-003, MOST 104-2311-B-003-001, MOST104-2311-B-038-002, and MOST105-2311-B-038-004-MY3).

ACKNOWLEDGMENTS

We would like to thank the Core Laboratory of Zebrafish, Office of R&D at Taipei Medical University, for providing wild-type fish. We are grateful to Dr. Christopher A. Loretz (University at Buffalo, Buffalo, NY, United States) for providing the CaSR antibodies.

REFERENCES

Adlimoghaddam, A., Weihrauch, D., and O'donnell, M. J. (2014). Localization of K+, H+, Na+ and Ca2+ fluxes to the excretory pore in *Caenorhabditis elegans*: application of scanning ion-selective microelectrodes. *J. Exp. Biol.* 217, 4119–4122. doi: 10.1242/jeb.112441

Alfadda, T. I., Saleh, A. M., Houillier, P., and Geibel, J. P. (2014). Calcium-sensing receptor 20 years later. *Am. J. Physiol. Cell Physiol.* 307, C221–C231. doi: 10.1152/ajpcell.00139.2014

Alharazneh, A., Luk, L., Huth, M., Monfared, A., Steyger, P. S., Cheng, A. G., et al. (2011). Functional hair cell mechanotransducer channels are required for aminoglycoside ototoxicity. *PLoS One* 6:e22347. doi: 10.1371/journal.pone.0022347

Bortolozzi, M., Brini, M., Parkinson, N., Crispino, G., Scimemi, P., De Siati, R. D., et al. (2010). The novel PMCA2 pump mutation *Tommy* impairs cytosolic calcium clearance in hair cells and links to deafness in mice. *J. Biol. Chem.* 285, 37693–37703. doi: 10.1074/jbc.M110.170092

Boudko, D. Y., Moroz, L. L., Linser, P. J., Trimarchi, J. R., Smith, P. J., and Harvey, W. R. (2001). In situ analysis of pH gradients in mosquito larvae using non-invasive, self-referencing, pH-sensitive microelectrodes. *J. Exp. Biol.* 204, 691–699.

Brown, E. M., and MacLeod, R. J. (2001). Extracellular calcium sensing and extracellular calcium signaling. *Physiol. Rev.* 81, 239–297. doi: 10.1152/physrev.2001.81.1.239

Brown, E. M., Pollak, M., and Hebert, S. C. (1998). The extracellular calcium-sensing receptor: its role in health and disease. *Annu. Rev. Med.* 49, 15–29. doi: 10.1146/annurev.med.49.1.15

Chattopadhyay, N., and Brown, E. M. (2006). Role of calcium-sensing receptor in mineral ion metabolism and inherited disorders of calcium-sensing. *Mol. Genet. Metab.* 89, 189–202. doi: 10.1016/j.ymgme.2006.07.003

Chattopadhyay, N., Ye, C. P., Yamaguchi, T., Kerner, R., Vassilev, P. M., and Brown, E. M. (1999a). Extracellular calcium-sensing receptor induces cellular proliferation and activation of a nonselective cation channel in U373 human astrocytoma cells. *Brain Res.* 851, 116–124.

Chattopadhyay, N., Ye, C. P., Yamaguchi, T., Vassilev, P. M., and Brown, E. M. (1999b). Evidence for extracellular calcium-sensing receptor mediated opening of an outward K+ channel in a human astrocytoma cell line (U87). *Glia* 26, 64–72.

Chen, Q., Mahendrasingam, S., Tickle, J. A., Hackney, C. M., Furness, D. N., and Fettiplace, R. (2012). The development, distribution and density of the plasma membrane calcium ATPase 2 calcium pump in rat cochlear hair cells. *Eur. J. Neurosci.* 36, 2302–2310. doi: 10.1111/j.1460-9568.2012.08159.x

Chow, J. Y., Estrema, C., Orneles, T., Dong, X., Barrett, K. E., and Dong, H. (2011). Calcium-sensing receptor modulates extracellular Ca2+ entry via TRPC-encoded receptor-operated channels in human aortic smooth muscle cells. *Am. J. Physiol. Cell Physiol.* 301, C461–C468. doi: 10.1152/ajpcell.00389.2010

Coffin, A. B., Reinhart, K. E., Owens, K. N., Raible, D. W., and Rubel, E. W. (2009). Extracellular divalent cations modulate aminoglycoside-induced hair cell death in the zebrafish lateral line. *Hear. Res.* 253, 42–51. doi: 10.1016/j.heares.2009.03.004

D'Silva, N. M., Patrick, M. L., and O'donnell, M. J. (2017). Effects of rearing salinity on expression and function of ion-motive ATPases and ion transport across the gastric caecum of Aedes aegypti larvae. *J. Exp. Biol.* 220, 3172–3180. doi: 10.1242/jeb.163170

Dumont, R. A., Lins, U., Filoteo, A. G., Penniston, J. T., Kachar, B., and Gillespie, P. G. (2001). Plasma membrane Ca2+-ATPase isoform 2a is the PMCA of hair bundles. *J. Neurosci.* 21, 5066–5078. doi: 10.1523/JNEUROSCI.21-14-05066.2001

Esterberg, R., Hailey, D. W., Coffin, A. B., Raible, D. W., and Rubel, E. W. (2013). Disruption of intracellular calcium regulation is integral to aminoglycoside-induced hair cell death. *J. Neurosci.* 33, 7513–7525. doi: 10.1523/JNEUROSCI.4559-12.2013

Farris, H. E., Wells, G. B., and Ricci, A. J. (2006). Steady-state adaptation of mechanotransduction modulates the resting potential of auditory hair cells, providing an assay for endolymph [Ca2+]. *J. Neurosci.* 26, 12526–12536. doi: 10.1523/JNEUROSCI.3569-06.2006

Faszewski, E. E., and Kunkel, J. G. (2001). Covariance of ion flux measurements allows new interpretation of *Xenopus laevis* oocyte physiology. *J. Exp. Zool.* 290, 652–661. doi: 10.1002/jez.1116

Fettiplace, R. (2009). Defining features of the hair cell mechanoelectrical transducer channel. *Pflugers. Arch.* 458, 1115–1123. doi: 10.1007/s00424-009-0683-x

Fettiplace, R. (2016). Is TMC1 the Hair Cell Mechanotransducer Channel? *Biophys. J.* 111, 3–9. doi: 10.1016/j.bpj.2016.05.032

Fettiplace, R., and Kim, K. X. (2014). The physiology of mechanoelectrical transduction channels in hearing. *Physiol. Rev.* 94, 951–986. doi: 10.1152/physrev.00038.2013

Flanagan, J. A., Bendell, L. A., Guerreiro, P. M., Clark, M. S., Power, D. M., Canario, A. V., et al. (2002). Cloning of the cDNA for the putative calcium-sensing receptor and its tissue distribution in sea bream (*Sparus aurata*). *Gen. Comp. Endocrinol.* 127, 117–127. doi: 10.1016/S0016-6480(02)00035-7

Froehlicher, M., Liedtke, A., Groh, K. J., Neuhauss, S. C., Segner, H., and Eggen, R. I. (2009). Zebrafish (*Danio rerio*) neuromast: promising biological endpoint linking developmental and toxicological studies. *Aquat. Toxicol.* 95, 307–319. doi: 10.1016/j.aquatox.2009.04.007

Gale, J. E., Marcotti, W., Kennedy, H. J., Kros, C. J., and Richardson, G. P. (2001). FM1-43 dye behaves as a permeant blocker of the hair-cell mechanotransducer channel. *J. Neurosci.* 21, 7013–7025. doi: 10.1523/JNEUROSCI.21-18-07013.2001

Garber, S. S., Messerli, M. A., Hubert, M., Lewis, R., Hammar, K., Indyk, E., et al. (2005). Monitoring Cl- movement in single cells exposed to hypotonic solution. *J. Membr. Biol.* 203, 101–110. doi: 10.1007/s00232-005-0735-x

Ghysen, A., and Dambly-Chaudiere, C. (2007). The lateral line microcosmos. *Genes Dev.* 21, 2118–2130. doi: 10.1101/gad.1568407

Giacomello, M., De Mario, A., Primerano, S., Brini, M., and Carafoli, E. (2012). Hair cells, plasma membrane Ca2+ ATPase and deafness. *Int. J. Biochem. Cell Biol.* 44, 679–683. doi: 10.1016/j.biocel.2012.02.006

Gillespie, P. G., and Muller, U. (2009). Mechanotransduction by hair cells: models, molecules, and mechanisms. *Cell* 139, 33–44. doi: 10.1016/j.cell.2009.09.010

Go, W., Bessarab, D., and Korzh, V. (2010). *atp2b1a* regulates Ca2+ export during differentiation and regeneration of mechanosensory hair cells in zebrafish. *Cell Calcium* 48, 302–313. doi: 10.1016/j.ceca.2010.09.012

Greenwood, M. P., Flik, G., Wagner, G. F., and Balment, R. J. (2009). The corpuscles of Stannius, calcium-sensing receptor, and stanniocalcin: responses to calcimimetics and physiological challenges. *Endocrinology* 150, 3002–3010. doi: 10.1210/en.2008-1758

Hackney, C. M., Mahendrasingam, S., Penn, A., and Fettiplace, R. (2005). The concentrations of calcium buffering proteins in mammalian cochlear hair cells. *J. Neurosci.* 25, 7867–7875. doi: 10.1523/JNEUROSCI.1196-05.2005

Haehnel, M., Taguchi, M., and Liao, J. C. (2012). Heterogeneity and dynamics of lateral line afferent innervation during development in zebrafish (*Danio rerio*). *J. Comp. Neurol.* 520, 1376–1386. doi: 10.1002/cne.22798

Herberger, A. L., and Loretz, C. A. (2013). Morpholino oligonucleotide knockdown of the extracellular calcium-sensing receptor impairs early skeletal development in zebrafish. *Comp. Biochem. Physiol. A. Mol. Integr. Physiol.* 166, 470–481. doi: 10.1016/j.cbpa.2013.07.027

Hirose, K., Westrum, L. E., Stone, J. S., Zirpel, L., and Rubel, E. W. (1999). Dynamic studies of ototoxicity in mature avian auditory epithelium. *Ann. N. Y. Acad. Sci.* 884, 389–409. doi: 10.1111/j.1749-6632.1999.tb08657.x

Ho, C., Conner, D. A., Pollak, M. R., Ladd, D. J., Kifor, O., Warren, H. B., et al. (1995). A mouse model of human familial hypocalciuric hypercalcemia and neonatal severe hyperparathyroidism. *Nat. Genet.* 11, 389–394. doi: 10.1038/ng1295-389

Hoenderop, J. G., Nilius, B., and Bindels, R. J. (2005). Calcium absorption across epithelia. *Physiol. Rev.* 85, 373–422. doi: 10.1152/physrev.00003.2004

Hofer, A. M., and Brown, E. M. (2003). Extracellular calcium sensing and signalling. *Nat. Rev. Mol. Cell Biol.* 4, 530–538. doi: 10.1038/nrm1154

Holt, J. R., Gillespie, S. K., Provance, D. W., Shah, K., Shokat, K. M., Corey, D. P., et al. (2002). A chemical-genetic strategy implicates myosin-1c in adaptation by hair cells. *Cell* 108, 371–381. doi: 10.1016/S0092-8674(02)00629-3

Horng, J. L., Chao, P. L., Chen, P. Y., Shih, T. H., and Lin, L. Y. (2015). Aquaporin 1 is involved in acid secretion by ionocytes of zebrafish embryos through facilitating CO2 transport. *PLoS One* 10:e0136440. doi: 10.1371/journal.pone.0136440

Hu, B. H. (2007). Delayed mitochondrial dysfunction in apoptotic hair cells in chinchilla cochleae following exposure to impulse noise. *Apoptosis* 12, 1025–1036. doi: 10.1007/s10495-006-0027-7

Hu, S. L., Du, P., Hu, R., Li, F., and Feng, H. (2014). Imbalance of Ca2+ and K+ fluxes in C6 glioma cells after PDT measured with scanning ion-selective electrode technique. *Lasers Med. Sci.* 29, 1261–1267. doi: 10.1007/s10103-014-1518-3

Huang, C., Sindic, A., Hill, C. E., Hujer, K. M., Chan, K. W., Sassen, M., et al. (2007). Interaction of the Ca2+-sensing receptor with the inwardly rectifying potassium channels Kir4.1 and Kir4.2 results in inhibition of channel function. *Am. J. Physiol. Renal Physiol.* 292, F1073–F1081. doi: 10.1152/ajprenal.00269.2006

Hubbard, P. C., Ingleton, P. M., Bendell, L. A., Barata, E. N., and Canario, A. V. (2002). Olfactory sensitivity to changes in environmental Ca2+ in the freshwater teleost *Carassius auratus*: an olfactory role for the Ca2+-sensing receptor? *J. Exp. Biol.* 205, 2755–2764.

Jaffe, L. F., and Nuccitelli, R. (1974). An ultrasensitive vibrating probe for measuring steady extracellular currents. *J. Cell Biol.* 63, 614–628. doi: 10.1083/jcb.63.2.614

Johnson, L. V., Walsh, M. L., and Chen, L. B. (1980). Localization of mitochondria in living cells with rhodamine 123. *Proc. Natl. Acad. Sci. U.S.A.* 77, 990–994. doi: 10.1073/pnas.77.2.990

Kazmierczak, P., and Muller, U. (2012). Sensing sound: molecules that orchestrate mechanotransduction by hair cells. *Trends Neurosci.* 35, 220–229. doi: 10.1016/j.tins.2011.10.007

Kong, S., Zhang, C., Li, W., Wang, L., Luan, H., Wang, W. H., et al. (2012). Stimulation of Ca2+-sensing receptor inhibits the basolateral 50-pS K channels in the thick ascending limb of rat kidney. *Biochim. Biophys. Acta* 1823, 273–281. doi: 10.1016/j.bbamcr.2011.10.007

Koseki, S., Tamplin, M. L., Bowman, J. P., Ross, T., and Mcmeekin, T. A. (2012). Evaluation of thermal inactivation of *Escherichia coli* using microelectrode ion flux measurements with osmotic stress. *Lett. Appl. Microbiol.* 54, 203–208. doi: 10.1111/j.1472-765X.2011.03194.x

Kwong, R. W., Auprix, D., and Perry, S. F. (2014). Involvement of the calcium-sensing receptor in calcium homeostasis in larval zebrafish exposed to low environmental calcium. *Am. J. Physiol. Regul. Integr. Comp. Physiol.* 306, R211–R221. doi: 10.1152/ajpregu.00350.2013

Lei, P., Pang, X., Feng, X., Li, S., Chi, B., Wang, R., et al. (2017). The microbe-secreted isopeptide poly-gamma-glutamic acid induces stress tolerance in *Brassica napus* L. seedlings by activating crosstalk between H2O2 and Ca2. *Sci. Rep.* 7:41618. doi: 10.1038/srep41618

Li, H., and Steyger, P. S. (2009). Synergistic ototoxicity due to noise exposure and aminoglycoside antibiotics. *Noise Health* 11, 26–32. doi: 10.4103/1463-1741.45310

Lin, C. H., and Hwang, P. P. (2016). The control of calcium metabolism in zebrafish (*Danio rerio*). *Int. J. Mol. Sci.* 17:1783. doi: 10.3390/ijms17111783

Lin, C. H., Su, C. H., and Hwang, P. P. (2014). Calcium-sensing receptor mediates Ca2+ homeostasis by modulating expression of PTH and stanniocalcin. *Endocrinology* 155, 56–67. doi: 10.1210/en.2013-1608

Lin, L. Y., Pang, W., Chuang, W. M., Hung, G. Y., Lin, Y. H., and Horng, J. L. (2013). Extracellular Ca2+ and Mg2+ modulate aminoglycoside blockade of mechanotransducer channel-mediated Ca2+ entry in zebrafish hair cells: an in vivo study with the SIET. *Am. J. Physiol. Cell Physiol.* 305, C1060–C1068. doi: 10.1152/ajpcell.00077.2013

Lin, Y. H., Hung, G. Y., Wu, L. C., Chen, S. W., Lin, L. Y., and Horng, J. L. (2015). Anion exchanger 1b in stereocilia is required for the functioning of mechanotransducer channels in lateral-line hair cells of zebrafish. *PLoS One* 10:e0117041. doi: 10.1371/journal.pone.0117041

Liu, C. H., Chang, H. K., Lee, S. P., and Shieh, R. C. (2016). Activation of the Ca2+-sensing receptors increases currents through inward rectifier K+ channels via activation of phosphatidylinositol 4-kinase. *Pflugers. Arch.* 468, 1931–1943. doi: 10.1007/s00424-016-1901-y

Loretz, C. A. (2008). Extracellular calcium-sensing receptors in fishes. *Comp. Biochem. Physiol. A. Mol. Integr. Physiol.* 149, 225–245. doi: 10.1016/j.cbpa.2008.01.037

Loretz, C. A., Pollina, C., Hyodo, S., and Takei, Y. (2009). Extracellular calcium-sensing receptor distribution in osmoregulatory and endocrine tissues of the tilapia. *Gen. Comp. Endocrinol.* 161, 216–228. doi: 10.1016/j.ygcen.2008.12.020

Loretz, C. A., Pollina, C., Hyodo, S., Takei, Y., Chang, W., and Shoback, D. (2004). cDNA cloning and functional expression of a Ca2+-sensing receptor with truncated carboxy terminal tail from the Mozambique tilapia (*Oreochromis mossambicus*). *J. Biol. Chem.* 279, 53288–53297. doi: 10.1074/jbc.M410098200

Lu, J. Y., Yang, Y., Gnacadja, G., Christopoulos, A., and Reagan, J. D. (2009). Effect of the calcimimetic R-568 [3-(2-chlorophenyl)-N-((1R)-1-(3-methoxyphenyl)ethyl)-1-propanamine] on correcting inactivating mutations in the human calcium-sensing receptor. *J. Pharmacol. Exp. Ther.* 331, 775–786. doi: 10.1124/jpet.109.159228

Ma, Y., Dai, X., Xu, Y., Luo, W., Zheng, X., Zeng, D., et al. (2015). COLD1 confers chilling tolerance in rice. *Cell* 160, 1209–1221. doi: 10.1016/j.cell.2015.01.046

Marcotti, W., Van Netten, S. M., and Kros, C. J. (2005). The aminoglycoside antibiotic dihydrostreptomycin rapidly enters mouse outer hair cells through the mechano-electrical transducer channels. *J. Physiol.* 567, 505–521. doi: 10.1113/jphysiol.2005.085951

Matsui, J. I., Gale, J. E., and Warchol, M. E. (2004). Critical signaling events during the aminoglycoside-induced death of sensory hair cells *in vitro*. *J. Neurobiol.* 61, 250–266. doi: 10.1002/neu.20054

Meyers, J. R., Macdonald, R. B., Duggan, A., Lenzi, D., Standaert, D. G., Corwin, J. T., et al. (2003). Lighting up the senses: FM1-43 loading of sensory cells through nonselective ion channels. *J. Neurosci.* 23, 4054–4065. doi: 10.1523/JNEUROSCI.23-10-04054.2003

Motoyama, H. I., and Friedman, P. A. (2002). Calcium-sensing receptor regulation of PTH-dependent calcium absorption by mouse cortical ascending limbs. *Am. J. Physiol. Renal Physiol.* 283, F399–F406. doi: 10.1152/ajprenal.00346.2001

Olt, J., Ordoobadi, A. J., Marcotti, W., and Trapani, J. G. (2016). Physiological recordings from the zebrafish lateral line. *Methods Cell Biol.* 133, 253–279. doi: 10.1016/bs.mcb.2016.02.004

Ou, H. C., Raible, D. W., and Rubel, E. W. (2007). Cisplatin-induced hair cell loss in zebrafish (*Danio rerio*) lateral line. *Hear. Res.* 233, 46–53. doi: 10.1016/j.heares.2007.07.003

Ou, H. C., Santos, F., Raible, D. W., Simon, J. A., and Rubel, E. W. (2010). Drug screening for hearing loss: using the zebrafish lateral line to screen for drugs that prevent and cause hearing loss. *Drug Discov. Today* 15, 265–271. doi: 10.1016/j.drudis.2010.01.001

Pan, T. C., Liao, B. K., Huang, C. J., Lin, L. Y., and Hwang, P. P. (2005). Epithelial Ca2+ channel expression and Ca2+ uptake in developing zebrafish. *Am. J. Physiol. Regul. Integr. Comp. Physiol.* 289, R1202–R1211. doi: 10.1152/ajpregu.00816.2004

Peng, A. W., Gnanasambandam, R., Sachs, F., and Ricci, A. J. (2016). Adaptation independent modulation of auditory hair cell mechanotransduction channel open probability implicates a role for the lipid bilayer. *J. Neurosci.* 36, 2945–2956. doi: 10.1523/JNEUROSCI.3011-15.2016

Radman, D. P., Mccudden, C., James, K., Nemeth, E. M., and Wagner, G. F. (2002). Evidence for calcium-sensing receptor mediated stanniocalcin secretion in fish. *Mol. Cell. Endocrinol.* 186, 111–119. doi: 10.1016/S0303-7207(01)00643-8

Ranieri, M., Tamma, G., Di Mise, A., Vezzoli, G., Soldati, L., Svelto, M., et al. (2013). Excessive signal transduction of gain-of-function variants of the calcium-sensing receptor (CaSR) are associated with increased ER to cytosol calcium gradient. *PLoS One* 8:e79113. doi: 10.1371/journal.pone.0079113

Riccardi, D., and Brown, E. M. (2010). Physiology and pathophysiology of the calcium-sensing receptor in the kidney. *Am. J. Physiol. Renal Physiol.* 298, F485–F499. doi: 10.1152/ajprenal.00608.2009

Ricci, A. (2002). Differences in mechano-transducer channel kinetics underlie tonotopic distribution of fast adaptation in auditory hair cells. *J. Neurophysiol.* 87, 1738–1748. doi: 10.1152/jn.00574.2001

Ricci, A. J., Bai, J. P., Song, L., Lv, C., Zenisek, D., and Santos-Sacchi, J. (2013). Patch-clamp recordings from lateral line neuromast hair cells of the living zebrafish. *J. Neurosci.* 33, 3131–3134. doi: 10.1523/JNEUROSCI.4265-12.2013

Ricci, A. J., and Fettiplace, R. (1998). Calcium permeation of the turtle hair cell mechanotransducer channel and its relation to the composition of endolymph. *J. Physiol.* 506(Pt 1), 159–173. doi: 10.1111/j.1469-7793.1998.159bx.x

Richardson, G. P., and Russell, I. J. (1991). Cochlear cultures as a model system for studying aminoglycoside induced ototoxicity. *Hear. Res.* 53, 293–311. doi: 10.1016/0378-5955(91)90062-E

Shabala, L., Ross, T., Mcmeekin, T., and Shabala, S. (2006). Non-invasive microelectrode ion flux measurements to study adaptive responses of microorganisms to the environment. *FEMS Microbiol. Rev.* 30, 472–486. doi: 10.1111/j.1574-6976.2006.00019.x

Shih, T. H., Horng, J. L., Liu, S. T., Hwang, P. P., and Lin, L. Y. (2012). Rhcgl and NHE3b are involved in ammonium-dependent sodium uptake by zebrafish larvae acclimated to low-sodium water. *Am. J. Physiol. Regul. Integr. Comp. Physiol.* 302, R84–R93. doi: 10.1152/ajpregu.00318.2011

Smajilovic, S., and Tfelt-Hansen, J. (2007). Calcium acts as a first messenger through the calcium-sensing receptor in the cardiovascular system. *Cardiovasc. Res.* 75, 457–467. doi: 10.1016/j.cardiores.2007.03.015

Smith, P. J., Hammar, K., Porterfield, D. M., Sanger, R. H., and Trimarchi, J. R. (1999). Self-referencing, non-invasive, ion selective electrode for single cell detection of trans-plasma membrane calcium flux. *Microsc. Res. Tech.* 46, 398–417. doi: 10.1002/(SICI)1097-0029(19990915)46:6<398::AID-JEMT8>3.0.CO;2-H

Stainier, D. Y. R., Raz, E., Lawson, N. D., Ekker, S. C., Burdine, R. D., Eisen, J. S., et al. (2017). Guidelines for morpholino use in zebrafish. *PLoS Genet* 13:e1007000. doi: 10.1371/journal.pgen.1007000

Stauffer, E. A., Scarborough, J. D., Hirono, M., Miller, E. D., Shah, K., Mercer, J. A., et al. (2005). Fast adaptation in vestibular hair cells requires myosin-1c activity. *Neuron* 47, 541–553. doi: 10.1016/j.neuron.2005.07.024

Toka, H. R., Al-Romaih, K., Koshy, J. M., Dibartolo, S. III, Kos, C. H., Quinn, S. J., et al. (2012). Deficiency of the calcium-sensing receptor in the kidney causes parathyroid hormone-independent hypocalciuria. *J. Am. Soc. Nephrol.* 23, 1879–1890. doi: 10.1681/ASN.2012030323

Uchida, K., Hasegawa, S., and Kaneko, T. (2002). Effects of a low-Ca2+ environment on branchial chloride cell morphology in chum salmon fry and immunolocalization of Ca2+-ATPase in chloride cells. *Can. J. Zool.* 80, 1100–1108. doi: 10.1139/z02-090

USGS Office of Water Quality (2017). *U.S. Geological Survey*. Available at: https://water.usgs.gov/owq/ (accessed January, 17).

VanHouten, J. N., Neville, M. C., and Wysolmerski, J. J. (2007). The calcium-sensing receptor regulates plasma membrane calcium adenosine triphosphatase isoform 2 activity in mammary epithelial cells: a mechanism for calcium-regulated calcium transport into milk. *Endocrinology* 148, 5943–5954. doi: 10.1210/en.2007-0850

Waguespack, J. R., and Ricci, A. J. (2005). Aminoglycoside ototoxicity: permeant drugs cause permanent hair cell loss. *J. Physiol.* 567, 359–360. doi: 10.1113/jphysiol.2005.094474

Weston, A. H., Absi, M., Ward, D. T., Ohanian, J., Dodd, R. H., Dauban, P., et al. (2005). Evidence in favor of a calcium-sensing receptor in arterial endothelial cells: studies with calindol and Calhex 231. *Circ. Res.* 97, 391–398. doi: 10.1161/01.RES.0000178787.59594.a0

Wu, S. C., Horng, J. L., Liu, S. T., Hwang, P. P., Wen, Z. H., Lin, C. S., et al. (2010). Ammonium-dependent sodium uptake in mitochondrion-rich cells of medaka (*Oryzias latipes*) larvae. *Am. J. Physiol. Cell Physiol.* 298, C237–C250. doi: 10.1152/ajpcell.00373.2009

Wu, Y. C., Ricci, A. J., and Fettiplace, R. (1999). Two components of transducer adaptation in auditory hair cells. *J. Neurophysiol.* 82, 2171–2181. doi: 10.1152/jn.1999.82.5.2171

Ye, C., Kanazirska, M., Quinn, S., Brown, E. M., and Vassilev, P. M. (1996). Modulation by polycationic Ca2+-sensing receptor agonists of nonselective cation channels in rat hippocampal neurons. *Biochem. Biophys. Res. Commun.* 224, 271–280. doi: 10.1006/bbrc.1996.1019

Ye, C. P., Yano, S., Tfelt-Hansen, J., Macleod, R. J., Ren, X., Terwilliger, E., et al. (2004). Regulation of a Ca2+-activated K+ channel by calcium-sensing receptor involves p38 MAP kinase. *J. Neurosci. Res.* 75, 491–498. doi: 10.1002/jnr.10875

15

Identification and characterization of mouse otic sensory lineage genes

Byron H. Hartman, Robert Durruthy-Durruthy, Roman D. Laske, Steven Losorelli and Stefan Heller**

Department of Otolaryngology, Head and Neck Surgery, Stanford University School of Medicine, Stanford, CA, USA

Edited by:
Andy Groves,
Baylor College of Medicine, USA

Reviewed by:
Ronna Hertzano,
University of Maryland School of Medicine, USA
Doris Wu,
National Institutes of Health, USA

***Correspondence:**
Byron H. Hartman and Stefan Heller, Department of Otolaryngology, Head and Neck Surgery, Stanford University School of Medicine, 300 Pasteur Drive, Edwards R213 Stanford, CA 94305, USA
byronh@stanford.edu;
hellers@stanford.edu

Vertebrate embryogenesis gives rise to all cell types of an organism through the development of many unique lineages derived from the three primordial germ layers. The otic sensory lineage arises from the otic vesicle, a structure formed through invagination of placodal non-neural ectoderm. This developmental lineage possesses unique differentiation potential, giving rise to otic sensory cell populations including hair cells, supporting cells, and ganglion neurons of the auditory and vestibular organs. Here we present a systematic approach to identify transcriptional features that distinguish the otic sensory lineage (from early otic progenitors to otic sensory populations) from other major lineages of vertebrate development. We used a microarray approach to analyze otic sensory lineage populations including microdissected otic vesicles (embryonic day 10.5) as well as isolated neonatal cochlear hair cells and supporting cells at postnatal day 3. Non-otic tissue samples including periotic tissues and whole embryos with otic regions removed were used as reference populations to evaluate otic specificity. Otic populations shared transcriptome-wide correlations in expression profiles that distinguish members of this lineage from non-otic populations. We further analyzed the microarray data using comparative and dimension reduction methods to identify individual genes that are specifically expressed in the otic sensory lineage. This analysis identified and ranked top otic sensory lineage-specific transcripts including *Fbxo2, Col9a2,* and *Oc90,* and additional novel otic lineage markers. To validate these results we performed expression analysis on select genes using immunohistochemistry and *in situ* hybridization. *Fbxo2* showed the most striking pattern of specificity to the otic sensory lineage, including robust expression in the early otic vesicle and sustained expression in prosensory progenitors and auditory and vestibular hair cells and supporting cells.

Keywords: cochlea, vestibular, microarray, inner ear, transcriptome

Introduction

The sensory and neuronal cells of the vertebrate inner ear arise from the otic vesicle (OV), a spheroid epithelial structure formed during midgestation embryogenesis through invagination of the otic placode. Of all the developmental lineages of the vertebrate embryo, the otic sensory lineage has the unique capacity to give rise to auditory and vestibular hair cells, supporting cells, and neurons, all of which are essential for hearing and balance function (**Figure 1A**). The otic placode is derived from posterior preplacodal non-neural ectoderm, specifically within the otic-epibranchial domain (Chen and Streit, 2013). The process of otic induction from preplacodal ectoderm is initiated around embryonic day 8 (E8) in mouse. By E10.5 otic vesicle invagination has encapsulated the otic placode epithelia into a vesicle where subsequent processes of morphogenesis and differentiation give rise to cell fates of the inner ear, including neural, sensory (hair cells and supporting cells) and non-sensory fates (**Figures 1B,C**). A progressive lineage bifurcation model of otic differentiation is consistent with experimental observations and illustrates how pan-otic progenitor cells of the otic vesicle could give rise to non-sensory, neural, supporting cell, and hair cell populations (**Figure 1C**). Several signaling pathways including Fgf, Notch, and Wnt have been shown to be involved in specification of the otic placode as well as subsequent specifications of neuronal and prosensory populations (Liu et al., 2003; Jayasena et al., 2008; Dominguez-Frutos et al., 2009; Hartman et al., 2010; Hammond and Whitfield, 2011; Chen and Streit, 2013; Vendrell et al., 2013; Schlosser, 2014). Evolutionarily conserved transcription factors such as Eya1, Six1, Gata3, and Pax2/8 are expressed in the early otic sensory lineage and have been implicated in its specification and development (Xu et al., 1999; Zheng et al., 2003; Hans et al., 2004; Lillevali et al., 2006; Zou et al., 2006; Barrionuevo et al., 2008; Freter et al., 2012). Despite the unique nature of the otic sensory lineage, there are no known markers that unambiguously discriminate this lineage from others persistently through the course of development. The goal of this study was to apply a transcriptome-wide comparison to find such markers. Systematic transcriptome-wide identification of otic lineage distinguishing genes would contribute to our understanding of transcriptional states and gene regulation in inner ear development and function. Furthermore, classification of genes that enable rigorous identification of otic sensory lineage cells would greatly benefit *in vitro* studies of inner ear development and regeneration, which currently rely on combinatorial expression of transient non-specific markers (Oshima et al., 2010; Koehler et al., 2013).

Here we compare transcriptional states in three branches of the otic sensory lineage (early otic progenitors, sensory hair cells and supporting cells) to those of tissues broadly representing non-otic lineages of vertebrate development. We

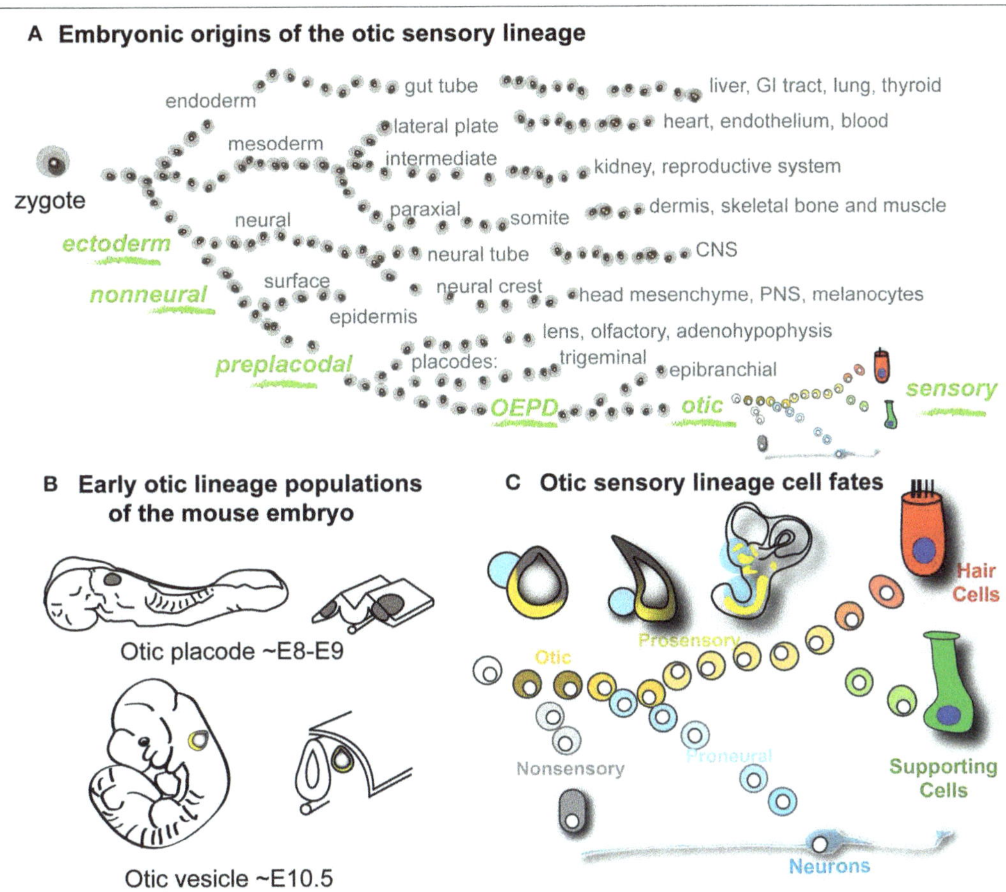

FIGURE 1 | Otic sensory development and project rationale. (A) Schematic of the major developmental lineages of the vertebrate embryo. The otic sensory lineage is derived from the non-neural preplacodal domain of the ectodermal germ lineage (green). The otic-epibranchial domain (OEPD) gives rise to the otic placode, which invaginates to form the epithelium of the otic vesicle, from which the otic sensory populations differentiate. **(B)** The locations of early otic lineage populations of the mouse embryo are depicted at the placode and vesicle stages with corresponding embryonic ages indicated. **(C)** Model of otic lineage differentiation. Through progressive lineage bifurcations, cells of the otic vesicle give rise to hair cells, supporting cells and neurons, as well as non-sensory epithelial cells of the inner ear.

used multivariate analysis methods to identify correlations across ~25,000 probe sets that distinguish the otic sensory lineage from non-otic populations. Otic consensus genes were identified based on differential expression between otic (otic vesicle, hair cell, and supporting cell) and non-otic groups (whole embryos with otic regions removed and periotic tissues). Otic consensus scores and rankings for each probe were devised as a reduction of enrichment values in each of the three otic categories to further aid in identification of lineage specific genes. Our analyses ranked top otic lineage-specific transcripts and identified many novel genes expressed in early otic progenitors as well as sensory hair cells and supporting cells. We performed additional expression analyses on select genes using immunohistochemistry and *in situ* hybridization, which revealed patterns that concurred with the array data. *Fbxo2* showed the most striking pattern of specificity to the otic sensory lineage, including robust expression in the early otic vesicle and sustained expression in prosensory progenitors, and subsequently in auditory and vestibular hair cells and supporting cells.

Materials and Methods

Mice

Embryos were collected from timed pregnant CD-1 dams (Charles River). Noon on the day of the vaginal plug was considered to be E0.5 and embryo ages were confirmed according to Theiler (Theiler, 1989). For postnatal mice, postnatal day 0 (P0) was defined as the day of birth. Mice were housed with the Stanford Department of Comparative Medicine and the Stanford University Administrative Panel on Laboratory Animal Care (APLAC) approved all procedures.

RNA Isolation from Otic and Non-Otic Tissue Populations from E10.5 Embryos

Three separate litters of E10.5 CD-1 embryos (Theiler Stage 16–17) were dissected in cold phosphate buffered saline (PBS) using fine forceps and separated into triplicate pools consisting of (1) 20 otic vesicles (OVs), (2) periotic tissue including mesenchyme and hindbrain, and (3) whole embryos minus the greater otic region (**Figures 2A,B**). RNA was isolated using the Nucleospin RNA XS Kit (Machery Nagel). RNA quality and concentrations were verified with Agilent BioAnalyzer RNA and Nanodrop spectrophotometer assays.

Gene Array Hybridization

Each of the nine RNA samples was amplified using the Ambion Illumina RNA amplification kit with biotin UTP labeling. The Ambion Illumina RNA amplification kit uses T7 oligo(dT) primer to generate single stranded cDNA followed by a second strand synthesis to generate double-stranded cDNA, which is then column purified. *In vitro* transcription was done to synthesize biotin-labeled cRNA using T7 RNA polymerase. The cRNA was then column purified and a total of 750 ng was hybridized for each array using standard Illumina protocols with streptavidin-Cy3 used for detection. The MouseRef-8 v2.0 Illumina beadchip targets ~25,600 annotated RefSeq transcripts, over 19,000 unique genes, and enables the interrogation of eight samples in parallel. For practical purposes we will refer to the *transcriptome-wide* scope of data from this assay, although technically it is limited because some transcripts are not represented and some probe sets will perform better than others. Slides were scanned on an Illumina Beadstation and analyzed using GenomeStudio (Illumina, Inc.). The data discussed in this publication were deposited in NCBI's Gene Expression Omnibus, accession number GSE65843 (accessible at http://www.ncbi.nlm.nih.gov/geo/).

Microarray Data Analysis

Differential microarray analysis was performed with the goal to identify genes enriched in early otic lineage cells as compared broadly to other developmental lineages. At E10.5 the mouse otic vesicle has fully invaginated from the head ectoderm and can be microdissected intact from the surrounding tissues (**Figure 2A**). Mouse embryos at E10.5 were dissected into three tissue groups, one otic and two non-otic. 20 otic vesicles were pooled for each OV sample and the remaining tissue of the embryos were dissected into two non-otic groups consisting of: (1) pooled periotic tissues including mesenchyme and dorsal neural tissue, and (2) whole embryos minus the greater otic regions (**Figures 2A,B**). We analyzed gene expression in triplicate samples for each group using MouseRef-8 v2.0 Expression Beadchip Microarrays (Illumina). To initially assess the quality of the data we performed principal component analysis (PCA) on all nine samples (**Figure 2C**). PCA reduces the high dimensionality of microarray data into a set of linearly uncorrelated variables called principal components, which are defined so that the first principal component retains the largest possible variance (Jollife, 2010). Projections on the first two principal components positioned samples of the same tissue origin in closer proximity with each other than samples from different origins (**Figure 2C**). As expected, transcriptome-wide expression profiles were more similar between replicates of each group. We also analyzed transcriptome-wide correlation between using Spearman's coefficients, which revealed intra-sample similarities and inter-sample differences (**Figure 2D**). Correlation coefficients and the structure of the associated dendrogram indicate that transcriptional profiles of otic vesicle cells are distinct from the two non-otic sample populations.

To compare gene expression in multiple otic sensory populations to non-otic populations, the data for the nine samples from E10.5 embryos described above were analyzed alongside equivalently generated array datasets for FACS-sorted neonatal cochlear hair cells and supporting cells generated in an earlier study (Sinkkonen et al., 2011). These included Illumina MouseRef-8 v2.0 datasets from P3 cochlear hair cells (HCs, $n = 4$, Atoh1-GFP+) and supporting cells (SCs, $n = 2$, Atoh1-GFP-/CD271L/CD146L/CD326+); NCBI Gene Expression Omnibus accession number GSE62582. GeneSpring 12.6 software and R 3.1.1 software packages (RStudio) were used for multivariate microarray data analysis. Data values were log2-transformed and quantile normalization was applied. Quantile normalization removes non-biological variance between arrays by making the distribution of probe intensities the same for each sample based on a normalization distribution chosen by averaging each quantile across all samples (Bolstad et al., 2003). Group

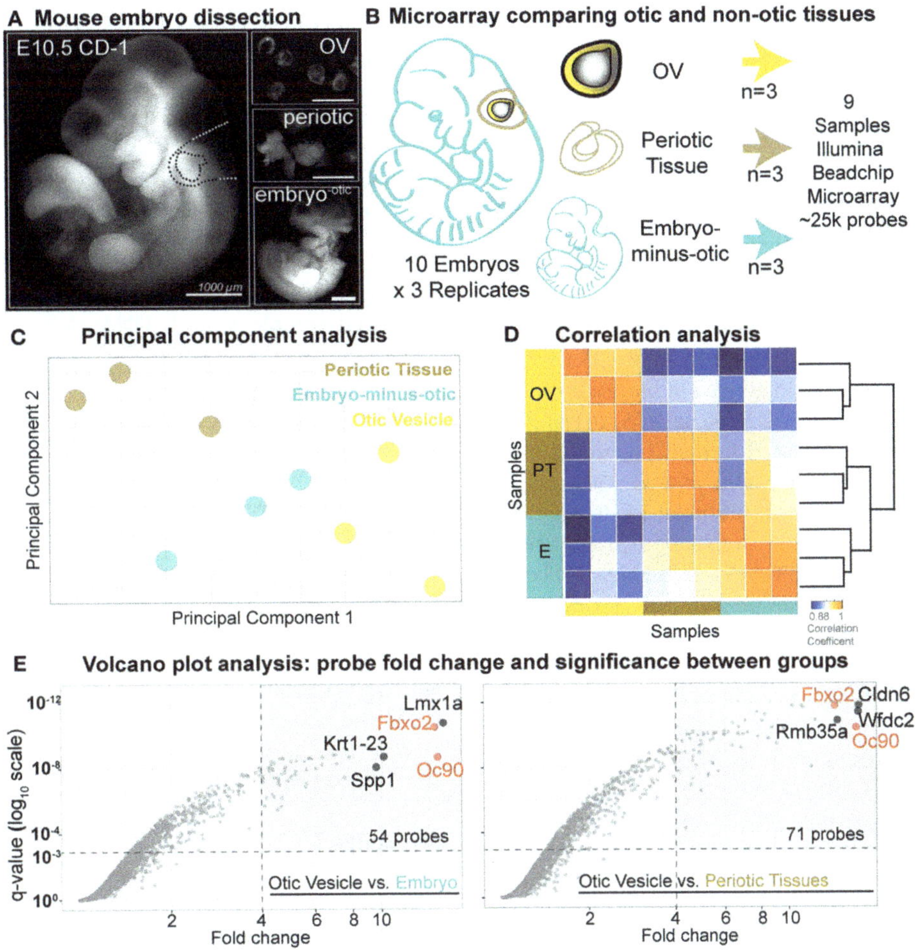

FIGURE 2 | Comparative early stage otic microarray. (A) E10.5 mouse embryos were dissected into OV, periotic, and the whole embryo minus greater otic region. **(B)** Dissected tissues were collected as indicated and nine samples were processed for microarray. **(C)** Score plot of principal component analysis. Individual replicates for each of the three populations (OV, periotic tissue, embryo minus greater otic region) are projected onto the first two principal components. Color-code corresponds to tissue origin. **(D)** Correlation analysis between samples using Spearman's correlation coefficients as a measure of similarity. Replicates within one group of samples show higher correlation with each other than with samples of other tissue populations. **(E)** Volcano plots display corrected *p*-values (*q*-values) for each probe set as a function of associated fold change values between OV and each non-otic group. Fold change values calculated based on log2-normalized probe intensity values. Horizontal dashed lines indicate statistical significance level of $q = 0.001$. Vertical dashed lines indicate fold change = 4.

means of expression and standard deviation (SD) were calculated for the five groups: E10.5 otic vesicle (OV), E10.5 periotic tissue, E10.5 embryo-minus-otic, and P3 hair cells (HCs) and supporting cells (SCs). Means of expression levels were compared between the otic groups and each of the two non-otic sample groups and fold change (fold Δ) values were calculated as the ratio of normalized mean intensities (for log2-transformed data, fold $\Delta = 2\text{^}(A - B)$, where A and B represent log2-transformed normalized intensity values for two different samples). All probes were ranked in three categories based on fold Δ in expression value in the OV, HC, and SC groups vs. the maximum expressing non-otic group (periotic or embryo-minus-otic) for the given probe. Calculated *p*-values (moderated *t*-test, Smyth, 2004) were corrected for multiple comparisons using Benjamini and Hochberg's false discovery rate algorithm (termed *q*-values, Benjamini and Hochberg, 1995; Benjamini and Yekutieli, 2005). The R packages *FactoMinerR* and *gplots* were used to perform principal component analysis and visualize correlation and expression data in heat map format.

To identify otic vesicle specific genes we compared expression values between the E10.5 OV and the two non-otic populations individually (periotic, and embryo-minus-otic groups). Use of different non-otic reference populations affects the fold change values for some genes more than others. This is illustrated by the differences in probes with high fold change (fold $\Delta > 4$) and high significance ($q < 0.001$) between comparisons (**Figure 2E**). For the OV vs. embryo-minus-otic comparison, 54 probes meet this cutoff, while 71 probes are found for the OV vs. periotic tissue. The probes with highest fold change in each category also change between comparisons, but some probes have high fold change in both, such as *Fbxo2* and *Oc90*, which are found in the top 5 probes for both comparisons. To rank genes based on the most conservative assessment of otic specificity, OV fold change values were determined using the highest non-otic intensity value for each probe (either the embryo-minus-otic, or the periotic tissue) (Supplemental File 1).

Whole Mount Fluorescent Immunohistochemistry

Whole embryos (E10.5–E12.5) or dissected neonatal cochlea tissues were fixed overnight at 4°C in either 4% paraformaldehyde (PFA) in phosphate-buffered saline at pH 7.4 (PBS), or *Glyofixx* (Thermo Fisher Scientific, Waltham, MA). Samples were washed in PBS then permeabilized with 2% TritonX100 in PBS for 1 h at room temperature. Samples were incubated in blocking solution (10% fetal bovine serum, 0.5% TritonX100, in PBS) overnight at 4°C. Primary antibodies were diluted in blocking solution and samples were incubated for three nights at 4°C with rocking. Samples were washed 4x in blocking solution for 1 h at room temperature, then overnight at 4°C, all with rocking. Species-specific Alexafluor 488-/568-/ or 633-conjugated secondary antibodies (Life Technologies) were diluted in blocking solution and samples were incubated for 2 nights at 4°C with rocking. Samples were washed twice at room temperature for 1 h in blocking solution, twice for 1 h in PBS, then overnight in PBS at 4°C, all with rocking. For optical clearing of whole embryos, samples were incubated at 4°C with rocking in Scale/A2 (Hama et al., 2011) for at least 5 days, with 2–3 changes of the Scale/A2 solution. For imaging, whole embryos were mounted in Scale/A2 between glass coverslips in imaging chambers consisting of 2–3 stacked 0.5 mm adhesive silicone spacers, modified from SecureSeal Hybridization Chambers (Grace Biolabs). Optically cleared embryos were imaged with a Zeiss LSM700 confocal microscope using a 10X or 20X objective to generate multiple z-stacks for coverage of the whole specimen. Maximum intensity z-projections were stitched together in Adobe Photoshop CS6 using the auto blend layers function.

Cryosection Fluorescent Immunohistochemistry

Embryonic heads or neonatal inner ears were fixed overnight at 4°C in 4% PFA in PBS. Samples were washed in PBS, then cryoprotected through graded sucrose in PBS (10% sucrose, 20% sucrose, 30% sucrose), then embedded in OCT (Tissue Tek), frozen in a bath of ethanol and dry ice, sectioned at 12 μm, and mounted on Superfrost+ slides (Fisher Scientific). Slides with cryosections were then washed briefly in PBS and incubated with blocking solution (10% fetal bovine serum, 0.5% TritonX100, in PBS). Primary antibodies were diluted in blocking solution and incubated overnight at 4°C. Slides were then washed in PBS 3 × 10 min and incubated in species-specific Alexafluor 488-/568-/ or 633-conjugated secondary antibodies (Life Technologies). After immunostaining, slides were coverslipped in Fluoromount G (Southern Biotechnology, Birmingham, AL, USA) and imaged on a Zeiss LSM700 confocal microscope.

Antibodies

The following primary antibodies were used for section and whole mount immunohistochemistry, at the dilutions indicated: rabbit anti-Fbx2 (1:300, Kato et al., 2005, gift of A. Kato and D. Bredt), goat anti-Sox2 (1:300, Santa Cruz Biotechnology, Sox2 Y-17, cat. no. SC-17320); goat anti-Sox10 (1:100, Santa Cruz Biotechnology, Sox10 N-20, SC-17342); mouse anti-Tuj1 (1:2000, Millipore, Ms X beta III tubulin, MAB5564); goat anti-Jag1 (1:300 Santa Cruz Biotechnology, Jag1 C-20, SC-6011); rabbit anti-COL9A2 (1:100, Atlas Antibodies, HPA056316), and rabbit anti-Pax2 (1:100, Covance).

Paraffin Section *in Situ* Hybridization

Digoxigenin-labeled probe was *in vitro* transcribed from a linearized complementary DNA clone corresponding to *Oc90* (MGC:59513 IMAGE:6334417). *In situ* hybridization was performed as previously described (Hartman et al., 2007). Briefly, whole embryos (E10.5 and E12.5) or half heads (E14.5 and older) were fixed overnight at 4°C in modified Carnoy's solution (60% ethanol, 11.1% formaldehyde (30% of 37% stock), 10% glacial acetic acid), dehydrated though an ethanol series, prepared for paraffin embedding, and sectioned at 10 μm. Slides were baked overnight at 68°C, dewaxed in xylene, rinsed in ethanol, and air-dried at room temperature. Overnight hybridization and subsequent washes were carried out at 68°C. Hybridized probe was detected using anti-digoxygenin alkaline phosphatase conjugated antibody (1:2000 dilution, Roche Biochemical, Indianapolis, IN, USA) and visualized with NBT/BCIP for a blue precipitate. After *in situ* hybridization, sections were postfixed in 4% PFA and coverslipped with Fluoromount G.

Results

Identification of Genes Distinguishing the Otic Vesicle from other Lineages of the Midgestation Embryo

OV fold Δ values (see Methods) for the top 100 OV probes range from about 15- to 3-fold, and 47 probes had OV fold Δ values greater than 4 (Supplemental File 1). Low q-values indicated high statistical significance ($q < 0.05$) for the vast majority of the probes that ranked in the top 200 based on OV fold Δ (**Table 1** and Supplemental File 1). Sensitivity and dynamic range are highly dependent on probe design and differ greatly between probes. This is reflected in the broad range of average OV intensity values among the top 30 OV probes (**Table 1**) and illustrates the necessity for differential comparison to reference populations. The MouseRef-8 Beadchip represents most genes with only a single probe (identified by Probe_ID, Supplemental File 1), however some genes are represented by more than one probe. The inclusion of two non-otic reference populations is useful for assessing dynamic range, estimating limit of detection and in some cases identification of the presence of non-otic expression sites. If an OV specific gene were not substantially expressed in other tissues then we would not expect to see differential expression between the two non-otic populations. Thus, periotic vs. embryo fold Δ values and statistical comparisons are included in **Table 1** and Supplemental File 1.

The top-ranking OV probe was for the *Oc90* gene, with an OV fold Δ of 15.32 (q = 2.08E-09), while the probe for *Fbxo2* had an OV fold Δ value of 14.62 (q = 1.74E−12) (**Figure 2E**, **Table 1**,

TABLE 1 | Top 30 probes ranked by OV fold Δ vs. maximum non-otic population.

Gene	E10.5 otic vesicle		Otic vesicle vs. Max non-otic			Periotic vs. Embryo	
	Mean intensity	*SD*	OV Fold Δ	*q*-value	OV rank	Fold Δ (abs)	UpReg (q > 0.05)
Oc90	**10.97366167**	**0.419246795**	**15.316797**	**2.08E-09**	**1**	**1.132771783**	**NS**
Fbxo2	**10.87404333**	**0.072690153**	**14.622012**	**1.74E-12**	**2**	**1.023630354**	**NS**
Lmx1a	11.06934217	0.056113649	11.061509	3.38E-04	3	1.448138913	Periotic
Krt1-23	10.25196333	0.288855995	10.184871	2.04E-09	4	1.220269579	NS
Spp1	9.971883833	0.332888479	8.454517	1.67E-10	5	1.136606365	NS
Cldn6	13.18188567	0.089216859	7.5281053	3.69E-08	6	2.35525402	Embryo
*Wfdc2**	13.53477267	0.213203	7.073592	5.33E-09	7	2.496286749	Embryo
Gata3	11.364921	0.142121662	7.0340185	1.49E-09	8	1.173139844	NS
Col9a2	**10.07369633**	**0.153509332**	**6.894713**	**1.49E-09**	**9**	**1.008878076**	**NS**
Arhgef19	9.768474333	0.09629171	6.341925	2.08E-09	10	1.218514062	NS
Rbm35a	12.29022383	0.143019237	6.3149257	6.10E-09	11	2.368308192	Embryo
Plekhb1	10.08439517	0.16829363	5.946511	6.30E-11	12	1.312607244	NS
Hs3st1	10.46399633	0.195136572	5.8575263	2.70E-09	13	1.048332013	No
Rgcc	10.77107167	0.161833702	5.628432	1.19E-08	14	1.990202734	Embryo
Tbx2	9.984906	0.297733516	5.626228	9.24E-08	15	1.702381408	Embryo
Prss8	10.105778	0.16620698	5.5848174	1.45E-07	16	1.290586405	NS
Sh3gl2	9.860674833	0.135098031	5.195888	8.67E-11	17	1.002118118	NS
*Wfdc2**	9.499769333	0.302036446	5.1527414	2.46E-08	18	1.227582286	NS
Marveld3	9.041756667	0.133118972	5.006034	3.82E-09	19	1.094974091	NS
Vwa2	9.691604	0.165306445	4.864665	5.78E-08	20	1.376504348	NS
Bdnf	9.836624667	0.178453967	4.78742	8.09E-09	21	1.246577778	NS
Espn	10.76721233	0.250324449	4.7623343	1.19E-08	22	2.301431921	Embryo
Plekha4	9.914148	0.299348822	4.7167573	8.07E-09	23	1.282688658	NS
Fgf10	10.70834767	0.021669661	4.700219	2.49E-09	24	2.193222734	Embryo
Car4	10.77693067	0.369327027	4.63751	2.23E-06	25	1.171838835	NS
Prr15	9.310321667	0.225649081	4.6330085	2.20E-08	26	1.146866527	NS
Col6a1	10.12810567	0.204186116	4.622068	2.27E-09	27	1.199047241	NS
Six1	11.91456133	0.035842889	4.5915775	2.49E-09	28	1.492275252	Embryo
Socs2	12.39277283	0.234257353	4.547705	2.49E-09	29	1.097722074	NS
Myo7a	9.023172167	0.481244122	4.538013	1.31E-07	30	1.027957463	NS

OV rank was determined based on fold Δ in mean OV intensity vs. that of the maximum expressing non-otic group for a given probe. Genes that appear more than once (*) are represented by multiple probe sets and those in bold are included in validation studies in later sections. OV, otic vesicle; SD, standard deviation; NS, not significant.

and Supplemental File 1). Both probes exhibited low non-otic group intensity values without significant differences between periotic and embryo-minus-otic samples (*Oc90* fold $\Delta = 1.13$, $q = 0.506$; *Fbxo2* fold $\Delta = 1.02$, $q = 0.946$, Supplemental File 1), suggesting that these two genes are otic-specific. Both of these genes were initially discovered based on high expression of RNA or protein in screens of rodent cochlea (Thalmann et al., 1997, 2003; Verpy et al., 1999). A probe for *Col9a2* (OV rank 9, OV fold $\Delta = 6.89$, $q = 1.49\text{E-}09$) also had nearly identical intensities between the two non-otic populations (periotic vs. embryo fold $\Delta = 1.01$, $q = 0.981$) suggestive of very low or undetectable expression in other lineages. Further discussion and analysis of expression patterns for *Oc90, Fbxo2,* and *Col9a2* are found below.

A difference in probe intensities between the two non-otic populations can be an indication of other regions of gene expression. For example, some probes had higher intensity in the periotic tissue group, which can indicate expression domains in the dorsal mesenchyme or neural tube. A probe for *Lmx1a* had a fold change in the OV vs. the rest of the embryo slightly higher than that of *Fbxo2*, however relatively high periotic tissue intensity put this probe in 3rd for the OV rankings (OV fold $\Delta = 11.06$, $q = 3.38\text{E-}04$). The difference between the periotic group and embryo-minus-otic group intensities for the *Lmx1a* probe (fold $\Delta = 1.45$, $q = 0.005$, Supplemental File 1) is consistent with the described expression of *Lmx1a* in OV as well as the dorsal midline (roof plate) of the developing neural tube (Failli et al., 2002; Nichols et al., 2008). Elevated probe intensity in the embryo-minus-otic group as compared to the periotic group was relatively common and is suggestive of gene expression in other ectodermal, endodermal, or mesodermal cell populations of the embryo. For example, *Cldn6, Wfdc2,* and *Rbm35a* (OV ranks: 6, 7, and 11, respectively), all have described expression patterns in the otic vesicle as well as endodermal tissues such as the branchial arches and pronephros (Kollmar et al., 2001;

Anderson et al., 2008; Tamplin et al., 2008; Ohazama et al., 2010). Expression in these domains is reflected as significantly elevated intensities in the embryo-minus-otic group vs. the periotic group for all of these probes (**Table 1** and Supplemental File 1). Two probes for *Fgf10* (OV ranks 24 and 37) were also elevated in the embryo-minus-otic group compared to the periotic group, reflective of *Fgf10* expression in the OV as well as limb bud mesoderm (Ohuchi et al., 1997; Mailleux et al., 2005). *Espn* (OV rank 22) was upregulated in the embryo compared to the periotic group, which is consistent with a well described pattern of Espin expression in early otic epithelia as well as brachial clefts, pharyngeal pouches and other embryonic epithelial tissues (Sekerkova et al., 2006).

Comparison to Neonatal Hair Cell and Supporting Cell Gene Array Data and Identification of Otic Consensus Genes

We next wanted to identify transcriptional features and individual genes that distinguish the otic sensory lineage from non-otic lineages throughout developmental time. To address this, we added two more otic populations to our comparative array analysis: hair cell (HC) and supporting cell (SC) RNA samples isolated from P3 mouse cochlea by dissociation and flow cytometry in an earlier study (Sinkkonen et al., 2011) (**Figure 3A**). We combined and normalized these P3 sample probe intensities [HC ($n = 4$) and SC ($n = 2$)] with those of our nine samples from E10.5 embryos described above (Supplemental File 1). We then performed principal component analysis to assess the transcriptome-wide similarities and differences between all of the samples (**Figure 3B**). Projection of the samples onto the first two principal components illustrates the inter-group relationship of otic sensory lineage populations and their segregation from non-otic samples.

To identify the most differentially expressed genes in the P3 hair cell and supporting cell populations, we compared individual probe intensity levels vs. the non-otic samples. The heat map of probe intensity values for the top 30 probes by OV rank across all samples shown in **Figure 3C** illustrates the diversity of gene expression profiles in these populations. As with the OV comparisons, HC fold Δ and SC fold Δ values were determined for each probe based on relative intensities between the HC or SC groups and the highest expressing non-otic group for a given probe (**Table 2** and Supplemental File 1). In general, probe intensities and fold Δ values for the HC and SC groups showed a much wider range than the OV samples. This is expected due to the more differentiated state of neonatal HCs and SCs as compared to OV progenitors, as well as the more homogeneous makeup of the FACS purified P3 samples (Sinkkonen et al., 2011). Both HC and SC fold Δ values across all probes ranged from about 300 fold up regulated to about 300 fold down regulated (0.003 fold Δ). 684 probes had HC fold Δ values greater than 4, while 565 probes had SC fold Δ values greater than 4 (Supplemental File 1).

We next sought to identify genes with consensus of specific expression in the OV as well as SC and HC groups. Probes were evaluated for otic consensus expression based on fold change and rankings in the three otic categories. As an initial approach, a fold change threshold was used to assign otic consensus expression groups, based on a minimum change vs. max non-otic of 4-fold (**Table 2** and Supplemental File 1). This analysis highlights the correlation of gene expression between the three otic populations and, in particular, shows that many genes strongly expressed in HCs and/or SCs are initially expressed quite early in otic development, showing elevated probe intensity in the OV. When we examined all probes ranked by OV fold Δ (Supplemental File 1) there is a notably high prevalence of probes with HC and/or SC consensus among the higher-ranked OV probes. Indeed, 17.4% of HC consensus probes and 25.5% of SC consensus probes (119/684 and 144/565 probes > 4-fold, respectively) are found within the top 500 probes by OV rank (Supplemental File 1). About half of the top 30-ranked OV probes shown in **Table 2** are designated as having consensus expression above the threshold in all three otic populations (OV/HC/SC). Other probes are designated as consensus only for one or two otic groups (i.e., OV, OV/HC, or OV/SC). For example, *Lmx1a, Spp1, Car4,* and *Col6a1* are enriched greater than 4-fold in OV, but not in HCs or SCs, suggesting down regulation of these genes in both HC and SC branches of the otic sensory lineage during development. Probes with OV/HC consensus expression are also indicated in **Table 2**, and include *Tbx2, Bdnf, Espn,* and *Myo7a*. OV/SC consensus probes include *Krt1-23, Cldn6, Wfdc2,* and *Vwa2*. This analysis shows how assignment of expression groups based on fold change and q-value cutoffs can be useful in identify genes with expression in the different branches of the otic sensory lineage. However, outcomes from this type of analysis are highly modulated by fold change and statistical cutoffs (Dalman et al., 2012) so interpretations will vary and multiple methods of comparison are necessary.

To address this, we calculated otic consensus scores for each probe as the sum of the three otic ranks. All probe sets were ranked by otic consensus score values, which ranged from 9 to 77,083 (Supplemental File 1). Otic consensus scores and ranks illustrate the relative differences between total otic vs. non-otic expression of genes. Lower otic consensus scores represent more "otic lineage-specific" genes. A representation of all probes positioned by OV rank vs. otic consensus score illustrates their distribution across the dataset and highlights top otic consensus genes *Fbxo2, Col9a2,* and *Oc90* (**Figure 3D**). The broad range of otic consensus ranks among the 30 top OV genes shown in **Table 2** is an indication of the diverse expression behavior of these genes in the later otic sensory lineages (HCs and SCs). The top 30 probes by OV consensus rank are listed in **Table 3**, with *Fbxo2, Col9a2,* and *Oc90* topping the list; all three with an OV rank less than 10 and OV consensus score below 50. Several of the probes in **Table 3** represent well-known otic genes and some are listed more than once due to having multiple probe sets similarly ranked. This analysis also highlights genes that are likely expressed in the OV but were not particularly noted earlier due to the relatively low range of fold change values across all probes in OV vs. non-otic samples. For example, probes for *Btbd14a, Otolin, Kai1, Gjb2,* and *Ush1c*, have OV rankings from about 100–380 and OV fold changes from 2.5 to 1.5-fold, but all ranked well by otic consensus due to high fold changes in HC and SC groups combined with a reasonably high OV rank.

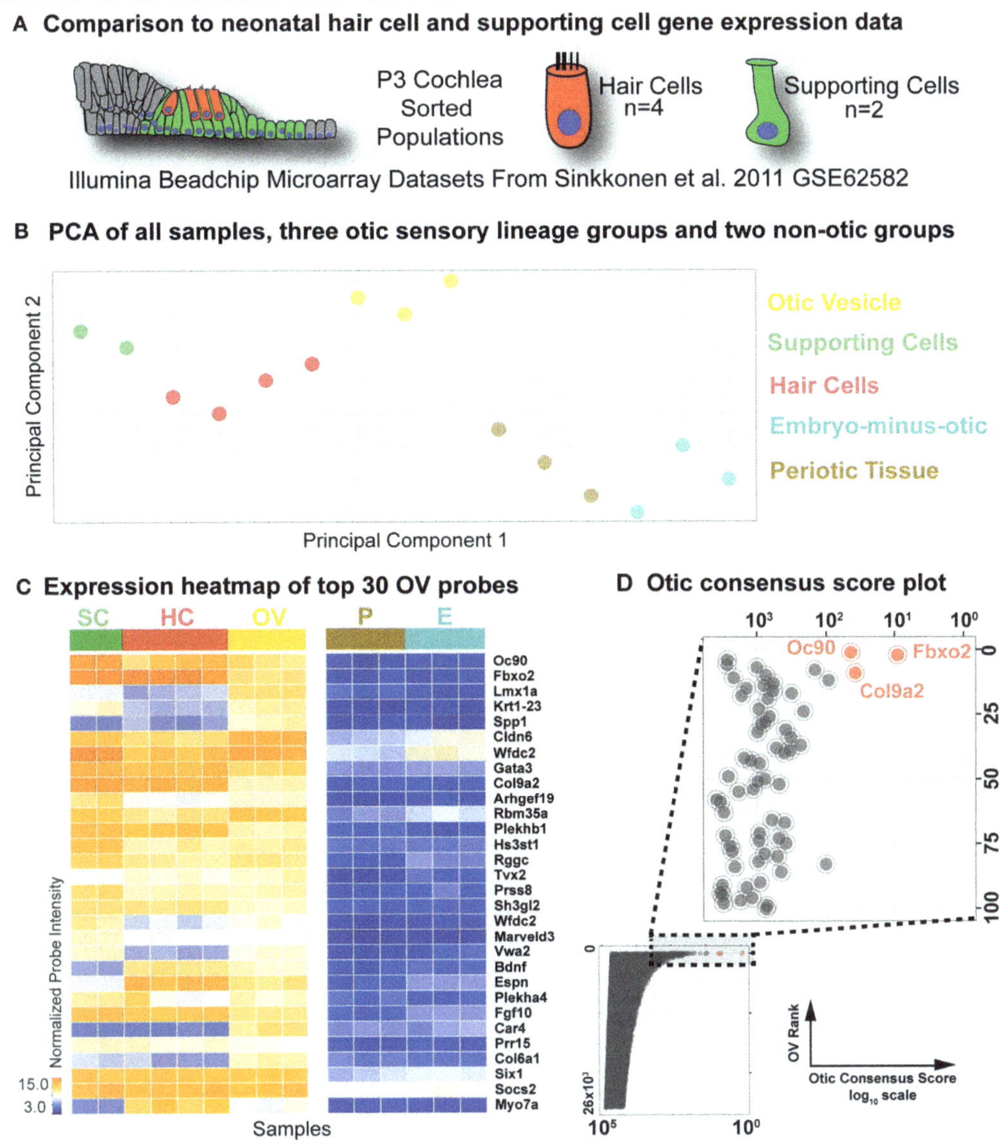

FIGURE 3 | Comparison to neonatal hair cell and supporting cell microarray data. (A) Differential comparison was extended to an existing microarray dataset (GSE62582, Sinkkonen et al., 2011) consisting of flow-sorted hair cell and supporting cell populations from P3 cochlea. **(B)** Principal component analysis score plot of all samples, color-coded as indicated on the right. **(C)** Probe intensity heat map of top 30 OV ranked probes in all samples, indicated by group color in the top bar. Genes are ordered according to **Table 1**. **(D)** Otic consensus score plotted against OV rank for all probes, with an enlargement of the top 100 OV probes in the inset. The top three probes are indicated in red.

Analysis of *Fbxo2*/Fbx2 Expression in the Developing Mouse

Fbxo2 was the highest-ranking gene based on otic consensus score and was in the top five probes for each of the otic rankings (rank 2 in OVs, 3 in SCs, and 4 in HCs). *Fbxo2* encodes the F-box ubiquitin ligase F-Box 2 (Fbx2) and previous studies have shown that this protein is strongly expressed in juvenile and adult mouse and guinea pig cochlea (Thalmann et al., 1997; Henzl et al., 2001, 2004; Nelson et al., 2007). Mice with targeted deletion of *Fbxo2* exhibit age-related cochlear degeneration with hearing loss beginning at 2 months, and the only deficiency observed is the inner ear phenotype, suggesting specificity (Nelson et al., 2007). These studies indicate that Fbx2 functions to ensure protein quality control required for cochlear homeostasis. While expression of Fbx2 was described in the mature cochlea in the above studies, the developmental expression pattern has not been reported. Thus, we used an antibody against mouse Fbx2 to assess expression in the developing mouse, with whole mount preparations as well as tissue sections. We labeled whole embryos at early stages of otic development with anti-Fbx2 and anti-Sox2, optically cleared samples with the Scale method (Hama et al., 2011), and generated confocal z-stacks to assess

TABLE 2 | Comparison of P3 hair cell and supporting cell expression intensities to non-otic populations.

Gene	HC/Max non-otic		SC/Max non-otic		Otic consensus expression groups fold Δ > 4	Otic consensus score: sum of three otic ranks	Otic consensus rank:
	HC fold Δ	HC rank	SC fold Δ	SC rank			
Oc90	**37.191532**	**36**	**133.68132**	**7**	**OV/HC/SC**	**44**	**3**
Fbxo2	**233.46231**	**3**	**209.10844**	**4**	**OV/HC/SC**	**9**	**1**
Lmx1a	1.071335	7460	2.1826358	1496	OV	8959	1220
Krt1-23	1.7182626	2426	7.448142	229	OV/SC	2659	259
Spp1	1.1694639	5352	1.0023074	16967	OV	22324	4802
Cldn6	1.8450933	2163	4.1609483	528	OV/SC	2697	264
*Wfdc2**	3.2619166	904	14.833333	88	OV/SC	999	85
Gata3	17.05958	99	22.630722	39	OV/HC/SC	146	6
Col9a2	**64.73929**	**16**	**99.665436**	**13**	**OV/HC/SC**	**38**	**2**
Arhgef19	4.2322383	639	14.127765	93	OV/HC/SC	742	49
Rbm35a	2.1024952	1724	4.913607	432	OV/SC	2167	206
Plekhb1	28.310795	56	33.40806	25	OV/HC/SC	93	4
Hs3st1	4.9308343	517	22.05582	44	OV/HC/SC	574	33
Rgcc	4.3943467	600	9.030337	175	OV/HC/SC	789	56
Tbx2	4.6268463	553	3.1064396	849	OV/HC	1417	119
Prss8	5.4411964	442	12.075007	123	OV/HC/SC	581	35
Sh3gl2	10.561689	174	11.849528	125	OV/HC/SC	316	10
*Wfdc2**	2.319336	1489	9.602433	161	OV/SC	1668	148
Marveld3	5.016969	502	9.084135	171	OV/HC/SC	692	45
Vwa2	1.0021158	10270	5.5677967	364	OV/SC	10654	1500
Bdnf	9.485823	208	1.0017089	19301	OV/HC	19530	3740
Espn	21.954702	79	1.1772411	5296	OV/HC	5397	653
Plekha4	4.1990533	647	6.789616	262	OV/HC/SC	932	75
Fgf10	13.839492	125	17.822388	64	OV/HC/SC	213	7
Car4	3.679346	25122	3.4888153	24946	OV	50093	18760
Prr15	6.245964	378	7.0138445	249	OV/HC/SC	653	42
Col6a1	1.2619317	21404	1.151628	5720	OV	27151	7232
Six1	5.8167586	403	5.891639	328	OV/HC/SC	759	52
Socs2	5.1087866	493	5.8204165	339	OV/HC/SC	861	64
Myo7a	28.857481	55	1.0124729	11440	OV/HC	11525	1651

The top 30 OV-ranked probes (as in ***Table 1****) are shown here with HC and SC Fold Δs and rankings, otic consensus group designations, and otic consensus scores and ranks. Genes that appear more than once (*) are represented by multiple probe sets and those in bold are included in validation studies in later sections.*

expression *in toto* (**Figures 4**, **5**). At E10.5, Fbx2 expression was robust throughout the OV including the Sox2+ prosensory and neurogenic domains and was undetectable in nearly all non-otic tissues (**Figures 4A–C″**). Sox2, which was not upregulated in the OV compared to the rest of the embryo based on the microarray, is broadly expressed in the developing central nervous system. An E11 otic vesicle stained for Fbx2 and Sox10 shows strong Fbx2 expression in the OV and lower levels of expression in delaminating cochleovestibular neuroblasts as well as the ninth cranial nerve ganglia (**Figures 4D–E″**). At E12.5, Fbx2 was detected only in the developing inner ear, where it was expressed throughout the membranous labyrinth (**Figures 5A,B″**), including prosensory epithelial regions that express Sox2 and contain Tuj1-labeled neurites (**Figures 5C–C″**). We stained for Fbx2 in tissue sections of embryos at E16.5 and E18.5 and co-labeled with antibodies to the prosensory/sensory domain markers Sox2 and Jag1 (**Figure 6**). Similar to earlier stages, expression of Fbx2 was strongly restricted to the otocyst-derived epithelium when compared broadly to the rest of the embryo in sagittal sections at E16.5 (**Figure 6A**). In the cochlea, Fbx2 was localized to the floor of the duct, including and flanking the sensory region marked by expression of Sox2 (**Figure 6B**) and Jag1 (**Figures 6C–C″**) and clearly expressed in both the young hair cells and supporting cells. In the vestibular epithelia including the saccule and crista, Fbx2 was also expressed in sensory regions, including hair cells and supporting cells (**Figures 6D–E″**).

Analysis of *Col9a2*/Col9a2 Expression in the Developing Mouse

Col9a2 held the second otic consensus rank, with OV/HC/SC ranks of 9, 16, and 13, respectively. *Col9a2* encodes collagen alpha-2(IX), one of the three essential alpha chains of the collagen IX protein. A loss of function mutation in *Col9a2* was

TABLE 3 | Top 30 probes by otic consensus rank.

Gene	OV/Max non-otic		HC/Max non-otic		SC/Max non-otic		Otic consensus		
	OV fold Δ	OV rank	HC fold Δ	HC rank	SC fold Δ	SC rank	Groups > 4-Fold Δ	Score: OV/SC/HC rank sum	Rank
Fbxo2	**14.62200927**	**2**	**233.462206**	**3**	**209.1084184**	**4**	**OV/HC/SC**	**9**	**1**
Col9a2	**6.894714915**	**9**	**64.73931483**	**16**	**99.66541579**	**13**	**OV/HC/SC**	**38**	**2**
Oc90	**15.31678675**	**1**	**37.19151468**	**36**	**133.6813688**	**7**	**OV/HC/SC**	**44**	**3**
Plekhb1	5.946512058	12	28.31080827	56	33.40807691	25	OV/HC/SC	93	4
S100a1	2.908877684	83	118.1935475	8	106.9791597	11	HC/SC	102	5
Gata3	7.034011368	8	17.05957342	99	22.63071352	39	OV/HC/SC	146	6
*Fgf10**	4.700220155	24	13.8394988	125	17.82238697	64	OV/HC/SC	213	7
*Fgf10**	4.314080209	37	13.59648272	128	16.99160918	71	OV/HC/SC	236	8
Btbd14a	2.583935277	107	12.9935202	138	24.78606653	34	HC/SC	279	9
Sh3gl2	5.195890282	17	10.56169338	174	11.84953165	125	OV/HC/SC	316	10
*Ap1m2**	4.401733497	34	16.98844137	100	8.629079783	190	OV/HC/SC	324	11
Cldn3	4.28578566	39	8.527481874	247	21.97050359	45	OV/HC/SC	331	12
Otolin	2.613673625	104	13.00452906	137	12.71711488	110	HC/SC	351	13
*Faah**	3.024489321	75	9.804033123	197	12.65490027	111	HC/SC	383	14
*Col2a1**	4.520159455	31	7.506419492	289	17.59092164	65	OV/HC/SC	385	15
Cd9	3.355323417	67	8.23098117	257	16.33853718	74	HC/SC	398	16
*Col2a1**	4.232269996	40	7.827652714	271	14.83067647	89	OV/HC/SC	400	17
Kai1	1.755355331	295	19.26278326	88	20.30006957	55	HC/SC	438	18
Matn1	2.017228994	189	8.875465831	229	39.5214772	21	HC/SC	439	19
Gal3st1	2.881826605	86	10.55670683	175	8.735986943	186	HC/SC	447	20
*Gjb2**	1.679839813	340	23.0501633	74	23.74169556	38	HC/SC	452	21
*Ap1m2**	3.920424836	52	13.46897818	132	6.465748986	291	HC/SC	475	22
Rab25	3.077388814	73	8.457112871	251	9.816023707	156	HC/SC	480	23
BC019731	2.606254615	105	24.07525961	68	6.247095999	308	HC/SC	481	24
Ush1c	1.613973622	381	21.22888215	83	33.21939745	26	HC/SC	490	25
Ltbp3	1.657999303	354	14.0823195	122	35.97926226	23	HC/SC	499	26
Cyb561	2.949823565	80	10.6399017	172	6.880909012	255	HC/SC	507	27
*Gjb2**	1.521293061	452	38.97023609	32	35.09867751	24	HC/SC	508	28
Kcnk1	4.298354088	38	6.723838937	332	10.01882675	151	HC/SC	521	29
*Faah**	2.569395243	109	8.469575034	250	9.13829701	168	HC/SC	527	30

Genes that appear more than once (*) are represented by multiple probe sets and those in bold are included in validation studies in later sections.

identified as a causative locus in autosomal recessive Stickler syndrome, characterized by hearing loss and ocular, skeletal, and orofacial abnormalities (Baker et al., 2011). Type IX collagen loss in mice (caused by absence of Col9a1, which leads to functional knockout of the entire collagen IX protein, Hagg et al., 1997), causes progressive hearing loss associated with abnormal integrity of collagen fibers in the tectorial membrane (Suzuki et al., 2005). The *Col9a1/2/3* genes were detected in adult mouse cochlea by RT-PCR and immunohistochemical analysis with a polyclonal antibody against type IX collagen indicated possible expression in the tectorial membrane (Asamura et al., 2005). Developmental expression of type IX collagen has not been investigated in the inner ear so we performed immunohistochemical analysis using a Col9a2-specific antibody to evaluate embryo-wide expression patterns (**Figure 7**). At E10.5, in a whole embryo preparation, Col9a2 immunofluorescence is prominent in the OV and is also visible in the branchial epithelia and pronephros (**Figures 7A–B′**). The signal is broad throughout most of the OV with reduced expression in the dorsal region (**Figures 7C,C′**). In P6 cochlea sections Col9a2 immunoreactivity is strong in the greater epithelial ridge (GER)/spiral limbus, tectorial membrane, organ of Corti, and spiral ligament (**Figures 7D–E″**). A closer look at the organ of Corti shows a strong signal in the basilar membrane as well as tunnel of Corti/pillar cell region and a less intense signal in hair cells (**Figures 7E–E″**).

Analysis of *Oc90* Expression in the Developing Mouse

Oc90 was the highest ranked probe by OV fold Δ and the third ranked by otic consensus score. *Oc90* (*Ocn-95, PLA2L*) encodes a 95-kDa secreted glycoprotein initially identified due to its abundant expression in the developing and adult inner ear and shown to be an essential organizer of the otoconial matrix (Wang et al., 1998; Verpy et al., 1999; Zhao et al., 2007, 2008). Consistent

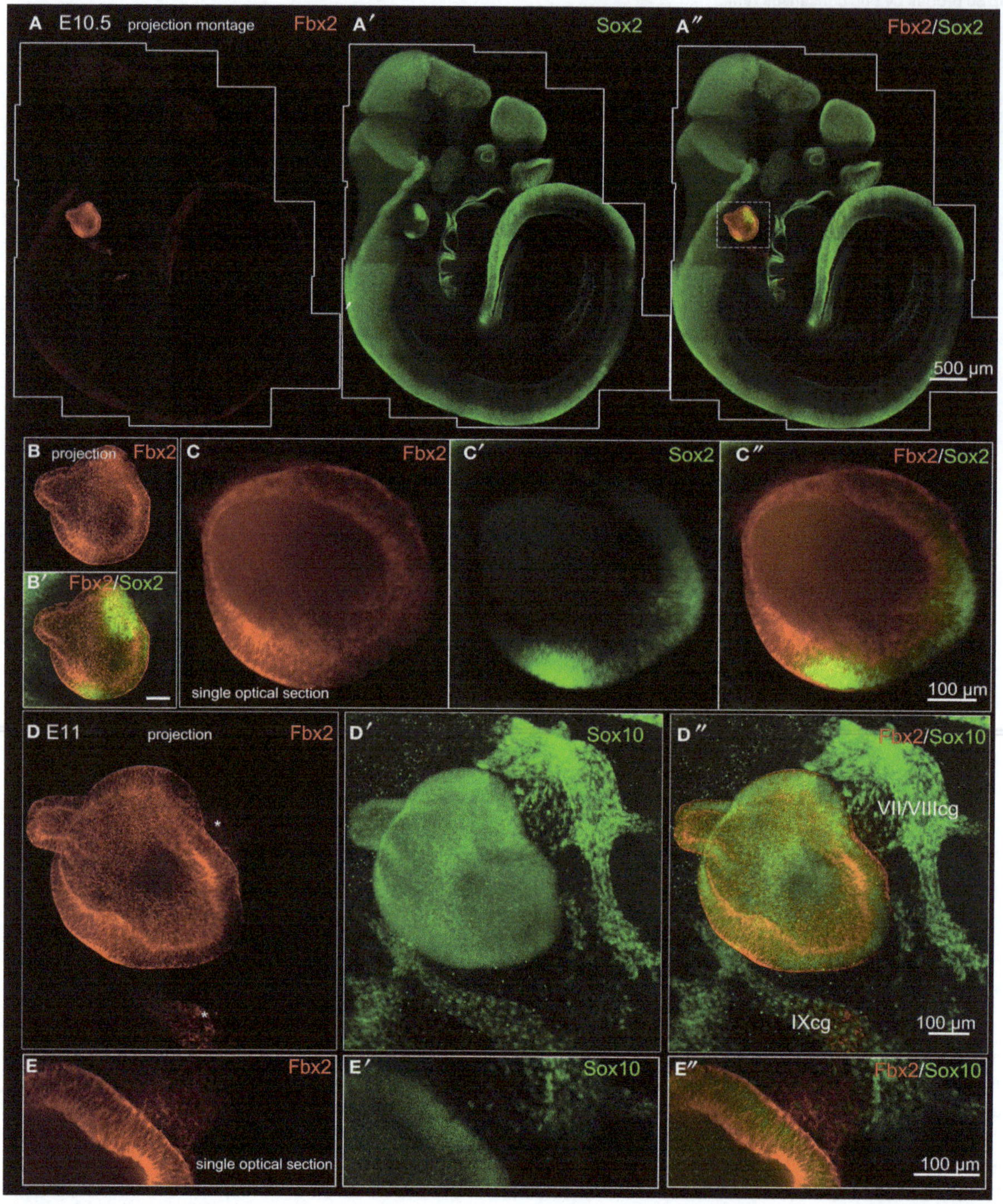

FIGURE 4 | *Fbxo2*/Fbx2 expression in whole embryos at E10.5–E11. Whole mount immunohistochemistry was performed with the antibodies indicated and embryos were imaged with confocal microscopy. Fbx2 expression is shown in red, with Sox2 at E10.5 **(A–C″)** and Sox10 at E11 **(D–E″)** in green. Fbx2 expression is strong in the otic vesicle epithelia and less intense expression is also noted (asterisks) in the neurons delaminating to the cochleovestibular and ninth cranial ganglia (VII/VIIIcg and IXcg).

with earlier reports (Verpy et al., 1999), our *in situ* hybridization expression analysis indicated that Oc90 is highly specific to the otic vesicle at E10.5 (**Figures 8A,B**). At E12.5 *Oc90* expression was present throughout most of the otocyst with a strong signal in the dorsal regions and less intense signal noted in the ventral domains (**Figures 8C,D**). In the cochlear duct at E16.5 and E18.5 we observed a wide dynamic range of *Oc90* expression, with very intense signal in the roof of the cochlear duct

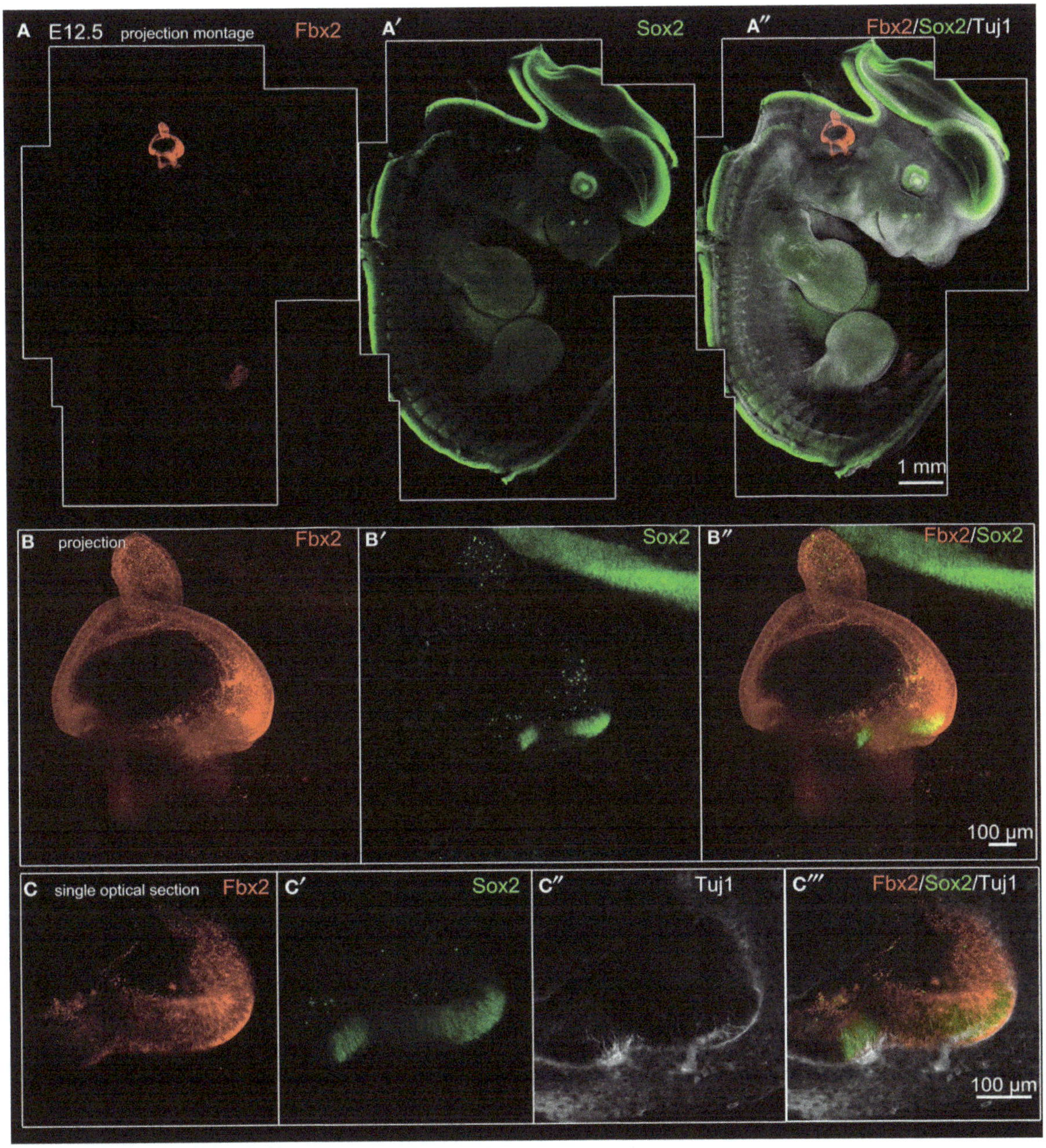

FIGURE 5 | *Fbxo2*/Fbx2 expression in whole embryos at E12.5. Whole mount immunohistochemistry was performed with the antibodies indicated and embryos were imaged with confocal microscopy. Fbx2 expression is shown in red, with Sox2 in green, and Tuj1 in white. **(A–A″)** Merged montages of maximum intensity z projections of confocal image stacks of a whole E12.5 embryo. **(B–B″)** show a projected stack of images through the otocyst region of the embryo shown in **(A)**. Sox2 expression is seen in two bright vestibular prosensory patches in the anterior region of the vestibule, while Sox2 expression in other prosensory domains (such as posterior vestibule or cochlea areas) are not visible in this projection due to lower intensity signal and attenuation from optical density of the tissue. **(C–C″)** Single optical sections through the anterior vestibular prosensory patches showing Fbx2-positive epithelia contain prosensory domains expressing bright Sox2 and containing Tuj1-labeled neurites.

(developing Reissner's membrane and stria vascularis) as well as weaker signal in the developing organ of Corti (**Figures 8E,F**). *In situ* hybridization is limited in capacity to evaluate expression signals across a wide dynamic range in regions of close proximity due to signal overdevelopment and saturation. Taken together with previous studies, our data suggest that expression of *Oc90* is high in the otic sensory lineage as compared to most genes. Within the inner ear, *Oc90* has a markedly higher expression in non-sensory otic cells, particularly in domains possibly derived from dorsal OV regions. The otic-specific expression and wide dynamic range of *Oc90* in the inner ear makes this an interesting gene for regulatory studies but its dominant expression is in

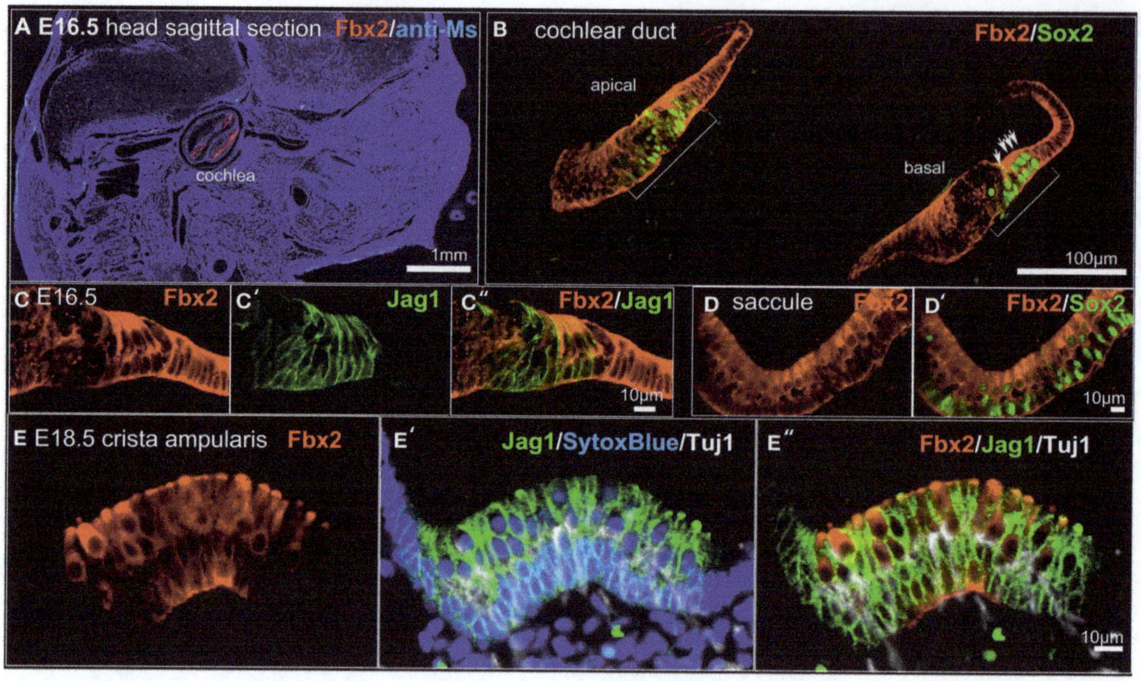

FIGURE 6 | *Fbxo2*/Fbx2 expression in tissue sections at E16.5–E18.5. Immunohistochemistry was performed with the antibodies indicated and embryos were imaged with confocal microscopy. Fbx2 expression is shown in red and additional antibodies or counter stains are shown in the colors indicated. **(A)** E16.5 sagittal head section immunolabeled for Fbx2 with anti-mouse IgG (blue) as a background stain. E16.5 cochlea **(B–C″)**, saccule **(D,D′)**, and E18.5 crista **(E–E″)** stained as indicated.

otic non-sensory domains, making it less useful for otic sensory lineage studies.

Discussion

We sought to systematically identify transcriptional features that distinguish the otic sensory lineage from other lineages of vertebrate development by employing a microarray approach to compare OV, HC, and SC populations with developmental non-otic tissues. Whole E10.5 embryos with the greater otic regions removed were used to represent a wide range of non-otic lineages from all three germ layers, and periotic tissues represented non-otic tissues proximally associated with the OV, such as dorsal neural tissues and periotic mesenchyme. The inclusion of two non-otic populations was effective for gauging dynamic range of probe intensity and identifying probes with expression domains outside of the inner ear. Multivariate analyses including PCA and Spearman's correlation demonstrated that samples from the three otic populations shared transcriptome-wide correlations in expression profiles that distinguish this lineage from non-otic populations. We further analyzed the microarray data to identify individual genes that are specifically expressed in the otic sensory lineage. Fold change comparisons of otic samples to the maximum expressing non-otic populations for each probe provided a conservative assessment of specificity and enabled ranking of probes across the dataset. Comparison of OV, HC, and SC fold changes for each probe allowed identification of otic consensus genes based on fold change thresholds. We developed otic consensus scores and rankings based on expression in individual otic categories to reduce the data to a single dimension to aid in identification of lineage-specific genes. The entire dataset is assembled in Supplemental File 1 as a searchable spreadsheet than can be sorted and further interrogated to suit the needs of individual readers.

A major motivation for this study was the previous lack of unambiguous otic sensory lineage markers, which has hindered advancement of regenerative and developmental studies. *In vitro* experiments aimed at producing otic progenitors and sensory epithelial cells from stem cells have had to rely on combinations of less specific markers to assay cell identities (Oshima et al., 2010; Koehler et al., 2013). Most current markers used to label potential early otic progenitor cells (i.e., Pax2/8, Gata3, Jag1, Sox2/9/10) are themselves transcription factors or signaling molecules involved in otic development. These highly conserved factors tend to be expressed in multiple embryonic lineages so coexpression of multiple markers has been used as an indication of otic identity. For example, Pax2 is expressed strongly in the otic vesicle at E10.5, but is also very abundant in the developing central nervous system and pronephros (**Supplemental Figure 1A**). On the other hand, Sox10 is expressed strongly in neural crest progenitors of the peripheral nervous system, but overlaps with Pax2 in the otic vesicle (**Supplemental Figures 1A–A″**). While coexpression of these two markers appears to be specific to the otic vesicle at this stage, this is a transient feature since Pax2 becomes downregulated in the otic sensory lineage soon after (Burton et al., 2004). Gata3 is one transcription factor that showed a high specificity to the otic sensory lineage based on our microarray analyses. This is consistent with the relatively

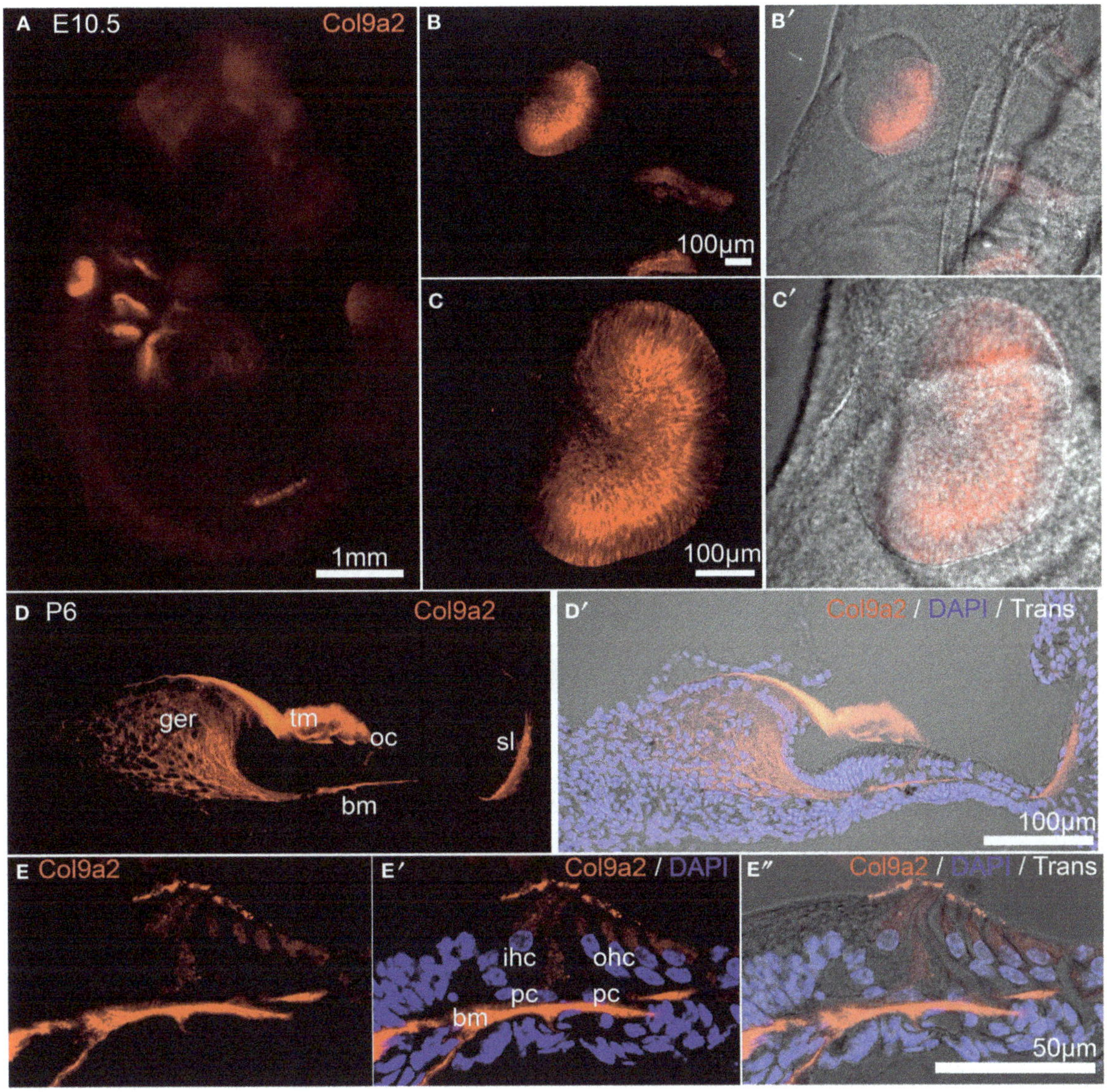

FIGURE 7 | Col9a2 expression in whole E10.5 embryo and neonatal cochlea. Col9a2 immunoreactivity is shown in red in E10.5 whole embryo **(A)**. Higher magnification views show the pattern of reactivity in the OV and surrounding tissues **(B–C′)**. **(D,D′)** A cochlea cryosection at P6 shows Col9a2 immunoreactivity in the tectorial membrane, greater epithelial ridge/spiral limbus, organ of Corti, and spiral ligament. **(E–E″)** A higher magnification view of a similar section of the organ of Corti with the tectorial membrane removed (to better image the lower intensity signal in the organ of Corti) shows the Col9a2 signal in the basilar membrane, pillar cells and the developing tunnel of Corti, and inner and outer hair cells. Abbreviations: ger, greater epithelial ridge; tm, tectorial membrane; oc, organ of Corti; sl, spiral ligament; bm, basilar membrane.

restricted pattern of Gata3 expression observed in E10.5 mouse embryos (**Supplemental Figure 1B**). While the non-otic expression of Gata3 is not as prominent as with Pax2 or Sox10, domains of varying intensities are present in the central nervous system and pronephros, though generally weaker than in the otic vesicle. Coexpression of Gata3 and Fbx2 occurs exclusively in the otic vesicle at E10.5 (**Supplemental Figures 1B–B″**) and these markers both persist in the otic sensory lineage through later stages of development (**Figure 6** and Luo et al., 2013).

Our study differs from most earlier microarray studies of the inner ear in its design as a comparative analysis of specific otic sensory lineage populations to a broad representation of non-otic lineages. Most of earlier analyses were conducted without comparative populations to other tissues. Many were designed to compare expression between wild type and mutant animals or between different tissues of the inner ear, such as at different ages or between the base and apex of the cochlea, or after insult (for review see Hertzano and Elkon, 2012). The most highly comprehensive microarray analysis of mouse inner ear morphogenesis included a total of 29 finely dissected inner ear samples in duplicate from E9 to E15 (Sajan et al., 2007). This study also included three samples designated as non-inner ear collected from areas in

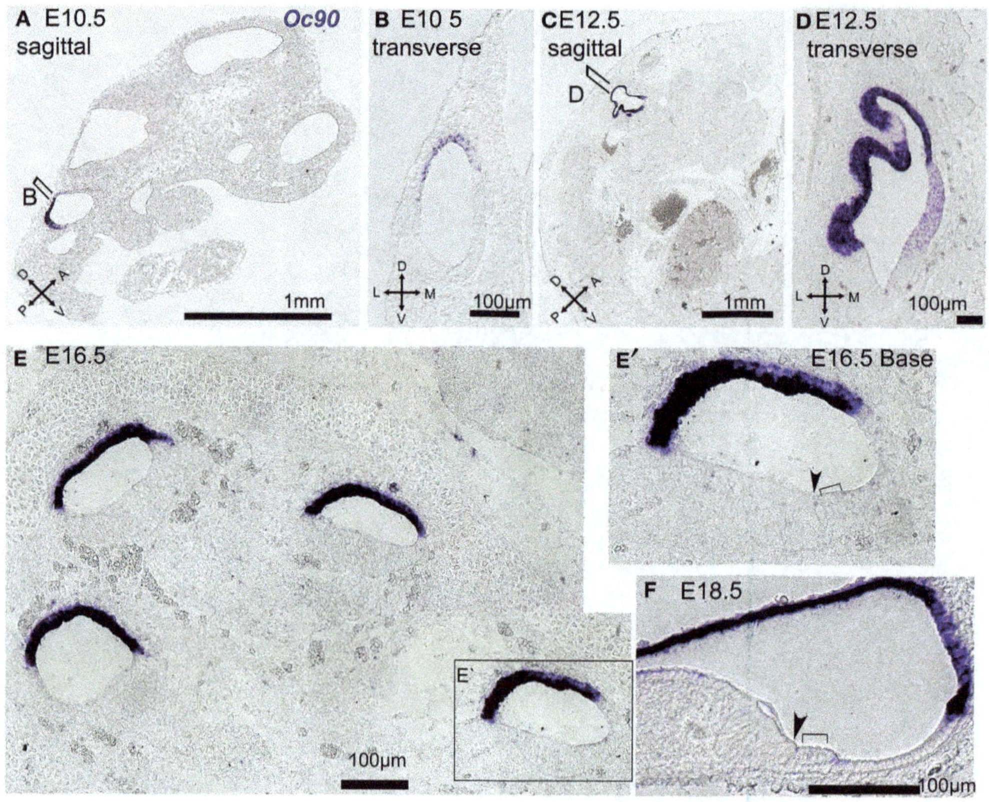

FIGURE 8 | *Oc90* expression in tissue sections at E10.5–E18.5. *In situ* hybridization was performed on paraffin sections at the indicated ages with antisense probe against *Oc90* (blue). E10.5 embryo specimens are shown in sagittal **(A)** and transverse views **(B)** and illustrate the dorsal and posterior expression domain of *Oc90* in the OV. At E12.5 the region of *Oc90* expression is expanded through most of the otic epithelium, save the most ventral region, as shown in sagittal **(C)** and transverse views **(D)**. **(E)** At E16.5 in a mid-modiolar section of the cochlea *Oc90* expression is strongest in the roof of the cochlear duct but is also present at lower signal levels in the thickened epithelium of the floor, as shown in higher magnification view in **(E′)**. **(F)** At E18.5 *Oc90* is strong in Reissner's membrane the stria vascularis and a lower level signal is also present in the organ of Corti and some non-sensory epithelial cells. In **(E′,F)**, inner hair cells are indicated with arrowheads and outer hair cells are indicated with brackets.

close proximity to the inner ear tissues pooled at E9, E9.5–10.5, and E11–15. These included neural tissue as well as mesenchyme, similar to the periotic tissue group used in this report. In another study aimed at identification of early otic-specific transcripts, cDNA subtractions of mouse otic vesicle against adult liver cDNA were used to identify candidate genes (Powles et al., 2004). Our use of whole embryos with the greater otic regions removed provided an inclusive representation of non-otic developmental lineages. While our findings indicate whole embryo-minus-otic tissue is an effective general non-otic reference population it has limitations in identifying genes expressed in smaller subsets of cells. We included periotic tissues as a separate non-otic population, which enabled us to gauge dynamic range of probes and evaluate the likelihood of non-otic expression domains based on differential expression between non-otic groups. Future studies may improve sensitivity of non-otic reference samples through further division of embryo tissue into a larger set of non-otic sample groups from smaller domains as well as from different stages of development.

Another feature distinguishing the current study is our use of data representing purified populations of HCs and SCs in combination with data from OV tissues to evaluate expression in distinct branches of the lineage before and after bifurcation of HC and SC fates. As the goal of this study was not to specifically search for genes that are exclusive for distinct otic lineages, we succeeded in the identification of markers that are much more restricted to the developing inner ear than those previously identified. The conditions that we chose for the top ranking genes were guided by restriction to the otic lineage at E10.5 and further by enrichment in hair cells and supporting cells in the neonatal cochlea.

Our analysis identified and ranked top otic sensory lineage-specific transcripts including *Fbxo2, Col9a2,* and *Oc90.* We verified otic-specific expression of these genes using immunohistochemistry and *in situ* hybridization, which revealed novel expression patterns and concurred with the array data. *Fbxo2*/Fbx2 showed the most striking pattern of specificity to the otic sensory lineage. Although Fbx2 expression has been reported in neuronal populations of the CNS (Eom et al., 2004) our analysis identified very few regions of expression outside of the inner ear and none with the robust intensity found in otic tissues. A likely explanation is that *Fbxo2* is expressed in some non-otic cell types, but at a very low level compared to the otic vesicle. The lack of any phenotype in *Fbxo2* null mice besides selective cochlear degeneration is evidence that this gene is functionally specific to the inner ear (Nelson et al., 2007). From our study it is clear that both at the transcript level and the protein level *Fbxo2* stands out from all other genes as a highly specific and robust marker of the otic sensory lineage. This feature elevates *Fbxo2* to an important gene for future studies of otic sensory lineage development and gene regulation. *Col9a2* also showed highly specific expression in the otic sensory lineage at both the transcript and protein levels. Compared to *Fbxo2* and *Oc90*, *Col9a2* is not as highly restricted to the otic sensory lineage as it is also expressed in branchial epithelia and pronephros (**Figures 7A–B′**). Col9a2 expression is initially robust in the OV epithelial cells and in the neonatal cochlea becomes organized largely in extracellular domains, including the tectorial and basilar membranes and the tunnel of Corti. We were unable to achieve adequate performance from a *Col9a2* probe for *in situ* hybridization in order to evaluate transcript levels in the organ of Corti, but this gene would be an interesting choice for future studies with a reporter mouse model. *Oc90* expression is highly specific to the inner ear and includes the sensory lineage populations but is actually expressed at even higher levels in non-sensory otic cells. The array data show *Oc90* at robust levels in the OV as well as HCs and SCs as compared to the non-otic samples. *In situ* hybridization also confirms highly specific expression of *Oc90* in the OV and, although expression is detectable in sensory progenitors of the organ of Corti, the strongest region of *Oc90* expression is found in non-sensory otic cells. This could be reflective of a very broad dynamic range of *Oc90* expression in the neonatal cochlea combined with a highly sensitive microarray probe, detecting the gene robustly in P3 HCs and SCs, and very low expression in the non-otic tissue groups resulting in a high rank for *Oc90* in HCs and SCs despite even higher expression of this gene in other cells. Beside *Fbxo2, Col9a2,* and *Oc90*, our analysis has revealed additional candidate novel otic sensory lineage genes and provided comparative expression data for quite a few well-known otic genes. Novel genes that show high-ranking consensus expression in the otic sensory lineage populations, such as *Plekhb1*, *Btbd14a*, *Ap1m2* *Kai1*, and *Faah*, would be excellent candidates for further studies of gene expression and function in this lineage. Additionally the results of this study will aid in the design of experiments that require carefully selected lists of genes to assay for cell identity. For example, we used these data to inform the design of the 96-gene expression assay applied in recent work using single cell analysis of individual OV cells to reconstruct the otocyst and early neuroblast lineages *in silico* (Durruthy-Durruthy et al., 2014).

Acknowledgments

We thank Andy Groves for consulting on this project, members of the Heller lab for constructive comments, Saku Sinkkonen and coauthors for P3 Cochlea array datasets (Sinkkonen et al., 2011), the Stanford DNA Microarray Core Facility for hybridization and scanning of the E10.5 tissue samples, and A. Kato and D. Bredt for Fbx2 antibodies. Imaging was performed at the Stanford OHNS Imaging Core Facility and supported by core grant P30DC010363-03. Funding was provided by NIH grants RO1DC006167 (SH), NRSA F32DC013210 (BH), and an NIH Pediatric Research LRP award (BH).

References

Anderson, W. J., Zhou, Q., Alcalde, V., Kaneko, O. F., Blank, L. J., Sherwood, R. I., et al. (2008). Genetic targeting of the endoderm with claudin-6CreER. *Dev. Dyn.* 237, 504–512. doi: 10.1002/dvdy.21437

Asamura, K., Abe, S., Imamura, Y., Aszodi, A., Suzuki, N., Hashimoto, S., et al. (2005). Type IX collagen is crucial for normal hearing. *Neuroscience* 132, 493–500. doi: 10.1016/j.neuroscience.2005.01.013

Baker, S., Booth, C., Fillman, C., Shapiro, M., Blair, M. P., Hyland, J. C., et al. (2011). A loss of function mutation in the COL9A2 gene causes autosomal recessive Stickler syndrome. *Am. J. Med. Genet. A* 155A, 1668–1672. doi: 10.1002/ajmg.a.34071

Barrionuevo, F., Naumann, A., Bagheri-Fam, S., Speth, V., Taketo, M. M., Scherer, G., et al. (2008). Sox9 is required for invagination of the otic placode in mice. *Dev. Biol.* 317, 213–224. doi: 10.1016/j.ydbio.2008.02.011

Benjamini, Y., and Hochberg, Y. (1995). Controlling the false discovery rate—a practical and powerful approach to multiple testing. *J. R. Stat. Soc. Ser. B Methodol.* 57, 289–300.

Benjamini, Y., and Yekutieli, D. (2005). False discovery rate-adjusted multiple confidence intervals for selected parameters. *J. Am. Stat. Assoc.* 100, 71–81. doi: 10.1198/016214504000001907

Bolstad, B. M., Irizarry, R. A., Astrand, M., and Speed, T. P. (2003). A comparison of normalization methods for high density oligonucleotide array data based on variance and bias. *Bioinformatics* 19, 185–193. doi: 10.1093/bioinformatics/19.2.185

Burton, Q., Cole, L. K., Mulheisen, M., Chang, W., and Wu, D. K. (2004). The role of Pax2 in mouse inner ear development. *Dev. Biol.* 272, 161–175. doi: 10.1016/j.ydbio.2004.04.024

Chen, J., and Streit, A. (2013). Induction of the inner ear: stepwise specification of otic fate from multipotent progenitors. *Hear. Res.* 297, 3–12. doi: 10.1016/j.heares.2012.11.018

Dalman, M. R., Deeter, A., Nimishakavi, G., and Duan, Z. H. (2012). Fold change and p-value cutoffs significantly alter microarray interpretations. *BMC Bioinformatics* 13(Suppl. 2):S11. doi: 10.1186/1471-2105-13-S2-S11

Dominguez-Frutos, E., Vendrell, V., Alvarez, Y., Zelarayan, L. C., Lopez-Hernandez, I., Ros, M., et al. (2009). Tissue-specific requirements for FGF8 during early inner ear development. *Mech. Dev.* 126, 873–881. doi: 10.1016/j.mod.2009.07.004

Durruthy-Durruthy, R., Gottlieb, A., Hartman, B. H., Waldhaus, J., Laske, R. D., Altman, R., et al. (2014). Reconstruction of the mouse otocyst and early neuroblast lineage at single-cell resolution. *Cell* 157, 964–978. doi: 10.1016/j.cell.2014.03.036

Eom, C. Y., Heo, W. D., Craske, M. L., Meyer, T., and Lehman, I. R. (2004). The neural F-box protein NFB42 mediates the nuclear export of the herpes simplex virus type 1 replication initiator protein (UL9 protein) after viral infection. *Proc. Natl. Acad. Sci. U.S.A.* 101, 4036–4040. doi: 10.1073/pnas.0400738101

Failli, V., Bachy, I., and Retaux, S. (2002). Expression of the LIM-homeodomain gene Lmx1a (dreher) during development of the mouse nervous system. *Mech. Dev.* 118, 225–228. doi: 10.1016/S0925-4773(02)00254-X

Freter, S., Muta, Y., O'Neill, P., Vassilev, V. S., Kuraku, S., and Ladher, R. K. (2012). Pax2 modulates proliferation during specification of the otic and epibranchial placodes. *Dev. Dyn.* 241, 1716–1728. doi: 10.1002/dvdy.23856

Hagg, R., Hedbom, E., Mollers, U., Aszodi, A., Fassler, R., and Bruckner, P. (1997). Absence of the alpha1(IX) chain leads to a functional knock-out of the entire collagen IX protein in mice. *J. Biol. Chem.* 272, 20650–20654. doi: 10.1074/jbc.272.33.20650

Hama, H., Kurokawa, H., Kawano, H., Ando, R., Shimogori, T., Noda, H., et al. (2011). Scale: a chemical approach for fluorescence imaging and reconstruction of transparent mouse brain. *Nat. Neurosci.* 14, 1481–1488. doi: 10.1038/nn.2928

Hammond, K. L., and Whitfield, T. T. (2011). Fgf and Hh signalling act on a symmetrical pre-pattern to specify anterior and posterior identity in the zebrafish otic placode and vesicle. *Development* 138, 3977–3987. doi: 10.1242/dev.066639

Hans, S., Liu, D., and Westerfield, M. (2004). Pax8 and Pax2a function synergistically in otic specification, downstream of the Foxi1 and Dlx3b transcription factors. *Development* 131, 5091–5102. doi: 10.1242/dev.01346

Hartman, B. H., Hayashi, T., Nelson, B. R., Bermingham-McDonogh, O., and Reh, T. A. (2007). Dll3 is expressed in developing hair cells in the mammalian cochlea. *Dev. Dyn.* 236, 2875–2883. doi: 10.1002/dvdy.21307

Hartman, B. H., Reh, T. A., and Bermingham-McDonogh, O. (2010). Notch signaling specifies prosensory domains via lateral induction in the developing mammalian inner ear. *Proc. Natl. Acad. Sci. U.S.A.* 107, 15792–15797. doi: 10.1073/pnas.1002827107

Henzl, M. T., O'Neal, J., Killick, R., Thalmann, I., and Thalmann, R. (2001). OCP1, an F-box protein, co-localizes with OCP2/SKP1 in the cochlear epithelial gap junction region. *Hear. Res.* 157, 100–111. doi: 10.1016/S0378-5955(01)00285-4

Henzl, M. T., Thalmann, I., Larson, J. D., Ignatova, E. G., and Thalmann, R. (2004). The cochlear F-box protein OCP1 associates with OCP2 and connexin 26. *Hear. Res.* 191, 101–109. doi: 10.1016/j.heares.2004.01.005

Hertzano, R., and Elkon, R. (2012). High throughput gene expression analysis of the inner ear. *Hear. Res.* 288, 77–88. doi: 10.1016/j.heares.2012.01.002

Jayasena, C. S., Ohyama, T., Segil, N., and Groves, A. K. (2008). Notch signaling augments the canonical Wnt pathway to specify the size of the otic placode. *Development* 135, 2251–2261. doi: 10.1242/dev.017905

Jollife, I. T. (2010). *Principal Component Analysis.* New York, NY: Springer.

Kato, A., Rouach, N., Nicoll, R. A., and Bredt, D. S. (2005). Activity-dependent NMDA receptor degradation mediated by retrotranslocation and ubiquitination. *Proc. Natl. Acad. Sci. U.S.A.* 102, 5600–5605. doi: 10.1073/pnas.0501769102

Koehler, K. R., Mikosz, A. M., Molosh, A. I., Patel, D., and Hashino, E. (2013). Generation of inner ear sensory epithelia from pluripotent stem cells in 3D culture. *Nature* 500, 217–221. doi: 10.1038/nature12298

Kollmar, R., Nakamura, S. K., Kappler, J. A., and Hudspeth, A. J. (2001). Expression and phylogeny of claudins in vertebrate primordia. *Proc. Natl. Acad. Sci. U.S.A.* 98, 10196–10201. doi: 10.1073/pnas.171325898

Lillevali, K., Haugas, M., Matilainen, T., Pussinen, C., Karis, A., and Salminen, M. (2006). Gata3 is required for early morphogenesis and Fgf10 expression during otic development. *Mech. Dev.* 123, 415–429. doi: 10.1016/j.mod.2006.04.007

Liu, D., Chu, H., Maves, L., Yan, Y. L., Morcos, P. A., Postlethwait, J. H., et al. (2003). Fgf3 and Fgf8 dependent and independent transcription factors are required for otic placode specification. *Development* 130, 2213–2224. doi: 10.1242/dev.00445

Luo, X. J., Deng, M., Xie, X., Huang, L., Wang, H., Jiang, L., et al. (2013). GATA3 controls the specification of prosensory domain and neuronal survival in the mouse cochlea. *Hum. Mol. Genet.* 22, 3609–3623. doi: 10.1093/hmg/ddt212

Mailleux, A. A., Kelly, R., Veltmaat, J. M., De Langhe, S. P., Zaffran, S., Thiery, J. P., et al. (2005). Fgf10 expression identifies parabronchial smooth muscle cell progenitors and is required for their entry into the smooth muscle cell lineage. *Development* 132, 2157–2166. doi: 10.1242/dev.01795

Nelson, R. F., Glenn, K. A., Zhang, Y., Wen, H., Knutson, T., Gouvion, C. M., et al. (2007). Selective cochlear degeneration in mice lacking the F-box protein, Fbx2, a glycoprotein-specific ubiquitin ligase subunit. *J. Neurosci.* 27, 5163–5171. doi: 10.1523/JNEUROSCI.0206-07.2007

Nichols, D. H., Pauley, S., Jahan, I., Beisel, K. W., Millen, K. J., and Fritzsch, B. (2008). Lmx1a is required for segregation of sensory epithelia and normal ear histogenesis and morphogenesis. *Cell Tissue Res.* 334, 339–358. doi: 10.1007/s00441-008-0709-2

Ohazama, A., Haworth, K. E., Ota, M. S., Khonsari, R. H., and Sharpe, P. T. (2010). Ectoderm, endoderm, and the evolution of heterodont dentitions. *Genesis* 48, 382–389. doi: 10.1002/dvg.20634

Ohuchi, H., Nakagawa, T., Yamamoto, A., Araga, A., Ohata, T., Ishimaru, Y., et al. (1997). The mesenchymal factor, FGF10, initiates and maintains the outgrowth of the chick limb bud through interaction with FGF8, an apical ectodermal factor. *Development* 124, 2235–2244.

Oshima, K., Shin, K., Diensthuber, M., Peng, A. W., Ricci, A. J., and Heller, S. (2010). Mechanosensitive hair cell-like cells from embryonic and induced pluripotent stem cells. *Cell* 141, 704–716. doi: 10.1016/j.cell.2010.03.035

Powles, N., Babbs, C., Ficker, M., Schimmang, T., and Maconochie, M. (2004). Identification and analysis of genes from the mouse otic vesicle and their association with developmental subprocesses through *in situ* hybridization. *Dev. Biol.* 268, 24–38. doi: 10.1016/j.ydbio.2003.11.024

Sajan, S. A., Warchol, M. E., and Lovett, M. (2007). Toward a systems biology of mouse inner ear organogenesis: gene expression pathways, patterns and network analysis. *Genetics* 177, 631–653. doi: 10.1534/genetics.107.078584

Schlosser, G. (2014). Early embryonic specification of vertebrate cranial placodes. *Wiley Interdiscip. Rev. Dev. Biol.* 3, 349–363. doi: 10.1002/wdev.142

Sekerkova, G., Zheng, L., Mugnaini, E., and Bartles, J. R. (2006). Differential expression of espin isoforms during epithelial morphogenesis, stereociliogenesis and postnatal maturation in the developing inner ear. *Dev. Biol.* 291, 83–95. doi: 10.1016/j.ydbio.2005.12.021

Sinkkonen, S. T., Chai, R., Jan, T. A., Hartman, B. H., Laske, R. D., Gahlen, F., et al. (2011). Intrinsic regenerative potential of murine cochlear supporting cells. *Sci. Rep.* 1, 26. doi: 10.1038/srep00026

Smyth, G. K. (2004). Linear models and empirical bayes methods for assessing differential expression in microarray experiments. *Stat. Appl. Genet. Mol. Biol.* 3, Article3. doi: 10.2202/1544-6115.1027

Suzuki, N., Asamura, K., Kikuchi, Y., Takumi, Y., Abe, S., Imamura, Y., et al. (2005). Type IX collagen knock-out mouse shows progressive hearing loss. *Neurosci. Res.* 51, 293–298. doi: 10.1016/j.neures.2004.12.001

Tamplin, O. J., Kinzel, D., Cox, B. J., Bell, C. E., Rossant, J., and Lickert, H. (2008). Microarray analysis of Foxa2 mutant mouse embryos reveals novel gene expression and inductive roles for the gastrula organizer and its derivatives. *BMC Genomics* 9:511. doi: 10.1186/1471-2164-9-511

Thalmann, R., Henzl, M. T., Killick, R., Ignatova, E. G., and Thalmann, I. (2003). Toward an understanding of cochlear homeostasis: the impact of location and the role of OCP1 and OCP2. *Acta Otolaryngol.* 123, 203–208. doi: 10.1080/0036554021000028100

Thalmann, R., Henzl, M. T., and Thalmann, I. (1997). Specific proteins of the organ of Corti. *Acta Otolaryngol.* 117, 265–268. doi: 10.3109/00016489709117784

Theiler, K. (1989). *The House Mouse: Atlas of Mouse Development.* New York, NY: Springer-Verlag.

Vendrell, V., Vazquez-Echeverria, C., Lopez-Hernandez, I., Alonso, B. D., Martinez, S., Pujades, C., et al. (2013). Roles of Wnt8a during formation and patterning of the mouse inner ear. *Mech. Dev.* 130, 160–168. doi: 10.1016/j.mod.2012.09.009

Verpy, E., Leibovici, M., and Petit, C. (1999). Characterization of otoconin-95, the major protein of murine otoconia, provides insights into the formation of these inner ear biominerals. *Proc. Natl. Acad. Sci. U.S.A.* 96, 529–534. doi: 10.1073/pnas.96.2.529

Wang, Y., Kowalski, P. E., Thalmann, I., Ornitz, D. M., Mager, D. L., and Thalmann, R. (1998). Otoconin-90, the mammalian otoconial matrix protein, contains two domains of homology to secretory phospholipase A2. *Proc. Natl. Acad. Sci. U.S.A.* 95, 15345–15350. doi: 10.1073/pnas.95.26.15345

Xu, P. X., Adams, J., Peters, H., Brown, M. C., Heaney, S., and Maas, R. (1999). Eya1-deficient mice lack ears and kidneys and show abnormal apoptosis of organ primordia. *Nat. Genet.* 23, 113–117. doi: 10.1038/12722

Zhao, X., Jones, S. M., Yamoah, E. N., and Lundberg, Y. W. (2008). Otoconin-90 deletion leads to imbalance but normal hearing: a comparison with other otoconia mutants. *Neuroscience* 153, 289–299. doi: 10.1016/j.neuroscience.2008.01.055

Zhao, X., Yang, H., Yamoah, E. N., and Lundberg, Y. W. (2007). Gene targeting reveals the role of Oc90 as the essential organizer of the otoconial organic matrix. *Dev. Biol.* 304, 508–524. doi: 10.1016/j.ydbio.2007.01.013

Zheng, W., Huang, L., Wei, Z. B., Silvius, D., Tang, B., and Xu, P. X. (2003). The role of Six1 in mammalian auditory system development. *Development* 130, 3989–4000. doi: 10.1242/dev.00628

Zou, D., Silvius, D., Rodrigo-Blomqvist, S., Enerback, S., and Xu, P. X. (2006). Eya1 regulates the growth of otic epithelium and interacts with Pax2 during the development of all sensory areas in the inner ear. *Dev. Biol.* 298, 430–441. doi: 10.1016/j.ydbio.2006.06.049

16

Changes in the regulation of the Notch signaling pathway are temporally correlated with regenerative failure in the mouse cochlea

*Juan C. Maass[1,2,3,4], Rende Gu[1], Martin L. Basch[1], Joerg Waldhaus[5], Eduardo Martin Lopez[1], Anping Xia[5], John S. Oghalai[5], Stefan Heller[5] and Andrew K. Groves[1,6,7]**

[1] Department of Neuroscience, Baylor College of Medicine, Houston, TX, USA, [2] Department of Otolaryngology, Hospital Clínico Universidad de Chile, Santiago, Chile, [3] Interdisciplinary Program of Physiology and Biophysics, ICBM Universidad de Chile, Santiago, Chile, [4] Department of Otolaryngology, Clínica Alemana de Santiago, Facultad de Medicina Clínica Alemana-Universidad del Desarrollo, Santiago, Chile, [5] Department of Otolaryngology —Head and Neck Surgery, Stanford University School of Medicine, Palo Alto, CA, USA, [6] Department of Molecular and Human Genetics, Baylor College of Medicine, Houston, TX, USA, [7] Program in Developmental Biology, Baylor College of Medicine, Houston, TX, USA

Edited by:
Qi Yuan,
Memorial University, Canada

Reviewed by:
Fernando Giraldez,
Universitat Pompeu Fabra, Spain
Nicolas Daudet,
University College London, UK
Jian Zuo,
St. Jude Children's Research Hospital, USA

***Correspondence:**
Andrew K. Groves, Department of Molecular and Human Genetics, Baylor College of Medicine, BCM295, 1 Baylor Plaza, Houston, TX 77030, USA
akgroves@bcm.edu

Sensorineural hearing loss is most commonly caused by the death of hair cells in the organ of Corti, and once lost, mammalian hair cells do not regenerate. In contrast, other vertebrates such as birds can regenerate hair cells by stimulating division and differentiation of neighboring supporting cells. We currently know little of the genetic networks which become active in supporting cells when hair cells die and that are activated in experimental models of hair cell regeneration. Several studies have shown that neonatal mammalian cochlear supporting cells are able to trans-differentiate into hair cells when cultured in conditions in which the Notch signaling pathway is blocked. We now show that the ability of cochlear supporting cells to trans-differentiate declines precipitously after birth, such that supporting cells from six-day-old mouse cochlea are entirely unresponsive to a blockade of the Notch pathway. We show that this trend is seen regardless of whether the Notch pathway is blocked with gamma secretase inhibitors, or by antibodies against the Notch1 receptor, suggesting that the action of gamma secretase inhibitors on neonatal supporting cells is likely to be by inhibiting Notch receptor cleavage. The loss of responsiveness to inhibition of the Notch pathway in the first postnatal week is due in part to a down-regulation of Notch receptors and ligands, and we show that this down-regulation persists in the adult animal, even under conditions of noise damage. Our data suggest that the Notch pathway is used to establish the repeating pattern of hair cells and supporting cells in the organ of Corti, but is not required to maintain this cellular mosaic once the production of hair cells and supporting cells is completed. Our results have implications for the proposed used of Notch pathway inhibitors in hearing restoration therapies.

Keywords: notch, hair cell, supporting cell, cochlea, regeneration

Introduction

The Notch signaling pathway is an evolutionarily ancient form of cell-cell communication. During Notch signaling, the binding of membrane-bound ligands of the Delta and Jagged/Serrate families to Notch receptors causes the cleavage of the receptor and release of an intracellular domain which travels to the nucleus and participates in transcriptional activation (Artavanis-Tsakonas et al., 1999; Ilagan and Kopan, 2007; Artavanis-Tsakonas and Muskavitch, 2010; Hori et al., 2013). Notch signaling is deployed in the development of many tissues, and can influence cell fate through lateral inhibition with feedback (Chitnis, 1995; Formosa-Jordan et al., 2013), inductive signaling (frequently to establish boundaries of different cell types) or by the asymmetrical inheritance of fate determinants that affect Notch signaling (Bray, 2006).

Notch signaling regulates many aspects of inner ear development (Kelley, 2003, 2006, 2007; Murata et al., 2012). During the induction of the otic placode, the anlagen of the inner ear, Jagged1 activation of Notch signaling acts to strengthen otic placode fate in response to FGF and Wnt signals (Jayasena et al., 2008; Groves and Fekete, 2012). As the first neuroblasts begin to differentiate and delaminate from the otocyst, Notch-Delta signaling regulates the proportion of progenitor cells that differentiate as neurons by lateral inhibition (Adam et al., 1998; Abelló et al., 2007; Daudet et al., 2007; Kiernan, 2013; Neves et al., 2013a). As the first sensory regions of the inner ear begin to develop, Notch-Jagged1 signaling helps maintain and promote the fate of vestibular sensory regions of the ear through lateral induction (Eddison et al., 2000; Daudet and Lewis, 2005; Kiernan et al., 2005a; Brooker et al., 2006; Daudet et al., 2007; Hartman et al., 2010; Pan et al., 2010, 2013; Neves et al., 2011, 2013a,b), although it is less clear if this mode of sensory induction also occurs in the cochlea (Basch et al., 2011; Yamamoto et al., 2011). Finally, as hair cell and supporting cells begin to differentiate from sensory progenitor cells in prosensory patches, hair cells begin to express the Notch ligands Delta1 and Jagged2 (Dll1, Jag2) on their cell surface, and signaling by these ligands through the Notch1 receptor on nascent supporting cells induces and maintains supporting cell fate though lateral inhibition. Accordingly, pharmacological or genetic disruption of Notch1, Dll1 or Jag2, singly or in combination, leads to a failure of Notch signaling and an increase in the number of hair cells at the expense of supporting cells, likely through loss of lateral inhibition (Kiernan et al., 2005a; Brooker et al., 2006). Mutation or knock-down of downstream transcriptional effectors of Notch signaling, such as members of the Hes and Hey gene families, also leads to an increase in hair cell numbers at the expense of supporting cells (Zheng et al., 2000; Zine et al., 2001; Hayashi et al., 2008; Li et al., 2008; Doetzlhofer et al., 2009; Tateya et al., 2011; Benito-Gonzalez and Doetzlhofer, 2014).

A number of studies suggest that Notch signaling between hair cells and supporting cells continues in the sensory end organs of the mammalian inner ear after birth (Zine et al., 2000; Murata et al., 2006; Yamamoto et al., 2006; Hartman et al., 2007, 2009; Hori et al., 2007; Batts et al., 2009; Doetzlhofer et al., 2009; Lin et al., 2011; Liu et al., 2012a,b). Downstream effectors of Notch signaling can be detected in the cristae and maculae of the vestibular system (Hartman et al., 2009; Wang et al., 2010; Lin et al., 2011; Slowik and Bermingham-McDonogh, 2013), and blockade of Notch signaling in the adult vestibular system can induce the formation of ectopic hair cells at the expense of supporting cells (Lin et al., 2011; Slowik and Bermingham-McDonogh, 2013). Similarly, inhibition of Notch signaling in the neonatal organ of Corti also down-regulates some downstream effectors of Notch signaling in supporting cells and leads to the rapid formation of extra hair cells (Doetzlhofer et al., 2009; Korrapati et al., 2013; Mizutari et al., 2013; Bramhall et al., 2014). In both the neonatal cochlea and adult vestibular system, the generation of hair cells has been proposed to occur through a direct trans-differentiation of supporting cells without cell division (Doetzlhofer et al., 2009; Lin et al., 2011; Bramhall et al., 2014), a mode of differentiation that has also been observed during hair cell regeneration in birds (Stone and Cotanche, 2007).

Recently, application of gamma secretase inhibitors that attenuate the Notch pathway to the noise-damaged cochlea has been shown to generate small numbers of new hair cells and a partial restoration of hearing (Mizutari et al., 2013), suggesting that the Notch pathway may still be active in the mature cochlea. However, two issues remain unaddressed by this study. First, it is not clear to what extent components of the Notch signaling pathway—Notch receptors, Notch ligands and their downstream effectors—are expressed in the maturing cochlea (Batts et al., 2009). Indeed, two studies examining the presence of the active cleaved intracellular portion of the Notch1 receptor found very little evidence for Notch activation in the cochlea 1 week after birth (Murata et al., 2006; Liu et al., 2013). Moreover, although gamma secretase inhibitors are known to inhibit cleavage and activation of Notch receptors, they also cleave many other membrane proteins, and so it is possible that their effects in the cochlea may not be specific to the Notch pathway (Kopan and Ilagan, 2004).

In the present study, we compared the effects of gamma secretase inhibitors or blocking antibodies to the Notch1 receptor on the patterning of hair cells and supporting cells in organ cultures of the neonatal cochlea. In each case, we found that inhibitor treatment causes an increase in hair cell numbers at the expense of supporting cells, suggesting that both inhibitors are likely causing supporting cell trans-differentiation through inhibition of the Notch pathway. However, we find a precipitous age-dependent decline in the ability of these inhibitors to cause supporting cell trans-differentiation into hair cells. This decline in response to Notch inhibition progresses in a basal-apical gradient along the organ of Corti, consistent with the gradient of cellular maturation in the cochlea, and by 6 days after birth, the organ of Corti is essentially unresponsive to Notch inhibition in culture. We combined *in situ* hybridization, Q-PCR quantitation and single cell Fluidigm analysis of Notch pathway components and showed that Notch receptors, ligands and effectors are down-regulated from the organ of Corti in basal-apical gradient during the first postnatal week, and are at least an order of magnitude lower in mature animals, even after noise damage. Our results suggest that the Notch signaling pathway is deployed to establish the pattern of hair cells and supporting cells in the cochlea, but is not required to maintain this pattern in the mature organ of Corti.

Materials and Methods

Mice

Atoh1$^{A1GFP/A1GFP}$ (MGI: *Atoh1*$^{tm4.1Hzo}$) knock-in mice and *Atoh1*^{GFP} transgenic reporter mice were generated as previously described (Lumpkin et al., 2003; Rose et al., 2009). ICR mice were used for Notch Intracellular Domain (NICD) immunostaining. Noise damage experiments were performed on wild type CBA/CaJ mice. Pillar cells and Deiters' cells were purified from *Fgfr3-iCreER*^{T2} (Young et al., 2010) mice mated with *Ai14:Rosa*^{tdTom} reporter mice (Jackson, #007908). All animal experiments were approved by the Baylor College of Medicine or Stanford University Institutional Animal Care and Use committees.

Cochlear Organ Culture

Cochleas were dissected in ice cold HBSS immediately after euthanasia. Briefly, the heads were bisected, the temporal bone was removed from the skull base and the otic capsule was removed with forceps until the intact membranous cochlea was separated from the bony structures. For P0 and P3 animals, the cochlear duct was peeled out from the modiolus and the medial structures (Kölliker and Corti's organs) were separated from the lateral wall, Reissner's membrane and the stria vascularis. For P6 mice, in order to preserve the structures in the organ of Corti, the cochlear duct was gently separated from the modiolus by cutting between them with forceps and the lateral wall, stria vascularis and Reissner's membrane were partially removed after cutting with 27 gauge needle. Immediately after dissection, the explants were placed on top of filter membranes with 1 μm pores (SPI-pore or Whatman) floating in DMEM/F12 (Hepes) supplemented with B27 supplements (Life Technologies), 1mM N-acetylcysteine (Sigma), 5 ng/ml EGF and 2.5 ng/ml FGF2 and 67 μg/ml penicillin. In some cultures DMEM/F12 medium was supplemented with N2 supplements (Life Technologies), N-acetylcysteine and penicillin. For Notch inhibition experiments, cultures were supplemented with 0.75–10 μM DAPT (Gamma secretase inhibitor IX, Calbiochem EMD) or DMSO 0.04% v/v (Life Technologies). Anti Notch1-specific antibodies and control IgD antibodies (Wu et al., 2010) were provided by Genentech and used at 2 μg/ml. The cultures were maintained for 1 h, 1, 2 or 3 days *in vitro* (DIV) at 37°C in 5% CO_2.

Immunostaining, Microscopy and Quantification

Whole cochlear explants were fixed in 4% paraformaldehyde, then permeabilized and blocked in 0.2% Triton X-100 and 10% donkey serum in PBS. The explants were incubated with primary antibodies overnight at 4°C, washed in PBST (0.1% Triton X-100 in PBS) and incubated with secondary antibodies for 2 h at room temperature, followed by 3 further washes in PBST and then incubated in 10 μg/ml DAPI for 10 min. Primary antibodies used were rabbit polyclonal anti-Myosin VIIa (1:500; Proteus Biosciences) and mouse monoclonal anti-GFP (1:200; Invitrogen). Secondary antibodies were Alexa Fluor 594 and 488 (Invitrogen). Images were obtained on an Axio Observer Zeiss microscope with an Apotome2 structured illumination attachment and analyzed in Axiovision 4.8 (Zeiss) and Image J (NIH) using Bioformat and the Cell Counter plugins. The cochlea was divided in five pieces: the tip, the apex, the middle, the base and the hook, and the center of each portion was analyzed, discarding the tip and the hook. Cell counts across different areas of the cochlea were normalized to cells per 100 μm and were expressed as a percentage increase with respect to control conditions. Significant differences were analyzed using a Mann-Whitney test for pairwise comparisons.

For NICD immunostaining in sections the protocol was modified from Morimoto et al. (2010). Briefly the heads of P0, P3 and P6 ICR mice were mounted in paraffin blocks and sectioned at 10 μm. The sections were rehydrated, bleached in H_2O_2 and boiled in a pressure cooker in antigen unmasking solution (Vectorlabs) for 20 min. The sections were then permeabilized, blocked and incubated with a cleaved Notch1 antibody (val1744; 1:100; Cell signaling) and anti- Myosin VIIa (1:500; Proteus Biosciences). The signal was amplified with Vectastain ABC Kit (rabbit IgG) (Vectorlabs) as indicated by manufacturer. The color was developed for 5–10 min with TSA Tyramide Cy3 Reagent (diluted 1:100 after reconstitution; Perkin Elmer) and then stained with DAPI. Images were obtained on a Zeiss Axio Observer microscope with an Apotome2 structured illumination attachment.

In Situ Hybridization

Digoxygenin-labeled *in situ* probe synthesis was performed on linearized plasmid DNA using standard protocols (Stern, 1998).The following mouse cDNA probes were used in the study and kindly provided by the investigators listed: *Notch1*, *Jag1*, *Dll1* (Gerry Weinmaster), *Notch3* (Urban Lendahl), *Hes5* (Ryoichiro Kageyama), *Hey1*, *Hey2*, *HeyL* (Manfred Gessler), and *Atoh1* (Huda Zoghbi). A cDNA clone for *Jag2* (BC010982) was purchased from open Biosystems. The *in situ* hybridization procedure for frozen sections was modified from previous protocols (Harland, 1991; Birren et al., 1993; Groves et al., 1995). Heads of perinatal mouse pups were fixed in 4% paraformaldehyde in PBS overnight at 4°C, cryoprotected in 30% sucrose in PBS at 4°C, embedded in OCT compound (Sakura Finetek), and cryosectioned at 14 μm. Sections were fixed in 4% paraformaldehyde in PBS, pH 7.2 for 10 min at room temperature, followed by three 5-min washes in DEPC-treated PBS. The sections were treated with 1 μg/ml Proteinase K in DEPC-PBS for 5 min at room temperature, followed by three 5-min washes in DEPC-PBS and re-fixation in 4% paraformaldehyde in PBS, pH 7.2 for 10 min at room temperature. Sections were acetylated in 0.25% acetic anhydride in 0.1 M triethanolamine, pH 8.0 for 10 min at room temperature, followed by three 5-min washes in DEPC-PBS. Slides were incubated in hybridization buffer (50% formamide, 5 × SSC, 50 μg/ml Yeast tRNA, 100 μg/ml Heparin, 1 × Denhardt's Solution, 0.1% Tween 20, 0.1% CHAPS, 5 mM EDTA) for 1–2 h at 65°C. 100 μl of digoxygenin-labeled probe (1 mg/ml) was added to each slide and the slides covered with glass coverslips. The slides were incubated in a chamber humidified with 5 × SSC, 50% formamide at 65°C overnight. Coverslips were removed by rinsing in 0.2 × SSC and the slides washed in 0.2 × SSC at 65°C for 1 h. The slides were then washed in 0.2 × SSC for 5 min at room temperature, followed by another 5-min wash in 0.1% Tween-20 in PBS (PTw). The slides were blocked in 10% lamb serum in PTw at room temperature for 1 h and then stained with anti-digoxygenin-alkaline phosphatase antibody (1:2000) for 1–3 h at room temperature in a humidified chamber. The slides were then washed three times for 5 min each in PTw and equilibrated with freshly-made alkaline phosphatase buffer (100 mM Tris pH 9.5, 50 mM $MgCl_2$, 100 mM NaCl, 0.1% Tween 20) for 10 min. The slides were developed in alkaline phosphatase buffer containing 0.33 mg/ml NBT and 0.18 mg/ml BCIP in the dark at room temperature until the purple reaction product had developed to a satisfactory degree. The reaction was stopped by washing the slides in PBS three times for 15 min each, followed by fixation in 4% paraformaldehyde in PBS, pH 7.2 for 30 min. The slides were then rinsed and mounted in 80% glycerol in PBS. Whole mount *in situ* hybridization was carried out as recently described in detail (Khatri and Groves, 2013).

RNA Isolation and Q-PCR

For each experimental condition, total RNA was extracted from 4 uncultured whole cochlear explants or 3 cultured cochlear explants using the RNeasy mini kit (Qiagen). RNA yield ranged from 480 to 1200 ng and was used for cDNA preparation using random primers and SuperScript III First-Strand Synthesis System (Invitrogen). qPCR reaction was performed with SYBRGreen PCR Master Mix in StepOnePlus RealTime PCR System (Applied Biosystems), using in the reaction cDNA at 0.3–0.6 ng/μl and primers at 50 nM (excepting 100 nM for the Hes5 reaction). Primers sequences are provided in **Table 1**. *GAPDH* and *L19* primers were used as reference genes. Significant differences were analyzed using a Mann-Whitney test for pairwise comparisons. Multiple comparisons or pairwise correction for multiple comparisons were not performed.

Single Cell Purification and Q-PCR Analysis

Triple transgenic mice heterozygote for Fgfr3-iCreER^{T2} (Young et al., 2010), Ai14:Rosa^{tdTom} (Jackson, #007908) and Sox2-EGFP (Jackson, #017592) were analyzed at P2, and double transgenic animals (Fgfr3-iCreER^{T2} and Ai14:Rosa^{tdTom}) were analyzed at P21. Animals were injected with 0.2 mg/g body weight tamoxifen at P0 and P19 respectively. Animals were euthanized 2 days after the tamoxifen injection and organs of Corti were dissected. Single cell dissociation, flow cytometry, RNA isolation and single cell qRT-PCR were performed as described in Durruthy-Durruthy et al. (2014) using the primers listed in **Table 2**. Briefly, expression of Actb or Gapdh at levels lower or higher than 3 standard deviations from the mean was used to exclude compromised cells/empty wells or possible doublets, respectively. Ai14-Control primers detect recombination within the Ai14-tdTomato reporter locus and cells with no detectable recombination were excluded from the analysis. Single cell expression data is presented as Log2Ex values, calculated by subtracting experimentally determined Ct-values from the median limit of detection calculated for all primers used in the study. Single cell data were normalized using the median Log2Ex values as recommended by Fluidigm.

TABLE 1 | Q-PCR primers for Figures 1, 3, 5, 7.

Gene	Forward primer	Reverse primer
Atoh1	5′-ATGCACGGGCTGAACCA-3′	5′-TCGTTGTTGAAGGACGGGATA-3′
Notch1	5′-GCCGCAAGAGGCTTGAGAT-3′	5′-GGAGTCCTGGCATCGTTGG-3′
Notch3	5′-GCACTTGCCGTGGTTACATG-3′	5′-CCTCACAACTGTCACCAGCATAG-3′
Hey1	5′-CACTGCAGGAGGGAAAGGTTAT-3′	5′-CCCCAAACTCCGATAGTCCAT-3′
Hey2	5′-AAGCGCCCTTGTGAGGAAA-3′	5′-TCGCTCCCCACGTCGAT-3′
HeyL	5′-GCGCAGAGGGATCATAGAGAA-3′	5′-TCGCAATTCAGAAAGGCTACTG-3′
Hes5	5′-GCACCAGCCCAACTCCAA-3′	5′-GGCGAAGGCTTTGCTGTGT-3′
Jag1	5′-AAAGACCACTGCCGTACCAC-3′	5′-GGGGACCACAGACGTTAGAA-3′
Jag2	5′-TGCGAACTAGAGTACGACAA-3′	5′-TTGGTTCACAGAGATCCATG-3′
Dll1	5′-TCCGATTCCCCTTCGGCTTCA-3′	5′-TCTGTTGCGAGGTCATCGGGA-3′
Dll3	5′-CCGCTTTCCCAGACGCTGAT-3′	5′-GGCCTGGCCCGAAAGAATGA-3′
Gapdh	5′-AGGTCGGTGTGAACGGATTTG-3′	5′-TGTAGACCATGTAGTTGAGGTCA-3′
Ll9	5′-GGTCTGGTTGGATCCCAATG-3′	5′-CCCGGGAATGGACAGTCA-3′

Noise Damage

Noise damage of six-week-old CBA/CaJ mice was performed as previously described (Liu et al., 2011). Briefly, a custom-built box contained six piezo horns (TW-125, Pyramid Car Audio, Brooklyn, NY, USA) inserted through the cover. Band-passed white noise (4–22 kHz) was generated digitally with RPvds software (Version 6.6, Tucker-Davis Technologies, Alachua, FL, USA), converted to analog by a digital-to-analog converter, and then transferred to the power amplifier (Servo 550, Sampson, Hauppauge, NY, USA) to drive the speakers. A cage containing the mice was placed inside the box and the mice were exposed to noise at 98 dB ± 2 dB for 4 h.

TABLE 2 | Q-PCR primers for Figure 6.

Gene	Forward primer	Reverse primer
Actb:	5′- CCCTAAGGCCAACCGTGAAA -3′	5′- CAGCCTGGATG GCTACGTAC -3′
Gapdh	5′- AGACGGCCGCATCTTCTT -3′	5′- TTCACACCGACC TTCACCAT -3′
Ai9-Control	5′- AGGAACTTCGTCGACATTTAAATCA -3′	5′- CTGCAGGTCGA GGGACCTAA -3′
Fgfr3	5′- AGGATTTAGACCGCATCCTCAC -3′	5′- CCTGGCGAGTAC TGCTCAAA -3′
Cdkn1b	5′- CAGTGTCCAGGGATGAGGAA -3′	5′- TTCGGGGAACCGTC TGAAA -3′
Sox2	5′- TGAAGGAGCACCCGGATTATA -3′	5′- CGGGAAGCGTGT ACTTATCC -3′
Jag1	5′- AACGACCGTAATCGCATCGTA -3′	5′- TCCACCAGCAAAGT GTAGGAC -3′
Jag2	5′- CTCGTCGTCATTCCCTTTCA -3′	5′- GGTGTCATTGTC CCAGTCC -3′
Hes1	5′- TGAAGCACCTCCGGAACC -3′	5′- CGCGGTATTTCC CCAACAC -3′
Hes5	5′- AAGAGCCTGCACCAGGACTA -3′	5′- GTGCAGGGTCAGG AACTGTAC -3′
Hey1	5′- ACGAGACCATCGAGGTGGAA -3′	5′- CGTTGGGGACAT GGAACACA -3′
Hey2	5′- ACTAGTGCCAACAGCTTTTGAA -3′	5′- TGTAGCCTGGAGC ATCTTCA -3′
LFng	5′- TCGATCTGCTGTTCGAGACC -3′	5′- CCTCCCCATCAG TGAAGATGAA -3′

Results

The Neonatal Cochlea Exhibits a Position-Dependent Variation of Supporting Cell Trans-Differentiation in Response to Gamma Secretase Inhibitors

A number of studies have demonstrated conversion or trans-differentiation of cochlear supporting cells into hair cells after treatment with gamma secretase inhibitors (Takebayashi et al., 2007; Hayashi et al., 2008; Doetzlhofer et al., 2009; Korrapati et al., 2013; Mizutari et al., 2013; Bramhall et al., 2014), although results in different studies have often been obtained with different gamma secretase inhibitors or at different concentrations of a given inhibitor. We confirmed these results in cochlear explant cultures from postnatal day 0 (P0) *Atoh1*$^{A1GFP/A1GFP}$ and *Atoh1-GFP* mice, using the gamma secretase inhibitor DAPT over a range of 0.75–10 μM. After 2 days in culture, we stained the cultures for Myosin VIIa and GFP to reveal the Atoh1-GFP fusion protein (*Atoh1*$^{A1GFP/A1GFP}$ mice) or GFP reporter (*Atoh1-GFP* mice). We observed a significant increase in the numbers of Myosin VIIa $^+$ hair cells at 2.5, 5 and 10 μM DAPT compared to DMSO vehicle (**Figures 1A,B**), but not at lower concentrations. We measured the levels of hair cell and supporting cell mRNAs in the *Atoh1-GFP* cultures and observed an increase of the hair cell markers *Atoh1* and *Jag2* and a decrease in the supporting cell markers *Jag1*, *Hey1* and *Hes5* (**Figure 1C**). As previously described (Doetzlhofer et al., 2009), *Hes5* was particularly sensitive to DAPT, with a strong reduction in mRNA levels being observed above 1 μM.

The organ of Corti differentiates in a broadly basal-apical direction, with the first differentiating Atoh1$^+$ hair cells appearing near the base of the cochlea, and a wave of hair cell and supporting cell differentiation spreading basally to the hook region and in an apical direction to the tip of the cochlea (Chen et al., 2002; Cai et al., 2013). Consequently at birth, hair cells and supporting cells in the basal region of the cochlea can be considered to be slightly more mature than their counterparts at the apex and tip. To determine whether these differences in maturity affected the response to gamma secretase inhibitors, we cultured whole P0 cochleas from Atoh1-GFP mice in 10 μM DAPT or DMSO vehicle for 1–3 days and counted the numbers of Atoh1-GFP or Myosin VIIa-expressing hair cells in the apical, middle and basal regions of the cochlea (**Figures 2A,B**; the approximate positions of the three regions are indicated in **Figure 2C**). We excluded from our counts the most basal hook region as it was more susceptible to variable damage during dissection and the most apical tip region because of its more variable behavior. We observed a clear effect of position on the number of supernumerary hair cells generated in the cultures over the 3 day culture period, with the apex producing 202% more hair cells after 3 days, whereas the base generated only 32% more hair cells in the same time period (**Figures 2A,B**). These results suggested that more mature supporting cells at the base of the cochlea were far less likely to trans-differentiate into hair cells in response to DAPT than their younger counterparts at the apex.

The Response of Supporting Cells to Gamma Secretase Inhibition or Notch Inhibition Declines Rapidly with Age

To test whether the response of cochlear supporting cells to DAPT was indeed age-dependent, we established cochlear cultures from newborn (P0), 3 and 6 day old mice and cultured them for 2 days in 5 μM DAPT. We quantified the number of supernumerary hair cells in the apical region. We saw significant numbers of supernumerary hair cells in DAPT-treated P0 cochlear cultures compared to DMSO vehicle, but observed no significant increase in hair cell numbers when either P3 or P6 cultures were treated with DAPT (**Figures 3A,B**).

Most experiments in which gamma secretase inhibitors have been used to promote supporting cell trans-differentiation into hair cells are interpreted on the assumption that the inhibitors are targeting the cleavage of Notch receptors in cochlear supporting cells. However, since gamma secretases cleave many other membrane proteins (Kopan and Ilagan, 2004), it is possible that some of the effects of gamma secretase inhibitors may be due to the inhibition of cleavage of other membrane proteins. To test this, we used specific blocking antibodies to the Notch1 receptor (Wu et al., 2010) at a concentration of 2 μg/ml, previously shown to effectively inhibit Notch1 signaling *in vitro* (Wu et al., 2010). Cochlear cultures from P0 animals showed similar age-dependent responses to Notch1 blocking antibodies (48%

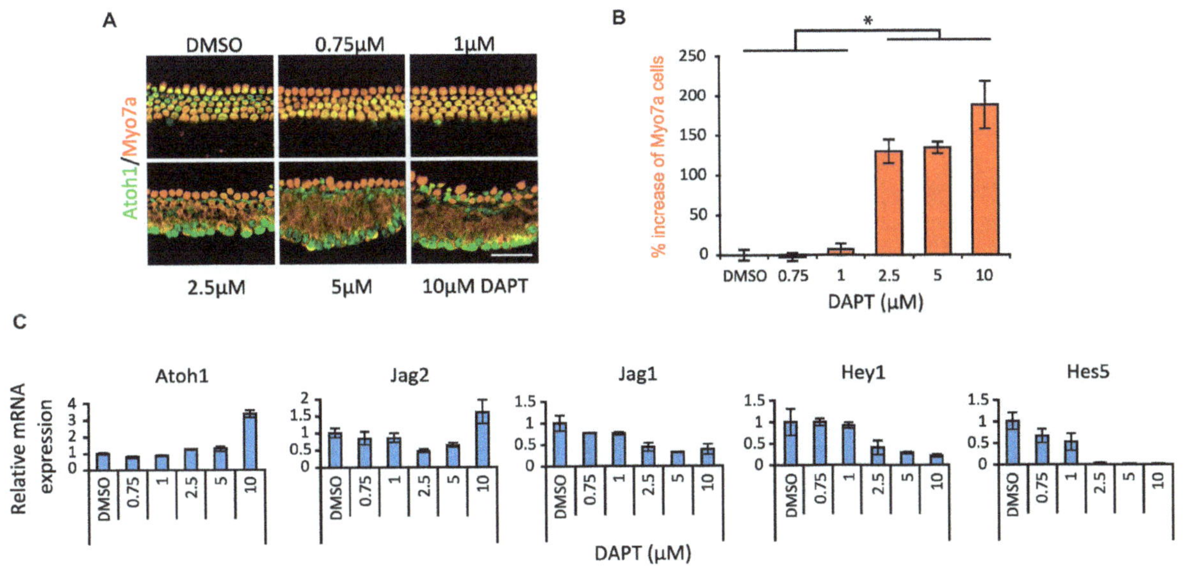

FIGURE 1 | Dose response of Notch inhibition in P0 cultures. **(A)** Immunostaining of apical portions of cochlear explants of newborn (P0) *Atoh1*$^{A1GFP/A1GFP}$ knock-in mice cultured 2 days *in vitro* (DIV) in DAPT from 0.75 to 10 µM or vehicle (DMSO). Atoh1: green. Myo7a: red. Scale 50 µm. **(B)** Quantitation of the increase in number of Myosin VIIa-labeled cells after different doses of DAPT compared to DMSO vehicle (same as shown in **A**). *N* = 4. *p = 0.030 (Mann-Whitney pairwise comparisons). Error bars: SEM. **(C)** mRNA amount of hair cell, supporting cell and Notch pathway genes obtained by QPCR in whole cochlear explants from P0 *Atoh1*^{GFP} transgenic reporter mice treated with DAPT compared to DMSO vehicle. *N* = 3. Error bars: SEM. Note that error bars are present for each condition but are very small in some cases.

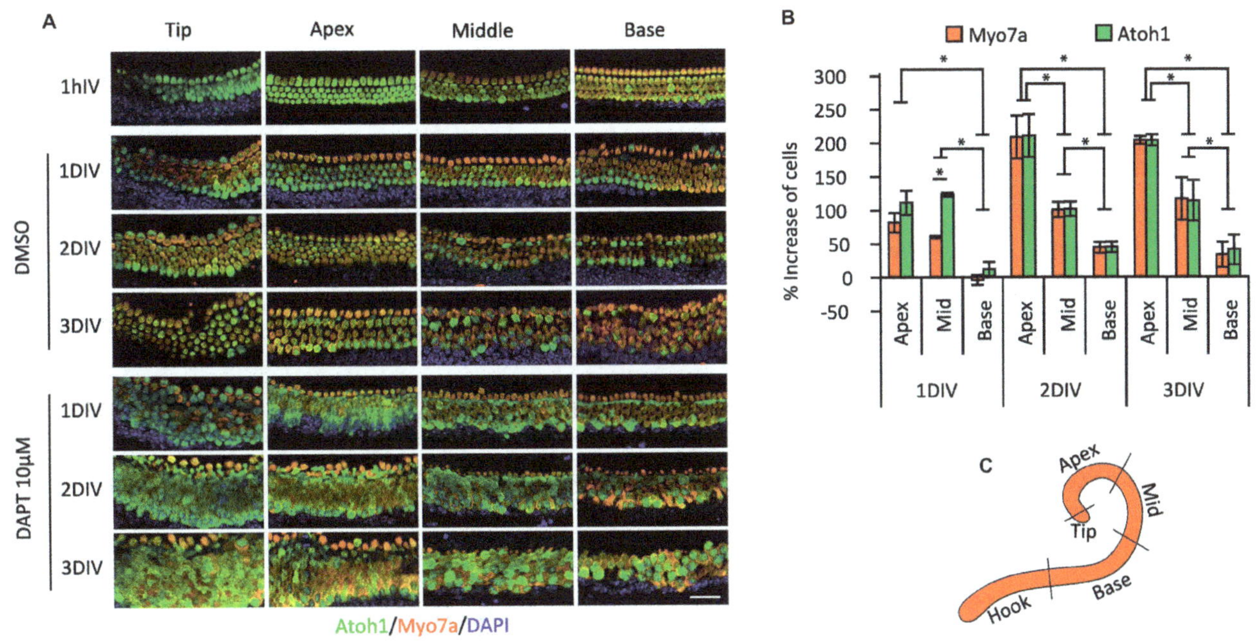

FIGURE 2 | Position-dependent effect of Notch inhibition in P0 cultures. **(A)** Immunostaining of different cochlear portions from newborn (P0) *Atoh1*$^{A1GFP/A1GFP}$ knock-in mice (shown in **C**) treated with 10 µM DAPT or vehicle (DMSO) for 1 h to 3 days *in vitro* (DIV). Atoh1: green. Myo7a: red. DAPI: Blue. **(B)** Percentage of increase in numbers of Myosin VIIa-labeled cells and GFP-labeled cells in the different regions of the cochlea after DAPT 10 µM treatment compared to vehicle (same as shown in **A**). *N* = 4. *p = 0.030 (Mann-Whitney pairwise comparisons). Error bars: SEM. **(C)** Schematic view of the cochlear portions evaluated in **(A,B)**.

increase in Myosin VIIa $^{+}$ hair cells) as cultures incubated for 2 days in 5 µM DAPT (41% increase) compared to control cultures containing DMSO or a control IgD (**Figures 3A,B**). However, we saw no significant response when P3 or P6

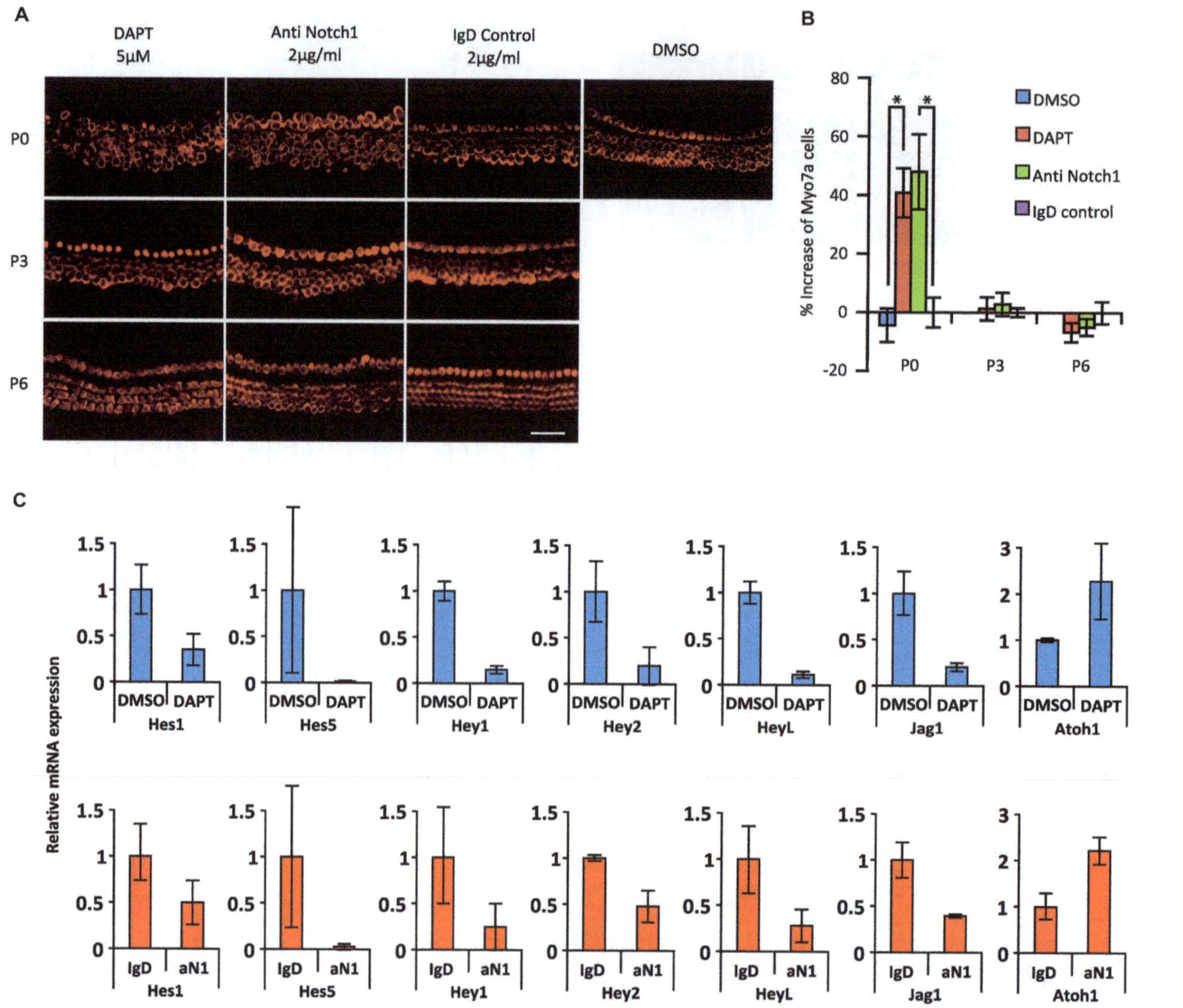

FIGURE 3 | Age-dependent decline in the effect of Notch inhibition on supporting cells in the presence of gamma secretase inhibitors or Notch1 blocking antibodies. (A) Immunostaining of apical portions of cochlear explants obtained at 0, 3 and 6 postnatal days (P0, P3 and P6) from *Atoh1*^{GFP} transgenic reporter mice treated with 5 μM DAPT, 2 μg/ml Notch1 antibodies (Anti Notch1), 2 μg/ml control IgD and DMSO cultured 2 days *in vitro* (DIV). Myo7a: red. Scale 50 μm. **(B)** The increase in numbers of Myosin VIIa-labeled cells in the apical portion of the cochleas shown in **(A)**. N = 6, 6 and 3 for P0, P3 and P6 respectively. $^{*}p$ = 0.0044 and 0.0045 for DMSO/DAPT and Anti Notch1/Control IgD comparisons respectively (Mann Whitney). Error bars: SEM. **(C)** mRNA amount of Notch pathway genes obtained by QPCR in whole cochlear explants of *Atoh1*^{GFP} transgenic reporter P0 newborn mice cultured in the presence of DAPT or DMSO and in Notch1 antibodies or control IgD antibodies. Blue columns (top): level of expression after DAPT treatment relative to DMSO. Red columns (bottom): level of expression after anti Notch1 antibodies (aN1) relative to control IgD antibodies. N = 3. Error bars: SEM. Note that error bars are present for each condition but are very small in some cases.

cultures were treated with blocking antibodies as we previously saw with 5 μM DAPT (**Figures 3A,B**). We also observed a comparable down-regulation of supporting cell-specific *Hes* and *Hey* genes and the supporting cell marker *Jag1* in P0 cultures treated with DAPT or Notch1 blocking antibodies, together with a comparable up-regulation of *Atoh1* (**Figure 3C**). These results suggest that the majority of the effects of the gamma secretase inhibitor DAPT on supporting cell trans-differentiation in neonatal cultures are likely specific to the Notch pathway.

Notch Pathway Genes are Down-Regulated in the Cochlea During the First Postnatal Week

The preceding results suggest that the Notch pathway is deployed to stabilize supporting cell fate of neonatal cochlear supporting cells, but that inhibition of the Notch pathway has no effect on supporting cell fate even a few days later. To determine out if this change in the response of supporting cells to Notch inhibition was related to changes in the endogenous activity of the Notch pathway, we examined the expression of mRNA for Notch receptors (*Notch1* and *Notch3*), ligands (*Dll1*, *Jag1*

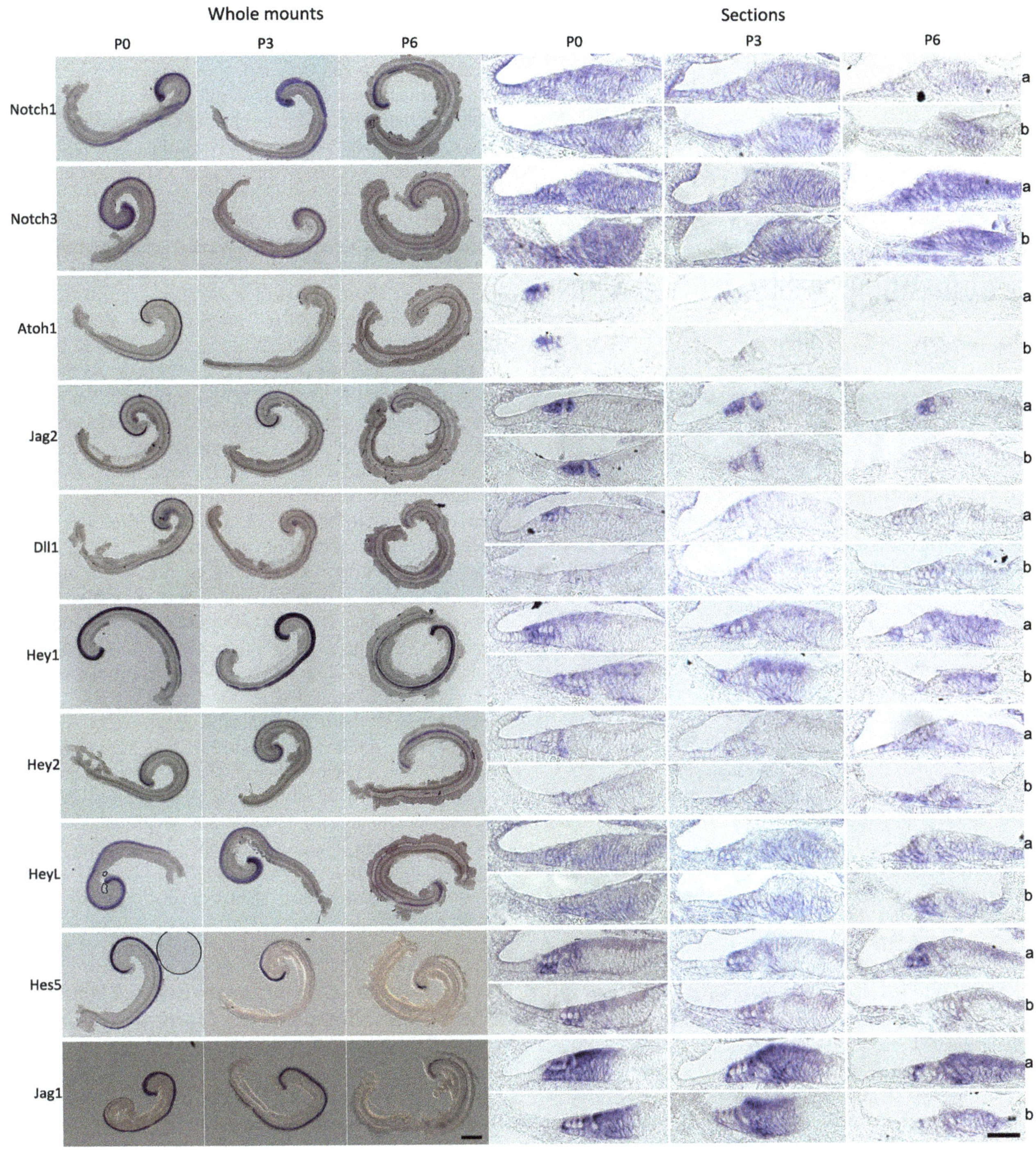

FIGURE 4 | Notch pathway components are down-regulated during the first postnatal week. *In situ* hybridization of Notch pathway genes in the cochlea at 0, 3 and 6 postnatal days (P0, P3 and P6). Left panels: Whole mount *in situs* of cochlear explants, with the samples curved clockwise from apex to base. Scale = 200 μm. Right panels: *In situ* hybridization of frozen sections; a: apex region, b: basal region. Scale 50 μm.

and *Jag2*) and downstream effectors of Notch signaling (*Hey1*, *Hey2*, *HeyL* and *Hes5*) in the cochlea from P0 to P6 by *in situ* hybridization on whole mount cochleas, sectioned cochleas and by Q-PCR of cochlear tissue (**Figures 4, 5A**). In general, all components of the Notch pathway evinced a down-regulation between P0 and P6 starting at the base and proceeding down to the apex. Specifically, *Notch1* and *Notch3* were expressed throughout the supporting cell layer and into Kölliker's organ

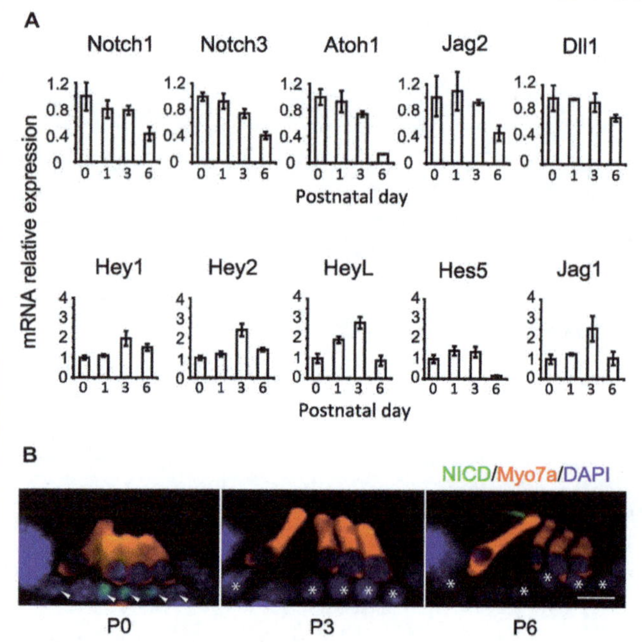

FIGURE 5 | Notch pathway components and Notch1 signaling activity decline during the first postnatal week. (A) Relative expression of some Notch pathway genes obtained by QPCR from whole cochlear explants at 1, 3 and 6 postnatal days relative to newborn (0 postnatal days). $N = 3$. Error bars: SEM. Note that error bars are present for each condition but are very small in some cases. **(B)** Notch1 intracellular domain (NICD) immunostaining in cochlear sections of ICR newborn mice, obtained at 0, 3 and 6 postnatal days (P0, P3 and P6 respectively). NICD: green. Myo7a: red. DAPI: blue. Arrow heads: supporting cells positive for NICD staining. Stars: same supporting cells pointed by arrow heads but negative for NICD staining. Scale = 20 μm.

and the outer sulcus, and both receptors showed a basal-apical down-regulation between P0 and P6. *Jag2* and *Dll1* were both down-regulated in hair cells between P0 and P6, along with the hair cell marker *Atoh1*. *Hey2* and *Hes5* were down-regulated from pillar cells and Deiters' cells respectively in a basal-apical gradient, whereas *Hey1*, *HeyL* and *Jag1* were expressed in all supporting cells and cells of Kölliker's organ, and down-regulated again in a basal-apical direction. The speed of down-regulation varied considerably from gene to gene—for example, *Dll1* was down-regulated in hair cells more quickly than *Jag2*, and *Hes5* was down-regulated much more quickly in supporting cells than *Hey1*. We also saw a general trend towards down-regulation of each gene by Q-PCR (**Figure 5A**), although the degree of down-regulation measured by this method was somewhat blunted as a result of including the entire basal-apical extent of the cochlear duct in each sample. To confirm that activation of the Notch1 receptor was also decreasing between P0 and P6, we immunostained cochlear sections with antibodies to the Notch1 intracellular domain (Notch1-ICD) which is released and localized to the nucleus after Notch activation (**Figure 5B**). We observed Notch1-ICD staining in Deiters' cells at P0, but could not detect staining in the supporting cells at later stages.

Although we did not see a significant increase in hair cells numbers at P3 or P6 after Notch inhibition in culture we did observe occasional isolated ectopic hair cells in our P3 (but not P6) cultures that may have been generated by trans-differentiation of supporting cells (**Figures 3A,B**) raising the possibility that a sub-population of supporting cells maintain Notch pathway expression at significant levels. To test whether small numbers of mature supporting cells maintain expression of some Notch pathway genes, we used the Fluidigm single cell handling system to compare gene expression in individual supporting cells purified from P2 and P21 mice. To label and purify pillar cells and Deiters' cells at P2, we injected triple transgenic mice (*FGFR3-iCreERT2/Ai14:Rosa*^{tdTom}*/Sox2-EGFP*) with tamoxifen at P0 and isolated TdTomato/EGFP double positive cells by flow cytometry. At this age, *FGFR3-iCreERT2* fate-labels pillar, Deiters', and outer hair cells, whereas EGFP is confined to all supporting cells. At P21, we used double transgenic (*FGFR3-iCreERT2/Ai14:Rosa*^{tdTom}) mice, injected with tamoxifen at P19, and sorted TdTomato-positive pillar and Deiters' cells, which were the only organ of Corti cell types labeled at this age. cDNA was prepared from individual P2 ($N = 162$) and P21 ($n = 123$) TdTomato cells using the Fluidigm single cell analysis system, and 96 genes analyzed from each sample by Q-PCR, including the Notch pathway genes *Jag1* and *2*, *Hes1* and *5*, *Hey1* and *2*, and the Notch target and ligand modulator *LFng* (**Figure 6**). In all cases, the numbers of cells with detectable amounts of Notch pathway genes declined from P2 to P21, (**Figure 6A**). The distribution in expression levels of Notch pathway genes in individual cells was visualized in violin plots and revealed a clear downward shift in expression across the population from P2 to P21 (**Figure 6B**), even when cells with undetectable levels of expression were removed from the analysis (**Figure 6C**). In some cases, we saw evidence for a small population of cells expressing high levels of a single Notch pathway gene at P21 (e.g., *Jag2*; **Figure 6C**), but we were unable to observe any single cells at P21 that co-expressed high levels of multiple Notch genes. These data suggest that the majority of P21 *FGFR3-iCreERT2* fate labeled supporting cells are unlikely to be transducing significant Notch signaling.

Notch Pathway Components are not Expressed at Significant Levels in the Normal and or Noise-Damaged Adult Organ of Corti

Several previous studies have suggested that some components of the Notch pathway may be re-activated in supporting cells following damage (Oesterle et al., 2008; Batts et al., 2009; Mizutari et al., 2013). However, these studies did not perform a direct quantitative comparison of message levels of Notch pathway components between neonatal animals (in which the Notch pathway is expressed and active) and mature animals before and after damage. We examined the expression of *Atoh1* and *Hes5* in cochleas isolated from cohorts of mice which received noise damage at P42 and were analyzed at one, three, or seven days later. Our controls were non-noise exposed cohorts of P0 and P49 mice. The level of noise we applied has been shown to be adequate to damage the cochlear epithelium and elicit changes in gene expression. In particular, it produces large temporary threshold

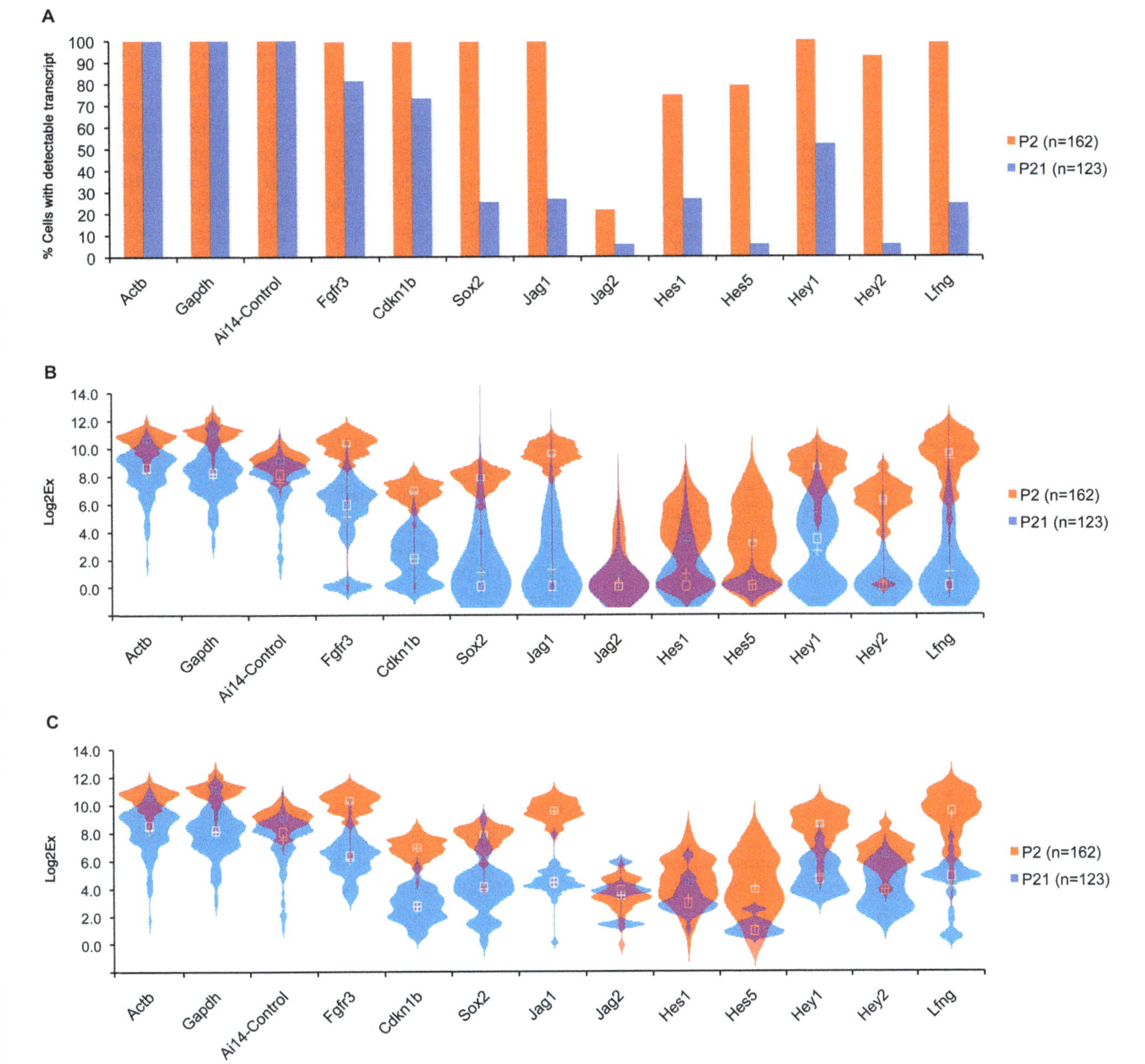

FIGURE 6 | Comparison of Notch pathway genes in P1 and P21 cochlea at the single cell level. Pillar and Deiters' cells were purified from P2 and P21 *FGFR3-CreER;ROSA-TdTomato* mice and RNA extracted from 162 (P2) and 123 (P21) single cells and subjected to QPCR analysis using the Fluidigm system (Durruthy-Durruthy et al., 2014) with primers for housekeeping genes and Notch pathway genes. **(A)** Graph showing the percentage of cells at each age that expressed detectable levels of each gene under analysis. **(B)** Violin plot showing the distribution of expression levels for each gene in all cells including the cells with no expression (Log2x = 0) presented in a combination of box plots and kernel density plots. White Crosses indicate the mean, white boxes the median expression levels. **(C)** Violin plot similar to **(B)**, excluding cells with undetectable levels of expression for each gene.

elevations, and mild permanent threshold shifts, 17% OHC loss and 3% IHC loss, and increases in prestin gene expression in residual OHCs (Wang et al., 2010; Xia et al., 2013). We found that levels of the hair cell-specific transcription factor *Atoh1* in 7 week old animals were less than 10% of their neonatal counterparts (**Figure 7**) and that these levels did not change significantly over a 7 day period after noise damage. Similar results were observed for *Hes5* (**Figure 7**). These data suggest that the Notch pathway remains down-regulated in the mature cochlea and that it is not significantly perturbed by noise damage.

Discussion

The Notch signaling pathway is deployed during the differentiation of hair cells and supporting cells and has been proposed to regulate the proportion of each cell type

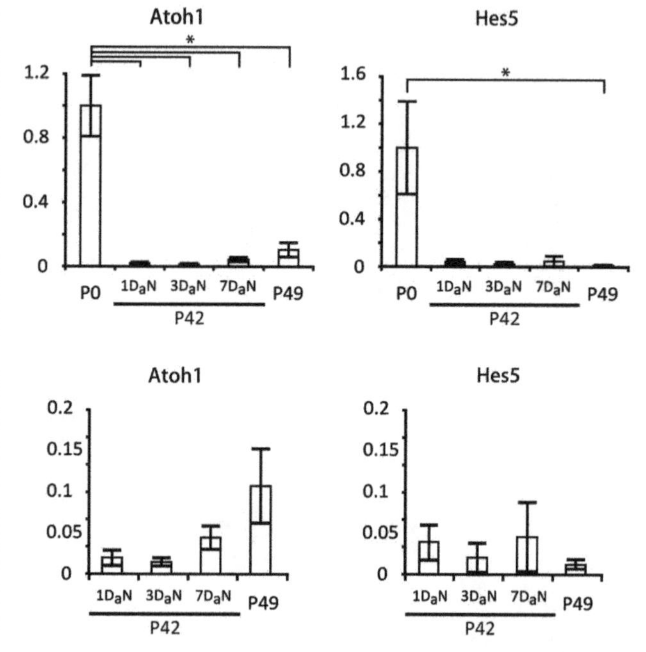

FIGURE 7 | Hes5 and Atoh1 remain expressed at very low levels in the mature organ of Corti, even after noise damage. Relative expression of *Atoh1* and *Hes5* obtained by QPCR in cochlear explants from neonatal (P0) and 6 to 7 week old mice exposed to noise. The mice exposed to noise on the 42nd postnatal day (P42) were evaluated after 1 (1D$_a$N), 3 (3D$_a$N), or 7 (7D$_a$N), days. As controls for the 7 day cohort we used 7 week old mice (P49) that had never been exposed to noise. The expression levels of *Atoh1* and *Hes5* were normalized to the level of expression at P0. $N = 3$ in all cases except P0, where $N = 6$. The values for adult animals are re-plotted on separate graphs; note that no significant changes occur in the adult samples. Error bars: SEM. $^*p = 0.03689$ (Mann-Whitney pairwise comparisons).

through lateral inhibition (Lewis, 1991; Eddison et al., 2000). The observation that inhibiting Notch signaling can generate ectopic hair cells at the expense of supporting cells (Takebayashi et al., 2007; Hayashi et al., 2008; Doetzlhofer et al., 2009; Korrapati et al., 2013; Mizutari et al., 2013; Bramhall et al., 2014), together with the observation that Notch signaling is re-deployed during avian hair cell regeneration (Stone and Rubel, 1999; Stone and Cotanche, 2007) has raised the possibility of targeting the Notch pathway in the damaged cochlea to effect hair cell replacement. However, results with Notch inhibitors in the adult cochlea have given variable results (Hori et al., 2007; Mizutari et al., 2013; Tona et al., 2014), prompting us to examine how this pathway is regulated as the cochlea matures. We show that the response of supporting cells to Notch inhibition drops dramatically in the first postnatal week, concomitant with a down-regulation of many components of the Notch signaling pathway.

Many studies have used gamma secretase inhibitors as a reagent to inhibit Notch signaling, despite the fact that gamma secretases are known to cleave scores of other transmembrane proteins in addition to Notch receptors (Kopan and Ilagan, 2004). Although it has generally been assumed that the conversion of supporting cells to hair cells in the presence of gamma secretase inhibitors is due to Notch inhibition, very few studies have tested this formally (Hayashi et al., 2008). We now show that the effects of the gamma secretase inhibitor DAPT on perinatal cochlear cultures—both in terms of the numbers of ectopic hair cells generated, in the down-regulation of Notch target genes and in the age-dependent response to these inhibitors—can be mimicked by blocking antibodies to the Notch1 receptor. While it remains formally possible that other gamma secretase-dependent signaling pathways are operating in perinatal supporting cells, our data suggest that the effect of inhibiting such pathways is negligible compared to their effect on Notch cleavage. We saw no evidence for supporting cell proliferation in our neonatal cultures treated with DAPT or Notch blocking antibodies (Doetzlhofer et al., 2009; data not shown). Conditional deletion of the Notch1 receptor, either at the otic placode stage (Kiernan et al., 2005a) or in neonatal mice (Li et al., 2015) has been reported to cause a small amount of supporting cell proliferation. Since these studies were both performed in intact animals, it is possible that the conditions used to establish organ cultures in our study militate against supporting cell proliferation when Notch signaling is blocked. Alternatively, it is possible that loss of a single allele in the *Sox2-CreER* and *Foxg1-Cre* knock-in lines used in these studies may interact genetically with *Notch1* mutants to cause abnormal proliferation. Indeed, haploinsufficiency of *Sox2* can modify the phenotype of $p27^{Kip1}$ mutants (Li et al., 2012), and *Foxg1-Cre* knock-in mice have been shown to have brain defects associated with proliferative defects on certain genetic backgrounds (Shen et al., 2006; Eagleson et al., 2007; Siegenthaler et al., 2008; see Cox et al., 2012 for further discussion).

We have characterized an age-dependent decline in the response of cochlear supporting cells to Notch inhibition in two ways. Our results from the most direct test of such age-dependence—treating cochlear tissue of different ages with Notch inhibitors (**Figure 3**)—are also supported by a careful analysis of basal-apical differences in the response of neonatal cochlear cultures to Notch inhibitors (**Figure 2**). Since hair cells and supporting cells in the mid-base of the cochlea differentiate at least 3 days before cells at the apex (Chen et al., 2002; Cai et al., 2013), analysis of whole cochlear explants allows us to directly compare different states of supporting cell differentiation in the same tissue. In P0 mice, we saw a higher proportion of ectopic outer hair cells vs. inner hair cells in the apex of the cochlea, and an even smaller proportion of ectopic inner hair cells at the base. Since inner hair cells begin to differentiate before outer hair cells in any given region of the cochlea (Chen et al., 2002; Cai et al., 2013), it is possible that these differences reflect a neural-abneural gradient of response to Notch inhibition as well as an apical-basal response. Alternatively, since different supporting cell types express different combinations of *Hes* and *Hey* genes (Zheng et al., 2000; Zine et al., 2001; Hayashi et al., 2008; Li et al., 2008; Doetzlhofer et al., 2009; Murata et al., 2009; Tateya et al., 2011), it is possible that these differences reflect the different sensitivities of these Notch target genes to Notch inhibition (Ong et al., 2006).

We observe a down-regulation of mRNA levels of Notch receptors, ligands and downstream effectors in the first postnatal week. The degree and rate of down-regulation varies, but analysis of Notch1 signaling in cochlear supporting cells over this time period (**Figure 5**; Murata et al., 2006; Basch et al., 2011) suggests that very little cleavage of the Notch1 receptor is occurring by the end of the first postnatal week. The mechanism of this down-regulation is currently not known, although given the absence of significant Notch pathway expression in the adult cochlea, it is possible that the loci of Notch pathway genes are becoming epigenetically modified and placed beyond use. It is also possible that this epigenetic silencing is accompanied by silencing of the direct targets of Notch effectors such as the Hes and Hey genes. However, it should be noted that the Notch pathway appears to be down-regulated in mature supporting cells in the chicken basilar papilla, as this sensory organ also fails to respond to gamma secretase inhibitors in the undamaged state (Daudet et al., 2009). Nevertheless, after damage, the Notch pathway is once again deployed in chicken supporting cells and the differentiating hair cells that they generate (Stone and Rubel, 1999; Daudet et al., 2009). It will therefore be of great interest to identify the epigenetic state of Notch pathway genes and their targets in mature mammalian supporting cells. It should also be noted that the co-expression of Jag1 and Sox2, which is seen in sensory patches from their first appearance (Kiernan et al., 2005b; Pan et al., 2010, 2013; Neves et al., 2011, 2012), is maintained in adult mouse supporting cells (Oesterle et al., 2008). It is thus formally possible that low levels of Notch signaling may persist in the adult cochlea and may maintain expression of these two genes by lateral induction. If this is the case, such signaling does not appear to confer competence for regeneration on supporting cells.

A recent study demonstrated that a small but significant number of new hair cells could be generated from supporting cells by treating noise-damaged animals with gamma secretase inhibitors (Mizutari et al., 2013), leading to a partial restoration of function. How can we reconcile these results with our data in the present study? First, it is possible that the Notch pathway can continue to regulate hair cell and supporting cell fate in the adult animal when expressed at significantly lower levels. We feel this is unlikely since binding of the Notch-ICD-MAML-RBPj complex to its target sites in the genome is likely to be severely compromised at low concentrations of Notch-ICD (Ong et al., 2006). Second, it is possible that a sub-population of supporting cells continue to express Notch pathway components at significant levels, but that these would not be detected when analyzing gene expression in the entire cochlea. In our single cell analysis of 123 P21 pillar cells and Deiters' cells, we were able to detect a very small number of cells in which Notch pathway components were expressed at comparable levels to their neonatal counterparts (**Figure 6**), and levels of *Hes5* and the hair cell marker *Atoh1* are more than 10-fold lower in the adult, even after noise damage (**Figure 7**). This suggests that if such cells persist in the adult cochlea, they are present in extremely small numbers. Finally, it is also possible that a second, Notch-independent pathway that can be targeted by gamma secretase inhibitors is operating in a small number of mature supporting cells. The effect of inhibiting this second pathway would be overshadowed by Notch inhibition in the neonatal cochlea, but might be uncovered in the adult cochlea when the Notch pathway is no longer active. It should also be noted that the noise damage protocol (Liu et al., 2011) used in our study—98 dB for 4 h—is significantly less severe than the protocol used by Mizutari et al. (116 dB for 2 h). However, the large and significant drop in *Atoh1* and *Hes5* levels we observe in undamaged adult tissue compared to neonatal animals still supports our observed down-regulation of Notch pathway genes in the first postnatal week.

In conclusion, our results suggest that the canonical Notch pathway is not active to any significant degree in the adult organ of Corti, and that the down-regulation of signaling occurs prior to the onset of hearing. The Notch pathway can therefore be viewed as a developmental scaffold for the organ of Corti—it is partly necessary for establishing the pattern and proportion of hair cells and supporting cells, but not necessary to maintain this pattern once it has been established. This suggests that inhibition of Notch signaling in the adult organ of Corti in the absence of other manipulations is unlikely to promote significant numbers of new hair cells, and that alternative or supplementary therapeutic interventions should be considered.

Acknowledgments

We thank Alyssa Crowder, Hongyuan Zhang and Huiling Li for excellent technical support. We thank Gerry Weinmaster, Urban Lendahl, Ryoichiro Kageyama and Manfred Gessler for gifts of cDNA probes. This work was supported by Department of Defense Grant DOD W81XWH-11-2-004 (AKG) and Hearing Restoration Project consortium grants from the Hearing Health Foundation (AKG and SH), NIH grant DC004563 (SH), NIH grant P30 DC010363 (SH, JSO), and NIH R01 DC014450 (JSO).

References

Abelló, G., Khatri, S., Giráldez, F., and Alsina, B. (2007). Early regionalization of the otic placode and its regulation by the Notch signaling pathway. *Mech. Dev.* 124, 631–645. doi: 10.1016/j.mod.2007.04.002

Adam, J., Myat, A., Le Roux, I., Eddison, M., Henrique, D., Ish-Horowicz, D., et al. (1998). Cell fate choices and the expression of Notch, Delta and Serrate homologues in the chick inner ear: parallels with Drosophila sense-organ development. *Development* 125, 4645–4654.

Artavanis-Tsakonas, S., and Muskavitch, M. A. (2010). Notch: the past, the present and the future. *Curr. Top. Dev. Biol.* 92, 1–29. doi: 10.1016/s0070-2153(10)92001-2

Artavanis-Tsakonas, S., Rand, M. D., and Lake, R. J. (1999). Notch signaling: cell fate control and signal integration in development. *Science* 284, 770–776. doi: 10.1126/science.284.5415.770

Basch, M. L., Ohyama, T., Segil, N., and Groves, A. K. (2011). Canonical Notch signaling is not necessary for prosensory induction in the mouse cochlea: insights from a conditional mutant of RBPjkappa. *J. Neurosci.* 31, 8046–8058. doi: 10.1523/jneurosci.6671-10.2011

Batts, S. A., Shoemaker, C. R., and Raphael, Y. (2009). Notch signaling and Hes labeling in the normal and drug-damaged organ of corti. *Hear. Res.* 249, 15–22. doi: 10.1016/j.heares.2008.12.008

Benito-Gonzalez, A., and Doetzlhofer, A. (2014). Hey1 and hey2 control the spatial and temporal pattern of mammalian auditory hair cell differentiation downstream of hedgehog signaling. *J. Neurosci.* 34, 12865–12876. doi: 10.1523/jneurosci.1494-14.2014

Birren, S. J., Lo, L., and Anderson, D. J. (1993). Sympathetic neuroblasts undergo a developmental switch in trophic dependence. *Development* 119, 597–610.

Bramhall, N. F., Shi, F., Arnold, K., Hochedlinger, K., and Edge, A. S. (2014). Lgr5-positive supporting cells generate new hair cells in the postnatal cochlea. *Stem Cell Reports* 2, 311–322. doi: 10.1016/j.stemcr.2014.01.008

Bray, S. J. (2006). Notch signalling: a simple pathway becomes complex. *Nat. Rev. Mol. Cell Biol.* 7, 678–689. doi: 10.1038/nrm2009

Brooker, R., Hozumi, K., and Lewis, J. (2006). Notch ligands with contrasting functions: Jagged1 and Delta1 in the mouse inner ear. *Development* 133, 1277–1286. doi: 10.1242/dev.02284

Cai, T., Seymour, M. L., Zhang, H., Pereira, F. A., and Groves, A. K. (2013). Conditional deletion of Atoh1 reveals distinct critical periods for survival and function of hair cells in the organ of corti. *J. Neurosci.* 33, 10110–10122. doi: 10.1523/JNEUROSCI.5606-12.2013

Chen, P., Johnson, J. E., Zoghbi, H. Y., and Segil, N. (2002). The role of Math1 in inner ear development: uncoupling the establishment of the sensory primordium from hair cell fate determination. *Development* 129, 2495–2505.

Chitnis, A. B. (1995). The role of Notch in lateral inhibition and cell fate specification. *Mol. Cell. Neurosci.* 6, 311–321. doi: 10.1006/mcne.1995.1024

Cox, B. C., Liu, Z., Lagarde, M. M., and Zuo, J. (2012). Conditional gene expression in the mouse inner ear using Cre-loxP. *J. Assoc. Res. Otolaryngol.* 13, 295–322. doi: 10.1007/s10162-012-0324-5

Daudet, N., Ariza-Mcnaughton, L., and Lewis, J. (2007). Notch signalling is needed to maintain, but not to initiate, the formation of prosensory patches in the chick inner ear. *Development* 134, 2369–2378. doi: 10.1242/dev.001842

Daudet, N., Gibson, R., Shang, J., Bernard, A., Lewis, J., and Stone, J. (2009). Notch regulation of progenitor cell behavior in quiescent and regenerating auditory epithelium of mature birds. *Dev. Biol.* 326, 86–100. doi: 10.1016/j.ydbio.2008.10.033

Daudet, N., and Lewis, J. (2005). Two contrasting roles for Notch activity in chick inner ear development: specification of prosensory patches and lateral inhibition of hair-cell differentiation. *Development* 132, 541–551. doi: 10.1242/dev.01589

Doetzlhofer, A., Basch, M. L., Ohyama, T., Gessler, M., Groves, A. K., and Segil, N. (2009). Hey2 regulation by FGF provides a Notch-independent mechanism for maintaining pillar cell fate in the organ of corti. *Dev. Cell* 16, 58–69. doi: 10.1016/j.devcel.2008.11.008

Durruthy-Durruthy, R., Gottlieb, A., Hartman, B. H., Waldhaus, J., Laske, R. D., Altman, R., et al. (2014). Reconstruction of the mouse otocyst and early neuroblast lineage at single-cell resolution. *Cell* 157, 964–978. doi: 10.1016/j.cell.2014.03.036

Eagleson, K. L., Schlueter Mcfadyen-Ketchum, L. J., Ahrens, E. T., Mills, P. H., Does, M. D., Nickols, J., et al. (2007). Disruption of Foxg1 expression by knock-in of cre recombinase: effects on the development of the mouse telencephalon. *Neuroscience* 148, 385–399. doi: 10.1016/j.neuroscience.2007.06.012

Eddison, M., Le Roux, I., and Lewis, J. (2000). Notch signaling in the development of the inner ear: lessons from Drosophila. *Proc. Natl. Acad. Sci. U S A* 97, 11692–11699. doi: 10.1073/pnas.97.22.11692

Formosa-Jordan, P., Ibañes, M., Ares, S., and Frade, J. M. (2013). Lateral inhibition and neurogenesis: novel aspects in motion. *Int. J. Dev. Biol.* 57, 341–350. doi: 10.1387/ijdb.120259jf

Groves, A. K., and Fekete, D. M. (2012). Shaping sound in space: the regulation of inner ear patterning. *Development* 139, 245–257. doi: 10.1242/dev.067074

Groves, A. K., George, K. M., Tissier-Seta, J. P., Engel, J. D., Brunet, J. F., and Anderson, D. J. (1995). Differential regulation of transcription factor gene expression and phenotypic markers in developing sympathetic neurons. *Development* 121, 887–901.

Harland, R. M. (1991). *In situ* hybridization: an improved whole-mount method for Xenopus embryos. *Methods Cell Biol.* 36, 685–695. doi: 10.1016/s0091-679x(08)60307-6

Hartman, B. H., Basak, O., Nelson, B. R., Taylor, V., Bermingham-Mcdonogh, O., and Reh, T. A. (2009). Hes5 expression in the postnatal and adult mouse inner ear and the drug-damaged cochlea. *J. Assoc. Res. Otolaryngol.* 10, 321–340. doi: 10.1007/s10162-009-0162-2

Hartman, B. H., Hayashi, T., Nelson, B. R., Bermingham-Mcdonogh, O., and Reh, T. A. (2007). Dll3 is expressed in developing hair cells in the mammalian cochlea. *Dev. Dyn.* 236, 2875–2883. doi: 10.1002/dvdy.21307

Hartman, B. H., Reh, T. A., and Bermingham-Mcdonogh, O. (2010). Notch signaling specifies prosensory domains via lateral induction in the developing mammalian inner ear. *Proc. Natl. Acad. Sci. U S A* 107, 15792–15797. doi: 10.1073/pnas.1002827107

Hayashi, T., Kokubo, H., Hartman, B. H., Ray, C. A., Reh, T. A., and Bermingham-Mcdonogh, O. (2008). Hesr1 and Hesr2 may act as early effectors of Notch signaling in the developing cochlea. *Dev. Biol.* 316, 87–99. doi: 10.1016/j.ydbio.2008.01.006

Hori, R., Nakagawa, T., Sakamoto, T., Matsuoka, Y., Takebayashi, S., and Ito, J. (2007). Pharmacological inhibition of Notch signaling in the mature guinea pig cochlea. *Neuroreport* 18, 1911–1914. doi: 10.1097/wnr.0b013e3282f213e0

Hori, K., Sen, A., and Artavanis-Tsakonas, S. (2013). Notch signaling at a glance. *J. Cell Sci.* 126, 2135–2140. doi: 10.1242/jcs.127308

Ilagan, M. X., and Kopan, R. (2007). SnapShot: notch signaling pathway. *Cell* 128, 1246.e1–1246.e2. doi: 10.1016/j.cell.2007.03.011

Jayasena, C. S., Ohyama, T., Segil, N., and Groves, A. K. (2008). Notch signaling augments the canonical Wnt pathway to specify the size of the otic placode. *Development* 135, 2251–2261. doi: 10.1242/dev.017905

Kelley, M. W. (2003). Cell adhesion molecules during inner ear and hair cell development, including notch and its ligands. *Curr. Top. Dev. Biol.* 57, 321–356. doi: 10.1016/s0070-2153(03)57011-9

Kelley, M. W. (2006). Regulation of cell fate in the sensory epithelia of the inner ear. *Nat. Rev. Neurosci.* 7, 837–849. doi: 10.1038/nrn1987

Kelley, M. W. (2007). Cellular commitment and differentiation in the organ of corti. *Int. J. Dev. Biol.* 51, 571–583. doi: 10.1387/ijdb.072388mk

Khatri, S. B., and Groves, A. K. (2013). Expression of the Foxi2 and Foxi3 transcription factors during development of chicken sensory placodes and pharyngeal arches. *Gene Expr. Patterns* 13, 38–42. doi: 10.1016/j.gep.2012.10.001

Kiernan, A. E. (2013). Notch signaling during cell fate determination in the inner ear. *Semin. Cell Dev. Biol.* 24, 470–479. doi: 10.1016/j.semcdb.2013.04.002

Kiernan, A. E., Cordes, R., Kopan, R., Gossler, A., and Gridley, T. (2005a). The Notch ligands DLL1 and JAG2 act synergistically to regulate hair cell development in the mammalian inner ear. *Development* 132, 4353–4362. doi: 10.1242/dev.02002

Kiernan, A. E., Pelling, A. L., Leung, K. K., Tang, A. S., Bell, D. M., Tease, C., et al. (2005b). Sox2 is required for sensory organ development in the mammalian inner ear. *Nature* 434, 1031–1035. doi: 10.1038/nature03487

Kopan, R., and Ilagan, M. X. (2004). Gamma-secretase: proteasome of the membrane? *Nat. Rev. Mol. Cell Biol.* 5, 499–504. doi: 10.1038/nrm1406

Korrapati, S., Roux, I., Glowatzki, E., and Doetzlhofer, A. (2013). Notch signaling limits supporting cell plasticity in the hair cell-damaged early postnatal murine cochlea. *PLoS One* 8:e73276. doi: 10.1371/journal.pone.0073276

Lewis, J. (1991). Rules for the production of sensory cells. *Ciba Found. Symp.* 160, 25–39; discussion 40–53.

Li, H., Collado, M., Villasante, A., Matheu, A., Lynch, C. J., Cañamero, M., et al. (2012). p27(Kip1) directly represses Sox2 during embryonic stem cell differentiation. *Cell Stem Cell* 11, 845–852. doi: 10.1016/j.stem.2012.09.014

Li, S., Mark, S., Radde-Gallwitz, K., Schlisner, R., Chin, M. T., and Chen, P. (2008). Hey2 functions in parallel with Hes1 and Hes5 for mammalian auditory sensory organ development. *BMC Dev. Biol.* 8:20. doi: 10.1186/1471-213X-8-20

Li, W., Wu, J., Yang, J., Sun, S., Chai, R., Chen, Z. Y., et al. (2015). Notch inhibition induces mitotically generated hair cells in mammalian cochleae via activating the Wnt pathway. *Proc. Natl. Acad. Sci. U S A* 112, 166–171. doi: 10.1073/pnas.1415901112

Lin, V., Golub, J. S., Nguyen, T. B., Hume, C. R., Oesterle, E. C., and Stone, J. S. (2011). Inhibition of Notch activity promotes nonmitotic regeneration of hair cells in the adult mouse utricles. *J. Neurosci.* 31, 15329–15339. doi: 10.1523/JNEUROSCI.2057-11.2011

Liu, C. C., Gao, S. S., Yuan, T., Steele, C., Puria, S., and Oghalai, J. S. (2011). Biophysical mechanisms underlying outer hair cell loss associated with a shortened tectorial membrane. *J. Assoc. Res. Otolaryngol.* 12, 577–594. doi: 10.1007/s10162-011-0269-0

Liu, Z., Liu, Z., Walters, B. J., Owen, T., Kopan, R., and Zuo, J. (2013). *In vivo* visualization of Notch1 proteolysis reveals the heterogeneity of Notch1 signaling activity in the mouse cochlea. *PLoS One* 8:e64903. doi: 10.1371/journal.pone.0064903

Liu, Z., Owen, T., Fang, J., Srinivasan, R. S., and Zuo, J. (2012a). *In vivo* Notch reactivation in differentiating cochlear hair cells induces Sox2 and Prox1 expression but does not disrupt hair cell maturation. *Dev. Dyn.* 241, 684–696. doi: 10.1002/dvdy.23754

Liu, Z., Owen, T., Fang, J., and Zuo, J. (2012b). Overactivation of Notch1 signaling induces ectopic hair cells in the mouse inner ear in an age-dependent manner. *PLoS One* 7:e34123. doi: 10.1371/journal.pone.0034123

Lumpkin, E. A., Collisson, T., Parab, P., Omer-Abdalla, A., Haeberle, H., Chen, P., et al. (2003). Math1-driven GFP expression in the developing nervous system of transgenic mice. *Gene Expr. Patterns* 3, 389–395. doi: 10.1016/s1567-133x(03)00089-9

Mizutari, K., Fujioka, M., Hosoya, M., Bramhall, N., Okano, H. J., Okano, H., et al. (2013). Notch inhibition induces cochlear hair cell regeneration and recovery of hearing after acoustic trauma. *Neuron* 77, 58–69. doi: 10.1016/j.neuron.2012.10.032

Morimoto, M., Liu, Z., Cheng, H. T., Winters, N., Bader, D., and Kopan, R. (2010). Canonical Notch signaling in the developing lung is required for determination of arterial smooth muscle cells and selection of Clara versus ciliated cell fate. *J. Cell Sci.* 123, 213–224. doi: 10.1242/jcs.058669

Murata, J., Ikeda, K., and Okano, H. (2012). Notch signaling and the developing inner ear. *Adv. Exp. Med. Biol.* 727, 161–173. doi: 10.1007/978-1-4614-0899-4_12

Murata, J., Ohtsuka, T., Tokunaga, A., Nishiike, S., Inohara, H., Okano, H., et al. (2009). Notch-Hes1 pathway contributes to the cochlear prosensory formation potentially through the transcriptional down-regulation of p27Kip1. *J. Neurosci. Res.* 87, 3521–3534. doi: 10.1002/jnr.22169

Murata, J., Tokunaga, A., Okano, H., and Kubo, T. (2006). Mapping of notch activation during cochlear development in mice: implications for determination of prosensory domain and cell fate diversification. *J. Comp. Neurol.* 497, 502–518. doi: 10.1002/cne.20997

Neves, J., Abelló, G., Petrovic, J., and Giraldez, F. (2013a). Patterning and cell fate in the inner ear: a case for Notch in the chicken embryo. *Dev. Growth Differ.* 55, 96–112. doi: 10.1111/dgd.12016

Neves, J., Parada, C., Chamizo, M., and Giráldez, F. (2011). Jagged 1 regulates the restriction of Sox2 expression in the developing chicken inner ear: a mechanism for sensory organ specification. *Development* 138, 735–744. doi: 10.1242/dev.060657

Neves, J., Uchikawa, M., Bigas, A., and Giraldez, F. (2012). The prosensory function of Sox2 in the chicken inner ear relies on the direct regulation of Atoh1. *PLoS One* 7:e30871. doi: 10.1371/journal.pone.0030871

Neves, J., Vachkov, I., and Giraldez, F. (2013b). Sox2 regulation of hair cell development: incoherence makes sense. *Hear. Res.* 297, 20–29. doi: 10.1016/j.heares.2012.11.003

Oesterle, E. C., Campbell, S., Taylor, R. R., Forge, A., and Hume, C. R. (2008). Sox2 and JAGGED1 expression in normal and drug-damaged adult mouse inner ear. *J. Assoc. Res. Otolaryngol.* 9, 65–89. doi: 10.1007/s10162-007-0106-7

Ong, C. T., Cheng, H. T., Chang, L. W., Ohtsuka, T., Kageyama, R., Stormo, G. D., et al. (2006). Target selectivity of vertebrate notch proteins. Collaboration between discrete domains and CSL-binding site architecture determines activation probability. *J. Biol. Chem.* 281, 5106–5119. doi: 10.1074/jbc.m506108200

Pan, W., Jin, Y., Chen, J., Rottier, R. J., Steel, K. P., and Kiernan, A. E. (2013). Ectopic expression of activated notch or SOX2 reveals similar and unique roles in the development of the sensory cell progenitors in the mammalian inner ear. *J. Neurosci.* 33, 16146–16157. doi: 10.1523/JNEUROSCI.3150-12.2013

Pan, W., Jin, Y., Stanger, B., and Kiernan, A. E. (2010). Notch signaling is required for the generation of hair cells and supporting cells in the mammalian inner ear. *Proc. Natl. Acad. Sci. U S A* 107, 15798–15803. doi: 10.1073/pnas.1003089107

Rose, M. F., Ren, J., Ahmad, K. A., Chao, H. T., Klisch, T. J., Flora, A., et al. (2009). Math1 is essential for the development of hindbrain neurons critical for perinatal breathing. *Neuron* 64, 341–354. doi: 10.1016/j.neuron.2009.10.023

Shen, L., Nam, H. S., Song, P., Moore, H., and Anderson, S. A. (2006). FoxG1 haploinsufficiency results in impaired neurogenesis in the postnatal hippocampus and contextual memory deficits. *Hippocampus* 16, 875–890. doi: 10.1002/hipo.20218

Siegenthaler, J. A., Tremper-Wells, B. A., and Miller, M. W. (2008). Foxg1 haploinsufficiency reduces the population of cortical intermediate progenitor cells: effect of increased p21 expression. *Cereb. Cortex* 18, 1865–1875. doi: 10.1093/cercor/bhm209

Slowik, A. D., and Bermingham-McDonogh, O. (2013). Hair cell generation by notch inhibition in the adult mammalian cristae. *J. Assoc. Res. Otolaryngol.* 14, 813–828. doi: 10.1007/s10162-013-0414-z

Stern, C. D. (1998). Detection of multiple gene products simultaneously by *in situ* hybridization and immunohistochemistry in whole mounts of avian embryos. *Curr. Top. Dev. Biol.* 36, 223–243. doi: 10.1016/s0070-2153(08)60505-0

Stone, J. S., and Cotanche, D. A. (2007). Hair cell regeneration in the avian auditory epithelium. *Int. J. Dev. Biol.* 51, 633–647. doi: 10.1387/ijdb.072408js

Stone, J. S., and Rubel, E. W. (1999). Delta1 expression during avian hair cell regeneration. *Development* 126, 961–973.

Takebayashi, S., Yamamoto, N., Yabe, D., Fukuda, H., Kojima, K., Ito, J., et al. (2007). Multiple roles of Notch signaling in cochlear development. *Dev. Biol.* 307, 165–178. doi: 10.1016/j.ydbio.2007.04.035

Tateya, T., Imayoshi, I., Tateya, I., Ito, J., and Kageyama, R. (2011). Cooperative functions of Hes/Hey genes in auditory hair cell and supporting cell development. *Dev. Biol.* 352, 329–340. doi: 10.1016/j.ydbio.2011.01.038

Tona, Y., Hamaguchi, K., Ishikawa, M., Miyoshi, T., Yamamoto, N., Yamahara, K., et al. (2014). Therapeutic potential of a gamma-secretase inhibitor for hearing restoration in a guinea pig model with noise-induced hearing loss. *BMC Neurosci.* 15:66. doi: 10.1186/1471-2202-15-66

Wang, G. P., Chatterjee, I., Batts, S. A., Wong, H. T., Gong, T. W., Gong, S. S., et al. (2010). Notch signaling and Atoh1 expression during hair cell regeneration in the mouse utricle. *Hear. Res.* 267, 61–70. doi: 10.1016/j.heares.2010.03.085

Wu, Y., Cain-Hom, C., Choy, L., Hagenbeek, T. J., de Leon, G. P., Chen, Y., et al. (2010). Therapeutic antibody targeting of individual Notch receptors. *Nature* 464, 1052–1057. doi: 10.1038/nature08878

Xia, A., Song, Y., Wang, R., Gao, S. S., Clifton, W., Raphael, P., et al. (2013). Prestin regulation and function in residual outer hair cells after noise-induced hearing loss. *PLoS One* 8:e82602. doi: 10.1371/journal.pone.0082602

Yamamoto, N., Chang, W., and Kelley, M. W. (2011). Rbpj regulates development of prosensory cells in the mammalian inner ear. *Dev. Biol.* 353, 367–379. doi: 10.1016/j.ydbio.2011.03.016

Yamamoto, N., Tanigaki, K., Tsuji, M., Yabe, D., Ito, J., and Honjo, T. (2006). Inhibition of Notch/RBP-J signaling induces hair cell formation in neonate mouse cochleas. *J. Mol. Med. (Berl)* 84, 37–45. doi: 10.1007/s00109-005-0706-9

Young, K. M., Mitsumori, T., Pringle, N., Grist, M., Kessaris, N., and Richardson, W. D. (2010). An Fgfr3-iCreER(T2) transgenic mouse line for studies of neural stem cells and astrocytes. *Glia* 58, 943–953. doi: 10.1002/glia.20976

Zheng, J. L., Shou, J., Guillemot, F., Kageyama, R., and Gao, W. Q. (2000). Hes1 is a negative regulator of inner ear hair cell differentiation. *Development* 127, 4551–4560.

Zine, A., Aubert, A., Qiu, J., Therianos, S., Guillemot, F., Kageyama, R., et al. (2001). Hes1 and Hes5 activities are required for the normal development of the hair cells in the mammalian inner ear. *J. Neurosci.* 21, 4712–4720.

Zine, A., Van De Water, T. R., and de Ribaupierre, F. (2000). Notch signaling regulates the pattern of auditory hair cell differentiation in mammals. *Development* 127, 3373–3383.

17

Numb is not a critical regulator of Notch-mediated cell fate decisions in the developing chick inner ear

Mark Eddison[1], Sara J. Weber[2], Linda Ariza-McNaughton[3], Julian Lewis[4†] and Nicolas Daudet[2]*

[1] Howard Hughes Medical Institute, Janelia Research Campus, Ashburn, VA, USA, [2] Ear Institute, University College London, London, UK, [3] Haematopoietic Stem cell Laboratory, Cancer Research UK, London Research Institute, London, UK, [4] Formerly of Vertebrate Development Laboratory, Cancer Research UK, London, UK

Edited by:
Andy Groves,
Baylor College of Medicine, USA

Reviewed by:
Fernando Giraldez,
Universitat Pompeu Fabra, Spain
Raj Ladher,
RIKEN Center for Developmental Biology, Japan

***Correspondence:**
Nicolas Daudet,
Ear Institute, University College London, 332 Gray's Inn Road, London WC1X 8EE, UK
n.daudet@ucl.ac.uk
† Deceased.

The Notch signaling pathway controls differentiation of hair cells and supporting cells in the vertebrate inner ear. Here, we have investigated whether Numb, a known regulator of Notch activity in *Drosophila*, is involved in this process in the embryonic chick. The chicken homolog of Numb is expressed throughout the otocyst at early stages of development and is concentrated at the basal pole of the cells. It is asymmetrically allocated at some cell divisions, as in *Drosophila*, suggesting that it could act as a determinant inherited by one of the two daughter cells and favoring adoption of a hair-cell fate. To test the implication of Numb in hair cell fate decisions and the regulation of Notch signaling, we used different methods to overexpress Numb at different stages of inner ear development. We found that sustained or late Numb overexpression does not promote hair cell differentiation, and Numb does not prevent the reception of Notch signaling. Surprisingly, none of the Numb-overexpressing cells differentiated into hair cells, suggesting that high levels of Numb protein could interfere with intracellular processes essential for hair cell survival. However, when Numb was overexpressed early and more transiently during ear development, no effect on hair cell formation was seen. These results suggest that in the inner ear at least, Numb does not significantly repress Notch activity and that its asymmetric distribution in dividing precursor cells does not govern the choice between hair cell and supporting cell fates.

Keywords: Numb, asymmetric cell division, Notch, lateral inhibition, inner ear, chick, hair cells

Introduction

In many tissues, the Notch pathway mediates lateral inhibition and thereby governs cell diversification: cells expressing high levels of Notch ligands activate Notch in neighboring cells and in this way force them to adopt a different fate. This process has been well studied in the developing mechanosensory bristles of *Drosophila*, and parallels between these insect sensillae and the mechanosensory epithelia of the vertebrate inner ear have guided our understanding of vertebrate ear development, and in particular of the role of Notch signaling in this process (Adam et al., 1998; Eddison et al., 2000).

Each insect bristle derives from a single sense-organ precursor (SOP) cell that undergoes a stereotyped sequence of asymmetric cell divisions. After each division, the two daughter cells adopt distinct cell fates that depend on the levels of Notch activation that they experience (Hartenstein and Posakony, 1990). In principle, the difference between the two cells could be generated through a feedback loop based on the ability of activated Notch to inhibit expression of Notch ligands (Chitnis, 1995; Heitzler et al., 1996). Such an effect, if present, means that neighboring cells will interact competitively, each tending to inhibit the other; and mathematical modeling shows that this competitive interaction can be sufficient to amplify any initial small difference between the cells and so to drive them along distinct paths of differentiation (Collier et al., 1996). In many cases, however, and in particular in insect bristle development, it appears that the interaction between sister cells is strongly biased from the outset by modulators of Notch signaling, such as Numb or Neuralized, which are asymmetrically localized in the parent cell and unequally distributed to the daughter cells after mitosis (see for reviews Roegiers and Jan, 2004; Schweisguth, 2004). The daughter cell that receives the favorable inheritance wins the competition and delivers overwhelming inhibition to its sister (and to other neighbors). In this paper, we focus on one of these modulators, Numb, and examine its role in the development of the sensory patches in the vertebrate inner ear. Does it act there, as it does in the insect bristle, to control choices of cell fate?

The *numb* gene takes its name from the *Drosophila* phenotype. Flies with loss-of-function mutations in this gene lack functional sensillae, because the daughters and grand-daughters of the SOP cells fail to diversify correctly: in place of a bristle consisting of a shaft cell, a socket cell, a neuron, and a neural sheath cell, the SOP generates a cluster of four socket cells. Conversely, artificial overexpression of *numb* can bias cell fate choices in an opposite way, causing the SOP cell (in extreme cases) to generate a cluster of four neurons (Uemura et al., 1989; Rhyu et al., 1994; Knoblich et al., 1995). The Numb gene product is a membrane-associated protein that has a conserved phosphotyrosine binding (PTB) domain and several conserved protein-protein interaction motifs in its proline-rich C-terminal region, representing binding sites for alpha-adaptin and a variety of other components of the machinery of clathrin-mediated endocytosis and ubiquitylation (Santolini et al., 2000). In the SOP lineage, Numb is asymmetrically localized at mitosis and influences cell fate decisions by reducing Notch activity in the cell that inherits it after an asymmetrical cell division (Frise et al., 1996; Guo et al., 1996; Spana and Doe, 1996; Bhalerao et al., 2005). Numb may exert its inhibitory effect by direct binding to the cytoplasmic domain of Notch (Guo et al., 1996; Zhong et al., 1996), by promoting the internalization and/or degradation of cell-surface Notch protein (Santolini et al., 2000; Berdnik et al., 2002; McGill and McGlade, 2003), by interfering with positive modulators of Notch signaling such as the transmembrane protein Sanpodo (O'Connor-Giles and Skeath, 2003; Hutterer and Knoblich, 2005; Couturier et al., 2012; Cotton et al., 2013), or by a combination of these actions.

The Notch pathway is a critical regulator of inner ear development, acting at different stages and through different ligands to control the differentiation of multiple cell types (Kiernan, 2013). Lateral inhibition regulates the production of otic neuroblasts at early stages of ear development (Adam et al., 1998; Haddon et al., 1998; Abello et al., 2007; Daudet et al., 2007), and controls hair cells vs. supporting cell fate decisions within the embryonic sensory patches (Adam et al., 1998; Lanford et al., 1999; Riley et al., 1999; Zine et al., 2000; Daudet and Lewis, 2005; Chrysostomou et al., 2012). The nascent hair cells express several Notch ligands: Delta1-like 1 (Dll1), Delta-like 3 (Dll3), and Serrate2/Jagged2 (Jag2) and activate Notch in their neighbors, which become supporting cells. The puzzling feature of the system is that the progenitor and supporting cells themselves express a Notch ligand, Jagged1 (Jag1, also known as Serrate1 in chick), which is positively regulated by Notch, a process defined as "lateral induction" (Adam et al., 1998; Lewis, 1998; Eddison et al., 2000). Jag1 contributes to the maintenance of Notch activity within progenitor cells (Neves et al., 2011), and this early phase of Notch activity is required for the maintenance, but not the initial specification, of the prosensory regions (Kiernan et al., 2001, 2006; Tsai et al., 2001; Brooker, 2006; Daudet et al., 2007; Hartman et al., 2010; Basch et al., 2011; Yamamoto et al., 2011). Although the levels of Notch activity elicited by Jag1 are thought to be relatively low compared to those resulting from Dll1 signaling (Petrovic et al., 2014), they still provide a potential obstacle to hair cell differentiation. Furthermore, direct contacts between immature hair cells or between immature hair cells and Dll1-expressing cells occur at least transiently during the development of the sensory epithelia (Goodyear and Richardson, 1997; Chrysostomou et al., 2012). How then, during normal development, do the nascent hair cells overcome Notch activation? In a previous study (Eddison et al., 2000), we reported that chicken Numb is expressed in the embryonic inner ear, and that its distribution makes it a plausible candidate to facilitate hair cell fate decisions. Because hair cells and supporting cells are derived from a common progenitor (Fekete et al., 1998; Lang and Fekete, 2001), they may perhaps be generated through asymmetric cell divisions analogous to those occurring in the insect bristle lineage.

Here, we have analyzed Numb expression pattern during chick inner ear development and have found that Numb is indeed sometimes inherited asymmetrically by the daughters of dividing precursor cells in the sensory patches. To test whether this is functionally significant, we have used *in ovo* electroporation of plasmid DNA to raise the levels of expression of Numb and analyzed the effects on hair cell fate decisions and on the endogenous levels of Notch activity. Our results indicate that Numb is not a strong inhibitor of Notch activity in the inner ear, and that it has no direct influence upon whether cells become hair cells or supporting cells. However, sustained Numb overexpression seems to impair hair cell differentiation, possibly by interfering with endocytosis or some other process important for hair cell maturation or survival.

Materials and Methods

Plasmids

We used RT-PCR to isolate from E6 chicken inner ear total RNA the full-length coding sequence of chicken Numb. In mammals, four Numb isoforms can be generated by alternative splicing (Dho et al., 1999; Verdi et al., 1999). From eight individual cloned cDNAs that we isolated by RT-PCR in the chick, one encoded an isoform with a 26 amino acid insert (LPSVIALDLSPLFLQERKFFKGFFGK) in the PTB domain, and was analogous to the human Numb isoform 2 (Verdi et al., 1999), although the chicken insert we isolated is 15 amino-acids longer than the human one and possibly represents a rare splicing variant. The remaining clones encoded an isoform that had no inserts in either the PTB or the C-terminal proline-rich region and resembled both the human Numb isoform 4 and the previously isolated chicken Numb (Wakamatsu et al., 1999). This chicken Numb isoform was almost perfectly identical to the peptide sequence ENSGALP00000015120, the product of the predicted Ensembl chicken *Numb* genomic sequence ENSGALG00000009300. The coding sequence of these two Numb isoforms (cNumb2 and cNumb4) have been deposited in Genbank (KP756695 and KP756696).

The full-length chicken Numb coding sequences were subcloned into RCAS(B) constructs (Morgan and Fekete, 1996), into the bicistronic pIRES2-EGFP expression vector (Clontech), or into Tol2 vectors enabling Tet-ON regulated gene expression (Freeman and Daudet, 2012; Freeman et al., 2012). Plasmid DNA solutions were prepared using a plasmid purification kit (Qiagen, United Kingdom) and diluted for electroporation to 0.8–1 μg/μl in water tinted with Fast Green for visualization.

Electroporation and Retroviral Infection of Embryonic Chick Inner Ear

Fertile white Leghorn eggs were incubated at 38°C and embryos were staged according to Hamburger–Hamilton (HH) tables. All procedures carried out on chicken embryos were approved by University College London and the UK Home Office. Micro-electroporation of the otic cup with plasmid DNA was performed at HH stages 13–15 (2–2.5 days of incubation) as described in Freeman et al. (2012). After electroporation, eggs were sealed with tape and returned to incubation at 38°C. Some embryos were further treated with Doxycyclin for *in ovo* induction of gene expression at E6 or E7. The numbers of positive embryos analyzed for each type of expression construct were as follows: RCAS-Numb: 35; RCAS-GFP: 12; Numb-IRES2-EGFP: 26; pTRE-Numb-FP635: 20; pTRE-FP635: 8.

Immunocytochemistry

Embryos were decapitated and their heads immersed in 4% paraformaldehyde in PBS at 4°C for 2–12 h. For whole-mount immunostaining, the membranous part of the inner ear was dissected out from the surrounding cartilage and incubated for 1 h in PBS containing 0.3% Triton X100 and 10% goat serum. All subsequent incubations and rinses were performed in PBS with 0.1% Triton X100 (PBT). Incubations with primary and secondary antibodies were carried out in PBT for 2 h at room temperature or overnight at 4°C. Antibodies and reagents used were: rabbit serum anti-Numb (Wakamatsu et al., 1999, 1/500), rabbit serum anti-GFP (Molecular Probes, 1/2000), mouse monoclonal IgG1 anti-Hair Cell Antigen (HCA, Bartolami et al., 1991, 1/100), mouse monoclonal IgG2a anti-HCS-1/Otoferlin (Gale et al., 2000, 1/100), mouse monoclonal IgG2b anti-TuJ1 (Covance, UK, 1/1000), Alexa 488-, 594-, and 633-conjugated goat IgG secondary antibodies (Molecular Probes, The Netherlands; 1/500 dilution), Alexa 633-conjugated phalloidin (Molecular Probes, 1/100). Nuclei were stained with either DAPI or Syto16. Specimens were mounted in Slowfade (Molecular Probes) and observed under a Zeiss LSM510 confocal microscope. For cryosectioning, embryo heads were fixed as described above, then immersed in a graded series of sucrose-PBS (5-10-20%), embedded in 1.7% agar with 5% sucrose, frozen at −20°C, and cryosectioned at 15 μm thickness.

Whole-Mount *In Situ* Hybridization

DIG-labeled RNA antisense probes were prepared from a plasmid encoding chick *Hes5.1* (a kind gift of Dr Domingos Henrique). Whole-mount in situ hybridization was performed as in Ariza-Mcnaughton and Krumlauf (2002) with minor modifications. DIG-labeled RNA probes were detected with an anti-DIG peroxidase-tagged antibody (diluted 1:100) and either the TSA-FITC or the TSA-Cy3 amplification system (Perkin Elmer). Following *in situ* hybridization, specimens were processed for Numb or TuJ1 immunostaining as described above.

Quantification of Fluorescence and Statistical Analysis

Samples co-transfected with the pT2-Hes5::nd2EGFP and either the pTRE-Numb-FP635 or the pTRE-FP635 (control) Tol2 plasmids were fixed for 2 h at room temperature and processed for immunostaining for MyoVIIa/HCA using Alexa 647-conjugated secondary antibody as described above. Confocal stacks (12 bits) were acquired within transfected sensory regions and the mean values of fluorescence intensity for the red ($Fluo_{Red}$) and green ($Fluo_{Green}$) channels within the nucleus of individual cells were collected using ImageJ and the Time Series Analyzer plugin (Schneider et al., 2012). For each confocal stack, mean values and standard deviation (S.D.) for the background levels of red fluorescence ($Fluo_{Bgd}$) were also collected from at least five untransfected cells. Cells with $Fluo_{Red} > (Fluo_{Bdg} + 2\times$ S.D $Fluo_{Bgd})$ were classified as induced cells. In order to compare data across experiments, Z-scoring values for $Fluo_{Red}$ and $Fluo_{Green}$ were computed for all the cells analyzed in each confocal stack. Statistical analysis of the data and graphs were made with the OriginPro 9.1 software (OriginLab Corporation).

Results

Numb is Expressed in Dividing Progenitor Cells in the Chick Inner Ear

The inner ear develops from the otic placode, a thickening of the head ectoderm visible from stage 10 (36 h of incubation) in the chick embryo. The placode invaginates to first form a cup, then a hollow epithelial sphere named the otic vesicle. At these early stages, Numb protein is detected throughout the otic epithelium, in both presumptive sensory and non-sensory regions (**Figures 1A,B**). As in the neural tube, Numb is expressed in the majority of cells and is strongly localized to the basal surface. At mitosis, when a cell moves its nucleus to the apical surface, Numb forms a characteristic crescent on the more basal side of the cell. This persistent basal localization of Numb is independent of the orientation of the cleavage plane. We found that cleavage planes were quite variable: some were perpendicular to the plane of the epithelium ("vertical"), producing two cells that lay side by side

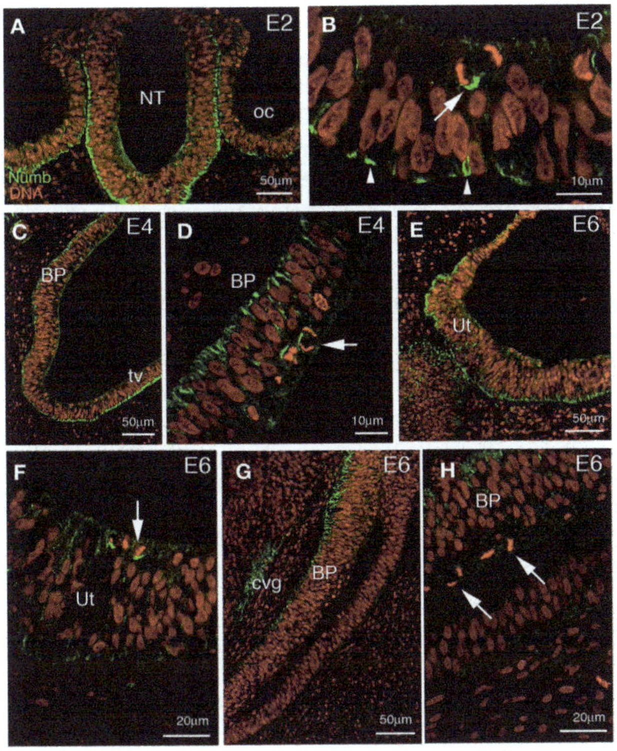

FIGURE 1 | Numb expression at early stages of chick inner ear development. Transverse sections through the hindbrain and parallel to the future longitudinal axis of the cochlea. **(A)** Low power picture at 2 days of incubation (E2) showing the hindbrain and adjacent otic vesicles. Numb is expressed throughout the otic epithelium and neuroepithelium. **(B)** Higher power views of the otic epithelium. The staining is predominantly basal (arrowheads) and remains on the basal side of cells rounded up for mitosis. Note the asymmetric division (arrow) where Numb is preferentially segregated into one of the two daughter cells. **(C)** At E4, Numb is expressed in all of the cells of the future basilar papilla (BP), and also in the non-sensory region (presumptive tegmentum vasculosum, tv). Basal Numb crescents can be seen in mitotic cells at the apical surface. **(D)** Detail of the same future basilar papilla, showing basal Numb crescents in mitotic cells (arrow). **(E)** Developing utricle (Ut) at E6. Numb is still expressed throughout the epithelium and is basal. **(F)** Detail of **(E)**; in the majority of utricular mitotic cells, basal Numb crescents can still be seen (arrow). **(G)** Developing basilar papilla (BP) at E6. Numb is basally localized in the epithelium, and is also seen in the cochleovestibular ganglion (cvg). **(H)** Detail of **(G)**; no Numb crescents are detected in the mitotic cells here (arrows).

in the epithelium; others were tilted (though rarely horizontal) such that a division produced one cell more apically and one cell more basally (**Figure 1B**). Because Numb is always basal, a vertical (symmetrical) cleavage will presumably entail that both daughters inherit Numb, while in a tilted (asymmetrical) cleavage only the basal daughter will do so.

As the otic vesicle grows, parts of the epithelium become specialized to form several sensory patches: three cristae and three maculae (the utricle, saccule, and the macula neglecta) in the vestibule, for balance; the basilar papilla, in the cochlea, for hearing; and the lagenar macula, at the tip of the cochlea, for balance. Within each sensory patch, progenitor cells divide repeatedly and give rise to hair cells and supporting cells. Both these differentiated cell types can arise from the same type of progenitor cell (Fekete et al., 1998; Stone and Rubel, 1999; Lang and Fekete, 2001), and the choice of cell fate depends on lateral inhibition mediated by Notch signaling, as discussed earlier. Thus, if asymmetric distribution of Numb influences the choice of cell fate, one might expect that Numb should be present in dividing progenitors at the time of the terminal mitoses that give rise to hair cells. In the vestibular patches, where hair cells begin to be born at E4, Numb crescents were indeed visible at this time (not shown), but they had become less prominent by E6 (3/9 mitotic cells from three separate embryos; **Figures 1E,F**) although hair cell production is then still in progress. In the basilar papilla, where hair cells are born at E5–E8 (Katayama and Corwin, 1989; Bartolami et al., 1991), Numb crescents were present at E4 (**Figures 1C,D**) but could no longer be detected at all in mitotic cells at E6 (12 mitotic cells from three separate embryos; **Figures 1G,H**).

By E7 many hair cells have differentiated in the vestibular patches, and a few hair cells can be detected in the basilar papilla. At this time, Numb expression is concentrated within the hair cells and it no longer has a basal location. Instead, it is expressed diffusely throughout the cytoplasm. This intracellular localization is consistent with previous reports indicating that Numb interacts with components of the endocytotic machinery (Offenhauser et al., 2000; Santolini et al., 2000; Berdnik et al., 2002; Nishimura et al., 2003). Within the supporting cells, there is no strong Numb expression, although some weak staining is apparent at the basal edge of the epithelium (not shown). At E10, this expression pattern is maintained in vestibular patches (**Figures 2A,B**), and it becomes more apparent in the basilar papilla (**Figures 2C,D**), which now has its full complement of hair cells (Katayama and Corwin, 1989). These results suggest that the hair cells and not the supporting cells either inherit Numb or switch on its expression at an increased level. The diffuse distribution of Numb in the hair cells persists in both vestibular and auditory patches until at least E12.

These observations leave open the possibility that high levels of Numb drive cells toward a hair-cell fate, possibly by an effect on Notch signaling.

Sustained Numb Overexpression Does Not Promote Commitment to a Hair-cell Fate

Several Numb isoforms have been reported in vertebrates (Dho et al., 1999; Verdi et al., 1999; Karaczyn et al., 2010), and we identified by RT-PCR two splice variants of the Numb gene in the E6 chicken inner ear, differing by the presence of a 26 amino-acid insert within the PTB domain (see Materials and Methods). These two isoforms exhibited the same membranous and vesicular subcellular localization in transfected chicken embryonic fibroblasts (data not shown) and produced an identical phenotype in our gain-of-function experiments, hence for clarity we will hereafter refer to either of these isoforms as Numb.

To test whether Numb indeed regulates commitment to a hair-cell fate, we investigated the consequences of overexpressing Numb in the developing chick inner ear. To overexpress Numb, we first used an RCAS-Numb proviral DNA that was transfected in the otic cup at stage HH 13–14 (E2). As a

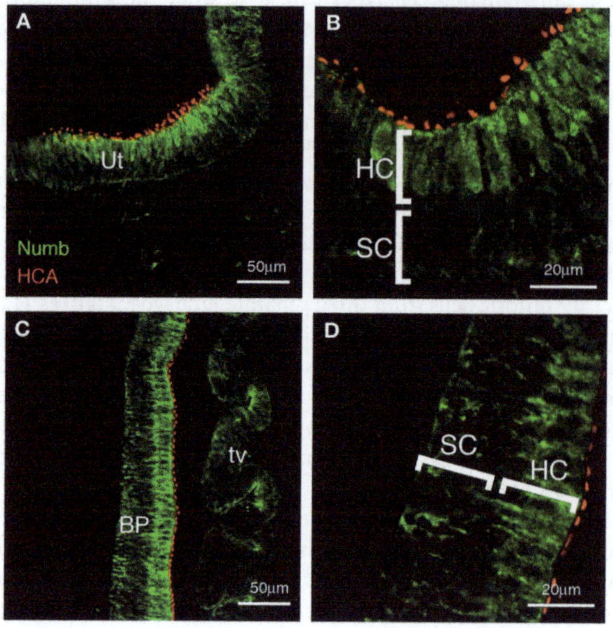

FIGURE 2 | Numb expression at late stages of chick inner ear development. Transverse sections (E10), showing expression of Numb (green) and HCA, marking the stereociliary bundles of hair cells (red). **(A,B)** Vestibular patches and **(C,D)** basilar papilla. Strong Numb expression is found only in the mature hair cells, and within these cells it is no longer localized but is diffuse throughout the cytoplasm. In the supporting cells (SC), Numb is absent or greatly reduced. Any Numb in these cells is basally located. Ut, utricle; BP, basilar papilla; HC, hair cells; SC, supporting cells; tv, tegmentum vasculosum.

control, some specimens were electroporated with RCAS-GFP plasmid DNA.

Following electroporation, the inner ear epithelium showed persistent long-term expression of the transgene carried by the plasmid—GFP or exogenous Numb as the case might be—as judged by anti-GFP or anti-Numb immunostaining. This was visible from 24 h until at least 10 days after electroporation (data not shown). The duration and extent of overexpression suggest that viral DNA had become integrated, giving rise to a spreading infection. Thus, we refer below to "infected" specimens even though RCAS plasmid electroporation, rather than RCAS viral particles, was used to initiate the process.

We took specimens at E10, 8 days after electroporation, and co-immunostained them for GFP and hair cell markers—either Hair-Cell Antigen (HCA, a protein tyrosine phosphatase receptor Q) (Bartolami et al., 1991; Goodyear et al., 2003) detected in the stereociliary bundle, or HCS1/otoferlin (Goodyear et al., 2010) expressed in the hair-cell cytoplasm. In the control specimens infected with RCAS-GFP, we saw GFP in both hair cells (approximately 25% of infected cells in the basilar papilla, $n = 4$ specimens analyzed) and supporting cells (**Figures 3A,B**). The levels of GFP immunostaining were quite variable from one cell to the other, but the differentiation of both hair cells and supporting cells appeared unaffected by the infection.

In RCAS-Numb infected specimens, the overall morphology of the inner ear was normal. Sixteen such specimens were examined at 8 days after electroporation, and 10 of these contained groups of cells or scattered cells overexpressing Numb protein within the sensory patches; large patches of infection were also frequently found outside the sensory patches (**Figure 3C**). The levels of expression of exogenous Numb protein were much higher than the levels of endogenous Numb in non-infected cells, and infected cells could be identified readily. The exogenous Numb was present at the cell membrane and in the cytoplasm, but not asymmetrically localized or concentrated at the basal ends of the infected cells. We looked closely at the cells overexpressing Numb within sensory patches, and we found, to our surprise, that none of them expressed the HCA or HCS1 hair-cell marker (**Figures 3D–F**). In the utricle of one specimen, we could find RCAS-Numb infected cells expressing HCS1 and HCA at a very low level, but with their cell bodies lying at the surface of the epithelium as if they had been expelled from it (**Figure 3G**). The majority of Numb-positive cells (88% out of over 140 infected cells counted in four different specimens) looked like typical supporting cells, intercalated between hair cells. A minority (12%) of infected cells, however, in both auditory and vestibular sensory patches, had a more cylindrical shape than typical supporting cells and had nuclei located at a more apical level than normal for supporting cells (**Figures 3H,I**).

From this we conclude that cells overexpressing Numb, far from becoming hair cells as predicted by the original hypothesis, predominantly become supporting cells: this is the most frequent fate, at least for cells that do not die and disappear from the epithelium. The minority that do not resemble normal supporting cells do not become normal hair cells either: they either fail to display normal hair-cell molecular markers, or express those markers weakly or seem to be extruded from the epithelium.

Early vs. Late Overexpression of Numb Differentially Affect Hair Cell Differentiation

The absence of hair cells overexpressing Numb could have various causes: Numb could, contrary to the initial hypothesis, block commitment to a hair-cell fate; hair cells might switch off expression of virus-encoded Numb so much more efficiently than supporting cells that they appear uninfected; the exogenous Numb might cause hair cells to die; or Numb overexpression might leave commitment unaffected, but block the subsequent process of differentiation. To distinguish among these possibilities, and to test for the effects of Numb at distinct stages of inner ear development, we used different vectors enabling either an early or a late pulse of Numb expression.

To test the effect of overexpressing Numb transiently and at a time when the first hair cell fate decisions occur, we electroporated the otic epithelium at E2 with a bi-cistronic Numb-IRES2-EGFP expression plasmid, driving conjoint expression of Numb and EGFP. Although the plasmid functions only transiently in the transfected cells, the GFP protein is very stable, thus allowing us to identify the transfected cells up to a week later using GFP immunostaining. We followed the time-course of Numb expression in these cells by immunostaining for Numb. At 2 days post-electroporation (E4), when cells in the vestibular patches are just beginning to undergo terminal mitosis and to become committed to a hair-cell fate, the majority of GFP-positive cells

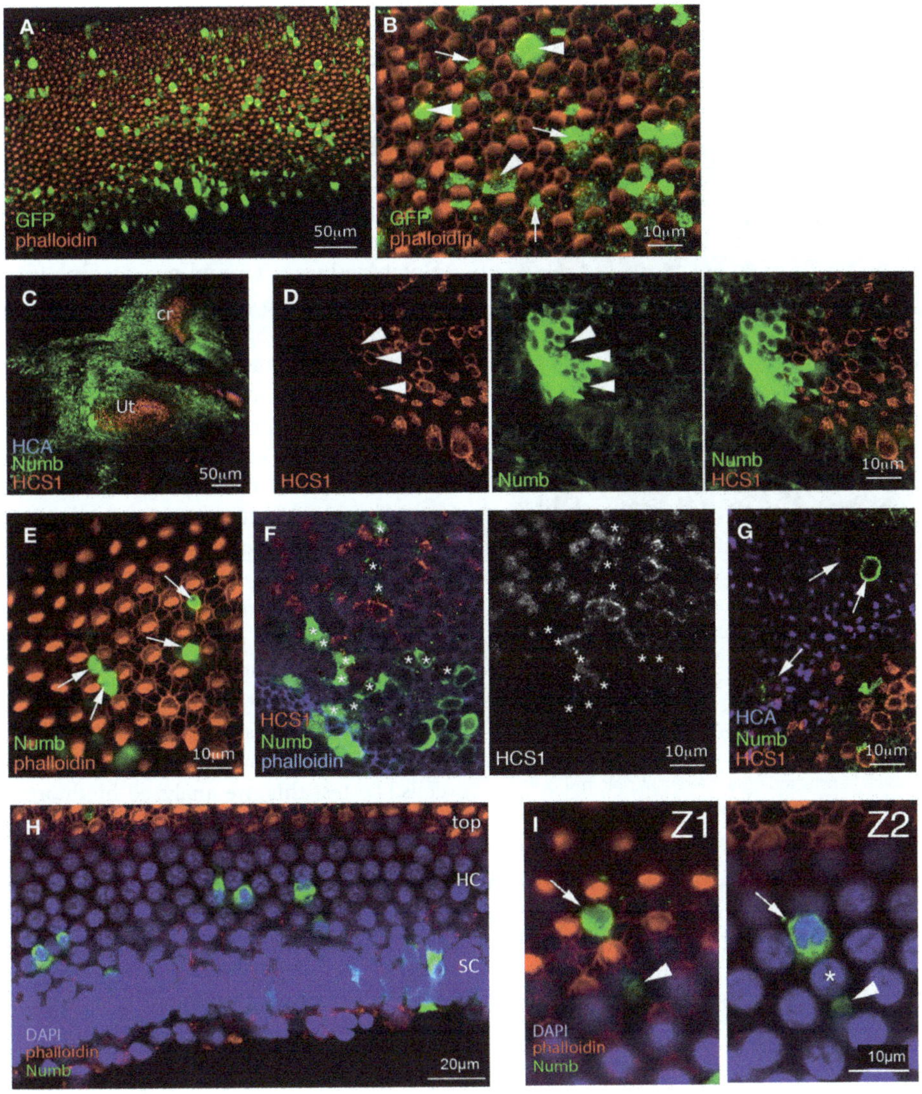

FIGURE 3 | Effects of sustained Numb overexpression using retroviral vectors. Specimens infected at E2 with RCAS-GFP **(A,B)** or with RCAS-Numb **(C–I)**, and fixed at 8 days post-electroporation (E10). **(A,B)** RCAS-GFP infected samples. Surface views of the basilar papilla show GFP expression in scattered cells. At high magnification, many of these GFP positive cells are seen to be hair cells (arrowheads), while others are supporting cells (arrows). **(C)** Low magnification view showing strong Numb overexpression (green) throughout the inner ear sensory and non-sensory regions (Ut, utricle; cr, crista). **(D)** Detail of the utricle shown in **(C)**, with a patch of infected cells overlapping the sensory patch. Within the infected patch, there are some HCS1-positive hair cells (arrowheads) but none of these are overexpressing Numb. **(E)** In the basilar papilla, the cells overexpressing Numb (arrows) lack hair bundles and occupy positions characteristic of supporting cells, intercalated between hair cells. **(F)** Infected sensory crista, seen in a confocal optical section passing obliquely through the hair cell layer. As in other sensory patches, the Numb-infected cells (asterisks) do not express hair-cell markers such as HCS1. **(G)** An infected utricle. Some of the Numb-infected cells lie above the surface of the epithelium (identified by the HCA staining) and appear to have been extruded from it. These cells have rounded cell bodies, and they display a faint HCS1 immunoreactivity (arrows). **(H)** A basilar papilla with Numb infected cells (green), seen in an oblique optical section. The apical most region of the epithelium is at the top of the micrograph (with the hair cell stereocilia visible, in red), and the basal region is at the bottom, and contains the supporting cell nuclei. Note that the apical, hair cell nuclei are regularly interspaced, and display less DAPI staining than the basal, supporting cell nuclei. **(I)** High magnification view of the specimen shown in **(H)**; Z1 corresponds to a more apical optical section than Z2. Some Numb-overexpressing cells have typical supporting cells morphologies (arrowheads) and extend their thin cellular processes in between the hair cells nuclei (asterisks), while some other (arrow) have a rounded appearance and a nucleus located in the hair-cell nuclei layer. The latter may correspond to hair cells that have failed to differentiate correctly. In the basilar papilla, they represent about 15% of the Numb-infected cells.

showed strong Numb expression (**Figure 4A**). However, at E6, almost all of them had ceased to overexpress Numb (**Figure 4B**), suggesting that production of Numb protein from the plasmid had ceased sometime between 2 and 4 days post-electroporation. In spite of the overexpression of Numb during the critical period for cell fate decisions, we saw no tendency of Numb-IRES2-EGFP transfected cells in the vestibular patches to differentiate into hair cells rather than supporting cells: at E8, approximately 22% of

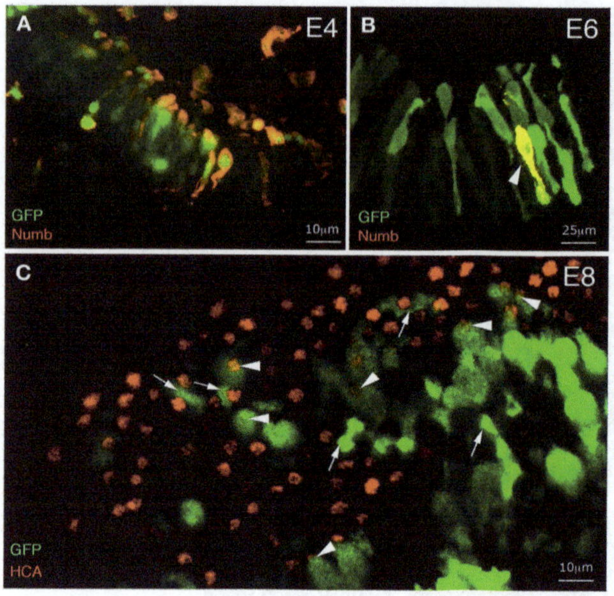

FIGURE 4 | Effects of early and transient Numb protein expression on hair cell differentiation. Whole-mount immunostaining of inner ear tissue from chick embryos electroporated at E2 with Numb-IRES2-EGFP. **(A)** At 2 days post-electroporation, most GFP-positive cells coexpress Numb. **(B)** At 4 days post-electroporation, only a few transfected cells maintain a strong expression of Numb (arrowhead). **(C)** Surface view of an utricular macula at 6 days post-electroporation. Some transfected cells differentiate into hair cells (arrowheads) and others into supporting cells (arrows).

the GFP-positive cells (out of $n = 290$ cells analyzed in seven different specimens) had differentiated into hair cells and 78% into supporting cells (**Figure 4C**). Thus, the two cell fate choices seemed to have been made with the normal relative probabilities, and to have been followed by normal differentiation of both cell types.

In order to test further the effects of Numb on late hair cell differentiation, we next used a Tol2 transposon vector enabling conditional induction of gene expression upon doxycycline (Dox) treatment (**Figure 5**). This construct, pTRE-Numb-FP635, contains a bi-directional promoter enabling co-expression of Numb and the red fluorescent protein Turbo-FP635 (FP635 thereafter) in order to identify induced cells (**Figure 5A**). Embryos transfected at E2 with the Tol2 transposase, a Tol2 plasmid driving expression of the rtTA "Tet-ON" transactivator, and pTRE-Numb-FP635 plasmids were left to develop until E7, at which point they were treated *in ovo* with 10 μg of Dox. The embryos were left to develop a further 48 h before their inner ear tissue was processed for immunostaining with Myo7A (expressed in hair cell cytoplasm) and HCA antibodies. The Numb-induced samples exhibited a phenotype very similar to that resulting from RCAS-Numb electroporation: none of the Numb-induced cells (identified by FP635 expression) expressed hair cell markers (**Figures 5B,C**). Furthermore, we noticed the presence of numerous cellular debris with strong FP635 fluorescence within transfected regions (**Figure 5C**), an observation further reinforcing the hypothesis that Numb overexpression causes cell death. From these data, we conclude that a transient and early pulse of Numb expression has no impact on hair cell vs. supporting cell fate decisions, but elevated levels of Numb expression could have a detrimental effect on hair cell survival.

Numb Overexpression Does Not Strongly Inhibit Notch Activity in the Ear

The preceding results imply that Numb does not control cell fate choices in the way that our original hypothesis would predict, but it remains possible that Numb regulates the activation of the Notch pathway. To find out, we first investigated the effects of exogenous Numb on expression of *Hes5.1*, a member of the *Hairy and Enhancer of Split* (*Hes*) family of genes, whose transcription is regulated by Notch activity and which thus serve as reporters of Notch activation in a number of tissues (Kageyama and Ohtsuka, 1999). In the mammalian cochlea and vestibule, *Hes1* and *Hes5* are expressed by supporting cells and their inactivation in knockout mice results in overproduction of hair cells (Shailam et al., 1999; Zine et al., 2001; Tateya et al., 2011). The chicken *Hes5.1* gene is an ortholog of the mammalian *Hes5* gene, and appears to be functionally equivalent (Fior and Henrique, 2005; Abello et al., 2007). In the developing inner ear, it is first expressed within the anterior region of the otic cup where neuroblasts delaminate, then within all inner ear sensory patches at the time of hair cell production (**Figure 6A** and Daudet et al., 2007).

If Numb blocks Notch activity as hypothesized, its overexpression should cause loss of *Hes5.1* expression in the infected cells. To test this, we analyzed by fluorescent *in situ* hybridization *Hes5.1* expression in inner ear sensory patches infected with RCAS-Numb and fixed at E6 and E8. At both stages, we found patches of infected cells ($n = 8$ infected patches in five embryos) located within ($n = 5$) or abutting ($n = 3$) sensory patches. As in the adjacent uninfected regions, some of these cells expressed *Hes5.1* and others did not; there was no obvious difference between the infected and uninfected regions, neither in the proportion of cells expressing *Hes5.1* nor in their levels of expression of *Hes5.1* (**Figure 6B**). This result suggests that Numb is not a negative regulator of Notch activity in the inner ear, but it remained difficult to precisely quantify at the cellular level the potential effects of Numb on Notch activity using *in situ* hybridization.

To test further the cell-autonomous effects of Numb on Notch signaling, we next used a Tol2 vector encoding a reporter of Notch activity, pT2-Hes5::nd2EGFP (Chrysostomou et al., 2012). In cells transfected with this construct, expression of a nuclear-localized and destabilized green fluorescent protein is regulated by the mouse Hes5 promoter (Takebayashi et al., 1995), providing a direct readout of the endogenous levels of Notch activity. In a previous study, we showed that this reporter is active within sensory progenitors and supporting cells of the chicken inner ear, and that it exhibits a rapid reduction in fluorescence levels following pharmacological blockade of Notch activity by the gamma-secretase inhibitor DAPT (Chrysostomou et al., 2012) or following induction of Sox21 expression (Freeman and Daudet, 2012). We co-transfected the chicken inner ear *in ovo* with the Hes5::nd2eGFP reporter and Dox-inducible Tol2 vectors driving expression of Numb-FP635, or FP635 alone as a control (**Figure 7A** and Figure S1). The embryos received Dox at E6,

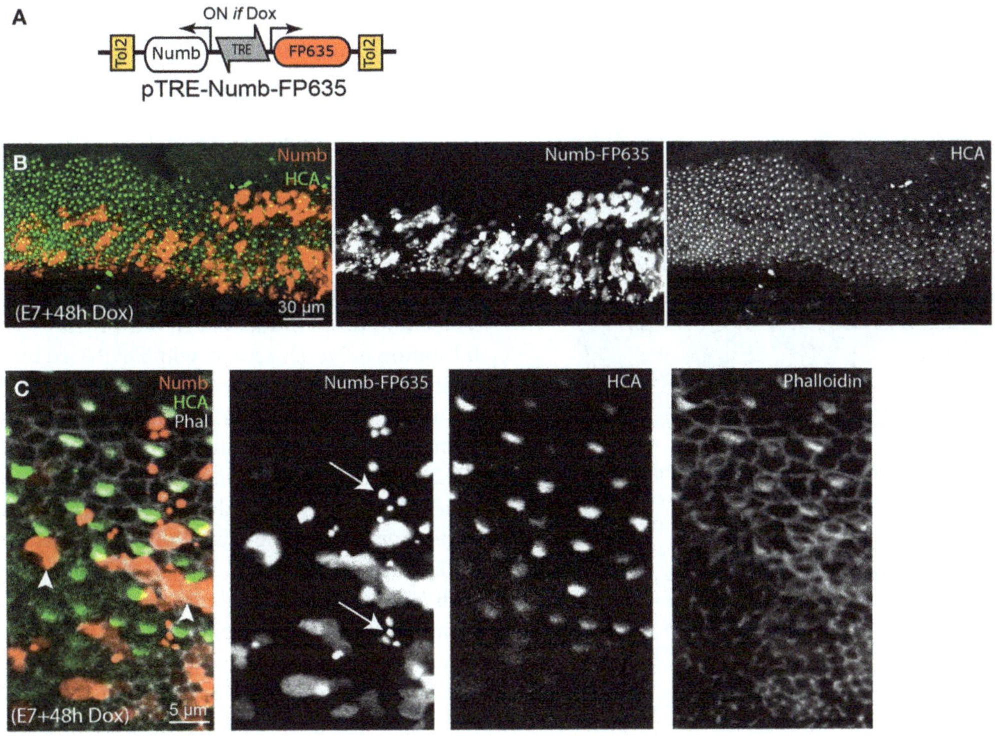

FIGURE 5 | Effects of conditional Numb overexpression at stages of hair cell differentiation. (A) Schematic representation of the pTRE-Numb-FP635 Tol2 Tet-on construct driving expression of Numb and the red fluorescent protein FP635 following Dox treatment *in ovo*. **(B)** Basilar papilla analyzed 48 h after Dox treatment at E6. A large number of Numb-induced cells, identified by FP635 expression, are present within the sensory epithelia. **(C)** High magnification view of the sample shown in **(B)**. None of the Numb-FP635 induced cells express HCA (arrowheads). Note also the presence of small vesicle-like structures with strong FP635 fluorescence (arrows) within transfected regions.

and their inner ear were fixed 24 or 48 h later then immunostained for HCA and Myo7A. The Hes5 reporter was active in cells with typical supporting cell and progenitor cell morphology, but not in differentiated hair cells (**Figure 7B** and data not shown). Probably owing to the mosaicism of transfection, only a subset of Hes5-positive cells were also FP635-positive in both control and Numb-induced cells. At 24 h post-induction, there was an important variability in the levels of Hes5::nd2EGFP fluorescence in the nucleus of both control (Figure S1) and Numb-positive cells, some of which clearly had high levels of Hes5 reporter fluorescence (**Figures 7B,C,F**). In contrast, at 48 h the levels of Hes5::nd2EGFP fluorescence appeared reduced in the majority of Numb-induced cells compared to non-induced cells (**Figures 7D,E**; Movie S1). A quantitative analysis of Hes5 reporter fluorescence in single (induced) cells (see Materials and Methods) showed that at both 24 and 48 h post-induction, there was a small reduction in the levels of Hes5::nd2EGFP fluorescence in Numb-induced cells compared to control, FP635-induced cells (**Figure 7G**). This reduction was not significant at 24 h (Mann–Whitney $U = 25981$; $p = 0.09278$) but significant at 48 h (Mann–Whitney $U = 43494$; $p = 2.07E\text{-}6$). We conclude from these results that Numb overexpression does induce a reduction in the intrinsic levels of Notch activity in the inner ear, but this effect is relatively mild and slow to develop, and Numb is therefore unlikely to significantly contribute to the regulation of hair cell fate decisions.

Discussion

Numb was identified in Drosophila as a critical regulator of Notch-dependent cell fate decisions during neurogenesis, acting as cell-intrinsic inhibitor of Notch activity during lateral inhibition. Although the vertebrate homologs of Numb were later proposed to have a similar function in vertebrates, some data suggested that they could also affect additional cellular processes. In this study, we set out to investigate Numb function in the embryonic chick inner ear using gain-of-function approaches. Our findings suggest that Numb is not a critical determinant of hair cell fate decisions and does not prevent the reception of lateral inhibition. Furthermore, high levels of Numb expression interfere with normal hair cell differentiation, an observation that hints at non-Notch dependent functions for Numb in the ear.

Numb does not Bias Hair Cell Fate Decisions in the Inner Ear

The molecular mechanisms regulating mechanosensory cell formation are evolutionary conserved. The vertebrate homolog of Atonal (Atoh1), a proneural bHLH transcription factor essential

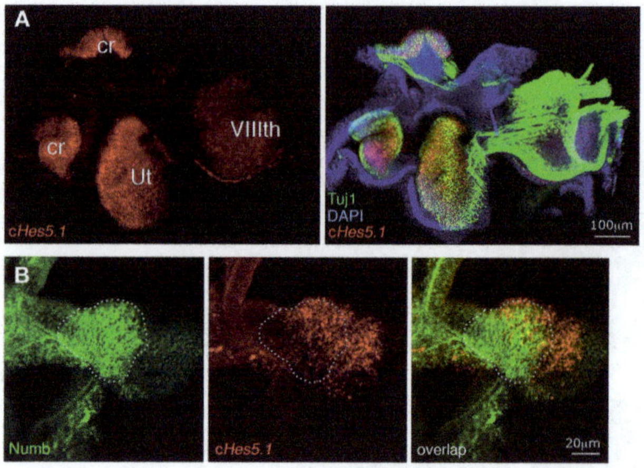

FIGURE 6 | Sustained Numb overexpression does not affect *Hes5.1* expression. (A) The Notch target gene *Hes5.1* (in red) is strongly expressed within inner ear sensory patches (ut, utricle; cr, crista). Beta-III tubulin (TuJ1) immunoreactivity (green) is intense in nerve fibers originating from the VIIIth ganglion and within sensory patches, coincident with the *Hes5.1* signal. **(B)** An RCAS-Numb infected sensory crista. Note that the levels of *Hes5.1* expression are unchanged in the infected region (dotted line) relative to the uninfected region, and that overexpression of Numb does not induce expression of *Hes5.1* outside of the sensory patch epithelium.

for the differentiation of the mechanosensory cells in flies, is required for hair cell differentiation in the inner ear (reviewed in Jarman and Groves, 2013). Furthermore, lateral inhibition mediated by the Notch pathway regulates cell fate diversification within the sensory organ precursor (SOP) lineage of *Drosophila* and in the inner ear (Eddison et al., 2000). Asymmetric cell division (reviewed in Zhong and Chia, 2008), which generates two daughter cells with unequal developmental potential at birth, is also an important contributor to cell diversification in the SOP lineage. Numb is one of the intrinsic factors asymmetrically inherited by one of the daughter cells, in which it inhibits Notch activity. As a consequence, the Numb-expressing cell gains a competitive advantage and is more able to deliver lateral inhibition to its sibling. In vertebrates, Numb has been proposed to have a similar function during neurogenesis (Wakamatsu et al., 1999; Shen et al., 2002; McGill and McGlade, 2003; Matsuda et al., 2005), where asymmetric cell divisions are thought to contribute at least partly to the control of neural differentiation.

In the embryonic chick inner ear, we found that Numb is initially expressed by all epithelial cells, including sensory progenitors, and analysis of fixed tissue suggest that Numb can be distributed asymmetrically in some dividing cells, as previously reported for neural progenitor cells. Numb then becomes enriched in differentiated hair cells, which have escaped Notch activation in order to commit to a hair cell fate. Our results, however, argue against the idea that Numb acts as a determinant of hair-cell fate decisions, either by blocking activation of Notch, or indeed by any other mechanism. Cells overexpressing Numb at either early or late stages of development are not biased toward a hair-cell fate, and they do not show altered expression of the Notch effector *Hes5.1*.

Using a genetically encoded fluorescent Hes5 reporter to quantify more precisely the effects of Numb on Notch activity, we found that Numb-induced cells do exhibit a significant reduction in the Hes5 reporter fluorescence levels 48 h after Dox treatment. Although this effect might suggest an interference with the reception of Notch signaling, several observations conflict with that interpretation. Firstly, the reduction in Hes5 reporter fluorescence in Numb-induced cells was very variable from cell to cell and did not appear to be correlated to the levels of expression of the Numb transgene in individual cells. Secondly, there was no significant reduction in the levels of Hes5 reporter fluorescence 24 h after Numb induction. In our previous work, we found that inhibition of Notch activity with DAPT led to an almost complete extinction of the same Hes5 reporter in less than 12 h (Chrysostomou et al., 2012), and Sox21 induction *in ovo* can result in a much stronger inhibition of this Hes5 reporter (Freeman and Daudet, 2012). By comparison, the reduction of Hes5 reporter fluorescence levels in Numb-induced cells is relatively modest and slow to develop, suggesting that Numb is neither directly nor strongly inhibiting Notch activity. Finally, the majority of cells transfected with Numb differentiated into supporting cells, and not hair cells as would be expected from a strong inhibition of Notch signaling. Altogether, these data suggest that Numb has little impact on intrinsic levels of Notch activity and is unlikely to act as a critical regulator of hair cell fate decisions. The reduction in Hes5 reporter fluorescence observed 48 h after Numb induction may reflect a weak and an indirect effect of Numb on Notch activity, but it may also be consecutive to some unspecific effect on the processing of the fluorescent reporter itself or some other aspect of cell metabolism that remains to be determined.

One surprising observation is that none of the Numb-overexpressing cells expressed hair cell markers, suggesting that Numb misexpression could interfere with normal hair cell differentiation and survival. A small fraction of the Numb-overexpressing cells also exhibited a mis-positioned nucleus in between the hair cell and supporting cell layers, suggesting a potential defect in their apico-basal polarity. It is possible that these merely reflect a non-specific toxic effect of the overexpressed protein, but Numb certainly has documented functions in other systems that might account for these abnormalities. In particular, Numb has been implicated in endocytosis (Santolini et al., 2000; Berdnik et al., 2002; Nishimura et al., 2003) as well as the maintenance of cell adhesion and apico-basal polarity (Rasin et al., 2007; Sato et al., 2011), and disturbance of both processes could interfere with hair-cell maturation. Numb is also expressed in terminally differentiated neurons (Zhong et al., 1997; Dooley et al., 2003), and it seems to be involved in neuronal maturation (Klein et al., 2004) and axonal growth (Nishimura et al., 2003; Huang et al., 2005). As it has been suggested in the context of neurogenesis, the changing localization of Numb in the developing ear could indicate that it may have different functions at different stages. Although we have not directly investigated these possibilities, Numb could have a role in the regulation of otic neurogenesis or cell proliferation. Numb functions, however, do not appear to include regulation of Notch activity in the context of hair cell fate decisions. One important caveat should be mentioned, however: we have performed overexpression experiments

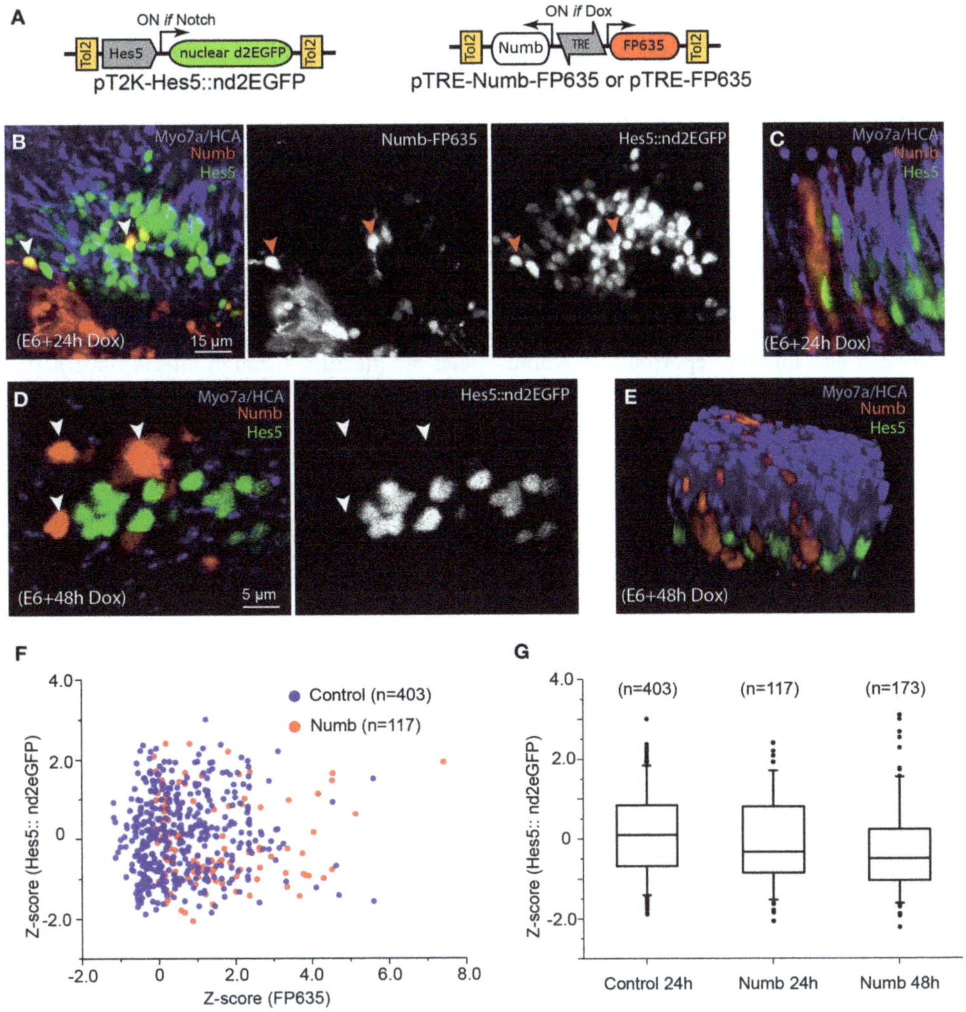

FIGURE 7 | Numb overexpression has a mild inhibitory effect on Notch activity. (A) Schematic representation of the Tol2 Numb-inducible construct and the Hes5 reporter used for the experiments. **(B)** Whole-mount preparation of a sensory crista with Numb-induced cells 24 h after Dox treatment. The sensory epithelium contains a large number of cells with variable levels of Hes5::nd2EGFP fluorescence in their cytoplasm. Note that some of the Numb-induced cells have high levels of Hes5 reporter fluorescence (red arrowheads), comparable to those of their neighboring, uninduced cells. **(C)** Another example of Numb-induced cells with Hes5 reporter fluorescence in their nuclei, seen from a transverse aspect. **(D)** At 48 h after Dox treatment, the Numb-induced cells appeared to have less Hes5 reporter fluorescence in their nuclei compared to non-induced cells but do not express the hair cell marker Myo7A. **(E)** A 3D rendering of the confocal stack from which the optical slice shown in **(D)** was selected, demonstrating that none of the Numb-induced cells expressed hair cell markers such as HCA or Myo7A (see also Movie S1). **(F)** Scatter plot of the Z-score for FP635 and Hes5::nd2EGFP fluorescence levels for individual cells positive for FP635 expression (see Methods) 24 h after Dox treatment, for control (FP635 alone) or Numb-FP635 induced cells. Note the absence of correlation between both parameters. **(G)** Box plot (box: 25–75% of cells, whiskers: 5–95% of cells, and dots: outliers) of the FP635-positive cells positive for control (24 h post-Dox), and Numb-induced conditions at 24 and 48 h after Dox treatment.

only, and have not been able to test the effects of eliminating Numb function in the chick inner ear. It is conceivable that a complete absence of Numb might alter Notch-regulated cell fate decisions, even though Numb overexpression does not do so.

The Functions of Numb in the Vertebrate Nervous System Cannot Be Explained Simply in Terms of Notch Regulation

Our findings add to the questions surrounding the proposed role of Numb as an asymmetrically inherited regulator of Notch activity in other vertebrate tissues, especially in the nervous system. As in *Drosophila*, neuroepithelial progenitor cells of the central nervous system of vertebrates can divide along different cleavage planes, and some studies suggest that the cleavage plane can be linked to the assignment of asymmetric daughter cell fates (Chenn and McConnell, 1995; Cayouette and Raff, 2003; Das et al., 2003; Das and Storey, 2012), although there is still some disagreement about this (Konno et al., 2008; reviewed in Zhong and Chia, 2008). There is, on the other hand, very strong evidence that a cell with Notch activated remains as a neural progenitor, whereas a cell that escapes Notch activation differentiates as a neuron. It is an obvious suggestion, therefore, that if there is a link between cell fate and the orientation of cell division, it could depend on an asymmetrically distributed factor that is inherited by the prospective neuron and inhibits Notch activity.

This notion was encouraged by the finding that vertebrate homologs of Numb are expressed by neural progenitor cells in chick and mammals (Zhong et al., 1996; Wakamatsu et al., 1999). However, despite a number of studies in both organisms, the role of Numb in vertebrate neurogenesis remains controversial. This is due in part to the fact that the subcellular localization of Numb in dividing neuroepithelial progenitors appeared to vary, depending on the species. In mice, it was initially reported that Numb accumulates at the apical pole of neuroepithelial cells and forms crescent-like structures in mitotic cells, and is therefore likely to be inherited by the cell that remains as a progenitor in the lumenal region of the neural tube after an apico-basal cell division (Zhong et al., 1996, 1997; Petersen et al., 2002, 2004). However a subsequent study reported that at least in the developing cortex, Numb is in fact enriched at the apical end-feet of interphase radial glial cells that are tightly surrounding mitotic cells (Rasin et al., 2007). In the chicken, Numb is clearly localized on the basolateral side of neuroepithelial cells in the neural tube, implying that after an apico-basal cell division it would be predominantly inherited by the basally located daughter cell, which is thought to migrate away from the proliferative zone and differentiate into a neuron (Wakamatsu et al., 1999). Thus, it has been proposed that in mice, Numb causes cells that inherit it to remain as progenitors, whereas in chick, it has been suggested that it has an opposite effect, causing them to differentiate as neurons.

Studies on cultured mouse cortical progenitor cells and in the mouse retina have demonstrated an involvement of Numb in asymmetric cell division, but with complex effects, including localization of Numb to the neuronal daughter cells in some circumstances (Cayouette et al., 2001; Shen et al., 2002; Cayouette and Raff, 2003). Mice with knockout mutations of *numb* show abnormalities of cortical and sensory neurogenesis (Zhong et al., 2000) and sensory neuron production (Zilian et al., 2001), but the mutant animals die at E11.5 from defects in neural tube closure. The early lethality can, however, be bypassed by means of conditional knockouts, which have been used to delete simultaneously both *numb* and the closely related *numblike* gene in the embryonic forebrain. Studies using different drivers for this double conditional knockout reported surprisingly different results, with apparently opposite effects on cell fate choices (Petersen et al., 2002, 2004; Li et al., 2003). Both sets of observations share one striking feature, however: the cytoarchitecture of the neural tube is disrupted and the dividing progenitors fail to stay in their proper location, in the ventricular zone. Likewise, deletion of *numb* and *numblike* in the embryonic retina leads to abnormal proliferation and severe defects in epithelial organization (Kechad et al., 2012).

Perhaps, therefore, the fundamental function of Numb in the vertebrate neuroepithelium is not to control cell fate decisions through effects on Notch signaling, but rather to control epithelial architecture through effects on cell polarity, cell adhesion, and the cytoskeleton. Indeed, there is growing evidence that Numb can have other functions apart from influencing cell fate choices: for example, mice with conditional knockout mutations of *numb* and *numblike* in their sensory ganglia have no deficit of neurogenesis, but show defects in axonal arborization (Huang et al., 2005). The different Numb isoforms can bind to a number of proteins of the endocytotic machinery (Krieger et al., 2013), hence the functions of Numb are expected to be highly context-dependent, affecting the intracellular trafficking of Notch receptors but also that of any other receptor or cell surface molecule directly or indirectly binding to Numb. Our findings are consistent with the view that Numb influences primarily cell structure and maturation rather than Notch-dependent cell fate choices in the inner ear. And if commitment to a hair-cell fate is after all regulated by an asymmetrically distributed factor that interferes with Notch signaling, that factor is not likely to be Numb.

Acknowledgments

We thank Jenny Corrigan for cryosectioning, and past members of the Lewis lab for their help and support. We are also indebted to Domingos Henrique for valuable discussions and advice, and Jeff Corwin, Guy Richardson, Weimin Zhong, Domingos Henrique, and Yoshio Wakamatsu for sharing reagents with us. This work was initiated in the Vertebrate Development Laboratory (Dr. Julian Lewis) with the support of Cancer Research UK. Work in ND lab is currently supported by the BBSRC (BB/L003163/1). SJW is a recipient of an Action on Hearing Loss PhD studentship (S29).

References

Abello, G., Khatri, S., Giraldez, F., and Alsina, B. (2007). Early regionalization of the otic placode and its regulation by the Notch signaling pathway. *Mech. Dev.* 124, 631–645. doi: 10.1016/j.mod.2007.04.002

Adam, J., Myat, A., Le Roux, I., Eddison, M., Henrique, D., Ish-Horowicz, D., et al. (1998). Cell fate choices and the expression of Notch, Delta and Serrate homologues in the chick inner ear: parallels with Drosophila sense-organ development. *Development* 125, 4645–4654.

Ariza-Mcnaughton, L., and Krumlauf, R. (2002). Non-radioactive *in situ* hybridization: simplified procedures for use in whole-mounts of mouse and chick embryos. *Int. Rev. Neurobiol.* 47, 239–250. doi: 10.1016/S0074-7742(02)47062-6

Bartolami, S., Goodyear, R., and Richardson, G. (1991). Appearance and distribution of the 275 kD hair-cell antigen during development of the avian inner ear. *J. Comp. Neurol.* 314, 777–788. doi: 10.1002/cne.903140410

Basch, M. L., Ohyama, T., Segil, N., and Groves, A. K. (2011). Canonical Notch signaling is not necessary for prosensory induction in the mouse cochlea: insights from a conditional mutant of RBPjkappa. *J. Neurosci.* 31, 8046–8058. doi: 10.1523/JNEUROSCI.6671-10.2011

Berdnik, D., Torok, T., Gonzalez-Gaitan, M., and Knoblich, J. (2002). The endocytic protein alpha-Adaptin is required for numb-mediated asymmetric cell division in Drosophila. *Dev. Cell* 3, 221–231. doi: 10.1016/S1534-5807(02)00215-0

Bhalerao, S., Berdnik, D., Torok, T., and Knoblich, J. (2005). Localization-dependent and -independent roles of numb contribute to cell-fate specification in Drosophila. *Curr. Biol.* 15, 1583–1590. doi: 10.1016/j.cub.2005.07.061

Brooker, R. (2006). Notch ligands with contrasting functions: Jagged1 and Delta1 in the mouse inner ear. *Development* 133, 1277–1286. doi: 10.1242/dev.02284

Cayouette, M., and Raff, M. (2003). The orientation of cell division influences cell-fate choice in the developing mammalian retina. *Development* 130, 2329–2339. doi: 10.1242/dev.00446

Cayouette, M., Whitmore, A., Jeffery, G., and Raff, M. (2001). Asymmetric segregation of Numb in retinal development and the influence of the pigmented epithelium. *J. Neurosci.* 21, 5643–5651.

Chenn, A., and McConnell, S. (1995). Cleavage orientation and the asymmetric inheritance of Notch1 immunoreactivity in mammalian neurogenesis. *Cell* 82, 631–641. doi: 10.1016/0092-8674(95)90035-7

Chitnis, A. (1995). The role of Notch in lateral inhibition and cell fate specification. *Mol. Cell. Neurosci.* 6, 311–321. doi: 10.1006/mcne.1995.1024

Chrysostomou, E., Gale, J. E., and Daudet, N. (2012). Delta-like 1 and lateral inhibition during hair cell formation in the chicken inner ear: evidence against cis-inhibition. *Development* 139, 3764–3774. doi: 10.1242/dev.074476

Collier, J. R., Monk, N. A., Maini, P. K., and Lewis, J. H. (1996). Pattern formation by lateral inhibition with feedback: a mathematical model of delta-notch intercellular signalling. *J. Theor. Biol.* 183, 429–446. doi: 10.1006/jtbi.1996.0233

Cotton, M., Benhra, N., and Le borgne, R. (2013). Numb inhibits the recycling of Sanpodo in Drosophila sensory organ precursor. *Curr. Biol.* 23, 581–587. doi: 10.1016/j.cub.2013.02.020

Couturier, L., Vodovar, N., and Schweisguth, F. (2012). Endocytosis by Numb breaks Notch symmetry at cytokinesis. *Nat. Cell Biol.* 14, 131–139. doi: 10.1038/ncb2419

Das, R. M., and Storey, K. G. (2012). Mitotic spindle orientation can direct cell fate and bias Notch activity in chick neural tube. *EMBO Rep.* 13, 448–454. doi: 10.1038/embor.2012.42

Das, T., Payer, B., Cayouette, M., and Harris, W. (2003). *In vivo* time-lapse imaging of cell divisions during neurogenesis in the developing zebrafish retina. *Neuron* 37, 597–609. doi: 10.1016/S0896-6273(03)00066-7

Daudet, N., Ariza-McNaughton, L., and Lewis, J. (2007). Notch signalling is needed to maintain, but not to initiate, the formation of prosensory patches in the chick inner ear. *Development* 134, 2369–2378. doi: 10.1242/dev.001842

Daudet, N., and Lewis, J. (2005). Two contrasting roles for Notch activity in chick inner ear development: specification of prosensory patches and lateral inhibition of hair-cell differentiation. *Development* 132, 541–551. doi: 10.1242/dev.01589

Dho, S., French, M., Woods, S., and McGlade, C. (1999). Characterization of four mammalian numb protein isoforms. Identification of cytoplasmic and membrane-associated variants of the phosphotyrosine binding domain. *J. Biol. Chem.* 274, 33097–33104. doi: 10.1074/jbc.274.46.33097

Dooley, C., James, J., Jane McGlade, C., and Ahmad, I. (2003). Involvement of numb in vertebrate retinal development: evidence for multiple roles of numb in neural differentiation and maturation. *J. Neurobiol.* 54, 313–325. doi: 10.1002/neu.10176

Eddison, M., Le Roux, I., and Lewis, J. (2000). Notch signaling in the development of the inner ear: lessons from Drosophila. *Proc. Natl. Acad. Sci. U.S.A.* 97, 11692–11699. doi: 10.1073/pnas.97.22.11692

Fekete, D., Muthukumar, S., and Karagogeos, D. (1998). Hair cells and supporting cells share a common progenitor in the avian inner ear. *J. Neurosci.* 18, 7811–7821.

Fior, R., and Henrique, D. (2005). A novel hes5/hes6 circuitry of negative regulation controls Notch activity during neurogenesis. *Dev. Biol.* 281, 318–333. doi: 10.1016/j.ydbio.2005.03.017

Freeman, S., Chrysostomou, E., Kawakami, K., Takahashi, Y., and Daudet, N. (2012). Tol2-mediated gene transfer and *in ovo* electroporation of the otic placode: a powerful and versatile approach for investigating embryonic development and regeneration of the chicken inner ear. *Methods Mol. Biol.* 916, 127–139. doi: 10.1007/978-1-61779-980-8_10

Freeman, S. D., and Daudet, N. (2012). Artificial induction of sox21 regulates sensory cell formation in the embryonic chicken inner ear. *PLoS ONE* 7:e46387. doi: 10.1371/journal.pone.0046387

Frise, E., Knoblich, J., Younger-Shepherd, S., Jan, L., and Jan, Y. (1996). The Drosophila Numb protein inhibits signaling of the Notch receptor during cell-cell interaction in sensory organ lineage. *Proc. Natl. Acad. Sci. U.S.A.* 93, 11925–11932. doi: 10.1073/pnas.93.21.11925

Gale, J. E., Meyers, J. R., and Corwin, J. T. (2000). Solitary hair cells are distributed throughout the extramacular epithelium in the Bullfrog's saccule. *J. Assoc. Res. Otolaryngol.* 1, 172–182. doi: 10.1007/s101620010037

Goodyear, R., and Richardson, G. (1997). Pattern formation in the basilar papilla: evidence for cell rearrangement. *J. Neurosci.* 17, 6289–6301.

Goodyear, R. J., Legan, P. K., Christiansen, J. R., Xia, B., Korchagina, J., Gale, J. E., et al. (2010). Identification of the hair cell soma-1 antigen, HCS-1, as otoferlin. *J. Assoc. Res. Otolaryngol.* 11, 573–586. doi: 10.1007/s10162-010-0231-6

Goodyear, R. J., Legan, P. K., Wright, M. B., Marcotti, W., Oganesian, A., Coats, S. A., et al. (2003). A receptor-like inositol lipid phosphatase is required for the maturation of developing cochlear hair bundles. *J. Neurosci.* 23, 9208–9219.

Guo, M., Jan, L., and Jan, Y. (1996). Control of daughter cell fates during asymmetric division: interaction of Numb and Notch. *Neuron* 17, 27–41. doi: 10.1016/S0896-6273(00)80278-0

Haddon, C., Jiang, Y. J., Smithers, L., and Lewis, J. (1998). Delta-Notch signalling and the patterning of sensory cell differentiation in the zebrafish ear: evidence from the mind bomb mutant. *Development* 125, 4637–4644.

Hartenstein, V., and Posakony, J. (1990). A dual function of the Notch gene in Drosophila sensillum development. *Dev. Biol.* 142, 13–30. doi: 10.1016/0012-1606(90)90147-B

Hartman, B. H., Reh, T. A., and Bermingham-McDonogh, O. (2010). Notch signaling specifies prosensory domains via lateral induction in the developing mammalian inner ear. *Proc. Natl. Acad. Sci. U.S.A.* 107, 15792–15797. doi: 10.1073/pnas.1002827107

Heitzler, P., Bourouis, M., Ruel, L., Carteret, C., and Simpson, P. (1996). Genes of the enhancer of split and achaete-scute complexes are required for a regulatory loop between Notch and Delta during lateral signalling in Drosophila. *Development* 122, 161–171.

Huang, E. J., Li, H., Tang, A. A., Wiggins, A. K., Neve, R. L., Zhong, W., et al. (2005). Targeted deletion of numb and numblike in sensory neurons reveals their essential functions in axon arborization. *Genes Dev.* 19, 138–151. doi: 10.1101/gad.1246005

Hutterer, A., and Knoblich, J. (2005). Numb and alpha-Adaptin regulate Sanpodo endocytosis to specify cell fate in Drosophila external sensory organs. *EMBO Rep.* 6, 836–842. doi: 10.1038/sj.embor.7400500

Jarman, A. P., and Groves, A. K. (2013). The role of Atonal transcription factors in the development of mechanosensitive cells. *Semin. Cell Dev. Biol.* 24, 438–447. doi: 10.1016/j.semcdb.2013.03.010

Kageyama, R., and Ohtsuka, T. (1999). The Notch-Hes pathway in mammalian neural development. *Cell Res.* 9, 179–188. doi: 10.1038/sj.cr.7290016

Karaczyn, A., Bani-Yaghoub, M., Tremblay, R., Kubu, C., Cowling, R., Adams, T. L., et al. (2010). Two novel human NUMB isoforms provide a potential link between development and cancer. *Neural Dev.* 5, 31. doi: 10.1186/1749-8104-5-31

Katayama, A., and Corwin, J. T. (1989). Cell production in the chicken cochlea. *J. Comp. Neurol.* 281, 129–135. doi: 10.1002/cne.902810110

Kechad, A., Jolicoeur, C., Tufford, A., Mattar, P., Chow, R. W. Y., Harris, W. A., et al. (2012). Numb is required for the production of terminal asymmetric cell divisions in the developing mouse retina. *J. Neurosci.* 32, 17197–17210. doi: 10.1523/JNEUROSCI.4127-12.2012

Kiernan, A. E. (2013). Notch signaling during cell fate determination in the inner ear. *Semin. Cell Dev. Biol.* 24, 470–479. doi: 10.1016/j.semcdb.2013.04.002

Kiernan, A. E., Ahituv, N., Fuchs, H., Balling, R., Avraham, K. B., Steel, K. P., et al. (2001). The Notch ligand Jagged1 is required for inner ear sensory development. *Proc. Natl. Acad. Sci. U.S.A.* 98, 3873–3878. doi: 10.1073/pnas.071496998

Kiernan, A. E., Xu, J., and Gridley, T. (2006). The Notch ligand JAG1 is required for sensory progenitor development in the mammalian inner ear. *PLoS Genet.* 2:e4. doi: 10.1371/journal.pgen.0020004

Klein, A., Zilian, O., Suter, U., and Taylor, V. (2004). Murine numb regulates granule cell maturation in the cerebellum. *Dev. Biol.* 266, 161–177. doi: 10.1016/j.ydbio.2003.10.017

Knoblich, J., Jan, L., and Jan, Y. (1995). Asymmetric segregation of Numb and Prospero during cell division. *Nature* 377, 624–627. doi: 10.1038/377624a0

Konno, D., Shioi, G., Shitamukai, A., Mori, A., Kiyonari, H., Miyata, T., et al. (2008). Neuroepithelial progenitors undergo LGN-dependent planar divisions to maintain self-renewability during mammalian neurogenesis. *Nat. Cell Biol.* 10, 93–101. doi: 10.1038/ncb1673

Krieger, J. R., Taylor, P., Gajadhar, A. S., Guha, A., Moran, M. F., and McGlade, C. J. (2013). Identification and selected reaction monitoring (SRM) quantification of endocytosis factors associated with Numb. *Mol. Cell. Proteomics* 12, 499–514. doi: 10.1074/mcp.M112.020768

Lanford, P. J., Lan, Y., Jiang, R., Lindsell, C., Weinmaster, G., Gridley, T., et al. (1999). Notch signalling pathway mediates hair cell development in mammalian cochlea. *Nat. Genet.* 21, 289–292. doi: 10.1038/6804

Lang, H., and Fekete, D. M. (2001). Lineage analysis in the chicken inner ear shows differences in clonal dispersion for epithelial, neuronal, and mesenchymal cells. *Dev. Biol.* 234, 120–137. doi: 10.1006/dbio.2001.0248

Lewis, J. (1998). Notch signalling and the control of cell fate choices in vertebrates. *Semin. Cell Dev. Biol.* 9, 583–589. doi: 10.1006/scdb.1998.0266

Li, H., Wang, D., Shen, Q., Schonemann, M., Gorski, J., Jones, K., et al. (2003). Inactivation of Numb and Numblike in embryonic dorsal forebrain impairs neurogenesis and disrupts cortical morphogenesis. *Neuron* 40, 1105–1118. doi: 10.1016/S0896-6273(03)00755-4

Matsuda, Y., Wakamatsu, Y., Kohyama, J., Okano, H., Fukuda, K., and Yasugi, S. (2005). Notch signaling functions as a binary switch for the determination of glandular and luminal fates of endodermal epithelium during chicken stomach development. *Development* 132, 2783–2793. doi: 10.1242/dev.01853

McGill, M. A., and McGlade, C. J. (2003). Mammalian numb proteins promote Notch1 receptor ubiquitination and degradation of the Notch1 intracellular domain. *J. Biol. Chem.* 278, 23196–23203. doi: 10.1074/jbc.M302827200

Morgan, B., and Fekete, D. (1996). Manipulating gene expression with replication-competent retroviruses. *Methods Cell Biol.* 51, 185–218. doi: 10.1016/S0091-679X(08)60629-9

Neves, J., Parada, C., Chamizo, M., and Giráldez, F. (2011). Jagged 1 regulates the restriction of Sox2 expression in the developing chicken inner ear: a mechanism for sensory organ specification. *Development* 138, 735–744. doi: 10.1242/dev.060657

Nishimura, T., Fukata, Y., Kato, K., Yamaguchi, T., Matsuura, Y., Kamiguchi, H., et al. (2003). CRMP-2 regulates polarized Numb-mediated endocytosis for axon growth. *Nat. Cell Biol.* 5, 819–826. doi: 10.1038/ncb1039

O'Connor-Giles, K. M., and Skeath, J. B. (2003). Numb inhibits membrane localization of Sanpodo, a four-pass transmembrane protein, to promote asymmetric divisions in Drosophila. *Dev. Cell* 5, 231–243. doi: 10.1016/S1534-5807(03)00226-0

Offenhauser, N., Santolini, E., Simeone, A., and Di Fiore, P. (2000). Differential patterns of expression of Eps15 and Eps15R during mouse embryogenesis. *Mech. Dev.* 95, 309–312. doi: 10.1016/S0925-4773(00)00363-4

Petersen, P. H., Zou, K., Hwang, J. K., Jan, Y. N., and Zhong, W. (2002). Progenitor cell maintenance requires numb and numblike during mouse neurogenesis. *Nature* 419, 929–934. doi: 10.1038/nature01124

Petersen, P., Zou, K., Krauss, S., and Zhong, W. (2004). Continuing role for mouse Numb and Numbl in maintaining progenitor cells during cortical neurogenesis. *Nat. Neurosci.* 7, 803–811. doi: 10.1038/nn1289

Petrovic, J., Formosa-Jordan, P., Luna-Escalante, J. C., Abello, G., Ibanes, M., Neves, J., et al. (2014). Ligand-dependent Notch signaling strength orchestrates lateral induction and lateral inhibition in the developing inner ear. *Development* 141, 2313–2324. doi: 10.1242/dev.108100

Rasin, M. R., Gazula, V. R., Breunig, J. J., Kwan, K. Y., Johnson, M. B., Liu-Chen, S., et al. (2007). Numb and Numbl are required for maintenance of cadherin-based adhesion and polarity of neural progenitors. *Nat. Neurosci.* 10, 819–827. doi: 10.1038/nn1924

Rhyu, M., Jan, L., and Jan, Y. (1994). Asymmetric distribution of numb protein during division of the sensory organ precursor cell confers distinct fates to daughter cells. *Cell* 76, 477–491. doi: 10.1016/0092-8674(94)90112-0

Riley, B., Chiang, M., Farmer, L., and Heck, R. (1999). The deltaA gene of zebrafish mediates lateral inhibition of hair cells in the inner ear and is regulated by pax2.1. *Development* 126, 5669–5678.

Roegiers, F., and Jan, Y. N. (2004). Asymmetric cell division. *Curr. Opin. Cell Biol.* 16, 195–205. doi: 10.1016/j.ceb.2004.02.010

Santolini, E., Puri, C., Salcini, A. E., Gagliani, M. C., Pelicci, P. G., Tacchetti, C., et al. (2000). Numb is an endocytic protein. *J. Cell Biol.* 151, 1345–1352. doi: 10.1083/jcb.151.6.1345

Sato, K., Watanabe, T., Wang, S., Kakeno, M., Matsuzawa, K., Matsui, T., et al. (2011). Numb controls E-cadherin endocytosis through p120 catenin with aPKC. *Mol. Biol. Cell* 22, 3103–3119. doi: 10.1091/mbc.E11-03-0274

Schneider, C. A., Rasband, W. S., and Eliceiri, K. W. (2012). NIH Image to ImageJ: 25 years of image analysis. *Nat. Methods* 9, 671–675. doi: 10.1038/nmeth.2089

Schweisguth, F. (2004). Regulation of Notch signaling activity. *Curr. Biol.* 14, R129–R138. doi: 10.1016/j.cub.2004.01.023

Shailam, R., Lanford, P., Dolinsky, C., Norton, C., Gridley, T., and Kelley, M. (1999). Expression of proneural and neurogenic genes in the embryonic mammalian vestibular system. *J. Neurocytol.* 28, 809–819. doi: 10.1023/A:1007009803095

Shen, Q., Zhong, W., Jan, Y., and Temple, S. (2002). Asymmetric Numb distribution is critical for asymmetric cell division of mouse cerebral cortical stem cells and neuroblasts. *Development* 129, 4843–4853.

Spana, E., and Doe, C. (1996). Numb antagonizes Notch signaling to specify sibling neuron cell fates. *Neuron* 17, 21–26. doi: 10.1016/S0896-6273(00)80277-9

Stone, J. S., and Rubel, E. W. (1999). Delta1 expression during avian hair cell regeneration. *Development* 126, 961–973.

Takebayashi, K., Akazawa, C., Nakanishi, S., and Kageyama, R. (1995). Structure and promoter analysis of the gene encoding the mouse helix-loop-helix factor HES-5. Identification of the neural precursor cell-specific promoter element. *J. Biol. Chem.* 270, 1342–1349. doi: 10.1074/jbc.270.3.1342

Tateya, T., Imayoshi, I., Tateya, I., Ito, J., and Kageyama, R. (2011). Cooperative functions of Hes/Hey genes in auditory hair cell and supporting cell development. *Dev. Biol.* 352, 329–340. doi: 10.1016/j.ydbio.2011.01.038

Tsai, H., Hardisty, R. E., Rhodes, C., Kiernan, A. E., Roby, P., Tymowska-Lalanne, Z., et al. (2001). The mouse slalom mutant demonstrates a role for Jagged1 in neuroepithelial patterning in the organ of Corti. *Hum. Mol. Genet.* 10, 507–512. doi: 10.1093/hmg/10.5.507

Uemura, T., Shepherd, S., Ackerman, L., Jan, L., and Jan, Y. (1989). numb, a gene required in determination of cell fate during sensory organ formation in Drosophila embryos. *Cell* 58, 349–360. doi: 10.1016/0092-8674(89)90849-0

Verdi, J. M., Bashirullah, A., Goldhawk, D. E., Kubu, C. J., Jamali, M., Meakin, S. O., et al. (1999). Distinct human NUMB isoforms regulate differentiation vs. proliferation in the neuronal lineage. *Proc. Natl. Acad. Sci. U.S.A.* 96, 10472–10476. doi: 10.1073/pnas.96.18.10472

Wakamatsu, Y., Maynard, T. M., Jones, S. U., and Weston, J. A. (1999). NUMB localizes in the basal cortex of mitotic avian neuroepithelial cells and modulates neuronal differentiation by binding to NOTCH-1. *Neuron* 23, 71–81. doi: 10.1016/S0896-6273(00)80754-0

Yamamoto, N., Chang, W., and Kelley, M. W. (2011). Rbpj regulates development of prosensory cells in the mammalian inner ear. *Dev. Biol.* 353, 367–379. doi: 10.1016/j.ydbio.2011.03.016

Zhong, W., and Chia, W. (2008). Neurogenesis and asymmetric cell division. *Curr. Opin. Neurobiol.* 18, 4–11. doi: 10.1016/j.conb.2008.05.002

Zhong, W., Feder, J., Jiang, M., Jan, L., and Jan, Y. (1996). Asymmetric localization of a mammalian numb homolog during mouse cortical neurogenesis. *Neuron* 17, 43–53. doi: 10.1016/S0896-6273(00)80279-2

Zhong, W., Jiang, M. M., Schonemann, M. D., Meneses, J. J., Pedersen, R. A., Jan, L. Y., et al. (2000). Mouse numb is an essential gene involved in cortical neurogenesis. *Proc. Natl. Acad. Sci. U.S.A.* 97, 6844–6849. doi: 10.1073/pnas.97.12.6844

Zhong, W., Jiang, M. M., Weinmaster, G., Jan, L. Y., and Jan, Y. N. (1997). Differential expression of mammalian Numb, Numblike and Notch1 suggests distinct roles during mouse cortical neurogenesis. *Development* 124, 1887–1897.

Zilian, O., Saner, C., Hagedorn, L., Lee, H. Y., Säuberli, E., Suter, U., et al. (2001). Multiple roles of mouse Numb in tuning developmental cell fates. *Curr. Biol.* 11, 494–501. doi: 10.1016/S0960-9822(01)00149-X

Zine, A., Aubert, A., Qiu, J., Therianos, S., Guillemot, F., Kageyama, R., et al. (2001). Hes1 and Hes5 activities are required for the normal development of the hair cells in the mammalian inner ear. *J. Neurosci.* 21, 4712–4720.

Permissions

All chapters in this book were first published in SHCDR, by Frontiers; hereby published with permission under the Creative Commons Attribution License or equivalent. Every chapter published in this book has been scrutinized by our experts. Their significance has been extensively debated. The topics covered herein carry significant findings which will fuel the growth of the discipline. They may even be implemented as practical applications or may be referred to as a beginning point for another development.

The contributors of this book come from diverse backgrounds, making this book a truly international effort. This book will bring forth new frontiers with its revolutionizing research information and detailed analysis of the nascent developments around the world.

We would like to thank all the contributing authors for lending their expertise to make the book truly unique.

They have played a crucial role in the development of this book. Without their invaluable contributions this book wouldn't have been possible. They have made vital efforts to compile up to date information on the varied aspects of this subject to make this book a valuable addition to the collection of many professionals and students.

This book was conceptualized with the vision of imparting up-to-date information and advanced data in this field. To ensure the same, a matchless editorial board was set up. Every individual on the board went through rigorous rounds of assessment to prove their worth. After which they invested a large part of their time researching and compiling the most relevant data for our readers.

The editorial board has been involved in producing this book since its inception. They have spent rigorous hours researching and exploring the diverse topics which have resulted in the successful publishing of this book. They have passed on their knowledge of decades through this book. To expedite this challenging task, the publisher supported the team at every step. A small team of assistant editors was also appointed to further simplify the editing procedure and attain best results for the readers.

Apart from the editorial board, the designing team has also invested a significant amount of their time in understanding the subject and creating the most relevant covers. They scrutinized every image to scout for the most suitable representation of the subject and create an appropriate cover for the book.

The publishing team has been an ardent support to the editorial, designing and production team. Their endless efforts to recruit the best for this project, has resulted in the accomplishment of this book. They are a veteran in the field of academics and their pool of knowledge is as vast as their experience in printing. Their expertise and guidance has proved useful at every step. Their uncompromising quality standards have made this book an exceptional effort. Their encouragement from time to time has been an inspiration for everyone.

The publisher and the editorial board hope that this book will prove to be a valuable piece of knowledge for researchers, students, practitioners and scholars across the globe.

List of Contributors

Litao Tao
Genetic, Molecular and Cellular Biology Program, University of Southern California, Los Angeles, CA, USA
Department of Stem Cell Biology and Regenerative Medicine, University of Southern California, Los Angeles, CA, USA

Neil Segil
Genetic, Molecular and Cellular Biology Program, University of Southern California, Los Angeles, CA, USA
Department of Stem Cell Biology and Regenerative Medicine, University of Southern California, Los Angeles, CA, USA

Department of Otolaryngology, University of Southern California, Los Angeles, CA, USA
Hongzhe Li, Allan Kachelmeier and Peter S. Steyger
Oregon Hearing Research Center, Oregon Health & Science University, Portland, OR, USA

David N. Furness
School of Life Sciences, Keele University, Staffordshire, UK

Jerry D. Monroe and Michael E. Smith
Department of Biology, Western Kentucky University, Bowling Green, KY, USA

Gopinath Rajadinakaran
Department of Genetics and Genome Sciences, University of Connecticut Health Center, Farmington, CT, USA

Elena I. Morgun and Ekaterina A. Vorotelyak
Laboratory of Cell Biology, Koltzov Institute of Developmental Biology of Russian Academy of Sciences, Moscow, Russia

Christine T. Dinh, Stefania Goncalves, Esperanza Bas and Thomas R. Van De Water
University of Miami Ear Institute, University of Miami Miller School of Medicine, Miami, FL, USA

Azel Zine
Integrative and Adaptive Neurosciences, Aix-Marseille Université, CNRS, UMR 7260, Marseille, France
Faculty of Pharmacy, Biophysics Department, University of Montpellier, Montpellier, France

Zhang
Research Center, Affiliated Eye and ENT Hospital of Fudan University, Shanghai, China
Key Laboratory of Hearing Medicine, Ministry of Health, Affiliated Eye and ENT Hospital of Fudan University, Shanghai, China
Institutes of Biomedical Sciences, Fudan University, Shanghai, China

Yan Chen, Luo Guo, Wen Li and Shan Sun
Research Center, Affiliated Eye and ENT Hospital of Fudan University, Shanghai, China
Key Laboratory of Hearing Medicine, Ministry of Health, Affiliated Eye and ENT Hospital of Fudan University, Shanghai, China

Wenli Ni and Xiaoling Lu
Department of Otorhinolaryngology, Affiliated Eye and ENT Hospital of Fudan University, Shanghai, China

Liman Liu
Key Laboratory of Hearing Medicine, Ministry of Health, Affiliated Eye and ENT Hospital of Fudan University, Shanghai, China

Lei Wang
Institutes of Biomedical Sciences, Fudan University, Shanghai, China

Huawei Li
Key Laboratory of Hearing Medicine, Ministry of Health, Affiliated Eye and ENT Hospital of Fudan University, Shanghai, China
Department of Otorhinolaryngology, Affiliated Eye and ENT Hospital of Fudan University, Shanghai, China
The State Key Laboratory of Medical Neurobiology, The Institutes of Brain Science and the Collaborative Innovation Center for Brain Science, Fudan University, Shanghai, China

Chao-Hui Yang
Department of Otolaryngology, Kresge Hearing Research Institute, University of Michigan, Ann Arbor, MI, USA
Division of Otology, Department of Otolaryngology, Kaohsiung Chang Gung Memorial Hospital, Chang Gung University College of Medicine, Kaohsiung, Taiwan

Thomas Schrepfer and Jochen Schacht
Department of Otolaryngology, Kresge Hearing Research Institute, University of Michigan, Ann Arbor, MI, USA

Paromita Majumder and Paulette A. Moore
UCL Ear Institute, University College London, London, UK

Guy P. Richardson
Sussex Neuroscience, School of Life Sciences, University of Sussex, Falmer, UK

Jonathan E. Gale
UCL Ear Institute, University College London, London, UK
Department of Cell and Developmental Biology, University College London, London, UK

Tejbeer Kaur, Keiko Hirose and Mark E. Warchol
Department of Otolaryngology, Washington University School of Medicine, St. Louis, MO, USA

Edwin W. Rubel
The Virginia Merrill Bloedel Hearing Research Center and Department of Otolaryngology - Head and Neck Surgery, University of Washington School of Medicine, Seattle, WA, USA

Paromita Majumder
UCL Ear Institute, University College London, London, UK

R. Duchen
Department of Cell and Developmental Biology, University College London, London, UK

Jonathan E. Gale
UCL Ear Institute, University College London, London, UK
Department of Cell and Developmental Biology, University College London, London, UK

Sofie Van Rossom
Department of Biomedical Sciences, Center of Medical Genetics, University of Antwerp, Antwerp, Belgium
Functional Biology, Department of Biology, KU Leuven, Heverlee, Belgium

Ken Op de Beeck and Guy Van Camp
Department of Biomedical Sciences, Center of Medical Genetics, University of Antwerp, Antwerp, Belgium

Vesna Hristovska and Joris Winderickx
Functional Biology, Department of Biology, KU Leuven, Heverlee, Belgium

Melissa M. McGovern, Luyi Zhou and Michelle R. Randle
Department of Pharmacology, School of Medicine, Southern Illinois University, Springfield, IL, United States

Brandon C. Cox
Department of Pharmacology, School of Medicine, Southern Illinois University, Springfield, IL, United States
Department of Surgery, Division of Otolaryngology, School of Medicine, Southern Illinois University, Springfield, IL, United States

Jinchao Lin, Xiaodong Zhang , Fengfang Wu and Weinian Lin
Department of Otolaryngology-Head and Neck Surgery, Quanzhou First Hospital Affiliated to Fujian Medical University, Quanzhou, Fujian, China

Li-Yih Lin and Ya-Hsin Yeh
Department of Life Science, National Taiwan Normal University, Taipei, Taiwan

Giun-Yi Hung
Department of Life Science, National Taiwan Normal University, Taipei, Taiwan
Department of Pediatrics, Taipei Veterans General Hospital, Taipei, Taiwan
Department of Pediatrics, Faculty of Medicine, National Yang-Ming University, Taipei, Taiwan

Chia-Hao Lin
Institute of Cellular and Organismic Biology, Academia Sinica, Taipei, Taiwan
Department of Anatomy and Cell Biology, School of Medicine, College of Medicine, Taipei Medical University, Taipei, Taiwan

Pung-Pung Hwang
Institute of Cellular and Organismic Biology, Academia Sinica, Taipei, Taiwan

Jiun-Lin Horng
Department of Anatomy and Cell Biology, School of Medicine, College of Medicine, Taipei Medical University, Taipei, Taiwan

Byron H. Hartman, Robert Durruthy-Durruthy, Roman D. Laske, Steven Losorelli and Stefan Heller
Department of Otolaryngology, Head and Neck Surgery, Stanford University School of Medicine, Stanford, CA, USA

Juan C. Maass
Department of Neuroscience, Baylor College of Medicine, Houston, TX, USA
Department of Otolaryngology, Hospital Clínico Universidad de Chile, Santiago, Chile
Interdisciplinary Program of Physiology and Biophysics, ICBM Universidad de Chile, Santiago, Chile
Department of Otolaryngology, Clínica Alemana de Santiago, Facultad de Medicina Clínica Alemana-Universidad del Desarrollo, Santiago, Chile

Rende Gu, Martin L. Basch and Eduardo Martin Lopez
Department of Neuroscience, Baylor College of Medicine, Houston, TX, USA

Joerg Waldhaus, Anping Xia, John S. Oghalai and Stefan Heller
Department of Otolaryngology —Head and Neck Surgery, Stanford University School of Medicine, Palo Alto, CA, USA

Andrew K. Groves
Department of Neuroscience, Baylor College of Medicine, Houston, TX, USA
Department of Molecular and Human Genetics, Baylor College of Medicine, Houston, TX, USA
Program in Developmental Biology, Baylor College of Medicine, Houston, TX, USA

Mark Eddison
Howard Hughes Medical Institute, Janelia Research Campus, Ashburn, VA, USA

Sara J. Weber and Nicolas Daudet
Ear Institute, University College London, London, UK

Linda Ariza-McNaughton
Haematopoietic Stem cell Laboratory, Cancer Research UK, London Research Institute, London, UK

Julian Lewis
Formerly of Vertebrate Development Laboratory, Cancer Research UK, London, UK

Index

O

P

R

S

T

W

Z

CPSIA information can be obtained
at www.ICGtesting.com
Printed in the USA
LVHW060853030122
707669LV00002B/120

9 781639 892495